Lecture Notes in Artificial Intelligence   3581

Edited by J. G. Carbonell and J. Siekmann

Subseries of Lecture Notes in Computer Science

Silvia Miksch   Jim Hunter
Elpida Keravnou (Eds.)

Artificial Intelligence in Medicine

10th Conference on Artificial Intelligence
in Medicine, AIME 2005
Aberdeen, UK, July 23-27, 2005
Proceedings

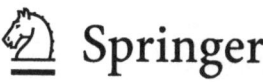 Springer

Series Editors

Jaime G. Carbonell, Carnegie Mellon University, Pittsburgh, PA, USA
Jörg Siekmann, University of Saarland, Saarbrücken, Germany

Volume Editors

Silvia Miksch
Vienna University of Technology
Institute of Software Technology and Interactive Systems
Favoritenstr. 9-11/E188, 1040 Vienna, Austria
E-mail: silvia@ifs.tuwien.ac.at

Jim Hunter
University of Aberdeen, King's College
Department of Computing Science
Aberdeen, AB24 3UE, UK
E-mail: jhunter@csd.abdn.ac.uk

Elpida Keravnou
University of Cyprus, Department of Computer Science
75 Kallipoleos Str., 1678 Nicosia, Cyprus
E-mail: elpida@turing.cs.ucy.ac.cy

Library of Congress Control Number: 2005929500

CR Subject Classification (1998): I.2, I.4, J.3, H.2.8, H.4, H.3

ISSN   0302-9743
ISBN-10 3-540-27831-1 Springer Berlin Heidelberg New York
ISBN-13 978-3-540-27831-3 Springer Berlin Heidelberg New York

This work is subject to copyright. All rights are reserved, whether the whole or part of the material is concerned, specifically the rights of translation, reprinting, re-use of illustrations, recitation, broadcasting, reproduction on microfilms or in any other way, and storage in data banks. Duplication of this publication or parts thereof is permitted only under the provisions of the German Copyright Law of September 9, 1965, in its current version, and permission for use must always be obtained from Springer. Violations are liable to prosecution under the German Copyright Law.

Springer is a part of Springer Science+Business Media

springeronline.com

© Springer-Verlag Berlin Heidelberg 2005
Printed in Germany

Typesetting: Camera-ready by author, data conversion by Scientific Publishing Services, Chennai, India
Printed on acid-free paper   SPIN: 11527770   06/3142   5 4 3 2 1 0

Preface

The European Society for Artificial Intelligence in Medicine (AIME) was established in 1986 with two main goals: 1) to foster fundamental and applied research in the application of Artificial Intelligence (AI) techniques to medical care and medical research, and 2) to provide a forum at biennial conferences for reporting significant results achieved. Additionally, AIME assists medical industrialists to identify new AI techniques with high potential for integration into new products. A major activity of this society has been a series of international conferences held biennially over the last 18 years: Marseilles, France (1987), London, UK (1989), Maastricht, Netherlands (1991), Munich, Germany (1993), Pavia, Italy (1995), Grenoble, France (1997), Aalborg, Denmark (1999), Cascais, Portugal (2001), Protaras, Cyprus (2003).

The AIME conference provides a unique opportunity to present and improve the international state of the art of AI in medicine from both a research and an applications perspective. For this purpose, the AIME conference includes invited lectures, contributed papers, system demonstrations, a doctoral consortium, tutorials, and workshops. The present volume contains the proceedings of AIME 2005, the 10th conference on Artificial Intelligence in Medicine, held in Aberdeen, Scotland, July 23-27, 2005.

In the AIME 2005 conference announcement, we encouraged authors to submit original contributions to the development of theory, techniques, and applications of AI in medicine, including the evaluation of health care programs. Theoretical papers were to include presentation or analysis of the properties of novel AI methodologies potentially useful to solving medical problems. Technical papers were to describe the novelty of the proposed approach, its assumptions, benefits, and limitations compared with other alternative techniques. Application papers were to present sufficient information to allow the evaluation of the practical benefits of the proposed system or methodology.

This year we received an all-time high number of very well-elaborated scientific paper submissions (148 paper submissions, 128% more than for AIME 2003). All papers were carefully evaluated by at least two independent reviewers from the program committee with support from additional reviewers. Submissions came from 32 different countries including 13 outside Europe. This emphasizes the international interest for an AI in medicine conference. The reviewers judged the originality, the quality, and the significance of the proposed research, as well as its presentation and its relevance to the AIME conference. All submissions were ranked on four aspects: the overall recommendation of each reviewer, the reviewer's confidence in the subject area of the paper, the quantitative scores obtained from all aspects of the detailed review, and the reviewer's detailed comments.

A small selection committee was established consisting of the AIME 2003 Program Chair Michel Dojat, the AIME 2003 Organizing Chair Elpida Keravnou, the AIME 2005 Program Chair Silvia Miksch, and the AIME 2005 Organizing Chair Jim Hunter. In the middle of April 2005 this committee met in Vienna to make the final decisions on the AIME 2005 program (scientific papers, doctoral consortium, tutorials, and workshops).

As a result we accepted 35 full papers (a 23.6% acceptance rate) for oral presentation. Each of them received a high overall ranking and two positive recommendations, of which at least one was highly positive. Ten pages were allocated to each full paper in this volume and 25 minutes of oral presentation during the conference. In addition, we accepted 34 short papers for poster presentation (a 23.0% acceptance rate). Each of them also received two positive recommendations. Five pages have been allocated to each short paper in this volume. The poster presenters had 5 minutes to present their papers, and their posters were shown throughout the main AIME 2005 conference to allow for fruitful discussions with the audience.

The papers and the sessions were organized according to the following themes: (1) Temporal Representation and Reasoning, (2) Decision Support Systems, (3) Clinical Guidelines and Protocols, (4) Ontology and Terminology, (5) Case-Based Reasoning, Signal Interpretation, Visual Mining, (6) Computer Vision and Imaging, (7) Knowledge Management, and (8) Machine Learning, Knowledge Discovery and Data Mining. These themes reflect the current interests of researchers in AI in medicine. The high quality of the papers selected in this volume demonstrates the vitality and diversity of research in Artificial Intelligence in Medicine.

Two invited speakers gave talks on two challenging topics in AIME. Frank van Harmelen (Vrije Universiteit Amsterdam, The Netherlands) spoke on ontology mapping and presented different approaches to ontology-mapping, covering linguistic, statistical and logical methods. Paul Lukowicz (University for Health Sciences, Medical Informatics and Technology, Hall in Tirol, Austria) introduced the topic of context-aware wearable systems with the focus on human computer interaction, and illustrated different ways forward within that research area. Two extended abstracts of these invited lectures are included in this volume.

An important new feature of the AIME conferences is the Doctoral Consortium (organized by Elpida Keravnou) held for the first time in the context of AIME. We would like to thank the eight students who presented their research work during the consortium and the participating faculty (Ameen Abu-Hanna, Riccardo Bellazzi, Carlo Combi, Michel Dojat, Peter Lucas, Silvana Quaglini, and Yuval Shahar) for their fruitful and constructive discussions and comments with the students.

AIME 2005 hosted two workshops: the Tenth IDAMAP Workshop on Intelligent Data Analysis in Medicine and Pharmacology and the Workshop on Biomedical Ontology Engineering. Four half-day tutorials were also offered: Evaluation of Prognostic Models; Evolutionary Computation Approaches to Mining Biomedical Data; Causal Discovery from Biomedical Data; and Applied Data Mining in Clinical Research.

We mourn the death of one of the members of the Program Committee – Barbara Heller died after a long illness during the reviewing process.

We would like to thank all the people and institutions who contributed to the success of the AIME 2005 conference: the authors, the members of the program committee as well as additional reviewers, all the members of the organizing committee, and the invited speakers Frank van Harmelen and Paul Lukowicz. Moreover, we would like to thank the organizers of the two workshops, John Holmes, Niels Peek, Jeremy Rogers, Alan Rector, and Robert Stevens and the presenters of the tutorials, Ameen Abu-Hanna, John Holmes, Subramani Mani, and Niels Peek. Finally, we would like to thank the University of Aberdeen for sponsoring and hosting the conference.

May 2005

Silvia Miksch
Jim Hunter
Elpida Keravnou

Organization

Program Chair: Silvia Miksch (Austria)
Organizing Chair: Jim Hunter (United Kingdom)
Tutorials & Workshops Chair: Jim Hunter (United Kingdom)
Doctoral Consortium Chair: Elpida Keravnou (Cyprus)

Program Committee

Ameen Abu-Hanna (The Netherlands)
Klaus-Peter Adlassnig (Austria)
Steen Andreassen (Denmark)
Giovanni Barosi (Italy)
Pedro Barahona (Portugal)
Robert Baud (Switzerland)
Riccardo Bellazzi (Italy)
Isabelle Bichindaritz (USA)
Enrico Coiera (Australia)
Carlo Combi (Italy)
Evert de Jonge (The Netherlands)
Michel Dojat (France)
Henrik Eriksson (Sweden)
John Fox (United Kingdom)
Catherine Garbay (France)
Arie Hasman (The Netherlands)
Reinhold Haux (Germany)
Barbara Heller (Germany)
Laurent Heyer (France)
Werner Horn (Austria)
Elpida Keravnou (Cyprus)
Nada Lavrač (Slovenia)
Peter Lucas (The Netherlands)
Neil McIntosh (United Kingdom)
Mark Musen (USA)
Mor Peleg (Israel)
Christian Popow (Austria)
Ian Purves (United Kingdom)
Silvana Quaglini (Italy)
Alan Rector (United Kingdom)
Stephen Rees (Denmark)
Rainer Schmidt (Germany)
Brigitte Séroussi (France)
Yuval Shahar (Israel)
Basilio Sierra (Spain)
Costas Spyropoulos (Greece)
Mario Stefanelli (Italy)
Vojtěch Svátek (Czech Republic)
Paolo Terenziani (Italy)
Samson Tu (USA)
Johan van der Lei (The Netherlands)
Dongwen Wang (USA)
Jim Warren (Australia)
Thomas Wetter (Germany)
Blaž Zupan (Slovenia)

Additional Reviewers

Wolfgang Aigner
Roberta Amici
Luca Anselma
Magnus Bång
Gleb Beliakov
Petr Berka
Elizabeth Black
Alessio Bottrighi
Jacques Bouaud
Umberto Castellani
Paolo Ciccarese
Jorge Cruz
Fulvia Ferrazzi
Ildiko Flesch
Susan George

Ranadhir Ghosh
Perry Groot
Arjen Hommersom
Yang Huang
Yannis Ioannidis
Ravi Jain
Karsten Jensen
Katerina Kabassi
Katharina Kaiser
Vangelis Karkaletsis
Stefania Montani
Barbara Oliboni
Dameron Olivier

Niels Peek
Stavros J. Perantonis
Ioannis Refanidis
Baud Robert
Kitty Rosenbrand
Rosalba Rossato
Patrick Ruch
Lucia Sacchi
Andreas Seyfang
Derek Sleeman
Jan Stanek
Rory Steele
Annette ten Teije

Evangelia Triantafyllou
Linda C. van der Gaag
Marcel van Gerven
Stefan Visscher
Frans Voorbraak
George Vouros
Floris Wiesman
Matt Williams
Jolanda Wittenberg
Roni F. Zeiger
Pierre Zweigenbaum

Workshops

IDAMAP-2005: Intelligent Data Analysis in Medicine and Pharmacology

Co-chairs: John Holmes, School of Medicine, University of Pennsylvania, USA
Niels Peek, Academic Medical Center, University of Amsterdam, The Netherlands

Biomedical Ontology Engineering

Co-chairs: Jeremy Rogers, University of Manchester, United Kingdom
Alan Rector, University of Manchester, United Kingdom
Robert Stevens, University of Manchester, United Kingdom

Tutorials

Evaluation of Prognostic Models

Ameen Abu-Hanna and Niels Peek, Academic Medical Center, University of Amsterdam, The Netherlands

Evolutionary Computation Approaches to Mining Biomedical Data

John Holmes, School of Medicine, University of Pennsylvania, USA

Causal Discovery from Biomedical Data

Subramani Mani, Department of Electrical Engineering and Computer Science, University of Wisconsin-Milwaukee, USA

Applied Data Mining in Clinical Research

John Holmes, School of Medicine, University of Pennsylvania, USA

Table of Contents

Invited Talks

Ontology Mapping: A Way Out of the Medical Tower of Babel?
Frank van Harmelen 3

Human Computer Interaction in Context Aware Wearable Systems
Paul Lukowicz 7

Temporal Representation and Reasoning

A New Approach to the Abstraction of Monitoring Data in Intensive Care
Samir Sharshar, Laurent Allart, Marie-Christine Chambrin 13

Learning Rules with Complex Temporal Patterns in Biomedical Domains
*Lucia Sacchi, Riccardo Bellazzi, Cristiana Larizza,
Riccardo Porreca, Paolo Magni* 23

Discriminating Exanthematic Diseases from Temporal Patterns of Patient Symptoms
Silvana Badaloni, Marco Falda 33

Probabilistic Abstraction of Multiple Longitudinal Electronic Medical Records
Michael Ramati, Yuval Shahar 43

Using a Bayesian-Network Model for the Analysis of Clinical Time-Series Data
Stefan Visscher, Peter Lucas, Karin Schurink, Marc Bonten 48

Data-Driven Analysis of Blood Glucose Management Effectiveness
Barry Nannings, Ameen Abu-Hanna, Robert-Jan Bosman 53

Extending Temporal Databases to Deal with Telic/Atelic Medical Data
*Paolo Terenziani, Richard Snodgrass, Alessio Bottrighi,
Mauro Torchio, Gianpaolo Molino* 58

Dichotomization of ICU Length of Stay Based on Model Calibration
*Marion Verduijn, Niels Peek, Frans Voorbraak, Evert de Jonge,
Bas de Mol* 67

Decision Support Systems

AtherEx: An Expert System for Atherosclerosis Risk Assessment
  Petr Berka, Vladimír Laš, Marie Tomečková 79

Smooth Integration of Decision Support into an Existing Electronic
Patient Record
  *Silvana Quaglini, Silvia Panzarasa, Anna Cavallini,
  Giuseppe Micieli, Corrado Pernice, Mario Stefanelli* 89

REPS: A Rehabilitation Expert System for Post-stroke Patients
  Douglas D. Dankel II, María Ósk Kristmundsdóttir 94

Clinical Guidelines and Protocols

Testing Asbru Guidelines and Protocols for Neonatal Intensive Care
  Christian Fuchsberger, Jim Hunter, Paul McCue 101

EORCA: A Collaborative Activities Representation for Building
Guidelines from Field Observations
  *Liliane Pellegrin, Nathalie Bonnardel, François Antonini,
  Jacques Albanèse, Claude Martin, Hervé Chaudet* 111

Design Patterns for Modelling Medical Guidelines
  *Radu Serban, Annette ten Teije, Mar Marcos, Cristina Polo-Conde,
  Kitty Rosenbrand, Jolanda Wittenberg, Joyce van Croonenborg* 121

Improving Clinical Guideline Implementation Through Prototypical
Design Patterns
  Monika Moser, Silvia Miksch 126

Automatic Derivation of a Decision Tree to Represent Guideline-Based
Therapeutic Strategies for the Management of Chronic Diseases
  Brigitte Séroussi, Jacques Bouaud, Jean-Jacques Vieillot 131

Exploiting Decision Theory for Supporting Therapy Selection in
Computerized Clinical Guidelines
  Stefania Montani, Paolo Terenziani, Alessio Bottrighi 136

Helping Physicians to Organize Guidelines Within Conceptual
Hierarchies
  Diego Sona, Paolo Avesani, Robert Moskovitch 141

MHB – A Many-Headed Bridge Between Informal and Formal
Guideline Representations
  *Andreas Seyfang, Silvia Miksch, Cristina Polo-Conde,
  Jolanda Wittenberg, Mar Marcos, Kitty Rosenbrand* 146

Clinical Guidelines Adaptation: Managing Authoring and Versioning
Issues
  *Paolo Terenziani, Stefania Montani, Alessio Bottrighi,
  Gianpaolo Molino, Mauro Torchio* 151

Open-Source Publishing of Medical Knowledge for Creation of
Computer-Interpretable Guidelines
  *Mor Peleg, Rory Steele, Richard Thomson, Vivek Patkar,
  Tony Rose, John Fox* 156

A History-Based Algebra for Quality-Checking Medical Guidelines
  *Arjen Hommersom, Peter Lucas, Patrick van Bommel,
  Theo van der Weide* 161

The Spock System: Developing a Runtime Application Engine for
Hybrid-Asbru Guidelines
  Ohad Young, Yuval Shahar 166

AI Planning Technology as a Component of Computerised Clinical
Practice Guidelines
  *Kirsty Bradbrook, Graham Winstanley, David Glasspool, John Fox,
  Richard Griffiths* 171

Gaining Process Information from Clinical Practice Guidelines Using
Information Extraction
  Katharina Kaiser, Cem Akkaya, Silvia Miksch 181

Ontology-Driven Extraction of Linguistic Patterns for Modelling
Clinical Guidelines
  *Radu Serban, Annette ten Teije, Frank van Harmelen, Mar Marcos,
  Cristina Polo-Conde* 191

Formalising Medical Quality Indicators to Improve Guidelines
  *Marjolein van Gendt, Annette ten Teije, Radu Serban,
  Frank van Harmelen* 201

Ontology and Terminology

Oncology Ontology in the NCI Thesaurus
  Anand Kumar, Barry Smith 213

Ontology-Mediated Distributed Decision Support for Breast Cancer
*Srinandan Dasmahapatra, David Dupplaw, Bo Hu, Paul Lewis,
Nigel Shadbolt* 221

Multimedia Data Management to Assist Tissue Microarrays Design
*Julie Bourbeillon, Catherine Garbay, Joëlle Simony-Lafontaine,
Françoise Giroud* 226

Building Medical Ontologies Based on Terminology Extraction from Texts: Methodological Propositions
Audrey Baneyx, Jean Charlet, Marie-Christine Jaulent 231

Translating Biomedical Terms by Inferring Transducers
Vincent Claveau, Pierre Zweigenbaum 236

Using Lexical and Logical Methods for the Alignment of Medical Terminologies
Michel Klein, Zharko Aleksovski 241

Latent Argumentative Pruning for Compact MEDLINE Indexing
*Patrick Ruch, Robert Baud, Johann Marty, Antoine Geissbühler,
Imad Tbahriti, Anne-Lise Veuthey* 246

A Benchmark Evaluation of the French MeSH Indexers
*Aurélie Névéol, Vincent Mary, Arnaud Gaudinat, Célia Boyer,
Alexandrina Rogozan, Stéfan J. Darmoni* 251

Populating an Allergens Ontology Using Natural Language Processing and Machine Learning Techniques
*Alexandros G. Valarakos, Vangelis Karkaletsis, Dimitra Alexopoulou,
Elsa Papadimitriou, Constantine D. Spyropoulos* 256

Ontology of Time and Situoids in Medical Conceptual Modeling
Heinrich Herre, Barbara Heller 266

The Use of Verbal Classification in Determining the Course of Medical Treatment by Medicinal Herbs
*Leonas Ustinovichius, Robert Balcevich, Dmitry Kochin,
Ieva Sliesoraityte* 276

Case-Based Reasoning, Signal Interpretation, Visual Mining

Interactive Knowledge Validation in CBR for Decision Support in Medicine
Monica Ou, Geoff A.W. West, Mihai Lazarescu, Chris Clay 289

Adaptation and Medical Case-Based Reasoning, Focusing on Endocrine
Therapy Support
    Rainer Schmidt, Olga Vorobieva 300

Transcranial Magnetic Stimulation (TMS) to Evaluate and Classify
Mental Diseases Using Neural Networks
    *Alberto Faro, Daniela Giordano, Manuela Pennisi,
    Giacomo Scarciofalo, Concetto Spampinato,
    Francesco Tramontana*... 310

Towards Information Visualization and Clustering Techniques for MRI
Data Sets
    *Umberto Castellani, Carlo Combi, Pasquina Marzola,
    Vittorio Murino, Andrea Sbarbati, Marco Zampieri* 315

Computer Vision and Imaging

Electrocardiographic Imaging: Towards Automated Interpretation of
Activation Maps
    Liliana Ironi, Stefania Tentoni 323

Automatic Landmarking of Cephalograms by Cellular Neural Networks
    *Daniela Giordano, Rosalia Leonardi, Francesco Maiorana,
    Gabriele Cristaldi, Maria Luisa Distefano* 333

Anatomical Sketch Understanding: Recognizing Explicit and Implicit
Structure
    *Peter Haddawy, Matthew Dailey, Ploen Kaewruen,
    Natapope Sarakhette*... 343

Morphometry of the Hippocampus Based on a Deformable Model and
Support Vector Machines
    Jeong-Sik Kim, Yong-Guk Kim, Soo-Mi Choi, Myoung-Hee Kim 353

Automatic Segmentation of Whole-Body Bone Scintigrams as a
Preprocessing Step for Computer Assisted Diagnostics
    Luka Šajn, Matjaž Kukar, Igor Kononenko, Metka Milčinski 363

Knowledge Management

Multi-agent Patient Representation in Primary Care
    Chris Reed, Brian Boswell, Ron Neville........................... 375

Clinical Reasoning Learning with Simulated Patients
Froduald Kabanza, Guy Bisson 385

Implicit Learning System for Teaching the Art of Acute Cardiac Infarction Diagnosis
Dmitry Kochin, Leonas Ustinovichius, Victoria Sliesoraitiene 395

Which Kind of Knowledge Is Suitable for Redesigning Hospital Logistic Processes?
Laura Măruşter, René J. Jorna 400

Machine Learning, Knowledge Discovery and Data Mining

Web Mining Techniques for Automatic Discovery of Medical Knowledge
David Sánchez, Antonio Moreno 409

Resource Modeling and Analysis of Regional Public Health Care Data by Means of Knowledge Technologies
Nada Lavrač, Marko Bohanec, Aleksander Pur, Bojan Cestnik, Mitja Jermol, Tanja Urbančič, Marko Debeljak, Branko Kavšek, Tadeja Kopač 414

An Evolutionary Divide and Conquer Method for Long-Term Dietary Menu Planning
Balázs Gaál, István Vassányi, György Kozmann 419

Human/Computer Interaction to Learn Scenarios from ICU Multivariate Time Series
Thomas Guyet, Catherine Garbay, Michel Dojat 424

Mining Clinical Data: Selecting Decision Support Algorithm for the MET-AP System
Jerzy Blaszczynski, Ken Farion, Wojtek Michalowski, Szymon Wilk, Steven Rubin, Dawid Weiss 429

A Data Pre-processing Method to Increase Efficiency and Accuracy in Data Mining
Amir R. Razavi, Hans Gill, Hans Åhlfeldt, Nosrat Shahsavar 434

Rule Discovery in Epidemiologic Surveillance Data Using EpiXCS: An Evolutionary Computation Approach
John H. Holmes, Jennifer A. Sager 444

Subgroup Mining for Interactive Knowledge Refinement
  *Martin Atzmueller, Joachim Baumeister, Achim Hemsing,
  Ernst-Jürgen Richter, Frank Puppe* 453

Evidence Accumulation for Identifying Discriminatory Signatures in
Biomedical Spectra
  *Adenike Bamgbade, Ray Somorjai, Brion Dolenko,
  Erinija Pranckeviciene, Alexander Nikulin, Richard Baumgartner* 463

On Understanding and Assessing Feature Selection Bias
  Šarunas Raudys, Richard Baumgartner, Ray Somorjai 468

A Model-Based Approach to Visualizing Classification Decisions for
Patient Diagnosis
  *Keith Marsolo, Srinivasan Parthasarathy, Michael Twa,
  Mark Bullimore* 473

Learning Rules from Multisource Data for Cardiac Monitoring
  Élisa Fromont, René Quiniou, Marie-Odile Cordier 484

Effective Confidence Region Prediction Using Probability Forecasters
  David G. Lindsay, Siân Cox 494

Signature Recognition Methods for Identifying Influenza Sequences
  Jitimon Keinduangjun, Punpiti Piamsa-nga, Yong Poovorawan 504

Conquering the Curse of Dimensionality in Gene Expression Cancer
Diagnosis: Tough Problem, Simple Models
  Minca Mramor, Gregor Leban, Janez Demšar, Blaž Zupan 514

An Algorithm to Learn Causal Relations Between Genes from Steady
State Data: Simulation and Its Application to Melanoma Dataset
  Xin Zhang, Chitta Baral, Seungchan Kim 524

Relation Mining over a Corpus of Scientific Literature
  *Fabio Rinaldi, Gerold Schneider, Kaarel Kaljurand, Michael Hess,
  Christos Andronis, Andreas Persidis, Ourania Konstanti* 535

Author Index 545

Invited Talks

Ontology Mapping: A Way Out of the Medical Tower of Babel?

(Summary of Invited Talk)

Frank van Harmelen

Vrije Universiteit Amsterdam, Dept. of Artificial Intelligence,
De Boelelaan 1081a, 1081HV Amsterdam, Netherlands
frank.van.harmelen@cs.vu.nl

The Problem

Integration of different information sources has been a problem that has been challenging (or perhaps better: plaguing) Computer Science throughout the decades. As soon as we had two computers, we wanted to exchange information between them, and as soon as we had two databases, we wanted to link them together.

Fortunately, Computer Science has made much progress on different levels:
Physical interoperability between systems has been all but solved: with the advent of hardware standards such as Ethernet, and with protocols such as TCP/IP and HTTP, we can nowadays walk into somebody's house or office, and successfully plug our computer into the network, giving instant world-wide physical connectivity.

Physical connectivity is not sufficient. We must also agree on the *syntactic form* of the messages we will exchange. Again, much progress has been made in recent years, with open standards such HTML and XML.

Of course, even syntactic interoperability is not enough. We need not only agree on the form of the messages we exchange, but also no the meaning of these messages. This problem of *semantic interoperability* is still wide open, despite its importance in many application areas, and despite decades of work by different disciplines within Computer Science.

It is clear that the problem of semantic interoperability is also plaguing Medical Informatics. Terminological confusion is plaguing the interoperability of data sources, and is hindering automatic support for document searches. [10] provides a study of synonymy and homonymy problems on gene-names in Medline. They established that genes have on the average 2-3 different names; cross-thesaurus homonymy is often up to 30%; and almost half of the of acronyms used to denote human genes also have another meaning in Medline entirely unrelated to human genes[1]. The conclusion of a report [8] by the same research group states:
"Information extraction and literature mining efforts will be strongly affected by this ambiguity, and solving this problem is essential for these research fields."

---

[1] My favorite example is PSA, (Prostate Specific Antigen), which also stands for Pot Smokers of America.

This problems is by no means unique to genomics. Perhaps the oldest taxonomy around is the Linneaus "Systema Naturae" [5]. The modern-day on-line version of this system[2] [1] lists 411 homonyms, with the same name used for birds as well as insects, and insect as well as fish.

Multiple Solutions

The problem of semantic interoperability has been the subject of research in different fields over many decades. Different variants of the problem received names such as "record linkage" (dating back to Newcombe's work on linking patient records [6], and surveyed in [11]), schema integration [7], and more recently ontology mapping (see [2] and [4] for recent surveys).

An important development in this historical progression is the move towards ever richer structure: the original record linkage problem was defined on simple strings that were names of record-fields; the schema-integration problem already had the full relational model as input; while ontology mapping problems are defined on full hierarchical models plus rich axiomatisations. Each step in this progress has all the solutions of the previous steps to its disposal (since each later model subsumes the earlier ones), plus new methods that can exploit the richer structures of the objects to be aligned.

Current approaches to ontology mapping deploy a whole host of different methods, coming from very different areas. We distinguish linguistic, statistical, structural and logical methods.

Linguistic Methods are directly rooted in the original record linkage work all the way back to the early 60's. They try to exploit the linguistic labels attached to the concepts in source and target ontology in order to discover potential matches. This can be as simple as basic stemming techniques or calculating Hamming distances, or can use specialised domain knowledge. An example of this would be that the difference between *Diabetes Melitus type I* and *Diabetes Melitus type II* are not an innocent difference to be removed by a standard stemming algorithm.

Statistical Methods typically use *instance data* to determine correspondences between concepts: if there is a significant statistical correlation between the instances of a source-concept and a target-concept, there is reason to belief that these concepts are strongly related (by either a subsumption relation, or perhaps even an equivalence relation). These approaches of course rely on the availability of a sufficiently large corpus of instances that are classified in both the source and the target ontology.

Structural Methods exploit the graph-structure of the source and target ontologies, and try to determine similarities between these structures, often in coordination with some of the other methods: if a source- and target-concept have

---

[2] http://www.taxonomicon.net/

similar linguistic labels, then dissimilarity of their graph-neighbourhoods can be used to detect homonym problems where purely linguistic methods would falsely declare a potential mapping.

Logical Methods are perhaps most specific to mapping *ontologies* (instead of mapping record-fields or database-schemata). After all, in the time-honoured phrase of [3], ontologies are *"formal specifications* of a shared conceptualisation" (my emphasis), and it makes sense to exploit this formalisation of both source and target structures. A particularly interesting approach is to use a third ontology as background knowledge when mapping between a source and a target ontology: if relations can be established between source (resp. target) ontology and different parts of the background knowledge, then this induces a relation between source and target ontologies. A serious limitation to this approach is that many practical ontologies are rather at the semantically lightweight end of Uschold's spectrum [9], and thus don't carry much logical formalism with them.

Where Are We Now?

Undoubtedly, the problem of semantic integration is one of the key problems facing Computer Science today. Despite many years of work, this old problem is still open, and has actually acquired a new urgency now that other integration barriers (physical, syntactic) have been largely removed.

Given the difficulty of the problem, and the amount of work already spent on it, it seems unlikely that the problem of ontology mapping will yield to a single solution. Instead, this seems more the kind of problem where many different partial solutions are needed.

Currently, our toolbox of such partial solutions is already quite well stocked, and is still rapidly growing. However, a theory of which combination of partial solutions to apply in which circumstances is still entirely lacking.

References

1. S.J. Brands. Systema naturae 2000. website, 1989–2005. http://www.taxonomicon.net/.
2. J. Euzenat (coord). State of the art on ontology alignment. Technical Report D2.2.3, Knowledge Web, 2004. http://knowledgeweb.semanticweb.org.
3. T.R. Gruber. A translation approach to portable ontologies. *Knowledge Acquisition*, 5(2):199–200, 1993.
4. Y. Kalfoglou and M. Schorlemmer. Ontology mapping: the state of the art. *Knowledge Engineering Review*, 18(1):1–31, 2003.
5. C. Linneaus. *Systema naturae per regna tria naturae, secundum classes, ordines, genera, species, cum characteribus, differentiis, synonymis, locis..* Holmiae (Laurentii Salvii), editio decima, reformata edition, 1758.
6. H.B. Newcombe, J.M. Kennedy, S.J Axford, and A.P. James. Automatic linkage of vital records. *Science*, 130:954–959, 1959.
7. Erhard Rahm and Philip A. Bernstein. A survey of approaches to automatic schema matching. *VLDB Journal: Very Large Data Bases*, 10(4):334–350, 2001.

8. M. Schuemie and J. Kors. Assessment of homonym problem for gene symbols. Technical report, Erasmus University Medical Center Rotterdam, 2004. Report D4.4 for the ORIEL project.
9. M. Uschold and M. Gruninger. Ontologies: principles, methods, and applications. *Knowledge Engineering Review*, 11(2):93–155, 1996.
10. M. Weeber, R.J.A. Schijvenaars, E.M. van Mulligen, B. Mons, R. Jelier, C.C. van der Eijk, and J.A. Kors. Ambiguity of human gene symbols in locuslink and medline: Creating an inventory and a disambiguation test collection. In *Proceedings of the American Medical Informatics Association (AMIA 2003)*, pages 704–708, 2003.
11. W. Winkler. The state of record linkage and current research problems. Technical report, Statistical Research Division, U.S. Bureau of the Census, Washington, DC, 1999.

Human Computer Interaction in Context Aware Wearable Systems

Paul Lukowicz

Institute for Computer Systems and Networks
UMIT- University for Health Sciences, Medical Informatics and Technology
Hall in Tirol, Austria
paul.lukowicz@umit.at

1 Introduction

Today access to computing power and communication has become nearly ubiquitous. Mobile computers and even mobile phones have computing power, storage and graphics capabilities comparable to PCs from a few years ago. With the advent of GPRS, UMTS, WLAN and other networking technologies high speed Internet access is possible nearly anywhere. At the same time an enormous amount of permanently updated information has become available online. In fact one can say that for nearly any situation there is guaranteed to be a piece of useful information somewhere on the network. This includes such trivial everyday things like restaurant menus and transportation delays but also information relevant to a variety of professional applications. The latter include building plans (relevant for rescue personnel), patient record (needed for example by emergency medics) and multimedia manuals (for maintenance and assembly work).

Thus in summary it can be said that in most settings mobile users have at their disposal both the relevant information and the means to access and process it. However currently they make only very limited use of it. In fact most people use their connected devices predominantly for conventional telephony, email access, scheduling and an occasional photograph. Despite a strong push by service providers accessing online information in a mobile environment is still the exception.

To a large degree the limited use of mobile connected devices can be attributed to the inadequacies of the current interaction paradigm. The most obvious problem is the user interface itself, which is based on standard desktop concepts emphasizing text, pointers, windows and menus. In addition network an application configuration and operation tend to be complex and time consuming.

Beyond these well known problems a new research direction has recently emerged: the development of proactive, so called context aware systems [1]. Such systems should automatically recognize the needs of the user and deliver the correct information at the correct time and place. Thus the idea is not just to provide a better interface, but to significantly reduce or even get rid of the need for explicit interaction. In the simplest case the context is just time and location.

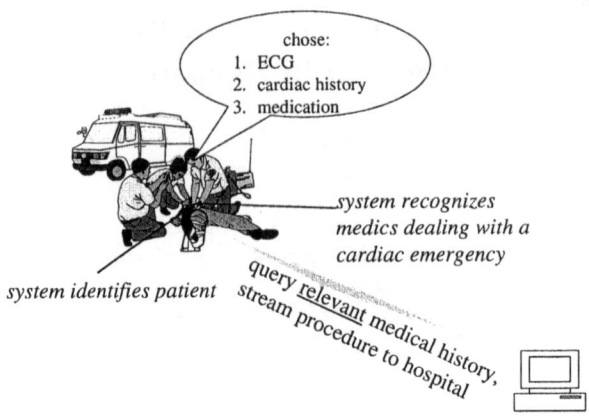

Fig. 1. An example scenario for context aware interaction

In more advanced applications it includes user activity (walking, standing, going to work, performing a particular maintenance task), environment state (e.g a meeting taking place) and background information such as the users schedule or habits.

2 Application Scenario

An example of context supported human computer interaction is shown in Figure 1. It envisions an emergency medical crew that attends to a heart attack patient on the street. Since time is critical the crew has little opportunity to access electronic information on the patient, look up advice on treatment, or transfer information back to the hospital. However if a computer system was able to automatically recognize what procedures the crew is performing and to identify the patient it could automatically deliver and collect the required information. Thus the system could contact a server, look up the medical history and automatically present the crew with information related to his cardiac history. For paramedics who might have problems dealing with a patient with a complex history action suggestions might also be provided. Finally the system might automatically record data from instruments and the paramedics actions and send them to the hospital to help prepare for the patients arrival.

Other health based scenarios [3, 4] include support of medical personnel in hospitals or lifestyle support for high risk patients and assisted living for the old and mentally handicapped. Other domains encompass office work [6] industrial assembly/maintenance scenarios [5], and consumer oriented systems. The office scenario has dealt with the automatic activity oriented annotation of multimedia meeting recordings. The industrial scenarios are part of the WearIT@Work project are car assembly, aircraft maintenance and emergency services (fire brigade) are being studied in real world environments.

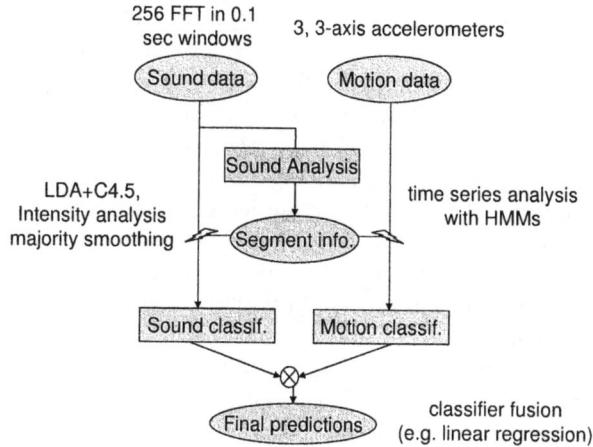

Fig. 2. Recognition method used in [5] to identify a set of wood workshop activities using three wearable 3-axis accelerometers and two microphones

What all the scenarios have in common is the fact that there are pieces of information available electronically that are not used today because finding and accessing them requires too much time and effort. A context sensitive system on the other hand can automatically identify what information the user needs, find it, and deliver it at the right moment and in the most appropriate form. Thus previously useless information suddenly becomes useful.

3 Recognition Methods

Context recognition, as defined in ubiquitous and wearable computing, builds on a many methods from classical AI and machine learning. However the problem that it addresses is significantly different from the classical AI vision. A typical context aware application can be described by a state machine. The states could be the individual steps of a surgical procedure or certain operations that need to be performed in an aircraft engine repair task. For each state a set of actions such as displaying a particular instructions or annotating a video recording is defined in the application. The aim of the context recognition process is to map a signal stream into this set of states. Thus context recognition neither aims to mimic human perception and cognitive processes nor does it really care about complex world models. In particular in the area of wearable computing much context recognition work refrains from using computer vision (with some exceptions e.g [7]) which is considered computationally to expansive and to unreliable in a mobile environment. Instead simple body worn sensors such as accelerometers, gyroscopes, ultrasonic positioning and microphones are used to track user's motions and his interaction with the environment. Since we assume the recognition to run on small embedded or mobile devices, strong emphasis is put achieving not just on optimal recognition rates, but also on the optimal tradeoff between recognition rates and resource consumption [2].

Figure 2 shows the principle of a recognition method used by our group in an experimental assembly scenario [5]. the scenario consisted of a series of procedures such as sawing, filing, taking something out of a drawer, drilling etc that were performed by 5 different subjects in a series of experiments. The subjects were outfitted with three accelerometers (one on each wrist and one on the upper arm of the right hand), and two microphones (one on the wrist and one on the chest). Based on the idea, that all activities can be associated with a characteristic sound the microphones were used to identify potentially interesting signal segments. To this end a combination of intensity analysis from the two microphones, simple sound recognition and smoothing was used. Time series analysis with Hidden Markov Models (HMM) was then applied to the accelerometer signals on the selected segments to classify the activity. The accelerometer classification was then compared with the sound classifier to weed out false positives and improve the overall accuracy.

Currently experiments with other sensors (e.g ultrasonic hand tracking, light sensors), instrumented environment and more complex scenarios are underway.

References

1. D. Abowd, A. K. Dey, R. Orr, and J. Brotherton. Context-awareness in wearable and ubiquitous computing. *Virtual Reality*, 3(3):200–211, 1998.
2. Holger Junker, Paul Lukowicz, Gerhard Tröster Using Information Theory to Design Context- Sensing Wearable Systems *to appear in the IEEE Monograph Sensor Network Operations*, edited by Shashi Phoha, Thomas F. La Porta and Christopher Griffin , IEEE Press, 2005
3. Paul Lukowicz, Tnde Kirstein, Gerhard Tröster, Wearable Systems for Health Care Applications, *Methods Inf Med* 3/2004
4. U. Anliker, J.A. Ward, P. Lukowicz, G. Trster, F. Dolveck, M. Baer, F. Keita, E. Schenker, F. Catarsi, L. Coluccini, A. Belardinelli, D. Shklarski, M. Alon, E. Hirt, R. Schmid, M. Vuskovic. AMON: A Wearable Multiparameter Medical Monitoring and Alert System, *IEEE Transactions on Information Technology in Biomedicine*, Vol. 8, No. 4, Dec. 2004, pages 415- 427
5. Paul Lukowicz, Jamie A Ward, Holger Junker, Mathias Stäger, Gerhard Tröster, Amin Atrash, Thad Starner , Recognizing Workshop Activity Using Body Worn Microphones and Accelerometers, Second International Conference on Pervasive Computing, Pervasive 04, Vienna Austria
6. N. Kern, B.Schiele, H. Junker, P.Lukowicz, G. Tröster Wearable Sensing to Annotate Meeting Recordings *Personal and Ubiquitous Computing*, October, 2003, vol 7, issue 5, Springer Verlag
7. T. Starner, B. Schiele, and A. Pentland. Visual contextual awareness in wearable computing. In *IEEE Intl. Symp. on Wearable Computers*, pages 50–57, Pittsburgh, PA, 1998.

Temporal Representation and Reasoning

A New Approach to the Abstraction of Monitoring Data in Intensive Care

S. Sharshar[1], L. Allart[2,*], and M.-C. Chambrin[1]

[1] EA 2689, Inserm IFR 114, Bat. Vancostenobel, CH&U de Lille,
59037 Lille Cedex, France
{sharshar, chambrin}@lille.inserm.fr
[2] EA 3614, Faculté de Pharmacie, 31, rue du Pr Laguesse, BP 83,
59006 Lille Cedex, France
lallart@pharma.univ-lille2.fr

Abstract. Data driven interpretation of multiple physiological measurements in the domain of intensive care is a key point to provide decision support. The abstraction method presented in this paper provides two levels of symbolic interpretation. The first, at mono parametric level, provides 4 classes (increasing, decreasing, constant and transient) by combination of trends computed at two characteristic spans. The second, at multi parametric level, gives an index of global behavior of the system, that is used to segment the observation. Each segment is therefore described as a sequence of words that combines the results of symbolization. Each step of the abstraction process leads to a visual representation that can be validated by the clinician. Construction of sequences do not need any prior introduction of medical knowledge. Sequences can be introduced in a machine learning process in order to extract temporal patterns related to specific clinical or technical events.

1 Introduction

The overall question of decision support in medical monitoring has been approached from two major perspectives. First, through signal processing based on the various measurements that can be obtained on patient's vital signs. Second, through methods to model knowledge, founded on medical experience and discourse. These approaches are the two extremes of a chain of processing linking the physiological signals, measured by sensors through monitors, to their interpretation by medical personnel. The median situation in this chain [1][2][3][4][5][6][7] mainly focuses on assistance to medical decision in Intensive Care and Anaesthesia, areas where monitoring makes the most intensive use of equipment and variables [8]. In a general manner, the approach to decision support can be expressed in terms of transformation of signals first into data, then into information, and last into knowledge [9]. The passage from one level of abstraction to the next

---

* The authors are grateful to François Douel who corrected the English manuscript.

requires the implementation of trans coding means, in order to switch from one system of representation (physiological signals) to another (medical knowledge) [8][10]. At present, systems of decision support in medical monitoring analyze physiological signals through a time frame and model patterns (such as trends and threshold changes). These temporal patterns describe and symbolize signal variations. The level of abstraction attained enables for instance to establish some pattern templates through which certain specific clinical situations can be recognized.

Extraction of Temporal Patterns. Several methods of extraction of temporal patterns from physiological signals can be found in existing literature. We will only mention here methods which have been used on signals acquired in ICU. *Avent and Charlton* [11] give a full review of the different techniques of extraction of trends used in the 80's. *Imhoff and al.*, [12] proposes either an auto-regressive model, or a non-linear model built from the phase space, which allow real time recognition of outliers and level changes. However, these models are less efficient in the detection of trends. *Makivirta and al.*, [13] proposes first a pre-processing of signals by median filtering, then obtains a qualitative trend from the sign of the slope of the regression line computed on a fixed time frame combined to a threshold change detector. The size of the time frame is set Òa prioriÓ. *Calvelo and al.*, [14] uses an original method of local trend extraction by determining, during a ÒlearningÓ period, the size of the time frame during which the linear approximation of the signal is statistically significant. The transformation allows to decompose each data stream into value, trend and stability. *Hau and Coiera* [15] propose an architecture to generate qualitative models which includes median filtering of the signal, followed by Gaussian filter for smoothing purpose. Then, the signal derivative is computed. A segmenter segments the signal at zero crossing of its derivative. The qualitative trend is given by the sign of the derivative within each interval. *Charbonnier and al.*, [16] uses a method of segmentation based upon gradual linear approximations of the signal ; the segments thus obtained are then aggregated in temporal forms by a classification algorithm. The construction of these segments and forms depends on the initial setting of various thresholds determined on a population of reference signals. *Salatian and Hunter* [17] abstract continuous data into trends by following three consecutive processes: first by median filtering, then by temporal interpolation which creates simple intervals between consecutive data points and finally temporal inference which iteratively merges intervals with similar characteristics into larger intervals. These multiple approaches bring two remarks to mind. First, linear approximation on a preset time interval or signal smoothing through a low-pass filter distort rapid variations of signal which it may be useful to track (such as threshold changes for instance). Second, according to the method used for the representation of trend, slow signal variations may not be taken into account. There are, simultaneously, the issues of the filtering step (which time scale should be used for the extraction of trend), and of the thresholds for reporting information considered as relevant (when should the signal be considered to rise or decrease locally ?).

Determining Pattern Templates. At the level of abstraction of the temporal pattern, it is possible to describe and recognize a certain number of specific clinical situations by pattern templates. A pattern template is a finite set of temporal patterns pre-established from medical knowledge and from the modelization of the variations of the different variables. *Haimowitz and al.,*[7] compares chronological data with pattern templates constructed from medical knowledge and different regression algorithms of signal value. This system, implemented under the name *TrendX*, has initially been developed to track and diagnose anomalies of the child's size-weight growth curve. It has only been applied on a single set of intensive care data for a unique patient. In *Vie-Vent* developed for the monitoring and therapeutic follow-up of artificially ventilated new-born, *Miksh and al.,* [4] proposes to define the trends from qualitative definitions set by medical doctors. The local temporal variation is then classified from exponential envelopes traced around the signal. *Lowe and al.,* [18] bases his works on *Steinmann*'s, and on the concept of Òfuzzy trendsÓ to develop *Sentinel*. ÒFuzzy Ó is defined by a membership relation which links signal to time. Various relationships are defined for each signal. The evolution of the signal is then analyzed by the degree of likelihood for a sample of signal values to belong to one or the other of fuzzy trends. The result is rendered in graphic form, overwriting in colors on each signal's trace the likelihood and the value of the trend detected by the system. *Sentinel* is a monitoring tool able to detect on-line a number of critical situations in anaesthesia area. All of these methods have different aims. For *TrendX* or *Vie-Vent*, the goal is clearly to provide an assistance to medical diagnosis. In the case of *Sentinel*, the goal is to provide visual support to medical decision. However, all of these methods have in common the construction Òa prioriÓ of pattern templates with their specific formalism, as well as the instantiation of these pattern templates through their recognition in the evolution of physiological signals. This last step can prove very complex in the recognition of non-trivial cases or in the recognition of degraded forms of the model.

Introduction of the Present Work. This short overview of the Òstate of the artÓ leaves a number of questions unresolved. At which level of temporal granularity extract the local information of signal variation ? What type of local information to acquire, and through what method of approximation ? Last, what information should be brought at the medical personnel's attention ? Each of these questions is far from having received a conclusive answer, and the multiplicity of methodological approaches used till now emphasizes the complexity of decision support in medical monitoring. The approach we have developed and which we present in this document brings some elements of answer.

1. The first element of answer is dictated by the great variability of signals for identical clinical situations, for a same patient or for different patients. In our approach, the pattern templates are replaced by *sequences* elaborated on-line from a temporal segmentation of signals. This segmentation is based on an analysis of the dynamics of all signals present in the observation. Each sequence is a structure composed of *words*. The words are built with an

alphabet built from the symbolization of the variation of each signal and of the contribution of this variation to the system's overall dynamics.
2. The second element of answer is that, in our opinion, the information given at each phase of the treatment to the medical personnel must for one part be explicit, and for another be easily integrated in a knowledge based system. Our method uses a simple formalism for the symbolization of signal local variation, for writing words, and uses ways of visual display of processing results adapted to medical Òdéjà-vuÓ.
3. The third element of answer is that the relevance of the local temporal pattern can only be established from the data themselves, taking into account their anteriority [13]. Our method uses adaptive thresholds which depend on the distribution of values to qualify signals.
4. Last, the level of temporal granularity chosen must allow to report both slow and fast components of each signal. We therefore analyze each signal on two separate time scales, the size of which is determined by the dynamics of the signal studied.

Our method uses the method described in [14] for the extraction of local trend. The different stages are presented in section 2 of the present document.

2 Methodology

W.L.T.A. or Windowed Linear Trend Analysis is a chain of abstraction which can be represented as a process composed of two levels: a uni varied processing of signals and a multi varied processing of signals. We will illustrate the presentation of information to medical personnel through results obtained on real signals. Finally the integration of knowledge of the domain will be presented in a perspective approach.

2.1 The Uni Varied Processing of Signals

Determination of Characteristic Spans. The whole process is extensively described in [14]. The computation of the characteristic span enables the decomposition of each data stream for any point of the signal into trend, given by the regression coefficient r, and stability, given by the standard deviation σ of the distribution of values within the determined time window. Different criteria are used to define the characteristic span. We used the two following ones: τ_f that is the length of the smallest span corresponding to a good local linear approximation and τ_z that is the overall good stepwise linear approximation.

Computation of the Gaussianity Index G. The gaussianity index proposes to quantify the signal's dynamic by studying the infra or supra gaussian character of the distribution of regression coefficients r, computed at each of the spans τ_f and τ_z, in a frame of observation of w points, displaced gradually on the whole duration of the signal. The gaussianity of the distribution is quantified by the

A New Approach to the Abstraction of Monitoring Data in Intensive Care

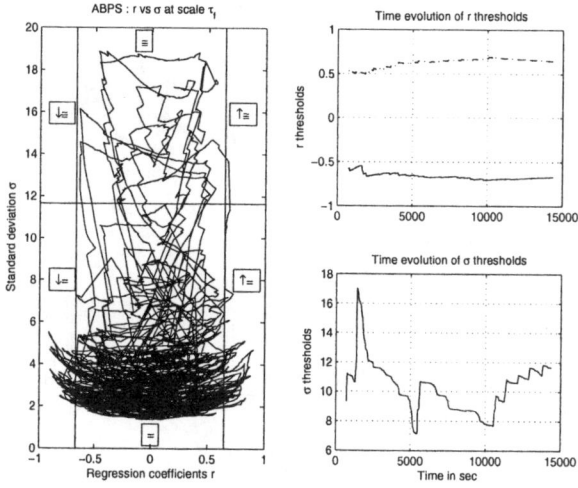

Fig. 1. Left panel : trend *vs* stability plane for systolic arterial blood pressure (ABPS) signal at span τ_f : dashed lines draw the boundaries of the partitioning for the last point t of the observation. Right top panel : temporal evolution of regression coefficients thresholds : plain line for negative threshold, dashed for positive one. Right bottom panel : temporal evolution of standard deviation threshold

kurtosis or flattening-coefficient K^1 which gives us for a span n equal to τ_f or τ_z:

$$G_n(t_i) = K(r_n(t)) \qquad t \in [t_{i-w}, t_i] \qquad (1)$$

Numeric → Symbolic Conversion. Conversion of the signals is done by partitioning the plane formed by the regression coefficients r and the standard deviations σ, as proposed in [14]. We chose to analyse the marginal distributions of r and σ, at each point t, to delineate six zones on the plane (Figure 1). The signal's symbolization is then obtained by applying at each point t, $t \in [t_0, t_{actual}]$, the following rules:

1. IF (zone $\cong$) at span τ_f AND (zone $\cong$) at span τ_z THEN symbol (T)ransient,
2. IF (zone $\downarrow\cong$ OR zone $\downarrow=$) at span τ_z THEN symbol (D)ecrease,
3. IF (zone $\uparrow\cong$ OR zone $\uparrow=$) at span τ_z THEN symbol incre(A)se,
4. IF none of the previous rules THEN symbol (C)onstant.

The result can be rendered in graphic form, overwriting in colors on each signal's trace the value of the symbol calculated by the system, but is presented on another graph for more legibility in black and white (Figure 2).

---

[1] For a set of values x of average μ and standard deviation s, the value of K is obtained from: $K(x) = \frac{\overline{x-\mu}^4}{s^4} - 3$

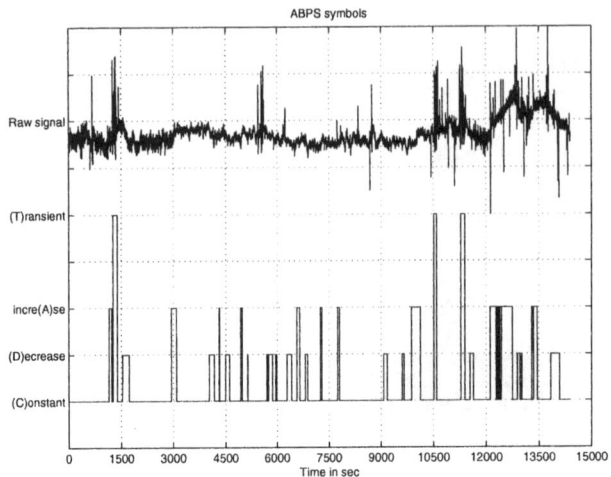

Fig. 2. Results of symbolization process for systolic arterial blood pressure (ABPS) signal

2.2 The Multi Varied Processing of Signals

The objective of the multi varied processing of the signals is first to analyze the behavior of the system (as observed starting from the recording of the physiological signals). This analysis seeks to highlight "states" of the dynamics. Then, the construction of sequences allows an "interpretation" of the states previously individualized.

Θ : *Indicator of System Behavior.* To define Θ we use a principal component analysis (PCA) [19] of the centered-reduced[2] values of the gaussianity indexes G previously defined in section 2.1. PCA is computed in a time frame of w points, displaced gradually on the whole duration of the signals. The average value μ of the projected values on the first component axis is calculated and positioned compared to the interval $[-1, +1]$. We then define a variable δ that takes value 0 when μ is included in the interval $[-1, +1]$ and value 1 if not, which gives us:

$$\Theta(t_i) = \frac{1}{(t_{i-w}) - t_i} \sum_{t=t_{i-w}}^{t_i} \delta(t) \qquad t \in [t_{i-w}, t_i] \qquad (2)$$

Plotting the value of θ by using a grey scale provides a simple visualisation of the behavior of the system. For instance, as shown on Figure 3, "dark" colors highlight the great episode of desaturation between 10333 and 13679 seconds. At this step of the process, Θ warns the medical personnel that "something occurs".

---

[2] for a set of values x of average m and standard deviation s, the value x_i expressed in centered-reduced coordinates is equal to $x_{i_c} = \frac{x_i - m}{s}$.

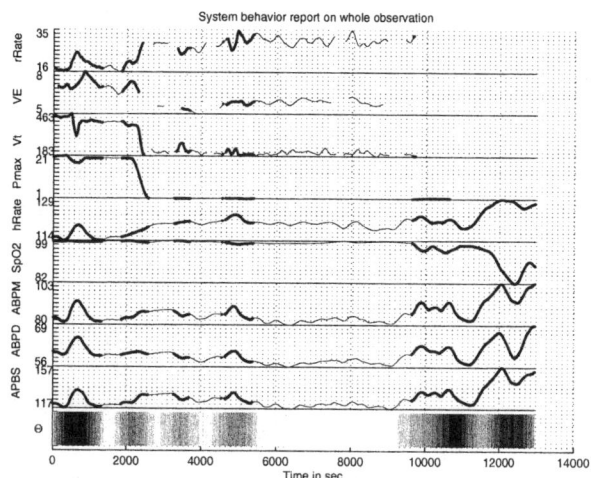

Fig. 3. Whole observation of an ICU patient under weaning of artificial ventilation procedure. Over lined parts of the signal's traces correspond to unstable states as defined by Θ threshold L_c

To go further, we have tested the clinical relevance of Θ's warnings on a set of signals corresponding to 44 hours/patient of recording. Medical expertise of the signals with the help of appended on-line clinical documentation was done. It was asked to the experts to classify the signals in two mutually exclusive states : "stable" or "unstable". Results of the expertise and Θ were therefore analysed by *Receiver Operating Characteristic* curve to evaluate the validity of Θ as a classifier and to define the threshold L_c from which it is considered that the system enters another state. The area under the curve (AUC) was 0.86 ± 0.12, sensitivity of θ was $81.1 \pm 11.1\%$, its specificity $83.4 \pm 15.7\%$ and the threshold L_c 0.31 ± 0.1. The introduction of L_c leads to a temporal subdivision of the signals as illustrated on Figure 3 by the over lined traces.

Building Sequences. Starting from the subdivision elaborated using Θ we can build sequences. Sequences are temporal structures composed of words. At each point t, a word concatenates symbols from an alphabet of four letters (C)onstant, (D)ecrease, incre(A)se, (T)ransient which are the results of the symbolization. At point t, each signal contributes the system's overall dynamics. However, the contribution of each signal is not the same. To take into account the hierarchy of the signals, we will integrate only in the word the symbol of the signals for which their contribution to the first component axis is greater than 60%. A sequence contains: the temporal order of the symbols forming the words, the number of occurrences of each word in the sequence, and the temporal order of the words in the sequences. Figure 4 illustrates the sequence built between 10333 and 13679 seconds that corresponds to an extubation followed by an oxygen desaturation. Visual analysis of the sequence shows that the most frequent word is decrease

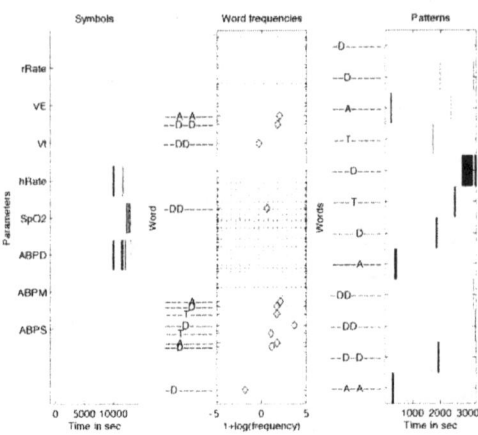

Fig. 4. Example of a sequence corresponding to the period from 10333 to 13679 seconds. Left panel: temporal localization of the symbols (from black to grey, values are (T)ransient, incre(A)se and (D)ecrease). Middle panel: word frequency : the number of occurrences p (in percent) of a word in the sequence is transformed using $wf = 1 + log(p)$. Right panel: the pattern. From left to right, the words include the value of the symbols corresponding to ABPS, ABPD, ABPM, SpO2, hRate,Vt, VE and rRate. Paw,max has not be included in the analysis. For more legibility, the (C)onstant values of the symbols are not represented

of SpO2. The preceding words are those showing modifications of arterial blood pressure (ABPD and ABPM) and heart rate (hRate).

3 Perspectives

Instead of the recognition of specific events or well established clinical situation, it could be interesting to link the sequences, determined by Θ but not labelled by clinical expertise, with actions that can be acquired automatically from the biomedical equipment (change in ventilatory therapy, drug therapy, alarm threshold, ...). The sequence output by the $W.L.T.A$ process describes clinical events or situations depending on the length of the sequence. The next step is to build a system recognizing first these sequences as events and situations, then the relations between these sequences. This recognition system will use the *Think!* formalism described in [20]. Containers will represent the words used in the sequences and the sequences themselves. Chains of processes will be dynamically constructed to represent the sequences, (as show in Figure 5, the sequence $m1 \rightarrow m2$ is built as $Seq1$), building a recognition network. Detection of sequences is done by the excitation of the containers describing the words (one after the other) and the transmission of these excitation along the chain describing the sequence. The use of special activation functions, in the processes taking into account the time delay between words, allows a fuzzy de-

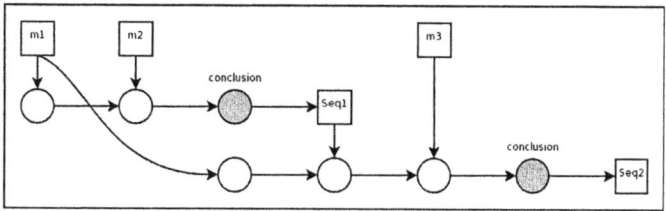

Fig. 5. Example of *Think!* network. This figure shows the network after the construction of two sequences ($m1 \to m2$ and $m1 \to m1 \to m2 \to m3$). A square represents a container, a circle represents a process and an arrow represents a tube. The conclusion process is filled in grey

tection of sequences : small differences between sequences will be ignored. The final detection process (conclusion) receives a number indicating the quality of detection. Construction is done by appending a tube-process combination to the currently built chain. The end of a sequence (conclusion) is done by a process exciting a container to label the sequence ($Seq1$). *Think!* network allows the simultaneous recognition of already learned sequences (already constructed chains) and the building of the new chain representing the current sequence. When an existing sequence is recognized during construction, the container representing this sequence is used for the new chain, as shown for the second chain in Figure 5 : $m1 \to m1 \to m2 \to m3$ is constructed as $m1 \to Seq1 \to m3$ as $m1 \to m2$ is recognized as $Seq1$ during construction. In fact, $m1 \to m1$ is built and when $m2$ arrives, it is simultaneously appended to the new sequence (building $m1 \to m1 \to m2$) as $Seq1$ is recognized by another part of the network . The process recognizing $Seq1$ transmits its detection to the process building the new chain (not represented in the figure). The building process then traces back the detected sequence and replaces its constituents in the new chain ($m1 \to m2$) by the conclusion of the recognized chain ($Seq1$). Advantages of the system are the simultaneous detection of learned sequences and their use in building the currently learned sequence, and the mixing of abstraction levels. The system could learn sequences with the associated actions, if any. The information provided to the clinician could then be to propose some actions according to the current sequence.

References

1. *Coll*: Improving Control of Patient Status in Critical Care: The IMPROVE Project. Computer Programs and Methods in Biomedicine **51** (1996) 1–130
2. Larsson, J., Hayes-Roth, B., Gaba, D.: Guardian : Final Evaluation. Technical Report KSL-96-25. Technical report, Knowledge Systems Laboratory, Stanford University (1996)
3. Manders, E., Davant, B.: Data Acquisition for an Intelligent Bedside Monitoring System. In: Proceedings of the 18th Annual International Conference of the IEEE Engineering in Medicine and Biology Society. (1996) 957–958

4. Miksch, S., Horn, W., Popow, C., Paky, F.: Utilizing Temporal Data Abstraction for Data Validation and Therapy Planning for Artificially Ventilated Newborn Infants. Artificial Intell. Med. **8** (1996) 543–576
5. Shahar, Y., Musen, M.: Knowledge-based Temporal Abstraction in Clinical Domains. Artificial Intell. Med. **8** (1996) 267–298
6. Dojat, M., Pachet, F., Guessoum, Z., Touchard, D., Harf, A., Brochard., L.: Neoganesh : a working System for the Automated Control of Assisted Ventilation in Icus. Artificial Intell. Med. **11** (1997) 97–117
7. Haimovitz, I., Kohane, I.: Managing Temporal Worlds for Medical Trend Diagnosis. Artificial Intell. Med. **8** (1996) 299–321
8. Coiera, E.: Automated Signal Interpretation. In: Monitoring in Anaesthesia and Intensive Care. W.B. Saunders Co Ltd (1994) 32–42
9. Calvelo, D.: Apprentissage de Modeles de la Dynamique pour l'Aide a la Decision en Monitorage Clinique. PhD thesis, Lille 1 (1999)
10. Mora, F., Passariello, G., Carrault, G., Pichon, J.P.L.: Intelligent Patient Monitoring and Management Systems : a Review. IEEE Eng. Med. Bio. **12** (1993) 23–33
11. Avent, R., Charlton, J.: A Critical Review of Trend-detection Methodologies for Biomedical Systems. Critical Reviews in Biomedical Engineering **17** (1990) 621–659
12. Imhoff, M., Bauer, M., Gather, U., Lohlein, D.: Statistical Pattern Detection in Univariate Time Series of Intensive Care Online Monitoring Data. Intensive Care Medicine **24** (1998) 1305–1314
13. Makivirta, A., Koski, E., Kari, A., Sukuwara, T.: The Median Filter as a Preprocessor for a Patient Monitor Limit Alarm System in Intensive Care. Computer Methods and Programs in Biomedicine **34** (1991) 139–144
14. Calvelo, D., Chambrin, M.C., Pomorski, D., Ravaux, P.: Towards Symbolization Using Data-driven Extraction of Local Trends for ICU Monitoring. Artificial Intell. Med. **1-2** (2000) 203–223
15. Hau, D., Coiera, E.: Learning Qualitative Models of Dynamics Systems. Machine Learning **26** (1997) 177–211
16. Charbonnier, S., Becq, G., Biot, L.: On Line Segmentation Algorithm for Continuously Monitored Data in Intensive Care units. IEEE Transactions on Biomedical Engineering **51** (2004) 484–492
17. Salatian, A., Hunter, J.: Deriving Trends in Historical and Real-time Continuously sampled Medical Data. Journal of Intelligence Information Systems **13** (1999) 47–71
18. Lowe, A., Jones, R., Harrison, M.: The graphical presentation of decision support information in an intelligent anaesthesia monitor. Artificial Intell. Med. **22** (2001) 173–191
19. Saporta, G.: Analyse en Composantes Principales. In: Probabilités, Analyse des Données et Statistiques. Technip (1990) 159–186
20. Vilhelm, C., Ravaux, P., Calvelo, D., Jaborska, A., Chambrin, M., Boniface, M.: Think!: a Unified Numerical - symbolic Knowledge Representation Scheme and Reasoning System. Artificial Intelligence **116** (2000) 67–85

Learning Rules with Complex Temporal Patterns in Biomedical Domains

Lucia Sacchi, Riccardo Bellazzi, Cristiana Larizza,
Riccardo Porreca, and Paolo Magni

Dipartimento di Informatica e Sistemistica, University of Pavia, via Ferrata 1,
27100 Pavia, Italy
lucia@aim.unipv.it
{riccardo.bellazzi, cristiana.larizza, paolo.magni}@unipv.it

Abstract. This paper presents a novel algorithm for extracting rules expressing complex patterns from temporal data. Typically, a temporal rule describes a temporal relationship between the antecedent and the consequent, which are often time-stamped events. In this paper we introduce a new method to learn rules with complex temporal patterns in both the antecedent and the consequent, which can be applied in a variety of biomedical domains. Within the proposed approach, the user defines a set of complex interesting patterns that will constitute the basis for the construction of the temporal rules. Such complex patterns are represented with a Temporal Abstraction formalism. An APRIORI-like algorithm then extracts precedence temporal relationships between the complex patterns. The paper presents the results obtained by the rule extraction algorithm in two different biomedical applications. The first domain is the analysis of time series coming from the monitoring of hemodialysis sessions, while the other deals with the biological problem of inferring regulatory networks from gene expression data.

1 Introduction

The application of data mining techniques to the medical and biological domain has gained great interest in the last few years, also thanks to the encouraging results that have been achieved in many fields [1,2]. One issue of particular interest in this area is represented by the analysis of temporal data, usually referred to as Temporal Data Mining (TDM) [3,4,5]. Within TDM, research usually focuses on the analysis of time series, collected measuring clinical or biological variables at different points in time. The explicit handling of time in the data mining process is extremely attractive, as it gives the possibility of deepening the insight into the temporal behavior of complex processes, and may help to forecast the future evolution of a variable or to extract causal relationships between the variables at hand.

An increasing number of TDM approaches is currently applied to the analysis of biomedical time series; in functional genomics, for example, clustering techniques have been largely exploited to analyze gene expression time series, in order to assess the function of unknown genes, relying on the assumption that genes with similar profiles may share similar function [6,7,8]. TDM has also been successfully used to study gene expression time series of particular cell lines which are crucial for understanding key molecular processes of clinical interest, such as the insulin actions in muscles [9] and the cell cycle in normal and tumor cells [10]. Several works have been proposed also for what concerns the representation and processing of time series coming from the monitoring of clinical parameters, collected for example during an ICU staying [11,12].

In this paper, we are interested into one of the most attractive applications of AI-based TDM: the extraction of temporal rules from data. Unlike association rules, temporal rules are characterized by the fact that the consequent is related to the antecedent of the rule by some kind of temporal relationship [13]; moreover, a temporal rule typically suggests a cause-effect association between the antecedent and the consequent of the rule itself. When applied to the biomedical domain, this could be of particular interest, for example in reconstructing gene regulatory networks or in discovering knowledge about the causes of a target event [4].

An interesting approach to the problem of extracting temporal rules has been presented in [14,15] where the authors, exploiting the ideas of Hoppner [13] and the well-known APRIORI algorithm [16], have defined a method for the discovery of both association and temporal rules to get an insight into the possible causes of non-adherence to therapeutic protocols in hemodialysis, through the analysis of a set of monitoring variables. The TDM approach relied basically on two phases, the first one concerning the time series representation while the second dealing with rule extraction. In particular, the time series are first summarized through qualitative patterns extracted with the technique of Temporal Abstractions; then, possible associations between those patterns and the non-adherence events are searched with an APRIORI-like procedure. The mentioned method, however, only treats rules with antecedents composed by the conjunction of simple patterns (i.e. patterns of the kind "increasing", "decreasing", ...), where the conjunction is interpreted as a co-occurrence relationship (i.e. "variable A increasing" occurs at the same time of "variable B decreasing"). If this conjunction temporally precedes another simple pattern, say "variable C increasing", sufficiently often, a rule of the kind "variable A increasing and variable B decreasing precedes variable C increasing" is generated.

In this paper, we propose an extension of the method described in [14,15] in order to extract rules with arbitrarily complex patterns as members of both the rule antecedents and consequents. The data miner can define in advance such patterns, or they might be automatically generated by a complex pattern extractor. This extension is able to deal with the search of relationships between complex behaviors, which can be particularly interesting in biomedical applications. For example, a drug is first absorbed and then utilized, so that its plasma distribution precedes its effect in the target tissue. In this case, it would be important to look for complex episodes of "up and down" type in the drug plasma concentration, to automatically extract temporal knowledge in the data. Therefore, the method that we propose in this paper enables the user to define episodes of interest, thus synthesizing the domain knowledge about a specific process, and to efficiently look for the specific temporal interactions between such complex episodes.

The paper is structured as follows: we first describe the new method for the extraction of complex temporal patterns from data; then, we introduce two different biomedical applications where the method is to provide interesting results on real data sets. Finally we discuss pros e cons of the proposed approach.

2 The Complex Temporal Rules Extraction Method

As shown in Figure 1, the method proposed in this paper develops following different steps that, starting from the raw time series and passing through different stages of representation, leads to the construction of a set of temporal rules, where both the antecedent and the consequent are made up of complex patterns.

2.1 A Formalism for Time Series Representation: The Technique of Temporal Abstractions

To be able to extract temporal rules from the data, we need first of all a suitable representation of the time series [13]. A convenient technique to extract a compact and meaningful representation of temporal data is to resort to Temporal Abstractions (TAs) [17].

TAs are an AI methodology characterized by the move from a time-stamped (quantitative) representation of temporal data to an interval-based qualitative one. In each interval, a specific pattern is verified in the data; such patterns represent a meaningful summary of the original data, and can be used to derive features that characterize the dynamics of the system under observation. Algorithms that, taking as input a time series, generate an interval series, with intervals corresponding to the time periods in which a specific pattern is present in the input, are referred to as TA *mechanisms*. TA mechanisms represent the fundamental step of TA-based analysis.

Within TAs, we can distinguish between two main categories: basic and complex abstractions. Basic TAs are used to detect simple patterns in numerical or symbolic time series. More precisely, we can extract *Trend* Temporal Abstractions, to capture increasing, decreasing or stationary courses in a numerical time series, and *State* TAs, to detect qualitative patterns corresponding to low, high or normal values in a numerical or symbolic time series. Complex TAs, on the other hand, correspond to intervals in which specific temporal relationships between basic or other complex TAs hold. These relationships are typically identified by the temporal operators defined in Allen algebra [18].

In our approach, we aim at representing the time series through a set of complex TAs, that will be denoted as *complex temporal events*; to obtain such representation, data are processed following two consecutive steps.

1. Raw time series are initially processed with a suitable TA mechanism [14] to describe the time course of a variable as a set of consecutive Basic *trend* TAs. The resulting representation is a label made up of simple qualitative elements of the kind [Increasing], [Decreasing], [Steady] (Figure 1 a) and b)).

2. The Basic TA description represents the basis for the creation of the final complex TA representation, that will be then used in the rule extraction algorithm. This representation is based on the definition of *complex temporal events*, that are complex abstractions defined as the time intervals in which specific interesting

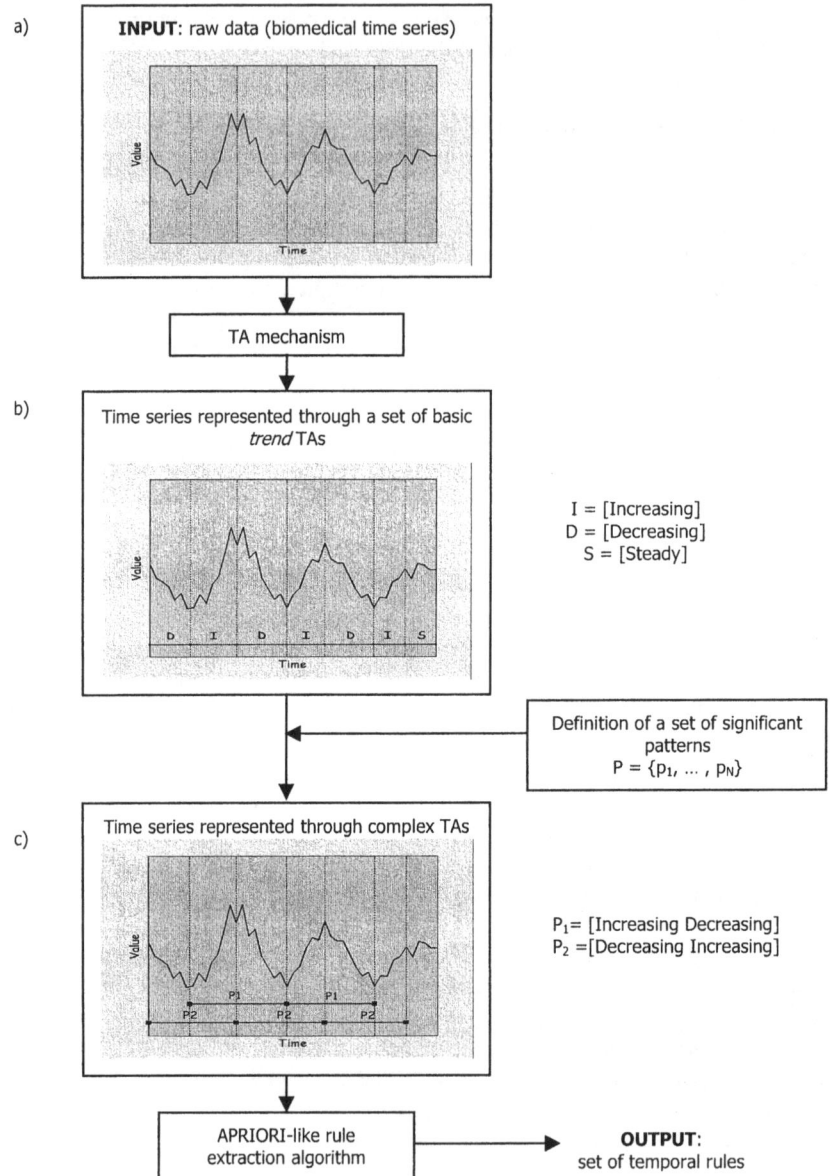

Fig. 1. The steps of the algorithm for temporal rules extraction

patterns occur in the input data. One of the core aspects of this phase is the definition of a set of significant patterns $P = \{p_1,...p_n\}$, where each p_i is made up by the composition of simple labels like [Increasing], [Decreasing], [Steady]. In general, the set P may be both user-defined or automatically suggested to the researcher after a pre-processing of the initial qualitative representation of the variables performed with an appropriate strategy, such as the one presented in [19]. Moreover, the definition of P clearly relies on the clinical/biological knowledge on the kind of relationships that may be useful to explore with respect to the analysis purposes. As an example, let us consider a situation in which there is interest to investigate if a particular peak in the dynamics of a variable V_1 is often related to an opposite peak of another variable V_2. We can formalize this problem by defining P as P={[Increasing Decreasing], [Decreasing Increasing]}. The rule extraction will then be performed only on those series that present the first pattern in V_1 and the second pattern in V_2; such rules will look for a temporal significant relationship between those two patterns.

The steps that lead from the raw data to the representation through *complex temporal events* are depicted in Figure 1 a), b) and c). The example reveals also that, in general, it is possible to find more than one example of the same pattern within a single time series and that the intervals that correspond to different patterns may overlap when dealing with the same profile.

2.2 Temporal Rules Extraction

Once we have derived a representation of the temporal profiles based on the definition of a set of complex TAs, the method for temporal rules extraction develops through a strategy which looks for both the antecedent and the consequent of the rule coming from the set of complex TAs that represent the time series. The rules extraction strategy will then look for rules in which a set of contemporaneous TAs (the antecedent) has a precedence temporal relationship with another TA (the consequent). Notice that, since temporal rules are derived through the combination of complex temporal abstractions on the basis of a temporal relationship, they can be considered themselves as complex TAs.

More formally, we consider temporal relationships expressed by the temporal operator PRECEDES, defined as follows: given two episodes, A and C, with time intervals $[a_1, a_2]$ and $[c_1, c_2]$, we say that A PRECEDES C if $a_1 \leq c_1$ and $a_2 \leq c_2$. Note that PRECEDES includes the Allen's temporal operators OVERLAPS, FINISHED-BY, MEETS, BEFORE, EQUALS and STARTS. Moreover, the PRECEDES relationship may be constrained by some parameters, that set some restrictions on the mutual position of the intervals involved [15]. These parameters are: the right shift (RS), defined as the maximum allowed distance between c_2 and a_2, the left shift (LS), defined as the maximum allowed distance between c_1 and a_1 and the gap, defined as the maximum distance between a_2 and c_1, when $c_1 > a_2$.

The search procedure is then aimed at defining rules of the kind $A \rightarrow_p C_i$, where A is a conjunction of complex TAs and constitutes the antecedent, while C_i is the consequent of the rule. The notation $\rightarrow_p$ defines the PRECEDES temporal relationship between A and C_i.

The search procedure develops following the ideas of [14,15], after having properly modified the definitions of the set from which to extract the antecedent and the consequent episodes. In more detail, in order to define confidence and support, we need first to introduce some quantities:

- TS: the time span, i.e. the total duration of the observation period in which the rule is derived;
- RTS: the rule time span, i.e. the time span corresponding to the union of the episodes in which both the antecedent and the consequent of the rule occur;
- NAT: the number of times (episodes) in which the antecedent occurs during the TS;
- NARTS : the number of times (episodes) in which the antecedent occurs during the RTS.

We can therefore define:

- Support (Sup) = RTS / TS[1];
- Confidence (Conf) = NARTS / NAT.

The strategy to extract temporal rules develops then as follows:

1. Put all the *complex temporal events* that represent the time series in the set A_0;
2. Fix the consequent as an episode $c_i \in A_0$;
3. Apply the PRECEDES operator between each a_i and c_i, where a_i is such that $a_i \in A_0 - \{c_i\}$ and a_i doesn't refer to the same time series as c_i. Put the results in the new set A_1 and set the counter k to 1. In general A_1 is formed by those rules that show a support greater then a fixed threshold;
4. Repeat:
   - Set k=k+1;
   - Generate the set A_k from A_{k-1} such that each rule in A_k has cardinality k (conjunction of k TAs in the antecedent) and verifies the PRECEDES relationship. Even in this case, it is possible to state a restriction for A_k based on a threshold on the support;

   Until: A_k is empty;
5. Put A= A_{k-1} and repeat from step 2 for another consequent $c_j \in A_0$.

3 Results

In this section we show the results obtained by applying the method to two different problems, the first in the clinical domain, while the other one concerning the biological problem of inferring gene regulatory networks from data. These examples allow to understand the wide spectrum of applicability of the proposed solutions.

3.1 Analysis of Time Series Coming from Haemodialysis Sessions Monitoring

The first application we introduce is about the use of the rule extraction algorithm to analyze time series coming from the monitoring of several variables during different dialysis sessions[2]. In particular, we have considered a single patient undergoing to 86

---

[1] Several definitions of support can be considered; in our case, we chose to consider the real time span of the episodes, in order to take into account low frequency episodes with long TS.
[2] The data have been made available by courtesy of the Dialysis Unit of the A.O. of Vigevano, Italy.

dialysis cycles, looking for the relationships occurring between arterial pressure and heart rate. In our study, we have considered systolic pressure (SP), diastolic pressure (DP) and heart frequency (HR). From a clinical point of view, it is interesting to look for temporal relationships that highlight a negative correlation between the pressure variables on one hand and the heart frequency on the other. Such relationships may be related to hypertension or hypotension episodes. Relying on this assumption, we have identified the set P as P = {[Increasing Steady Decreasing], [Decreasing Steady Increasing]}. The rule extraction algorithm searches for rules that satisfy the PRECEDES operator between opposite *complex temporal events* in the antecedents with respect to the consequents (e.g. [Increasing Steady Decreasing] vs [Decreasing Steady Increasing]). Table 1 shows the results we obtained fixing a threshold for the confidence, Conf ≥ 0.7, and for the support, Sup ≥ 0.1. We have been able to derive rules with complex patterns involving one or more variables. The first rule extracts a contemporaneous pattern for Systolic and Diastolic pressure, in which an up and down pattern is followed by a down and up pattern of the Heart Rate; the rule has confidence 0.7 and is verified in 10 dialysis over 86. Other two similar rules, which relate Heart Rate with Systolic and Diastolic pressures are also found. In both cases the number of dialysis in which the rule is verified is 24. These episodes are clinically relevant, since they correspond to the patient response to hypertension, probably due to vasoconstriction.

Table 1. The rules derived from the analysis of the haemodialysis data ([ISD]= [Increasing Steady Decreasing], [DSI] = [Decreasing Steady Increasing])

RULE (OPERATOR: PRECEDES) P={[Increasing Steady Decreasing], [Decreasing Steady Increasing]}					
Antecedent		Consequent		Confidence	Support
Variable	Pattern	Variable	Pattern		
SP	[ISD]	HR	[DSI]	0.706	0.156
DP	[ISD]				
HR	[DSI]	DP	[ISD]	0.755	0.398
HR	[DSI]	SP	[ISD]	0.8	0.407

3.2 Analysis of Gene Regulatory Networks Through Gene Expression Data

The second study regards the attractive biological problem of inferring genetic regulatory networks starting from gene expression data. In this domain, our algorithm could be particularly suited since it allows to describe patterns of synchronization and precedence in gene expressions; such patterns might be the evidence of a close relationships between genes. Moreover, by highlighting the relationships between synchronized gene sets, we can gain insight into the temporal sequence of macro-processes, potentially suggesting cause-effect relationships between the involved genes.

In this paper we have analysed the data coming from DNA microarray experiments on human cell cycle, presented in [10] and available at http://genome-www.stanford.edu/Human-CellCycle/Hela/. From the whole dataset, we extracted 5 time series of 47 samples that correspond to some of the human genes which are known to regulate cell cycle [20]. We have considered the rules characterized by pattern P={[Increasing Decreasing], [Decreasing Increasing]}. This pattern is useful to highlight the synchronization and phase shifts between genes during the cell cycle. The rules have been derived with confidence Conf =1 and support Sup ≥ 0.7. Rather interestingly, the most important known relationships between genes are automatically derived by the algorithm. Table 2 and Figure 2 show some examples related to the gene for Cyclin E, the protein which regulates the transition from the phase G1 to S. Protein P27, a Cyclin E repressor, is always in opposition to Cyclin E; this is expressed by a precedence relationship, where a peak of one gene always precedes the peak of the other. Moreover, Cyclin A and B regulate transition from phase S to G2 and M, and CDC25 is a protein which favors the transition from G2 to M. Such genes are always find to be synchronized, and their complex pattern periodically precedes Cyclin E.

Table 2. Examples of the Rules extracted from the analysis of gene expression data of human cell cycle ([ID] = [Increasing Decreasing], [DI] = [Decreasing Increasing])

RULE (OPERATOR: PRECEDES) P = {[Increasing Decreasing] [Decreasing Increasing]}					
Antecedent		Consequent		Confidence	Support
Gene	Pattern	Gene	Pattern		
P27	[ID]	Cyclin E	[DI]	1	0.915
Cyclin A Cyclin B	[ID] [ID]	Cyclin E	[ID]	1	0.745
CDC25C Cyclin A	[ID] [ID]	Cyclin E	[ID]	1	0.745

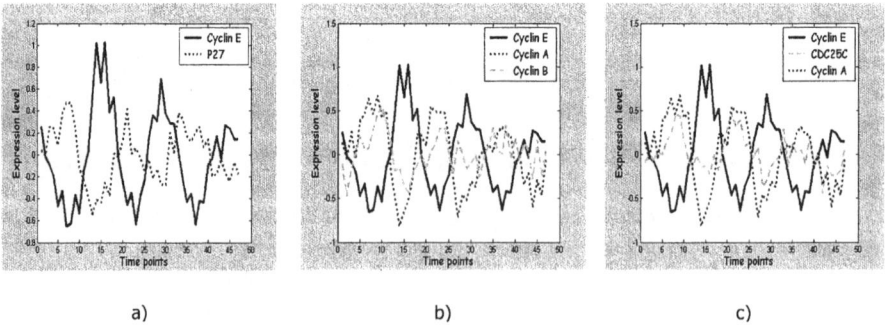

a) b) c)

Fig. 2. The time series corresponding to the temporal rules reported in Table 2. Protein P27 is always in opposition to Cyclin E (a); Cyclin A, Cyclin B and CDC25 are synchronized; their complex pattern periodically precedes Cyclin E (b,c)

4 Discussion

In this paper we have presented a new method for the automated generation of temporal rules which involve complex patterns in both the antecedent and the consequent. This algorithm is particularly suited for exploring the temporal relationships between the variables collected in different kind of biomedical data bases. It is important to note that the method performs a knowledge-based search in the data set. Knowledge is required to the domain expert to specify the parameters of the temporal abstraction mechanisms, such as the minimum slope of the trends used to define the simple patterns; moreover, additional knowledge is needed to select the interesting temporal complex patterns and to completely specify the precede temporal relationship. Finally, the rules are extracted after the choice of support and confidence. Such a knowledge-intensive procedure can be considered both a strength and a weakness of the approach. It is a strength, since it allows the extraction of results which are driven by background knowledge in an explicit way. This facilitates explanation and user control on the output. It is a weakness, since the degrees of freedom of the users are high, so that the results may be difficult to reproduce if all the parameters are not clearly reported in the data analysis process; moreover it requires a workload to the user in knowledge elicitation. In our opinion, it can be used as a useful instrument to complement data-driven approaches to gain insight in complex temporal behaviours, which are common in biomedical domains.

Given the great flexibility that characterizes the algorithm, immediate extensions may lead to consider both Trend and State TAs for the representation of the temporal profiles; moreover also different relationships between the events may be taken into account. As a future development we are including in the algorithm a strategy to automatically propose to the user the most relevant complex patterns in the data; moreover, we are working on a technique for result visualization through a semantic network of temporal relationships.

References

1. Li, L., Tang, H., Wu, Z., Gong, J., Gruidl, M., Zou, J., Tockman, M., Clark, R.A.: Data mining techniques for cancer detection using serum proteomic profiling. Artif Intell Med 32 (2004) 71-83.
2. Golub, T.R., Slonim, D.K., Tamayo, P., Huard, C., Gaasenbeek, M., Mesirov, J.P., Coller, H., Loh, M.L., Downing, J.R., Caligiuri, M.A., Bloomfield, C.D., Lander, E.S.: Molecular classification of cancer: class discovery and class prediction by gene expression monitoring. Science 286 (1999) 531-537
3. Augusto, J.C.: Temporal reasoning for decision support in medicine. Artif Intell Med. 33 (2005) 1-24
4. Roddick, J.F., Spiliopoulou, M.: A survey of temporal knowledge discovery paradigms and methods. IEEE Transactions on Knowledge and Data Engineering 14 (2002) 750-767
5. Lin, W., Orgun, M.A., Williams, G.J.: An overview of temporal data mining. In: Simeoff, S., Williams, G., Hegland, M. (eds.): Proceedings of the 1st Australian Data Mining Workshop (ADM02), (2002) 83-90
6. Eisen, M., Spellman, P.T., Botstein, D., Brown, P.O.: Cluster analysis and display of genome-wide expression patterns. Proc Natl Acad Sci 95 (1998)14863-14868

7. Ramoni, M., Sebastiani, P., Cohen, P.: Bayesian clustering by dynamics. Machine Learning 47 (2002) 91-121
8. Hvidsten, T.R., Lægreid, A., Komorowski, J.: Learning rule-based models of biological process from gene expression time profiles using Gene Ontology. Bioinformatics 19 (2003)1116-1123
9. Di Camillo, B., Sreekumar, R., Greenlund, L.J., Toffolo, G., Cobelli, C., Nair, S.K.: Selection of insulin regulated genes based on array measurement error. In: Proceedings of Genomics of Diabetes and Associated Diseases in the Post Genome Era, (2003) 113
10. Whitfield, M.L., Sherlock, G., Saldanha, A.J., Murray, J.I., Ball, C.A., Alexander, K.E., Matese, J.C., Perou, C.M., Hurt, M.M., Brown, P.O., Botstein, D.: Identification of genes periodically expressed in the human cell cycle and their expression in tumors. Mol Biol Cell 13 (2002) 1977-2000
11. Salatian, A., Hunter, J.R.W.: Deriving Trends in Historical and Real-Time Continuously Sampled Medical Data. Journal of Intelligent Information Systems 13 (1999) 47-71
12. Salatian, A.: Interpreting Historical ICU Data Using Associational and Temporal Reasoning. In: ICTAI (2003) 442-450
13. Höppner, F.: Discovery of temporal patterns-learning rules about the qualitative behaviour of time series. In: Proceedings of the Fifth PPKDD, LNAI (2001) 192-203
14. Bellazzi, R., Larizza, C., Magni, P., Bellazzi, R.: Quality assessment of hemodialysis services through temporal data mining. In: Dojat, M., Keravnou, E., Barahona, P. (eds.): Artificial Intelligence in Medicine. Ninth Conference on Artificial Intelligence in Medicine in Europe, LNAI 2780. Springer-Verlag (2003) 11-20
15. Bellazzi, R., Larizza, C., Magni, P., Bellazzi, R.: Temporal data mining for the quality assessment of hemodialysis services. Artificial Intelligence in Medicine, May 2005.
16. Agrawal, R., Srikant, R.: Fast algorithms for mining association rules in large databases. In: Proceedings of the International Conference on Very Large Databases. Morgan Kaufmann (1994) 478-499
17. Shahar, Y.: A framework for knowledge-based temporal abstraction. Artificial Intelligence 90 (1997) 79-133
18. Allen, J.F.: Towards a general theory of action and time. Artificial Intelligence 23 (1984) 123-154
19. Sacchi, L., Bellazzi, R., Larizza, C., Magni, P., Curk, T., Petrovic, U., Zupan, B.: Clustering gene expression data with temporal abstractions. In: Medinfo. (2004) 798-802
20. Tyson, J.J., Chen, K., Novak, B.: Network dynamics and cell physiology. Nat Rev Mol Cell Biol 2 (2001) 908-916

Discriminating Exanthematic Diseases from Temporal Patterns of Patient Symptoms

Silvana Badaloni and Marco Falda

Dept. of Information Engineering, University of Padova,
Via Gradenigo 6/B - 35131 Padova, Italy
{silvana.badaloni, marco.falda}@unipd.it

Abstract. The temporal dimension is a characterizing factor of many diseases, in particular, of the exanthematic diseases. Therefore, the diagnosis of this kind of diseases can be based on the recognition of the typical temporal progression and duration of different symptoms. To this aim, we propose to apply a temporal reasoning system we have developed. The system is able to handle both qualitative and metric temporal knowledge affected by vagueness and uncertainty. In this preliminary work, we show how the fuzzy temporal framework allows us to represent typical temporal structures of different exanthematic diseases (e.g. Scarlet Fever, Measles, Rubella et c.) thus making possible to find matches with data coming from the patient disease.

1 Introduction

The necessity for the recruitment of symbolic approach to solve medical problems arises from the understanding that medical problems are often too complex to be modeled analytically [21].

An important contribution to symbolic approach is given by fuzzy methodologies that can be regarded as a formalism particularly suitable to deal with the imprecision intrinsic to many medical problems and useful to build models for biological systems when a precise model doesn't exist or it is difficult to realize [16].

The claim that fuzzy logic is a useful theoretical, methodological, and design tool for addressing some of the problems found in developing intelligent patient supervision systems can be widely found in the literature concerning medical AI [9,1]. In [9] where a patient supervision system for intensive and coronary care units is described, the role of fuzzy logic is strongly emphasized. In fact, uncertainty and impreciseness pervade system input information as well as the representation of knowledge, and the *modus operandi* of human expert. The model proposed for developing this supervision system allows the integration of knowledge on the evolution of a set of parameters into a knowledge representation scheme in which time plays a fundamental role [9,13].

More in general, taking into account also the temporal dimension, the development of hybrid systems combining the two notions of fuzziness and time makes possible to perform fuzzy temporal reasoning particularly useful in many medical applications [22, 15]. Medical diagnosis is a field in which imprecise information about symptoms and events can appear; for example this happens when the physician must interpret the description of a patient, or when a new disease appears and typical patterns have to be discovered.

Moreover, there are diseases characterized by a typical temporal evolution and duration of different symptoms such as fever, appearance of skin rush et c., that is the occurrence of symptoms follows a typical temporal behavior. In these cases, the study of the temporal evolution of a set of physical parameters may be a way for discriminating among a set of diseases. Then the diagnosis can be based on the recognition of typical temporal structures. This is the case of exanthematic diseases.

This paper deals with representation and reasoning on information concerning the evolution of physical parameters by means of a model based on Fuzzy Temporal Constraint Networks [12, 14]. Temporal information coming from the domain may be both qualitative such as "the interval I_1 with fever precedes the interval I_2 with skin rush" or metric such as "fever lasts one day" or mixed such as "symptom m_2 follows symptom m_1 and starts at 8pm". Moreover the information is often affected by imprecision and uncertainty. For this reason, crisp relations both qualitative and metric are not adequate and fuzzy temporal relations have to be introduced [15, 22].

The aim of this paper is the application of our system capable of handling fuzzy temporal knowledge in a very general way [5] to recognize different patterns typical of diseases in order to build a first step towards an automated tool for medical diagnosis to be applied in all those cases in which these temporally-based features are relevant.

2 Qualitative and Quantitative Fuzzy Temporal Constraints

The most famous approach to deal with qualitative temporal constraints is the Allen's Interval Algebra [2]; in this algebra each constraint is a binary relation between a pair of intervals, represented by a disjunction of *atomic relations*:

$$I_1 \ (rel_1, \ldots, rel_m) \ I_2$$

where each rel_i is one of the 13 mutually exclusive atomic relations that may exist between two intervals (such as *equal, before, meets* etc.).

Allen's Interval Algebra has been extended in [3, 4, 7] with the Possibility Theory by assigning to every atomic relation rel_i a degree α_i, which indicates the *preference degree* of the corresponding assignment among the others

$$I_1 \ R \ I_2 \text{ with } R = (rel_1[\alpha_1], \ldots, rel_{13}[\alpha_{13}])$$

where α_i is the preference degree of rel_i ($i = 1, \ldots, 13$); preferences can be defined in the interval $[0, 1]$. If we take the set $\{0, 1\}$ the classic approach is obtained.

Intervals are interpreted as ordered pairs $(x, y) : x \leq y$ of $\Re^2$, and soft constraints between them as fuzzy subsets of $\Re^2 \times \Re^2$ in such a way that the pairs of intervals that are in relation rel_k have membership degree α_k.

Temporal metric constraints have been extended to the fuzzy case starting from the traditional TCSPs [11] in many ways [17, 14]. To represent fuzzy temporal metric constraints we adopt trapezoidal distributions [5], since they seem enough expressive and computationally less expensive than general semi-convex functions [19].

Each trapezoid is represented by a 4-tuple of values describing its four characteristic points plus a degree of consistency α_i denoting its height.

$$T_k = \ll a_k, b_k, c_k, d_k \gg [\alpha_k]$$

with $a_k, b_k \in \Re \cup \{-\infty\}$, $c_k, d_k \in \Re \cup \{+\infty\}$, $\alpha_k \in (0, 1]$, $\ll$ is either (or [and $\gg$ is either) or].

The points b_k and c_k determine the interval of those temporal values which are likely, whereas a_k and d_k determine the interval out of which the values are absolutely impossible.

The effective translation of $\ll$ and $\gg$ is not completely arbitrary, but it is constrained to well defined rules that lead to build well-formed trapezoids [5].

As an example, let's consider the following sentence:

"In disease d_1 the symptom m_1 occurs always after about a day. The symptom m_2 follows m_1 rather commonly; it uses to last between 2 to 4 days, though other less possible cases range from 1 day as the lowest bound to a week as the uppest one."

We can model the sentence as shown in Figure 1 and express it as

$$m_1 : \{(0.5, 1, 1, 1.5)\}$$
$$m_2 : \{(1, 2, 4, 7)[0.7]\}$$

in the first constraint an uncertainty of half a day has been added and its degree of preference has been omitted because it is 1.

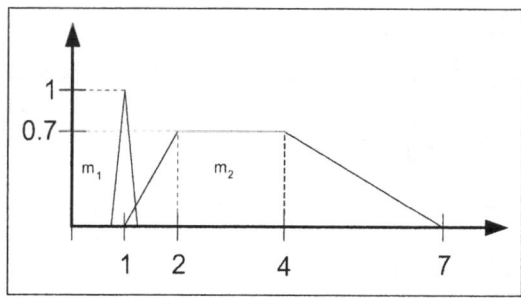

Fig. 1. example of metric constraint

The generalized definition of trapezoid extreme increases the expressivity of the language, therefore the range of allowed trapezoids is augmented with respect to e.g. [8]; for instance, the following trapezoids can be modeled:

$$\text{open triangle:} (a_i, a_i, a_i, d_i)[\alpha_i]$$

$$\text{open trapezoid:} (-\infty, -\infty, c_i, d_i)[\alpha_i]$$

$$\text{closed left semiaxis:} (-\infty, -\infty, d_i, d_i)[\alpha_i]$$

Besides, these trapezoids allow us to integrate qualitative constraints.

As far as operations between metric constraints are concerned, the usual operations i.e. inversion, conjunctive combination, disjunctive combination and composition have been defined.

2.1 About the Integration

Dealing with classical crisp constraints a qualitative algebra QA that includes all the combinations that can occur in composition operation between points and intervals is defined in [18]. Considering all the algebrae PA, PI, IP and IA referring to point-point, point-interval, interval-point and interval-interval relations, we have defined the corresponding fuzzy extensions PA^{fuz}, PI^{fuz}, IP^{fuz} and IA^{fuz} [5,6,7]. In order to integrate different kinds of fuzzy temporal constraints in a general framework we extend to the fuzzy case the composition operation [18] as shown in Table 1; here the symbol "$\oslash$" denotes illegal combinations. We have defined the fuzzy extension of the involved algebrae IA, PA, IP and PI (tables $T'_1, \ldots, T'_4$), thus obtaining the qualitative algebra QA^{fuz}.

Table 1. Transitivity table of QA^{fuz}

	PA^{fuz}	PI^{fuz}	IP^{fuz}	IA^{fuz}
PA^{fuz}	$[T_{PA^{fuz}}]$	$[T'_1]$	$[\oslash]$	$[\oslash]$
PI^{fuz}	$[\oslash]$	$[\oslash]$	$[T'_2]$	$[T'_4]$
IP^{fuz}	$[T'^T_1]$	$[T'_3]$	$[\oslash]$	$[\oslash]$
IA^{fuz}	$[\oslash]$	$[\oslash]$	$[T'^T_4]$	$[T_{IA^{fuz}}]$

This way, we can manage temporal networks where nodes can represent both points and intervals, and where edges are accordingly labeled by qualitative and quantitative fuzzy temporal constraints.

In particular, we maintain point to point constraints in their metric form, while interval to interval, point to interval, interval to point constraints are qualitative and are given by IA^{fuz}, PI^{fuz} and IP^{fuz} relations.

Moreover, the operations to translate a fuzzy metric constraint C_1 into a fuzzy qualitative one C_2 and vice versa have been defined.

More detailed description of our integrated framework can be found in [5].

2.2 Algorithms

The notions of local consistency have been extended too [6, 5]. In particular, local consistency has been expressed as the degree of satisfaction which denotes the acceptability of an assignment with respect to the soft constraints involved in the relative sub-network. According to [12], this degree of satisfaction corresponds to the least satisfied constraint.

Moreover, Path-Consistency and Branch & Bound algorithms have been generalized to the fuzzy case adding some relevant refinements that improve their efficiency. Path-consistency allows to prune significantly the search space while having a polynomial computing time.

In our integrated system embedding both qualitative and metric constraints composition and conjunction operations used in the algorithms depend on the type of operands, therefore they change according to the kind of constraints to be processed (qualitative or metric).

3 Temporal Patterns of Diseases

Dealing with an application in the medical domain we focus our attention on the temporal aspects rather than on the atemporal ones.

Let us consider a set of disorders having the manifestations presented by a patient in common but with different temporal progressions and durations. For this, we examine three exanthematic diseases, namely Measles, Rubella and the Sixth Disease (*Exanthema subitum*, also called *Roseola infantum*), analyzing three characteristic periods (incubation, fever and exanthemata) and the contagion period.

The main idea is to use the temporal evolution of the manifestations which is typical of the disease to select the disease itself in a set of diseases and hence to deduce important advices about the quarantine period.

The sequence can be modeled in a graph whose vertices, labelled by a number, represent:

1. starting of the incubation period;
2. ending of the incubation period;
3. starting of the fever;
4. ending of the fever period;
5. starting of the exanthemata period;
6. ending of the exanthemata period;
7. starting of the contagion period;
8. ending of the contagion period.
9. incubation period.
10. fever period.
11. contagion period.

In the following we report the timelines of the three diseases and the most significant constraints defined for the first networks. In a similar way, the other two networks can be represented. The time unit is hour, and an uncertainty of 33% with respect to the duration is assumed. The possible contagion period is represented by the gray area.

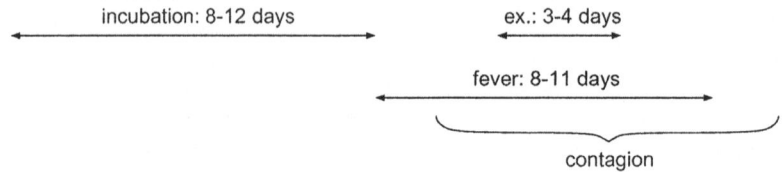

Fig. 2. Measles

3.1 Measles (Paramyxovirus)

– the fever starts when the incubation period ends
$$2\{equals\}3$$
– the **incubation** period lasts 8-12 days
$$1\{(160.0, 192.0, 288.0, 320.0)\}2$$
– the **fever** lasts 8-11 days
$$3\{(168.0, 192.0, 264.0, 288.0)\}4$$
– the **exanthemata** appear 3-4 days after the fever begins and vanish in 3-4 days; they appear after about 14 days
$$3\{(64.0, 72.0, 96.0, 104.0)\}5, 3\{b\}5$$
$$5\{(64.0, 72.0, 96.0, 104.0)\}6$$
$$1\{(240.0, 264.0, 336.0, 360.0)\}5$$
– the **contagion** period begins 1-2 days before the exanthemata and ends 4-5 days after their vanishing
$$7\{(16.0, 24.0, 48.0, 56.0)\}5, 5\{a\}7$$
$$6\{(88.0, 96.0, 120.0, 128.0)\}8$$
$$10\{during\}11$$

3.2 Rubella (Rubivirus)

– the fever starts when the incubation period ends;
– the **incubation** period lasts 14-21 days;
– the **fever** lasts 1-3 days;
– the **exanthemata** last 2-5 days and begin 0-2 days after the fever begins;
– the **contagion** period begins 2-6 days before the exanthemata and ends a week after their vanishing.

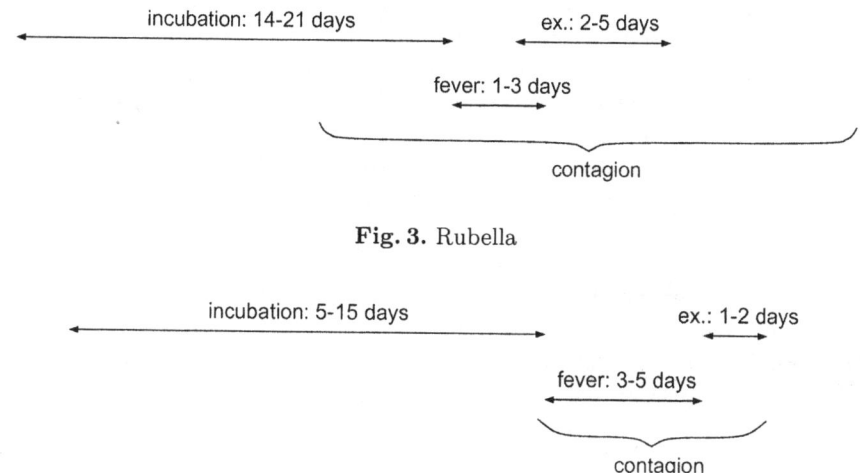

Fig. 3. Rubella

Fig. 4. Sixth Disease

3.3 Sixth Disease (Herpesvirus)

- the fever starts when the incubation period ends;
- the **incubation** period lasts 5-15 days;
- the **fever** lasts 3-5 days;
- then appears the **exanthemata** that last 1-2 days and begin at the end of the fever;
  the **contagion** period is almost during the fever and the exanthemata.

4 Diagnostic Task

In order to do a diagnosis of these types of diseases we can now represent the report of a patient presumably affected by an exanthematic disorder in terms of temporal information about patient symptoms.

By adding new information from the report into the networks built on the basis of standard disease data, the network consistency can be confirmed or it can be lost. The analysis of the changes of the consistency in the networks constitutes a first approach to diagnostic task for exanthematic diseases. In particular, we study how changes the consistency of the three temporal networks by inserting new constraints about the symptoms progression and duration coming from a patient. This kind of model can be very useful since human memory is often little precise about time.

Let's see with an example. If the patient had symptoms that continued for more than a week, the constraint to be added in each of the three networks is:

$$3\{(152.0, 192.0, 312.0, 352.0)\}6$$

By applying the Path-Consistency algorithm, only the Measles network results consistent, while the other two become inconsistent. Setting the present of the patient at the end of the symptoms period, it is also possible to foresee that she/he should stay in quarantine during the next 5-9 days, that is till to the end of the contagion period.

On the other hand, if the patient had symptoms that vanished almost certainly in less than a week, by inserting the constraint

$$3\{(24.0, 48.0, 120.0, 144.0)[0.6]\}6$$

the Rubella network becomes consistent and the Measles one inconsistent. The problem is that in this case also the Sixth Disease network is now consistent. Therefore, in order to make a diagnosis, another clue is needed; this clue must be about time, because the system deals with temporal information. Then, to discriminate between Rubella and the Sixth Disease, further information has to be acquired from the patient asking her/him if the exanthemata appeared shortly after the fever or a few days after. In the first case the Sixth Disease can be diagnosed, while in the latter case Rubella can be identified.

At the moment the system is used to verify at each step the consistency of the constraint networks. Indeed, the system can calculate the degree of consistency of different possible solutions of the networks. This information could be useful to manage more sophisticated and more refined diagnoses.

5 Related Works and Conclusions

An approach which is more directly related with ours is the one proposed in [22] where a system that incorporates fuzzy temporal reasoning within diagnostic reasoning is presented. Disorders are described as a dynamic set of manifestations and fuzzy intervals are used to model their ill-known location in time. As in our case, this approach is based on the work of [14] about FCN (Fuzzy Constraint Networks) and it addresses the problem of diagnosis including not only temporal infomation but also categorical and intensity information. In the present paper we are not concerned with the atemporal aspects of the domain. As far as temporal information is concerned, our system extends the FCN model by allowing multiple constraints that can also be non normalized differently from [22]. Moreover, it allows the integration of fuzzy metric constraints with fuzzy qualitative constraints based on Allen's Interval Algebra [2].

Other works present fuzzy extensions of Allen's Interval Algebra (e.g. [10]) where, instead of attaching preference degrees to qualitative temporal relations as we have done, the indeterminacy of temporal information relative to the patient therapeutic history is dealt with by considering the indeterminacy of period bounds. Even if limited, this method works well for restoring the therapeutic history from prescription data and could be a good basis for an automatic system.

A causal-temporal-action model for clinical diagnoses is proposed in [15] where threee types of ATG (Abstract Temporal Graph) are considered. This model accounts also for uncertainty and for causal links. Again, our work is only devoted to deal with temporal aspects of the domain. Moreover the problem of integration of different types of constraints is tackled in our work in the line of Meiri's classical approach [18].

In this paper we have shown an application of our temporal constraint solver in a medical domain; this application could support the physician to make a diagnosis of the exanthematic diseases on the basis of their temporal patterns. Our solver extends the classic temporal constraints by allowing to specify uncertainty and vagueness; this is fundamental in all those applications where data are gathered from noisy environments or natural language descriptions.

In order to make the system more useful a first enhancement will be the management of constraint classes; in this way, it will be possible to reason about several diseases in parallel.

Moreover, as in [22, 15], a real diagnosis expert system should consider also atemporal aspects of diseases. As future work we intend to enrich our system by addressing also these aspects.

As a final remark, an automated reasoning tool can be useful to find matches against typical patterns of known diseases, but is also interesting the opposite deduction, that is the discovery of the temporal evolution of a disease from the patient data; such an application could be useful for characterizing new diseases, like for example SARS.

References

1. Abbod M.F, von Keyserlinngk, D.G., A, L.D., Mahfouf, M.: Survey of utilization of fuzzy technology in medicine and healthcare. Fuzzy Sets and Systems **120** (2001) 331–349
2. Allen, J.F.: Maintaining knowledge about temporal intervals. Communications of the ACM **26** (1983) 832–843
3. Badaloni, S., Giacomin, M.: A fuzzy extension of Allen's interval algebra. In Verlag, S., ed.: LNAI. Volume 1792. (2000) 1555–165
4. Badaloni, S., Giacomin, M.: Flexible temporal constraints. In: Proc. of IPMU 2000, Madrid, Spain (2000) 1262–1269
5. Badaloni, S., Falda, M., Giacomin, M.: Integrating quantitative and qualitative constraints in fuzzy temporal networks. AI Communications **17** (2004) 183–272
6. Badaloni, S., Giacomin, M.: Fuzzy extension of interval-based temporal sub-algebras. In: Proc. of IPMU 2002, Annecy, France (2002) 1119–1126
7. Badaloni, S., Giacomin, M.: The algebra IA^{fuz}: a framework for qualitative fuzzy temporal reasoning. To appear (2005)
8. Barro, S., Marín, R., Mira, J., Paton, A.: A model and a language for the fuzzy representation and handling of time. Fuzzy Sets and Systems **175** (1994) 61–153
9. Barro, S., Marín, R., Palacios, F., Ruiz, R.: Fuzzy logic in a patient supervision system. Artificial Intelligence in Medicine **21** (2001) 193–199
10. Bouaud, J., Séroussi, B., Touzet, B.: Restoring the patient therapeutic history from prescription data to enable computerized guideline-based decision support in primary care. In: Proc. Medinfo 2004. (2004) 120–124
11. Dechter, R., Meiri, I., Pearl, J.: Temporal constraint networks. Artificial Intelligence **49** (1991) 61–95

12. Dubois, D., Fargier, H., Prade, H.: Possibility theory in constraint satisfaction problems: Handling priority, preference and uncertainty. Applied Intelligence **6** (1996) 287–309
13. Félix, P., Barro, S., Marín, R.: Fuzzy constraint networks for signal pattern recognition. Artificial Intelligence **148** (2003) 103–140
14. Godo, L., Vila, L.: Possibilistic temporal reasoning based on fuzzy temporal constraints. In: Proc. of IJCAI95. (2001) 1916–1922
15. Keravnou, E.T.: Temporal constraints in clinical diagnosis. Journal of Intelligent and Fuzzy Systems **12** (2002) 49–67
16. Mahfouf, M., F., A.M., A., L.D.: A survey of fuzzy logic monitoring and control utilization in medicine. Artificial Intelligence in Medicine **21** (2001) 27–42
17. Marín, R., Cárdenas, M.A., Balsa, M., Sanchez, J.L.: Obtaining solutions in fuzzy constraint network. International Journal of Approximate Reasoning **16** (1997) 261–288
18. Meiri, I.: Combining qualitative and quantitative constraints in temporal reasoning. Artificial Intelligence **87** (1996) 343–385
19. Rossi, F., Sperduti, A., Venable, K.B., Khatib, L., Morris, P., Morris, R.: Learning and solving soft temporal constraints: An experimental study. In: CP 2002, Ithaca, NY, Springer Verlag (2002)
20. Schwalb, E., Dechter, R.: Processing temporal constraint networks. Artificial Intelligence **93** (1995) 29–61
21. Steimann, F.: On the use and usefulness of fuzzy sets in medical AI. Artificial Intelligence in Medicine **21** (2001) 131–137
22. Wainer, J., Sandri, S.: Fuzzy temporal/categorical information in diagnosis. Journal of Intelligent Information Systems **11** (1999) 9–26

Probabilistic Abstraction of Multiple Longitudinal Electronic Medical Records

Michael Ramati and Yuval Shahar

Medical Informatics Research Center, Department of Information Engineering,
Ben-Gurion University, P.O.B. 653, 84105 Beer-Sheva, Israel
{ramatim, yshahar}@bgu.ac.il

Abstract. Several systems have been designed to reason about longitudinal patient data in terms of abstract, clinically meaningful concepts derived from raw time-stamped clinical data. However, current approaches are limited by their treatment of missing data and of the inherent uncertainty that typically underlie clinical raw data. Furthermore, most approaches have generally focused on a single patient. We have designed a new probability-oriented methodology to overcome these conceptual and computational limitations. The new method includes also a practical parallel computational model that is geared specifically for implementing our probabilistic approach in the case of abstraction of a large number of electronic medical records.

1 Introduction

The commonly occurring task of Temporal Abstraction (TA) was originally defined as the problem of converting a series of time-oriented raw data (e.g., a time-stamped series of chemotherapy-administration events and various hematological laboratory tests) into interval-based higher-level concepts (e.g., a pattern of bone-marrow toxicity grades specific to a particular chemotherapy-related context) [1]. Former solutions [1-4], although being evaluated as fruitful, maintained several unsolved subproblems. These subproblems seem common to some of other methods suggested for solving the TA task as well as closely related systems applied in the clinical domain (e.g., [5-7]). Thus, Considering these challenging subproblems suggests an additional method.

At least three subproblems in the former methods can be pointed out, which we propose to solve through the method discussed in this paper. First, raw clinical data, to which the temporal reasoning is being applied, are assumed as certain – that is, typically no mechanism is suggested for handling the inherent impreciseness of the laboratory tests taken to obtain the clinical data. Second, current mechanisms used for completing missing data in an electronic medical record are typically not sound and are incomplete. For example, in the case of the KBTA method, a knowledge-based interpolation mechanism is used [8]. However, completion of missing values is supported only for bridging gaps between two intervals, in which the proposition (e.g., anemia level) had the same value (e.g., moderate anemia). Furthermore, the value concluded by inference is too crisp, and a threshold is used for computing it with absolute certainty, eliminating uncertainty and leading to potentially unsound conclusions. Third, no special mechanism has been devised for multiple patient abstraction. That is, so far temporal abstraction was performed on a single patient only.

The proposed method, *Probabilistic Temporal Abstraction* (PTA), decomposes the temporal abstraction task into three subtasks, that solve the case of a single patient, and two more subtasks that solve the case of multiple patients.

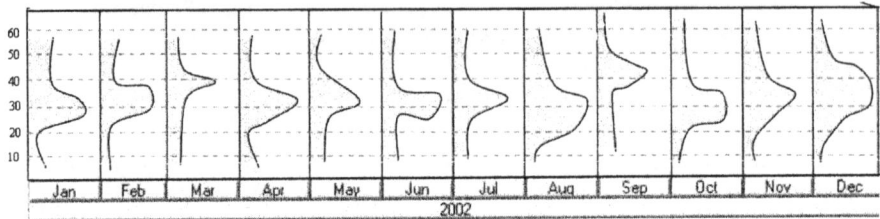

Fig. 1. A typical instance of using the PTA method: the value (*vertical axis*) distribution of a certain medical concept appears for different (in this case consecutive) periods along the time axis. The medical concept, which can be either raw or abstract, and the specification of the set of periods (including the time granularity) are determined by the application using the PTA method

2 The PTA Method

The main computational concept in our methodology is the PTA chain. A *PTA chain* is defined as the application of any subset of the following composition of subtasks, while preserving the relative order among them:

$$Coarsen \circ Correlate \circ Aggregate \circ Transform \circ Interpolate\,(data)\,. \qquad (1)$$

These subtasks are introduced below using the following known notions in probability theory. A *stochastic process* $\{X(t): t \text{ in } T\}$ is a set of random variables, and may represent a clinical observation, a medical intervention, or an interpretation context of some clinical protocol. The index is often interpreted as time, and thus $X(t)$ is referred as the *state* of the process at time t. The set T is called the *index set* of the process.

2.1 The PTA Property and Temporal Interpolation

The central property of the PTA method is based on the notion of *temporal field*, as explicated below. Following this definition, the property states, that each unobserved state of some stochastic process is a linear combination of the temporal fields of the observed states of the process. Thus, the unobserved distribution of bone-marrow toxicity grades is a linear combination of all of the observed distributions, before and after it. An observed state is distributed as a function of the reliability or precision of the clinical test taken (variance) and the value sampled (mean), and induces a *field*[1] over its temporal environment, expressing the temporal knowledge about the stochastic process in question, such as a *periodic* behavior, *monotonic* change, or *persistence*.

---

[1] In the sense of an electromagnetic field.

For example, suppose a stochastic process with a periodic behavior and cycle length c. The temporal field of an observed state of such stochastic process could be as follows:

$$(field_{\bar{X}}(t_s))(t_i) = \sin\left(\frac{\pi}{c} \cdot (|t_i - t_s| \mod c)\right) \cdot X_{t_s}. \qquad (2)$$

Having multiple fields induced over an unobserved state necessitates the use of weights, to express the notion that the closer-in-time the observed state is – the more relevant it is. Therefore, there is a need to choose a monotonic decreasing function of absolute time differences between a dependent state and its inducing observed states. A natural choice for the monotonic decreasing weighting function would be a normal density, where its variance (σ^2) determines the temporal tolerance of observed states of the stochastic process. Thus, w may hold:

$$w_{\bar{X}}(\Delta t) = f_W(\Delta t) \ , \ W \sim Normal(0, \sigma^2). \qquad (3)$$

The *Temporal Interpolation* subtask is aimed at estimating the distribution of a stochastic process state, given the distributions of some of its other states. For example, estimating the distribution of raw hematological data or derived concepts (such as bone-marrow toxicity grades) during a week in which raw data were not measured, using the distribution of values before and after that week. Applying the interpolation subtask does not increase the abstraction level of the underlying stochastic process, but rather serves the role of a core operation that enables the application of actual temporal abstraction. The subtask of interpolation is solved by the application of the PTA property. Thus, the subset of sampled states which participate in the calculation of each unobserved state determines the precision of its distribution, and could be determined given the temporal weighting function. If we interpolate in t_i and know all sampled values t_s (where s=-∞ stands for prior distribution), then:

$$X_{t_i} = \frac{1}{\sum_{t_s} w_{\bar{X}}(t_i - t_s)} \sum_{t_s} w_{\bar{X}}(t_i - t_s) \cdot (field_{\bar{X}}(t_s))(t_i). \qquad (4)$$

For the case in which updates to the underlying clinical data occur, we consider a hierarchical system of states, where each unobserved state has a set of observed parent states, as depicted by Pearl [9]. In case the sample is updated, propagating the new piece of evidence we are viewing as the perturbation that propagated through a Bayesian network via message-passing between neighboring processors.

2.2 Other Subtasks and Their Mechanisms

Temporal abstraction for a single patient requires one basic subtask, temporal interpolation, and the two interpolation-dependent subtasks explicated below. The *Temporal Coarsening* subtask is aimed at the calculation of a stochastic process at a coarser time granularity, according to the following formula:

$$X_{[t_i,t_j]} = \frac{1}{j-i+1} \cdot \sum_{k=i}^{j} X_{t_k}. \tag{5}$$

The *Temporal Transformation* subtask is aimed at the generation of a stochastic process, given stochastic processes of a lower abstraction level, according to the following formula:

$$Y_t = (g(\vec{X_1},\ldots,\vec{X_n}))(t). \tag{6}$$

For example, deriving bone-marrow toxicity grade distribution, given the distributions of the raw white blood cell and platelet counts. A special transformation function is:

$$(change(\vec{X}))(t_i) = X_{t_i} - X_{t_{i-1}}. \tag{7}$$

Applying the TA task to multiple patients requires extra subtasks, such as the ones explicated below. However, these subtasks fit also sophisticated needs of abstraction for a single patient. The *Temporal Aggregation* subtask is aimed at the application of an aggregation function (such as minimum, maximum, average, etc.) to temporally corresponding states of stochastic processes of the same sample space and independent patients. In the case of a single patient, the aggregated states are taken from the same process. The *Temporal Correlation* subtask is intended to mainly compare two patient populations, but should work the same when comparing different time periods of the same patient, resulting in a series of correlation factors between corresponding states of the given stochastic processes. An example for a single patient would be the contemporaneous correlations between height and weight or correlation of height during different periods for the same person.

3 Parallel Implementation

The computational model used to compute a PTA chain is *goal-driven, bottom-up* and *knowledge-based*. That is, the main algorithm is required to compute the result of a PTA chain (the goal), given the transformation and interpolation functions (the temporal knowledge) as well as the access to the clinical data, beginning at the raw (lowest abstraction level) clinical data. The computational model is parallelized (and hence *scalable* [10]) in three orthogonal aspects: (1) Time, during the calculation of the PTA chains' states; (2) Transformation, during the calculation of the transformation arguments; and (3) Patient, during the calculation of the PTA chains for multiple patients.

The PTA architecture is in the process of being fully implemented using is the C++ programming language, the Standard Template Library (STL), and the MPICH2 implementation of the Message-Passing Interface (MPI)[2], an international parallel programming standard. The implementation is thus object-oriented and platform-independent. The implementation is in the process being integrated into the IDAN system [11], which satisfies the need to access medical knowledge and clinical data sources.

---

[2] http://www.mpi-forum.org/

4 Discussion

The new probabilistic method has removed several limitations of former methods. First, the use of PTA chains enables the expression of uncertainty in the underlying clinical data. Second, two mechanisms were developed for temporal abstraction of the clinical data of multiple patients. Third, the interpolation mechanism was shown to be sound and complete. However, observed clinical data are assumed to be independently distributed. This assumption could be easily removed, given the necessary domain-specific conditional distribution functions.

The Markovian property (i.e., the conditional distribution of any future state, given the present state and all past states, depends only on the present state) is not assumed by the PTA method, where past states may be relevant in computing future states. The interpolation in the PTA model is performed at the lowest abstraction level only, as opposed to being repeatedly performed at every abstraction level as in the KBTA method [1]. Finally, the components of the PTA method are highly modular and do not assume, for example, a particular temporal representation.

References

1. Y. Shahar: A Framework for Knowledge-Based Temporal Abstraction. Artificial Intelligence (1997) 90:79-133
2. M.J. O'Connor, W.E. Grosso, S.W. Tu, M.A. Musen: RASTA: A Distributed Temporal Abstraction System to facilitate Knowledge-Driven Monitoring of Clinical Databases. MedInfo, London (2001)
3. A. Spokoiny, Y. Shahar: A Knowledge-based Time-oriented Active Database Approach for Intelligent Abstraction, Querying and Continuous Monitoring of Clinical Data. MedInfo (2004) 84-88
4. M. Balaban, D. Boaz, Y. Shahar: Applying Temporal Abstraction in Medical Information Systems. Annals of Mathematics, Computing & Teleinformatics (2004) 1(1):54-62
5. M.G. Kahn: Combining physiologic models and symbolic methods to interpret time varying patient data. Methods of Information in Medicine (1991) 30(3):167-178
6. I.J. Haimowitz, I.S. Kohane: Automated trend detection with alternate temporal hypotheses. Proceedings of the Thirteenth International Joint Conference on Artificial Intelligence. Morgan Kaufmann, San Mateo (1993) 146-151
7. A. Salatian, J. Hunter: Deriving trends in historical and real-time continuously sampled medical data. Journal of intelligent information systems (1999) 13:47-71
8. Y. Shahar: Knowledge-Based Temporal Interpolation. Journal of Experimental and Theoretical Artificial Intelligence (1999) 11:123-144
9. J. Pearl: Probabilistic Reasoning in Intelligent Systems: Networks of Plausible Inference. Morgan Kaufmann Publishers (1987)
10. K. Hwang, Z. Xu: Scalable Parallel Computing, WCB McGraw-Hill (1998)
11. D. Boaz, Y. Shahar: A Framework for Distributed Mediation of Temporal-Abstraction Queries to Clinical Databases: Artificial Intelligence in Medicine (in press)

Using a Bayesian-Network Model for the Analysis of Clinical Time-Series Data

Stefan Visscher[1], Peter Lucas[2], Karin Schurink[1], and Marc Bonten[1]

[1] Department of Internal Medicine and Infectious Diseases,
University Medical Center Utrecht, The Netherlands
{S.Visscher, K.Schurink, M.J.M.Bonten}@azu.nl
[2] Institute for Computing and Information Sciences,
Radboud University Nijmegen, The Netherlands
peterl@cs.ru.nl

Abstract. Time is an essential element in the clinical management of patients as disease processes develop in time. A typical example of a disease process where time is considered important is the development of ventilator-associated pneumonia (VAP). A Bayesian network was developed previously to support clinicians in the diagnosis and treatment of VAP. In the research described in this paper, we have investigated whether this Bayesian network can also be used to analyse the temporal data collected in the ICU for patterns indicating development of VAP. In addition, it was studied whether the Bayesian network was able to suggest appropriate antimicrobial treatment. A temporal database with over 17700 patient days was used for this purpose.

1 Introduction

Diagnosing infections in critical ill patients is a challenging task, as when an infection is missed, and thus treatment is delayed this may actually be the cause of death of a patient. Diagnosing an infection may also be difficult if only few signs and symptoms are specific, especially when it occurs infrequently. This is the situation with ventilator-associated pneumonia, or VAP for short. VAP is a form of pneumonia that occurs in patients whom are mechanically ventilated in critical care units and involves infection of the lower respiratory tract. This has implications for patient management. Diagnosing VAP is difficult and therefore some form of decision support could be helpful. As diagnosing an infection in medicine involves reasoning with uncertainty, we used a Bayesian network as our primary tool for building a decision-support system [3]. The construction of the Bayesian network was done in cooperation with two infectious-disease specialists. The development of VAP is a time-based process, involving colonisation of the patient by microorganisms. Clinical time series were analysed in order to find optimal treatment for patients who were admitted to the ICU using this Bayesian network.

2 Bayesian Networks in Biomedicine

Health care institutions collect large amounts of information about patients' state and interventions performed by physicians and nursing staff, such as therapies. The use of these 'rough' process data is still limited for scientific and patient management purposes [1]. However, the interest has grown to analyse these data collections for management purposes. For understanding the complex decision-making processes in health-care it is important to reason about them. Since these processes often include uncertainty, Bayesian-network models are constructed to support decision-making in real-life practice as a Bayesian network is an excellent tool for reasoning with uncertainty [4].

Formally, a Bayesian network $\mathcal{B} = (G, \mathrm{Pr})$ is a directed acyclic graph $G = (V(G), A(G))$ with set of vertices $V(G) = \{V_1, \ldots, V_n\}$, representing stochastic variables, and a set of arcs $A(G) \subseteq V(G) \times V(G)$, representing statistical dependences and independences among the variables. On the set of stochastic variables, a joint probability distribution $\mathrm{Pr}(V_1, \ldots, V_n)$ is defined that is factorised respecting the (in)dependences represented in the graph:

$$\mathrm{Pr}(V_1, \ldots, V_n) \prod_{i=1}^{n} \mathrm{Pr}(V_i \mid \pi(V_i))$$

where $\pi(V_i)$ stands for the variables corresponding to the parents of vertex V_i.

3 Patient Data

A temporal database of 17710 records was used. Each record represents data of a patient in the ICU during a period of 24 hours. The database contains 2424 admissions to the ICU. For 157 of the 17710 episodes, VAP was diagnosed by two infectious-disease specialists (See Table 1 for a description of the patients' data). There is no gold standard for diagnosing VAP. Important entities that are related to the development of VAP include *body temperature*, amount and of *sputum*, *signs* on the chest X-ray, the duration of *mechanical ventilation* and

Table 1. Data description

Diagnosis	VAP $n = 157$	no VAP $n = 17553$
abn. temperature	62%	32%
mech. ventilation (mean)	271h	268h
abn. leukocytes	65%	49%
abn. sputum amount	76%	42%
positive X-chest	68%	24%
positive culture	32%	6%

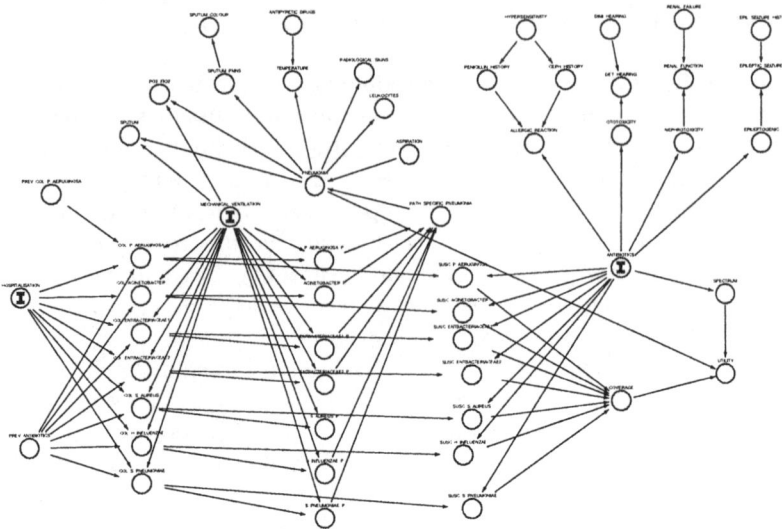

Fig. 1. Bayesian network for Ventilator-Associated Pneumonia

the amount of *leukocytes*, i.e. white blood cells [5]. These symptoms and signs involve the diagnostic part of the Bayesian network for VAP.

ICU patients become colonised by bacteria present in the ICU environment. When colonisation of the lower respiratory tract occurs within 2–4 days after intubation, this is usually caused by antibiotic-sensitive bacteria. When VAP is diagnosed after 4 days of intubation, often antibiotic-resistant bacteria are involved. Such infections are more difficult to treat and immediate start of appropriate treatment is important. [2]. Duration of hospital stay and severity of illness are associated with an increased risk on colonisation and infection with Gram-negative bacteria. We modelled bacterial species each as one vertex in the Bayesian network (See Fig. 1). Also, for each modelled microorganism, the pathogenicity, i.e. the influence of the microorganism on the development of VAP, was included in the model. The presence of certain bacteria is influenced by antimicrobial therapy. Each microorganism is susceptible to some particular antibiotics. Susceptibility, in this case, is stated as the sensitivity to or degree to which a microorganism is effected by treatment with a specific antibiotic. The susceptibility of each microorganism was taken into account while constructing the model. Our infectious-disease experts assigned utilities to each combination of microorganism(s) and antimicrobial drug(s) using a decision-theoretic model [3]. These variables belong to the therapeutic part of the Bayesian network for VAP.

4 The Role of Time in the Colonisation Process

The development of VAP is a time-based process. By including the variable *mechanical ventilation* in the Bayesian network, we modelled the influence of time.

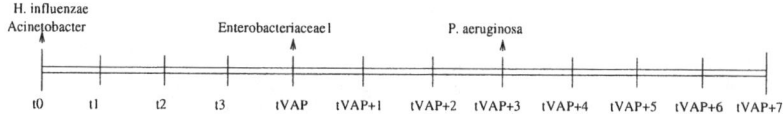

Fig. 2. Timeline for patient 3

Table 2. Bayesian network versus ICU physicians: judged by ID-specialists

Patient	ICU Physician	Bayesian Network	IDS Judgement
1	cefpirom	meropenem	spectrum too broad
2	cefpirom	clindamycin+aztreonam	not the same, but correct
3	augmentin, ceftriax.	meropenem	spectrum too broad
4	cefpirom	meropenem	not the same, but correct
5	augmentin	meropenem	spectrum too broad
6	pipcil, ciproxin	clindamycin+ciproflox.	not the same, but correct
7	tazocin	ceftriaxone	not the same, but correct
8	ceftriaxon	cotrimoxazol	not the same, but correct

Also, the node 'hospitalisation' represents a certain notion of time. The first 48 hours a patient is mechanically ventilated, the probability of colonisation is low. After a period of two days, this probability is higher and as a result, the probability of developing a VAP is also higher. Our database represents the situation for several patients from admission to discharge. We consider the period from admission to discharge of the patient as a *time series* $\langle X_t \rangle$, $t = 0, \ldots, n_p$, where $t = n_p$ is the time of discharge of patient p. For each record, we collected the output of the Bayesian network, i.e., the best possible antimicrobial treatment. This antimicrobial treatment is based on the utility, i.e. the preference - according to the experts, and the overall-susceptibility of the microorganisms, i.e. the coverage. The optimal coverage is computed by varying therapy choice, and selecting the therapies with maximum expected utility. Prescribing antibiotics is a trade-off between *maximising coverage and minimising broadness of spectrum*. When a patient is known to be colonised with a particular microorganism, the antimicrobial spectrum should be as narrow as possible, as this creates the lowest selection pressure. The therapeutic performance of the network, thus far, was somewhat poor: on days when no microorganism was found, the advised antibiotic spectrum was too small and otherwise, the spectrum was too broad. Therefore, improvement was needed.

As inference of the network is time-consuming when varying therapy advice, we (randomly) selected only 8 patients with VAP. During the period of seven days from timepoint of diagnosis, the patient is treated with antibiotics. For each of the 8 patients, a timeline was drawn which shows colonisation information and the timepoint VAP was diagnosed. As mentioned before, it is not clinically relevant to look at the data of one particular patient day. To judge a patient's condition, we have to look at the data of more than one day, therefore we considered the time window $[t, t + 7]$, also taking into account information about (previous) colonisation, since this has direct influence on the choice of antimicrobial therapy. We took the *minimal set* of the advised antibiotics as the Bayesian network's output. This advice was compared to actually prescribed antibiotics, and agreement or disagreement between the two advices was judged by the infectious disease specialists (IDS). For patient 3, the colonisation process is shown by a timeline in Fig. 2. The present microorganisms are depicted. The therapy advice of the Bayesian network and the antibiotics that were prescribed, are presented together with the judgement of the IDS, in Table 2.

5 Conclusions and Future Work

Since the development of ventilator-associated pneumonia is a time-based process involving uncertainty, we have analysed temporal patient data using a Bayesian network. In this paper, we have only analysed time-series data of 8 patient with VAP. One of the most important processes in VAP is the colonisation by microorganisms. The results show that for 3 of the 8 patients, the antibiotic spectrum was too broad. Compared to the method to compute the best appropriate treatment that was used before, i.e. taking into account patient's characteristics of the day of interest without considering the days preceding, we improved the therapeutic performance of the network. Thus, we made a step forward in our search for prescribing optimal treatment for critically ill patients using a Bayesian network.

References

1. Riccardo Bellazzi, Christiana Larizza, Paolo Magni, and Roberto Bellazi. Temporal data mining for the quality assessment of hemodialysis services. *Artificial Intelligence in Medicine*, in press.
2. Michael T. Brenman, Farah Bahrani-Mougeot, Philip C. Fox, Thomas P. Kennedy, Sam Hopkins, Rcihard C. Boucher, and Peter B. Lockhart. The role of oral microbial colonization in ventilator-associated pneumonia. *Oral Medicine*, 98(6), 2004.
3. Peter J.F. Lucas, Nicolette C. de Bruijn, Karin Schurink, and Andy Hoepelman. A probabilistic and decision-theoretic approach to the management of infectious disease at the icu. *Artificial Intelligence in Medicine*, 19(3):251–279, 2000.
4. Peter J.F. Lucas, Linda C. van der Gaag, and Ameen Abu-Hanna. Bayesian networks in biomedicine and health-care. *Artificial Intelligence in Medicine*, 30(3):201–214, 2004.
5. Bonten MJM, Kollef MH, and Hall JB. Risk factors for ventilator-associated pneumonia: from epidemiology to patient management. *Clinical Infectious Diseases*, 38(8), 2004.

Data-Driven Analysis of Blood Glucose Management Effectiveness

Barry Nannings[1], Ameen Abu-Hanna[1], and Robert-Jan Bosman[2]

[1] Academic Medical Center, Universiteit van Amsterdam,
Department of Medical Informatics, PO Box 22700,
1100 DE Amsterdam, The Netherlands
[2] Department of Intensive Care, Onze Lieve Vrouwe Gasthuis,
1e Oosterparkstraat 279, PO box 10550, 1090 HM Amsterdam, The Netherlands

Abstract. The blood-glucose-level (BGL) of Intensive Care (IC) patients requires close monitoring and control. In this paper we describe a general data-driven analytical method for studying the effectiveness of BGL management. The method is based on developing and studying a clinical outcome reflecting the effectiveness of treatment in time. Decision trees are induced in order to discover relevant patient and other characteristics for influencing this outcome. By systematically varying the start and duration of time intervals in which the outcome behavior is studied, our approach distinguishes between time-related (e.g. the BGL at admission time) and intrinsic-related characteristics (e.g. the patient being diabetic).

1 Introduction

Monitoring a patient's state and intervening over time is quite common in clinical practice. For example the disordered metabolism of Intensive Care Unit (ICU) patients requires the close monitoring and control of their blood-glucose-level (BGL) by taking blood samples for measuring the patients' BGL and adjusting the insulin infusion rate accordingly. The focus of this paper is scrutinizing and refining the treatment based on data that is generated from the BGL management process.

In this study we use data generated from the BGL management of the ICU of the OLVG hospital in Amsterdam. The BGL management follows a locally developed guideline [10]. Based on past values of BGL, the guideline advices on the insulin amount to be administered and on the time interval between the current and the next measurement. An important medical study in 2002 [3] has reported that maintaining the patients' BGL in ranges lower than was the case in conventional treatment, was highly significant in reducing mortality and improving patient co-morbidity. The OLVG incorporated this knowledge in their guideline, but the resulting average BGL turned out to be too high. It is unclear why this happens and how to improve BGL management.

Our approach to refining BGL management is based on measuring the effectiveness of the treatment in time. The approach can be sketched as follows.

First, a measurable outcome indicating effectiveness is defined, for example the rate of reduction in some entity in time. A judgment on the outcome's value, for example using a threshold on its value, is then suggested in order to distinguish between those who respond well to the treatment and those who do not. Second, the approach requires defining clinically relevant time intervals in which the outcome is to be studied. For a given interval, decision trees are used to discriminate between patients that respond well to therapy and those who do not. This provides a set of discriminating variables. In the section below we explain how we applied this method to the OLVG data.

2 Materials and Methods

Data. Our data is an extract of data that has been collected by the OLVG ICU patient data management system between April and September of 2003. Patients were included when they were treated using the guideline described above. This resulted in a total of 700 patients. The patient data consist of two types: static data and temporal data. Table 1 presents a small but important sample of a total of 117 attributes that form the static data. The temporal data consists of measurement times, BGL measurements and insulin pump settings at these times.

Table 1. Descriptive statistics of static data

Attribute	Description	Mean±sd	Median
Age	-	66.46±13.82	69.5
BMI	Body Mass Index	26.47±5.25	25.61
Diabetes	-	0.29±0.46	-
First.gluc	First glucose measurement (mmol/l) at ICU admission	9.58±5.20	8.45

Approach. To assess treatment effectiveness, it is important to define an outcome measure that reflects the degree in which the treatment achieves its goal. The goal of the treatment of our case-study is to keep the patient's BGL between 4.4 and 6.1 mmol/l. Given the situation in the OLVG we want our outcome measure to distinguish between patients that have an appropriate mean BGL and patients that have a mean BGL that is too high. The outcome we used classified patients based on the percentage of time in which their BGL was above 8.5 mmol/l.

To account for temporal aspects we systematically shifted the start and the duration of the time intervals in which the outcome measure was determined. Eventually this resulted in two types of analysis each using a different type of outcome. The 6 outcome measures are described in Table 2. The last column in this table includes different thresholds on the percentage of time spent in a

Table 2. Summary of the outcome measures. From left to right: 1. minimum amount of length of stay required for outcome determination, 2. start of the time interval for the outcome, 3. end of the time interval, 4. number of measurements in a hypoglycemic state leading to exclusion of the patient and 5. percentage of time required in a high state to be classified as not responsive to treatment

ID	Minimal ICU length of stay	Interval start	Interval end	Exclusion due to hypoglycemia	Time required above 8.5
a	36 hours	0	12	> 0	61 %
b	36 hours	12	24	> 0	25 %
c	36 hours	24	36	> 0	18 %
d	24 hours	0	discharge	> 1	32 %
e	24 hours	12	discharge	> 1	23 %
f	24 hours	24	discharge	> 1	18 %

"bad" state in order to ensure sufficient number of patients for the analysis. Decisions regarding these outcomes have been made after consulting a domain expert.

Construction of Decision Trees. For the induction of decision trees we used the Rpart (recursive partitioning) module under the S-plus statistical package. Rpart induces binary decision trees and is an implementation of the CART (classification and regression trees) algorithm [4]. Rpart was run in the following setting: splits were based on information gain; cross-validation had 10 folds; pruning was based on minimizing the cross-validated error. For constructing the decision trees we included all predictor variables in the static database. We specified the 6 outcomes defined above to be the outcome in the decision trees.

3 Results

Figure 1 displays the decision trees based on outcomes defined in Table 2. Although we discuss these results in the discussion and conclusion section, there are things worth pointing out here, regarding alternative primary splits and surrogate splits that are also provided by the Rpart algorithm. It is worth noting that in tree b, first.gluc is closely followed by other attributes such as paco2 (arterial CO_2 pressure), urine.24 and some categorical attributes related to the patients admission source and the referring specialism. In tree c resprate.max is very closely followed by diabetes (not having diabetes seems to help to respond well to the therapy). Surprisingly none of the trees make use of BMI, and BMI could not even be found when looking at the top 5 primary and surrogate splits for each of the trees. In the final three trees it is worth noting that BMI is still not chosen, but BMI has been identified as of the best surrogate splits for diabetes. Also worth noting is that although not chosen in the actual trees, first.gluc is

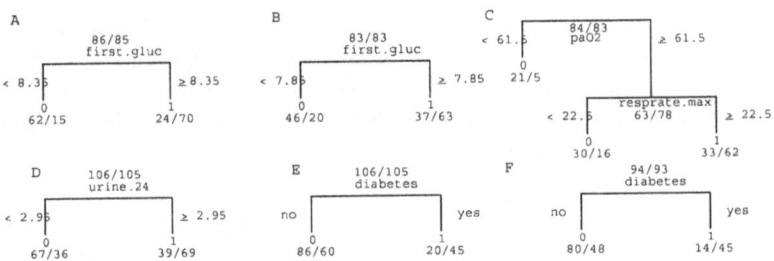

Fig. 1. The resulting decision trees

still present in the top 5 of primary splits in trees d and e. It is however, not present in tree f.

4 Discussion and Conclusion

The trees based on 12 hour interval outcomes clearly show the importance of the first.gluc attribute during the first 24 hours. It seems that the guideline, or at least the actual treatment, has trouble lowering these patients' BGL. It is only later that intrinsic attributes such as diabetes become part of the decision trees. One way of refining the treatment is by performing more frequent measurements, and hence actions, or a higher dosage of insulin for these patients. The current guideline is a control-system: it checks the current BGL and decides on decreasing or increasing insuline. This characteristic of the guideline makes the physicians at the OLVG believe that it should work for both diabetic and non-diabetic patients. However, the results show that diabetics still have a higher mean BGL, suggesting that the guideline does not adequately deal with diabetic patients. Possibly the guideline can be refined for these types of patients.

In the literature there is much related work on BGL management especially in diabetic patients [9], [2], [6], [11]. Decision support systems have been devised such as HumaLink [1], and DIAS [5] which providing insulin dosage advice for diabetic patients. The major difference between this work and ours is the aim. These systems are often predictive systems aiming at providing individual patients with advice about insulin dosage. Our research is explorative and aims at understanding a process, and using this understanding to refine a guideline. Also the methods that are used by these systems can not simply be directly applied for IC patients because of differences in population. IC patients have a continuous food intake and perform no physical activities, and often their BGL is not well controlled. Therefore IC patients will not have the same types of cycles of BGL transitions that are often present in home-based diabetes patients and that are used for making predictions by decision support systems.

Further work includes applying our method on a yet larger dataset and using new outcome measures such as the measure proposed in [13]. This outcome measure reflects the surface between the BGL curve in time and a minimum clinically relevant threshold. Another possibility is performing the analysis in a new domain that shows similarity to the BGL management domain. An interesting application of our method is to use it to perform a comparison between guidelines or treatments used in different hospitals. Finally it is worth studying the role of frequent temporal patterns and including them in the outcome measures.

References

1. A.M. Albisser, R.H. Harris, S. Sakkal, et al., Diabetes intervention in the information age. Med. Inf. (1996) 21: 297-316.
2. R. Bellazzi, C. Larizza, P. Magni, et al., Intelligent analysis of clinical time series: an application in the diabetes mellitus domain. Artif Intell. Med. (2001) 20(1): 37-57.
3. G. Van den Berghe, P. Wouters, F. Weekers, et al. Intensive Insulin Therapy in Critically Ill Patients, NEJM 2001; 345: 1359-67
4. L. Breiman, J. H. Friedman, R. A. Olsen, et al., Classification and Regression Trees. Belmonst, CA: Wadsworth International Group, 1984.
5. D.A. Cavan, O.K. Hejlesen, R. Hovorka, et al., Preliminary experience of the DIAS computer model in providing insulin dose advice to patients with insulin dependent diabetes, Comp. Methods Programs Biom. (1998) 56: 157-164.
6. T. Deutsch, T. Gergely, V. Trunov, A computer system for interpreting blood glucose data, Comp. Methods Programs Biom. 2004
7. B.C. James, M.E. H. H. Hammond, The Challenge of Variation in Medical Practice, Arch. Path. Lab. Med. (200) 124: 1001-1003
8. W.A. Knaus, E.A. Draper, et al., APACHE II: A severity of disease classification system. Crit. Care Med. (1985) 13: 818-829.
9. E. D. Lehmann, Application of computers in clinical diabetes care, Diab. Nutr. Metab. (1997) 10: 45-59.
10. E. Rood, R.J. Bosman, J.I. Van der Spoel, et al., Use of a computerized guideline for glucose regulation in the ICU improved both guideline adherence and glucose regulation, preprint, 2004, JAMIA preprint sever: http://www.jamia.org/cgi/reprint/M1598v1/.
11. Y. Shahar, M.A. Musen, Knowledge based temporal abstractions in clinical domain, Artif. Intell. Med. (1996) 8: 267-208.
12. Y. Shahar, S. Miksch, P. Johnson, The Asgaard project: a task-specific framework for the application and critiquing of time-oriented clinical guidelines, Artif. Intell. Med. (1998) 14: 29-51
13. M. Vogelzang, I. C. C. van der Horst, M. W. N. Nijsten, Hyperglycaemic index as a tool to assess glucose control: a retrospective study, Crit. Care (2004) 8(3): 122-127.
14. J. Weeks, D.G. Pfister, Outcomes research studies, Oncology (1996) 10(11):29-34

Extending Temporal Databases to Deal with Telic/Atelic Medical Data

Paolo Terenziani[1], Richard T. Snodgrass[2], Alessio Bottrighi[1], Mauro Torchio[3], and Gianpaolo Molino[3]

[1] DI, Univ. Piemonte Orientale "A. Avogadro", Via Bellini 25, Alessandria, Italy
terenz@mfn.it, alessio@unipmn.it
[2] Department of Computer Science, University of Arizona, Tucson, AZ 85721, USA
rts@cs.arizona.edu
[3] Lab. Informatica Clinica, Az. Ospedaliera S. G. Battista, C.so Bramante 88, Torino, Italy
{mtorchio, gmolino}@molinette.piemonte.it

Abstract. In the area of Medical Informatics, there is an increasing realization that temporal information plays a crucial role, so that suitable database models and query languages are needed to store and support it. In this paper we show that current approaches developed within the database field have some limitations even from the point of view of the data model, so that an important class of temporal medical data cannot be properly represented. We propose a new three-sorted model and a query language that overcome such limitations.

1 Introduction

Time plays a very important role in many real-world phenomena. For example, in the area of medicine, an explicit management of the time when symptoms took place and clinical actions were taken is needed to model the patients' status (e.g., for diagnostic or therapeutic purposes [12]). Thus several data models used to capture clinical data provide suitable supports to explicitly deal with time (consider, e.g., [18], [13], [14], [7]). Over the last two decades, the database community has devised many different approaches to model the validity time of data (i.e., the time when the data holds [20]). In particular, many temporal extensions to the standard relational model were developed, and more than 2000 papers on temporal databases have published (see the cumulative bibliography in [28] and recent surveys [17], [5], [16], [11]). Recently, the TSQL2 approach has consolidated many years of results into a single "consensus" approach [21], which in revision as SQL/Temporal [22]) has been proposed to the ISO and ANSI standardization committees. Such database approaches are domain-independent, so that they can be profitably exploited also to model temporal data in medical applications. However, recently, some papers pointed out that the lack of specific supports makes the task of managing medical temporal data quite complex. For instance, O'Connor et al. implemented Chronus II, a temporal extension of the standard relational model and query language with specific features to make the treatment of clinical data more natural and efficient [15].

In this paper, we focus on temporal relational models and query languages, showing that current approaches have some limitations from the data model point of view, so that relevant temporal phenomena in the medical field cannot be adequately modeled. We then propose a three-sorted model and a query language that overcome such a limitation.

2 Data Models and Data Semantics

As mentioned, many different database approaches have been devised in order to provide specific support to the treatment of time. Although there are remarkable differences between the alternative approaches, basically all of them adopt the same data semantics: the data in a temporal relation is interpreted as a sequence of states (with each state a conventional relation: a set of tuples) indexed by points in time, with each state independent of every other state (see, e.g., the discussions in [9], [10], [17][22], [27]). We will call such a semantics *point-based*, in accordance with the terminology adopted in artificial intelligence, linguistics and mathematical logic (but not in the database area, where "point-based semantics" has a different interpretation [27], [5] and is often used in relation to the semantics of the *query language* [26]).

It is important to clarify that in this paper we focus on *data semantics*, and we sharply distinguish between *semantics* and *representation language*; our distinction is analogous to the distinction between *concrete* and *abstract* databases emphasized by [6]. For instance, in many approaches, such as SQL/Temporal, TSQL2, TSQL, HQL, and TQuel, and Gadia's [8] Homogeneous Relational Model, a *temporal element* (a set of time intervals) is associated with each temporal tuple (or attribute), but this is only a matter of representation language, while the semantics they adopt is point based [27]. However, a model based on a point-based interpretation of temporal data has severe expressive limitations. In section 3, we will substantiate this claim by considering an example in the medical field. We take TSQL2 as a representative example, but analogous problems arise in the other temporal relational approaches in the DB literature (since all these approaches assume a point-based semantics).

3 Limitations of Data Models Grounded on the Point-Based Semantics

We illustrate these problems with an example, but we stress that the same problem arises whenever data models using the *point-based* semantics are utilized to model a whole class of data (namely, Aristotle's class of *telic* data [1]; see the discussion below).

Let us consider, e.g., drug intravenous infusion (henceforth, "i.v." for short). In some cases, the administration event might stop suddenly (e.g., if the i.v. line falls out) and be resumed immediately. In other cases, two successive i.v. (to be distinguished) of a given drug may be prescribed to the same patient, with no time gap between them. In both cases, the two different i.v. infusions (again, with no temporal gap between them) must be recorded, since the process of restoring a phleboclysis requires medical staff intervention and is costly. On the other hand, notice that the biological effect of the drug is only slightly (if at all) influenced by a short interruption of the i.v. (except in few well-known cases). This is the reason why, at the level of granularity of minutes (that we choose for the whole clinical sample database), we model interruptions as instantaneous events (i.e., the interruption is simply expressed by stating that the i.v. ends on a time granule and re-starts in the next one).

From a technical point of view, if a patient X had two i.v. infusions of the drug Y, one starting at 10:00 and ending at 10:50, and the other from 10:51 to 11:30 (all extremes included), we cannot say that:

(i) X had a (complete) i.v. at time 10:31 (that is, a particular minute; thus, *downward inheritance* [19] does not hold);
(ii) X had a one-hour-and-a-half-long i.v. of drug X (thus, *upward inheritance* [19] does not hold);
(iii) X had just one i.v. (i.e., i.v. events are *countable*, and must be kept distinct one from another)

In accordance with Aristotle [1] and with the linguistic literature, we term **telic facts** those facts that have and *intrinsic goal* or *culmination*, so that the three above properties do **not** hold, and **atelic** facts (e.g., *"patient X having a high temperature"*) facts for which all the three implications (i)-(iii) above hold [8]. The importance of properly dealing with telic facts have been widely recognised in many different areas, spanning from artificial intelligence to philosophy, from cognitive science to linguistics [26].

Now, let us use a standard (i.e., point-based) temporal DB model to deal with therapies. For concreteness, we use the bitemporal conceptual data model (BCDM) [10] (which is the model upon which TSQL2 is based [21]), in which the validity time is denoted with sets of time points. (As an aside, even if we chose to use time intervals in the *representation* language, as in Figure 3, the problem discussed below would still occur, due to the point-based semantics, as we'll discuss shortly. Hence, the use of BCDM is not restrictive: the same problem arises for any data model that is based on the point-based semantics.)

For example, let us model the afore-mentioned patient X, who is named John. Consider the following temporal relation PHLEBO[A], modeling also the facts that John had an i.v. of drug Z from 17:05 to 17:34, that Mary had two i.v. infusions of Z, one from 10:40 to 10:55 and the other from 10:56 to 11:34, and finally that Ann had an i.v. from 10:53 to 11:32.

PHLEBO[A]

P_code	Drug	VT
John	Y	{10:00,10:01,...,10:50,10:51,...,11:30}
John	Z	{17:05, 17:06, ..., 17:34}
Mary	Z	{10:40,...,10:55,10:56,...,11:34}
Ann	Z	{10:53, 10:34, ..., 11:32}

Fig. 1. Relation PHLEBO[A]

This relation captures, among other facts, the fact that the drug Y was given by i.v. to John from 10:30 to 11:30. Formally, this semantics can be modeled as a function from time points to the tuples holding over such time points (see Figure 2).

```
10:00      →     <John, Y>
10:01      →     <John, Y>
......
```

Fig. 2. Point-based semantics of the relation PHLEBO^A in Figure 1

On the other hand, this relation does not capture other relevant information, namely, the fact that there were two distinct i.v. infusions, one ending at 10:50 and another starting at 10:51. Such a loss of information becomes clear and explicit if temporal queries are considered. The most important problems arise, in our opinion, in case of queries involving *upward inheritance* and *countability* of tuples. Again, we will use the TSQL2 query language, just to be concrete, but we stress that such a choice is not restrictive.

(1) Upward inheritance holds on all data models based on point-based semantics. Since the semantics implies the validity of tuples over each point in the validity time, it implies the validity on the whole time interval covering all of them[1]. This is not correct when dealing with telic facts such as i.v. Consider the following query over the relation PHLEBO^A in Figure 1, where a relational table based on point-based semantics is used to model telic facts.

(Q1) *Who had one i.v. of Y lasting more than 1 hour?*
SELECT P_CODE
FROM PHLEBO^A (**PERIOD**) **AS** P
WHERE CAST(P **AS INTERVAL HOUR**) > 1
          AND Drug = 'Y'
Answer_1: {<John ┆ {10:00, ..., 11:30}>}

Since John's two i.v. infusions of Y cannot be distinguished at the semantic level, their validity time is "merged together", so that the above tuple is reported as output. Analogous problems when considering qualitative temporal constraints between validity times, such as, e.g., the *"after"* predicate in Q2, following.

(Q2) *Who had an i.v. starting after one of the i.v. infusions of Y to John?*
SELECT P2.P_CODE
FROM PHLEBO^A (**PERIOD**) **AS** P, P **AS** P2
WHERE P.P_CODE='John' **AND** P.Drug='Y'
          AND P **PRECEDES** P2
Answer_2: <John ┆ {17:05, ..., 17:34}>

Notice that since the tuples <John ┆ {[10:51,..,11:30]}>, <Mary ┆ {[10:56,...,11:34]}> and <Ann ┆ {[10:53,...,11:32]}> are not reported as output, even if they follow one of John's infusions (the one which ended at 10:50).

---

[1] From the technical point of view, within temporal Databases approaches, upward hereditary is introduced by performing *temporal coalescing* [4] over value-equivalent tuples.

(2) Countability. Since there is no way to distinguish, at the semantic level, temporally contiguous value-equivalent tuples, contiguous telic facts are "merged together", and one loses the correct count. Consider the following query.

(Q3) *How many i.v. did John have?*
SELECT COUNT(P)
FROM PHLEBO^A (**PERIOD**) **AS** P
WHERE P_CODE='John'
Answer_3: 2

In fact, in the point-based semantics, {[10:00,...,10:50], [10:51,...,11:30]} is interpreted as the set of points {10:00,...,11:30}.

It is important to notice that these problems are not related to the *representation* language, but to the underlying (point-based) *semantics*. Indeed, several alternative implementations (*representations*) are possible, each maintaining the same (point-based) semantics [21]. The same consideration also concerns the adoption of first normal form [21], in which each timestamp is restricted to be a period, with timestamps associated with tuples. As long as the underlying semantics is point-based, *each possible representation* of the (telic) event that John had two i.v. infusions of Y, one from 10:00 to 10:50 and the other from 10:51 to 11:30, is equivalent to the first tuple in PHLEBO^A, and conveys the same content shown in Figure 2, i.e., that John had an i.v. of Y in each time point within the whole span of time starting at 10:00 and ending at 11:30.

4 A Three-Sorted Model

Notice once again that the above appear whenever a *telic* event (roughly speaking: an event which behaves as described by points (i)-(iii) in section 3: it has *no downward* and *upward hereditary* properties and it is *countable*) is modeled through a DB data model and query language which are based on the *point-based semantics* [23]. In order to deal with *telic* events (which respect the particular intervals, even if adjacent), a new data model and query language are needed, based on *interval-based semantics*[2].

PHLEBO^T

P_code	Drug	VT
John	Y	{[10:00-10:50],[10:51,11:30]}
John	Z	{[17:05-17:34]}
Mary	Z	{[10:40-10:55],[10:56-11:34]}
Ann	Z	{[10:53-11:32]}

Fig. 3. Relation PHLEBO^T

---

[2] This point, initially risen by [2], is now generally accepted within the linguistic and the AI communities (see, e.g., [8]).

Definition. *Interval-based semantics for relational data:* each *tuple* in a temporal relation is associated with a set of time intervals, which are the temporal extents in which the fact described by the tuple occurs. In this semantics time intervals are atomic primitive entities, in the sense that they cannot be decomposed.

As an example, the relation in Figure 3 shows a telic relation PHLEBO^T (i.e., a relation based on interval semantics) modelling our example.

Notice that the difference between PHLEBO^A and PHLEBO^T is not one of *syntax* (in the latter, time intervals are explicitly represented), but rather one of semantics. If an interval-based semantics is adopted, each interval is interpreted as an atomic (indivisible) one (see Figure 4). Thus, e.g., the tuple <John, Y ¦ {[10:00-10:50], [10:51-11:30]} does *not* imply that John had a administration at 10:05.

[10:00-10:50]   →   <John, Y>
[10:51-11:30]   →   <John, Y>
......

Fig. 4. Interval-based semantics of the relation PHLEBO^T in Figure 3

On the other hand, *atelic* events (e.g., *"patient Y having very high temperature"*; roughly speaking: events for which *downward* and *upward inheritance* hold, and which are not *countable*) are correctly coped with by "standard" point-based-semantics relational approaches. Moreover, in most medical applications, also standard *atemporal* relations (i.e., relations where time has not to be coped with) are very useful. Thus, our extended temporal model consists of relations of three sorts: "standard" *atemporal* relations, *atelic* relations (with the "usual" *point-based semantics*) and *telic* relations (with an *interval-based semantics*).

5 Query Language

The preceding sections focused on extensions to a temporal model to add support for both telic and atelic tables. We now show how these concepts can be added to an SQL-based temporal query language. As we'll see, only a few new constructs are needed. The specifics (such as using TSQL2) are not as important; the core message is that incorporating the distinction between telic and atelic data into a user-oriented query language is not difficult.

The first change is to support the definition of telic tables (the default is designated as atelic). This can be done with an "**AS TELIC**" clause in the TSQL2 **CREATE TABLE** statement.

For telic queries, we prepend the keyword "TELIC". For example, the three queries Q1, Q2, and Q3 could all be correctly written as TELIC SELECT ... Q1 would then return the empty relation, as no single i.v. period was longer than an hour. Q2 would return two infusions for John, one starting at 10:51 and one starting at 17:05, as well as one i.v. for Mary (starting at 10:56) and one for Ann, starting at 10:53. The third query would return a count of 3.

Furthermore, in the queries, *coercion* functions are useful in order to convent tables of the different sorts.

(Q4) Who had one (complete) i.v., while John was having an Y i.v.?

As shown in Section 3, i.v. should be regarded as telic facts. However, when stating *"while John was having an i.v. of Y"* we look inside the fact, *coercing* it into an atelic one. Thus, this query involves two different ways of looking at the tuples in relation PHLEBO^T. First, John's i.v. infusions must be interpreted as atelic facts, since we are not looking for i.v. infusions that occurred during *one* of John's infusions, but, more generally, *while John was having an i.v.* (i.e., we are interested in i.v. infusions occurred during [10:00-11:30]). On the other hand, the i.v. infusions we are asking for must be interpreted as telic facts, since we look for *each complete occurrence* of them which is fully contained in [10:00-11:30]. For example, we want Ann in our output, since she had an i.v. from 10:40 to 10:55, regardless of the fact that she also had another i.v. from 10:56 to 11:34. We thus need more flexibility: although each base relation must be declared as telic or atelic, we need coercion functions (**TELIC** and **ATELIC**) to allow switch from one interpretation to the other at query time.

TELIC SELECT P2.P_CODE
FROM PHLEBO^A (**ATELIC PERIOD**) **AS** P,
      PHLEBO^A (**PERIOD**) **AS** P2
WHERE P.P_CODE='John' **AND** P.Drug='Y'
      AND P **CONTAINS** P2

6 Conclusions

In this paper, we have argued that current database approaches have some limitations, so that an important class of temporal medical data (i.e., *telic* data) cannot be properly represented, and we have proposed a new three-sorted model and a query language that overcome such limitations. While the data model has been already presented in [26], where we also proposed an extended three-sorted temporal algebra coping with both telic and atelic relations, and with coercion functions, , in this paper we considered the impact of the telic/atelic distinction on medical data, and extended the TSQL2 query language to cope with it.

Before concluding, we think that it is worth remarking that, although in this paper we showed the impact of neglecting the telic/atelic distinction on a specific medical example, problems such as the ones discussed in section 3 arise whenever *value-equivalent* tuples (i.e., tuples which are equal in their data part) concerning telic data have temporal extents that meet or intersect in time. This phenomena can occur in *primitive* relations, such as PHLEBO^A in figure 1, but also, and more frequently, in *derived* relations. For example, projection of a relation on a subset of its attributes (e.g., projecting the PHLEBO^A relation over the *Drug* attribute) usually generates several value-equivalent tuples. Also, switching from a finer to a coarser *temporal granularitiy* in the validity time (e.g., from minutes to hours, or days; consider, e.g., [3]) can originate temporal intersections that where not present in the primitive data.

As regards future work, we envision the possibility of extending also the conceptual level (e.g., the *entity-relationship* model) to properly cope with *telic* (and *atelic*) facts. Moreover, we want to implement our approach and apply in GLARE (Guide-Line Acquisition, Representation and Execution), a manager of clinical guidelines which strictly interacts with different databases [24],[25].

Finally, we plan to investigate the impact of considering other semantic features of temporal data (such as, e.g., the ones addressed in [19] or in [3]).

References

[1] Aristotle, The Categories, on Interpretation. Prior Analytics. Cambridge, MA, Harvard University Press.
[2] Bennet, M., Partee, B.: Tense and Discourse Location In Situation Semantics. Indiana University Linguistics Club, Bloomington (1978)
[3] Bettini, C., Wang, X.S., Jajodia, S., Temporal Semantic Assumptions And Their Use In Databases. IEEE Transactions on Knowledge and Data Engineering 10(2) (1998)
[4] Böhlen, M. H. , Snodgrass, R. T., Soo, M.: Coalescing in Temporal Databases. Proc. of the International Conference on Very Large Databases (1996) 180–191
[5] Böhlen, M. H., Busatto, R., Jensen C. S.: Point- Versus Interval-Based Data Models. Proc. of the IEEE Int'l Conference on Data Engineering (1998) 192–200
[6] Chomicki, J.: Temporal Query Languages: A Survey. Proc. of the International Conference on Temporal Logic, Springer-Verlag (LNAI 827) (1994) 506–534
[7] Combi, C.: Modeling Temporal Aspects of Visual and Textual Objects in Multimedia Databases. Proc. TIME'00 (2000) 59-68
[8] Dowty, D.: The effects of the aspectual class on the temporal structure of discourse. Tense and Aspect in Discourse, Linguistics and Phylosophy 9(1) (1986) 37-61
[9] Gadia, S. K.: A homogeneous relational model and query languages for temporal databases. ACM Transactions on Database Systems 13(4) (1988) 418-448
[10] Jensen, C. S., Snodgrass, R. T.: Semantics of Time-varying information. Information Systems 21(4) (1996) 311-352
[11] Jensen, C. S., Snodgrass, R. T.: Temporal Data Management. IEEE Transactions on Knowledge and Data Engineering 11(1) (1999) 36-44
[12] Keravnou, E.T.: Special issue: Temporal Reasoning in Medicine. Artificial Intelligence 8(3) (1996)
[13] Keravnou, E.T.: A Multidimensional and Multigranular Model of Time for Medical Knowledge-Based Systems. J. Intell. Inf. Syst. 13(1-2) (1999)73-120
[14] Nguyen, J. H., Shahar, Y., Tu, S. W., Das, A. K., Musen, M. A.: Integration of Temporal Reasoning and Temporal-Data Maintenance into a Reusable Database Mediator to Answer Abstract, Time-Oriented Queries: The Tzolkin System. J. Intell. Inf. Syst. 13(1-2) (1999) 121-145
[15] O'Connor, M. J., Tu, S. W., Musen, M. A.: The Chronus II Temporal Database Mediator. JAMIA, Symposium Supplement, AMIA Fall Symposium, Isaak S. Kohane ed. (2002) 567-571
[16] Özsoyoglu, G., Snodgrass, R. T.: Temporal and real time databases: a survey, IEEE Transaction On Data and Knowledge Engineering 7(4) (1995) 513-532
[17] Roddick, J. F., Patrick, J. D.: Temporal semantics in information systems: a survey. Information Systems 17(3) (1992) 249-267
[18] Shahar, Y., Musen, M.: Knowledge-based temporal abstraction in clinical domains. Artificial Intelligence in Medicine 8(3) (1996) 267-298

[19] Shoham, Y.: Temporal Logics in AI: Semantical and Ontological Considerations, Artificial Intelligence 33 (1987) 89–104
[20] Snodgrass, R. T., Ahn, I.: Temporal databases. IEEE Computer 19(9), 35-42, (1986)
[21] I. Ahn, G. Ariav, D. Batory, J. Clifford, C. Dyreson, R. Elmasri, F. Grandi, C. S. Jensen, W. Kafer, N. Kline, K. Kulkarni, C. Leung, N. Loretzos, J. Roddick, A. Segev, M. Soo, S.M. Sripada: in R. T. Snodgrass (ed.) The Temporal Query Language TSQL2, Kluwer Academic, (1995)
[22] Snodgrass, R. T., Böhlen, M. H., Jensen, C. S., Steiner, A.: Transitioning temporal support in TSQL2 to SQL3, in O. Etzion, S. Jajodia, and S. Sripada (eds.): Temporal Databases: Research and Practice, LNCS 1399, Springer Verlag, 150-194, 1998.
[23] Terenziani. P.: Is point-based semantics always adequate for temporal databases?. Proc. TIME 2000, Cape Breton,Canada IEEE Press (2000) 191-199
[24] Terenziani, P., Molino, G., Torchio, M.: A Modular Approach for Representing and Executing Clinical Guidelines. Artificial Intelligence in Medicine 23 (2001) 249-276
[25] Terenziani, P., Montani, S., Bottrighi, A., Torchio, M., Molino, G., Correndo, G.: A context-adaptable approach to clinical guidelines. Proc. MEDINFO'04, M. Fieschi et al. (eds), Amsterdam, IOS Press (2004) 169-173
[26] Terenziani, P., Snodgrass, R. T.: Reconciling Point-based and Interval-based Semantics in Temporal Relational Databases: A Treatment of the Telic/Atelic Distinction. IEEE Transactions on Knowledge and Data Engineering 16(5) (2004) 540-551
[27] D. Toman: "Point-based temporal extensions of SQL and their efficient implementation", in O. Etzion, S. Jajodia, and S. Sripada (eds.): Temporal Databases: Research and Practice, LNCS 1399, Springer Verlag (1998) 211-237
[28] Y. Wu, S. Jajodia, and X. S. Wang: "Temporal Database Bibliography Update," 338-366, in O. Etzion, S. Jajodia, and S. Sripada (eds.): Temporal Databases: research and practice, Lecture Notes in Computer Science, Vol. 1399, Springer Verlag (1998).

Dichotomization of ICU Length of Stay Based on Model Calibration

Marion Verduijn[1,4], Niels Peek[1], Frans Voorbraak[1], Evert de Jonge[2], and Bas de Mol[3,4]

[1] Dept. of Medical Informatics, Academic Medical Center,
University of Amsterdam (AMC UvA), Amsterdam, The Netherlands
[2] Dept. of Intensive Care Medicine, AMC UvA, Amsterdam, The Netherlands
[3] Dept. of Cardio-thoracic Surgery AMC UvA, Amsterdam, The Netherlands
[4] Dept. of Biomedical Engineering, Eindhoven University of Technology,
Eindhoven, The Netherlands

Abstract. This paper presents a method to choose the threshold for dichotomization of survival outcomes in a structured fashion based on data analysis. The method is illustrated with an application to the prediction problem of the outcome *length of stay at Intensive Care Unit* (ICU LOS). Threshold selection is based on comparing the calibration of predictive models for dichotomized outcomes with increasing threshold values. To quantify model calibration a measure insensitive to class unbalance is used. The threshold value for which the associated predictive model has superior calibration is selected, and the corresponding model is used in practice. Using this method to select the threshold for ICU LOS, the best model calibration is found at a threshold of five days.

1 Introduction

Outcomes that describe the time until a specific event occurs are important in medicine. Examples of these outcomes are time until death, length of hospitalization, and length of mechanical ventilation. In medical prediction problems, these *survival* outcome variables are often dichotomized, e.g., [1,2,3]. Dichotomization is performed by using a *threshold*, after which a prognostic model is developed for the dichotomized outcome. In this approach, potentially valuable information about the problem that is contained in the data is lost. However, this loss may be compensated for by increased possibilities to build a prognostic model, because it opens a much larger array of data analysis techniques that may be applied to solve the prediction problem.

When a clear clinical question underlies model development (e.g., Which patients have high risk to be mechanically ventilated longer than 24 hours?), the threshold for dichotomization is given, and threshold selection is no question. However, in practice, clinical questions are often less specific (e.g., Which patients have high risk of prolonged mechanical ventilation?). Selection of a threshold value is then required.

Generally, two approaches can be distinguished for threshold selection. First, a dichotomous variable can be defined based on *knowledge of practitioners*. The threshold value that is used in this case is for instance a breakpoint that is generally agreed upon in the field of application, or inferred from the decision-making policy that is pursued in the field of application. As these methods rely on consensus among practitioners and the existence of clean decision-making policy, they may fail to work in practice when these are lacking. Second, a threshold can be selected based on *data analysis*. In the literature on prognostic models in medicine, dichotomization is often based on *percentiles* of the sample distribution of the outcome variable, e.g., [3, 4, 5]. The choice of the percentiles is generally arbitrary, because no relation needs to exist with the natural separation (if existent) of the outcome classes.

This paper describes a method to select the optimal threshold in a structured fashion based on *calibration* of predictive models that are to be used in clinical practice. We used this method to dichotomize the outcome *length of stay at the Intensive Care Unit* (ICU LOS). However, the method can be applied to similar dichotomization problems, that could precede model development.

The paper is organized as follows. First, the prediction problem of ICU LOS is described in Section 2. Subsequently, we describe the method for threshold selection based on model calibration in Section 3. The method for threshold selection is applied to ICU data that are described in Section 4; Section 5 describes the results. We conclude the paper with some discussion and conclusions.

2 Prediction of ICU Length of Stay

Cardiac surgery patients can be seen as a relatively homogeneous subgroup of ICU patients with a high morbidity risk. During the first hours after the operation, that involves coronary artery bypass grafting (CABG), and repair or replacement of heart valves, many physiological disturbances are commonly found in patients. For this reason, each patient is monitored and mechanically ventilated at the ICU. In a normal (uncomplicated) recovery process though, a stable condition is reached within 24 hours; then the recovery process is completed at the nursing ward.

However, several postoperative complications may occur in different organs or organ systems, which make longer intensive care inevitable. For that reason, the ICU LOS can be seen as a 'proxy' for the degree of complication and therefore, as a measure of the quality of delivered care. So, the identification of patient groups that are likely to have a complicated recovery process are useful for determining policy of care and benchmark purposes. Furthermore, if the cardiac surgical patients form a relatively large part of the ICU population, the staff of ICUs is often interested in the prediction of this outcome for case load planning.

The development of models to predict ICU LOS is complicated, though. The outcome ICU LOS is primarily determined by the patient's condition at ICU admission and the complications that occur during ICU stay. But, beside these patient-related factors, a number of interfering factors exist that influence the ICU LOS, such as discharge policy, workload and available facilities at the medium care unit and nursing ward. Furthermore, a short ICU LOS can be related to a fast recovery process, but also to a quick death. For these latter patients, the ICU LOS is censored. Therefore, it is difficult to predict the ICU LOS.

When developing predictive models for this outcome, dichotomization is frequently applied to estimate a patient's risk on long ICU LOS. The threshold value is often chosen "arbitrarily" (3 days [6]), without motivation (threshold of 2 days [7] and 10 days [8]), or based on simple statistics such as median (threshold of 7 days [5]) or 90% percentile (threshold of 3 days [9] and 6 days [4]). The differences in selected threshold values are largely caused by differences in the distribution of ICU LOS which depends on patient population and types of cardiac surgery. However, in these studies, no systematic investigation is done to select the threshold value. This is unfortunate as suboptimal threshold selection can lead to an inaccurate model that is developed for the dichotomized outcome and to restricted insight into the structure of the prediction problem.

In the next section, we describe our method to select the optimal threshold in a structured fashion. The predictive model for ICU LOS is intended to be used for estimation at the level of patient groups and populations, rather than for estimation at the level of individual patients. Therefore, the model should be well calibrated (i.e., the estimated class-conditional probabilities should be close to the true class-conditional probabilities). For that reason, we selected the threshold for dichotomization based on model calibration.

3 Threshold Selection Based on Model Calibration

In this section, we describe the method that we used to select the threshold value to dichotomize the outcome ICU LOS. The method is based on optimization of the prediction problem of ICU LOS in terms of model calibration, and consists of three consecutive parts. For outcomes that are dichotomized using threshold values of 2 up to and including 12 days, 1) predictive models are developed and 2) their calibration is determined. Based on the evaluation of the models in terms of calibration, 3) the threshold value that defines the dichotomized outcome for which the model has maximal calibration is finally selected to dichotomize ICU LOS. The following sections describe how we determine model calibration.

3.1 Model Calibration Statistic

Let Y_t denote the survival outcome ICU LOS dichotomized using threshold t, and let $\mathbf{x}$ denote the vector of covariates that is used to predict the value of Y_t. The concept of model calibration concentrates on the difference between true class-conditional probabilities $P(Y_t = 1|\mathbf{x})$ and probabilities $M(Y_t = 1|\mathbf{x})$ estimated by model M [10]. Other terms used for this concept are *reliability* [11] and *precision* [12]. A predictive model is perfectly calibrated if these probabilities are equal for each element $\mathbf{x}$ of the feature space F. The larger the average difference between these probabilities is, the worse the predictive model is calibrated.

We use the MALOR statistic [13] to quantify the difference between the estimated model M and the true model P. For notational brevity, we assume

Table 1. Comparison of the MALOR statistic to the squared error (se) and Kullback-Leibler distance (KL)

$M_\mathbf{x}$	$P_\mathbf{x}$	$d_{\text{ALOR}}(M_\mathbf{x}, P_\mathbf{x})$	$d_{\text{se}}(M_\mathbf{x}, P_\mathbf{x})$	$d_{\text{KL}}(M_\mathbf{x}, P_\mathbf{x})$
0.1	0.15	0.4626	0.0025	0.0122
0.01	0.015	0.4105	0.000025	0.00109
0.001	0.0015	0.4060	0.00000025	0.000108

that the dichotomization threshold t is given, and write $P_\mathbf{x}$ for the probability value $P(Y_t = 1|\mathbf{x})$, and $M_\mathbf{x}$ for its estimate $M(Y_t = 1|\mathbf{x})$. The MALOR statistic is a distance measure and is defined as follows:

$$D_{MALOR}(M, P) = \int_{\mathbf{x} \in F} |\ln(\frac{O_M(\mathbf{x})}{O_P(\mathbf{x})})| p(\mathbf{x}) \, dx, \quad (1)$$

where $O_M(\mathbf{x}) = \frac{M_\mathbf{x}}{1-M_\mathbf{x}}$ and $O_P(\mathbf{x}) = \frac{P_\mathbf{x}}{1-P_\mathbf{x}}$, and $0 < M_\mathbf{x} < 1$ and $0 < P_\mathbf{x} < 1$.

This statistic is called *MALOR* as it is the Mean value of the Absolute Log-Odds Ratio for all elements $\mathbf{x} \in F$. We refer to [13] for an extensive explanation of the MALOR statistic and its properties. The important property of the MALOR statistic for our purpose is that it takes relative differences between probabilities into account. This is best explained by temporarily assuming that the feature space F contains only a single element. The models are than determined by a single probability value, and the MALOR statistic reduces to the following distance measure on probabilities, which we call the *ALOR* distance.

$$d_{ALOR}(M_\mathbf{x}, P_\mathbf{x}) = |\ln(\frac{\frac{M_\mathbf{x}}{1-M_\mathbf{x}}}{\frac{P_\mathbf{x}}{1-P_\mathbf{x}}})|. \quad (2)$$

In [13] it is shown that the MALOR statistic satisfies a property called *approximate proportional equivalence*, which essentially means that the distance between two small probabilities stays approximately constant if both probabilities are reduced by the same factor. Table 1 shows this property for three pairs of $M_\mathbf{x}$ and $P_\mathbf{x}$ (first and second column). The three pairs have equal relative differences, while the absolute differences become progressively smaller. The ALOR distance (third column) is approximately equal when reducing both probabilities using the same factor, and this 'equivalence' increases as the probabilities become smaller. The fourth and fifth column show that this property does not hold for well-known distance measures such as the *squared error* (and related measures such as the absolute error and the Euclidean distance), and the *Kullback-Leibler distance* (also known as relative entropy). The squared error and Kullback-Leibler distance become steadily smaller as the probabilities get smaller, so these two distance measures will always value the model for the most unbalanced problem to be best calibrated.

Because of the property of approximate proportional equivalence, the MALOR statistic is insensitive to class unbalance; its values are therefore comparable for different prediction problems. So, when selecting the optimal threshold for dichotomization based on model calibration, the MALOR statistic is suitable to quantify the calibration of predictive models that have been developed for outcomes dichotomized using increasing thresholds.

3.2 Model Calibration Assessment

To select the threshold value for dichotomization of ICU LOS, we developed predictive models for outcomes that are dichotomized using increasing threshold values (2 up to and including 12 days), and used the regression tree method for model development. The regression tree method belongs to the family of recursive partitioning techniques, and is one of tree-building methodologies in *Classification and Regression Trees* (CART) that is described by L. Breiman et al. [14]. Based on the tree structure, it is easy to determine which subgroup patients belong to and what the related outcome estimations are. Furthermore, the tree structure supports the identification of high risk groups. Therefore, these models are useful in clinical practice.

The calibration is determined for all regression tree models, in order to select the threshold that defines the dichotomized outcome for which the model has maximal calibration. As described in the previous section, model calibration is determined by the difference between the estimated class-conditional probabilities $M(Y_t = 1|\mathbf{x})$ and the true class-conditional probabilities $P(Y_t = 1|\mathbf{x})$, and the MALOR statistic is a suitable measure to quantify this difference. However, model calibration can only be assessed when the true probabilities are known, which is in practice not the case. For the purpose of calibration assessment of the regression tree models, we approximated the true class-conditional probabilities by *ensemble learning*, using bootstrap aggregation or *bagging* [15].

An ensemble learner is an aggregated predictor existing of a collection of predictive models. These models are developed based on bootstrap samples [16] that are sampled from the data set with replacement. The prediction of the ensemble is an average of the prediction that is delivered by the individual predictive models, thereby reducing its variance. We developed tree ensembles that exist of a collection of regression tree models. The regression tree method is known to be an unstable method that tends to benefit substantially from this bagging procedure; it leads to improvements in the model accuracy [15, 17]. Tree ensembles consist of an aggregation of models; the relation between predictors and outcome is therefore complex and not transparent. Therefore, tree ensembles are not very useful in clinical practice. The improvement of predictions that is realized by the bagging procedure makes this method suitable to approximate the true probabilities for calibration assessment of the regression tree models.

4 Data and Methods

We have selected the threshold for dichotomization of ICU LOS using a data set from cardiac operations conducted at the Academic Medical Center, Amsterdam, in the years 1997–2002. The data set contains 144 data items including patient characteristics such as age and gender, details of the surgical procedure, such as surgery type, and indicators of the patient's state during the first 24 hours at the ICU such as blood and urine values for 4453 patients. Because of including these latter data items, we excluded all patients who left the ICU within one day. Furthermore, 27 patients were excluded because of the large amount of missing ICU data; the median ICU LOS of these patients is 2.0 days (range 1.0-8.7), no patient died. We developed tree models for dichotomized outcomes of ICU LOS based on data of the remaining 2327 patients; the median ICU LOS of these patients is 2.2 days (1.0-153.8), 122 of these patients died at the ICU (5,2%).

We dichotomized ICU LOS using thresholds of 2 days up to and including 12 days. We decided to allocate all 122 patients who died to the group of patients with an ICU LOS above the threshold value, because death censors the outcome ICU LOS informatively. The patients who die are probably more similar to patients who stay long at the ICU than to quickly recovered patients. So, two outcome categories have been created: *short LOS*, and *long LOS or death*.

The data set was randomly divided into a training set and test set, that contain respectively 1540 patients and 787 patients. For each LOS threshold value, we developed a regression tree and a tree ensemble based on the training set, using the S-plus library *Rpart* [18], which is an implementation of CART [14]. In Rpart, the optimal tree size was determined based on minimization of the 10-fold cross-validation squared error. The tree ensembles were composed of 25 regression trees. To increase the stability of the regression tree models, we performed univariate tree analyses for feature selection beforehand. For each threshold value, all features that explained at least three percent of the variation in the outcome were selected with development of the regression tree. This feature selection procedure was not performed for tree ensemble development.

We quantified the performance of the regression tree models and the tree ensembles based on the training set by calculating the Brier score [19]; we used 10-fold cross-validation to avoid an optimistic bias. In addition, we calculated the calibration of the regression trees using the MALOR statistic. The MALOR statistic was calculated without cross-validation, because it quantifies the difference between the estimated class-conditional probabilities provided by the regression tree and the tree ensemble, without relating this to the observed outcome class. Finally, the threshold value for which the computed MALOR statistic was minimal, was selected to dichotomize the outcome variable ICU LOS, with the corresponding regression tree as predictive model to be used in clinical practice. We used the paired t-test to investigate whether the minimal MALOR value differs significantly from the MALOR values of the other threshold values.

Based on the independent test set, we determined the unbiased performance of the regression tree for the selected threshold value using the Brier score and the area under the ROC curve (AUC) [20].

5 Results

The results are summarized in Table 2. Each table row first lists the threshold that is used for dichotomization. The second column shows the proportion of cases with an ICU LOS higher than the threshold value, or death, within the training set. The Brier scores of the tree ensemble and regression tree are shown in the third and fourth column. The fifth column shows the MALOR statistic, that quantifies the distance between the predictions of both model types.

As appears from the third and fourth column, the tree ensembles provide more accurate predictions than the regression trees at all threshold values. We note that the Brier scores cannot be compared for the different prediction problems, as these scores become steadily lower as the prediction problem becomes more unbalanced. The MALOR statistic takes relatively low values at low thresholds, and reaches its minimum value at a threshold of five days (fifth column). This value is not significantly different to the value of the MALOR statistic at the thresholds of two and three days (p-values of 0.069 and 0.095, respectively), in contrast to the MALOR values of the other thresholds (all p-values < 0.0001).

Figure 1 shows the regression tree for the outcome *ICU LOS longer than 5 days or death*. Each node is labeled with the estimated probability of the outcome and the number of relevant observations. Four variables have been selected as important predictors for this outcome: type of cardiac surgery, and three variables measured during the first 24 hours ICU stay (*maximal creatinine, minimal bicarbonate,* and *fraction inspired oxygen*). Based on these variables, the probability of *ICU LOS longer than 5 days or death* can be estimated for cardiac surgical patients. The tree models for the threshold of two and three days are quite different in tree structure and selected predictors.

We determined the unbiased performance of this regression tree based on the independent test set; the Brier score of the model is 0.330, and the AUC is 0.718.

Table 2. Evaluation of the tree ensembles (TE) (Brier score) and the regression trees (RT) (Brier score and MALOR statistic) for dichotomized outcomes of ICU LOS based on the training set

threshold	proportion events †	Brier score ‡		MALOR
		TE	RT	
2 days	0.548	0.415	0.475	0.492
3 days	0.390	0.366	0.418	0.490
4 days	0.292	0.312	0.348	0.516
5 days	0.245	0.280	0.293	0.468
6 days	0.207	0.251	0.280	0.534
7 days	0.182	0.232	0.274	0.575
8 days	0.167	0.212	0.242	0.618
9 days	0.156	0.206	0.230	0.616
10 days	0.141	0.193	0.232	0.765
12 days	0.129	0.181	0.216	0.709

†events: patients with ICU LOS higher than the threshold value, or death
‡determined using 10-fold cross-validation

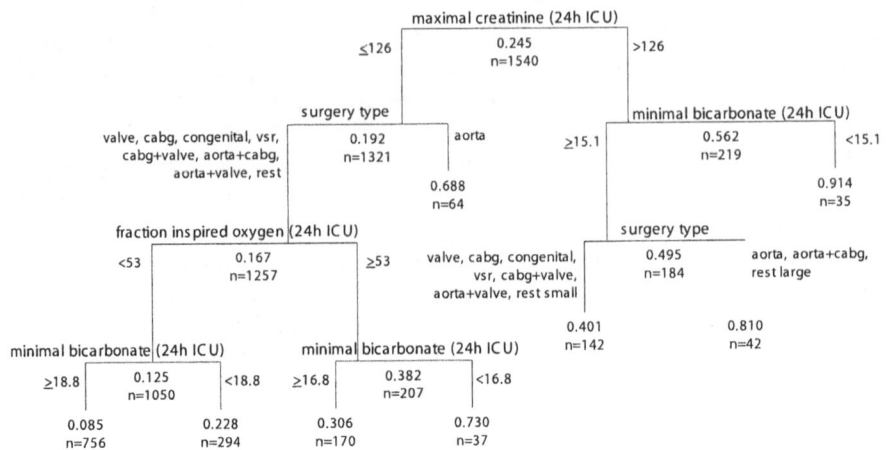

Fig. 1. The regression tree model for prediction of the outcome *ICU LOS>5 days or death*. The variables *maximal creatinine value*, *fraction inspired oxygen* and *minimal bicarbonate value* are variables of the first 24 hours of ICU stay

6 Discussion and Conclusions

The main contribution of this paper is the introduction of a procedure to select the threshold value for dichotomization of survival outcomes, such as ICU LOS, in a structured fashion. The procedure is data-driven and selects the threshold for which the corresponding model has minimal calibration loss, and combines threshold selection with model development. In addition to threshold selection, a direct result of applying the method is a predictive model that can be used in clinical practice for the outcome defined using the optimal threshold.

Application of the proposed procedure for threshold selection to the prediction problem of ICU LOS, the threshold value of five days is selected to dichotomize this outcome. As we found that the value of the MALOR statistic is not significantly different for those values for the thresholds of 2 and 3 days, these threshold values are also good candidates to dichotomize ICU LOS.

The choice of methods to develop a predictive model for survival outcome variables is not trivial. Development of a Cox proportional hazards model [21] is the standard approach. Furthermore, methods have been developed to perform tree-structured survival analysis [22]. A completely different approach to handle (possibly informatively censored) survival outcomes is dichotomization of the survival outcome prior to model development. Comparison of these different approaches to model survival outcomes is a interesting topic for further research.

We used the regression tree method for development of models to be used in clinical practice. Due to the tree structure, the modeled relationship between predictors and outcome is comprehensible for clinicians. This factor is of importance for the clinical reliability of predictive models [23]. For this purpose, we were willing to give up some performance. Good performance is generally obtained for predictive models that are developed by powerful methods such as ensemble learning. However, these models have a black box nature, and are therefore suitable when only the predictions are important. For this reason, we developed tree ensembles only for approximation of the true probability values in order to assess the calibration of the regression trees.

If consensus among practitioners about the threshold value for dichotomization is lacking, an arbitrary choice of a threshold value can be avoided by performing threshold selection based on data analysis. We note that this approach does not necessarily yield a threshold value with a high clinical relevance. However, clinical knowledge can be combined with the procedure to avoid the selection of clinically irrelevant thresholds, for instance, by limiting the search to threshold values that are considered to be clinically relevant.

We have shown that several well-known measures to quantify model performance are sensitive to differences in the outcome distribution (e.g., the mean squared error and the Brier score). These performance measures are often used in the literature on evaluation of predictive models. For the purpose of model selection for a single prediction problem, these performance measures are perfectly suitable. As a result of their sensitivity to class unbalance, however, general performance standards cannot be based on these measures ('a good Brier score'). This fact even holds for the standardized mean squared error R^2 [24]. In contrast to these measures, the underlying distance measure of the MALOR statistic is insensitive to class unbalance. Therefore, its values are comparable for different prediction problems.

Acknowledgments

Niels Peek receives a grant from the Netherlands Organization of Scientific Research (NWO) under project number 634.000.020.

References

1. Dunning, J., Au, J., Kalkat, M., Levine, A.: A Validated Rule for Predicting Patients Who Require Prolonged Ventilation Post Cardiac Surgery. European Journal of Cardio-Thoracic Surgery 24 (2003) 270–276
2. Kern, H., Redlich, U., Hotz, H., von Heymann, C., Grosse, J., Konertz, W., Kox, W.J.: Risk Factors for Prolonged Ventilation after Cardiac Surgery using APACHE II, SAPS II, and TISS: Comparison of Three Different Models. Intensive Care Medicine 27 (2001) 407–415
3. Marcin, J.P., Slonim, A.D., Pollack, M.M., Ruttimann, U.E.: Long-stay Patients in the Pediatric Intensive Care Unit. Critical Care Medicine 29 (2001) 652–657
4. Tu, J.V., Jaglal, S.B., Naylor, C.D., the Steering Committee of the Provincial Adult Cardiac Care Network of Ontario: Multicenter Validation of a Risk Index for Mortality, Intensive Care Unit Stay, and Overall Hospital Length of Stay after Cardiac Surgery. Circulation 91 (1995) 677–684
5. Stein, P.K., Schmieg, R.E., El-Fouly, A., Domitrovich, P.P., Buchman, T.G.: Association between Heart Rate Variability Recorded on Postoperative Day 1 and Length of Stay in Abdominal Aortic Surgery Patients. Critical Care Medicine 29 (2001) 1738–1743

6. Christakis, G.T., Fremes, S.E., Naylor, C.D., Chen, E., Rao, V., Goldman, B.S.: Impact of Preoperative Risk and Perioperative Morbidity on ICU Stay following Coronary Bypass Surgery. Cardiovascular Surgery **4** (1996) 29–35
7. Hugot, P., Sicsic, J., Schaffuser, A., Sellin, M., Corbineau, H., Chaperon, J., Ecoffey, C.: Base Deficit in Immediate Postoperative Period of Coronary Surgery with Cardiopulmonary Bypass and Length of Stay in Intensive Care Unit. Intensive Care Medicine **29** (2003) 257–261
8. Bashour, C.A., Yared, J., Ryan, T.A., Rady, M.Y., Mascha, E., Leventhal, M.J., Starr, N.J.: Long-term Survival and Functional Capacity in Cardiac Surgery Patients after Prolonged Intensive Care. Critical Care Medicine **28** (2000) 3847–3853
9. Janssen, D.P.B., Noyez, L., Wouters, C., Brouwer, R.M.H.J.: Preoperative Prediction of Prolonged Stay in the Intensive Care Unit for Coronary Bypass Surgery. European Journal of Cardio-Thoracic Surgery **25** (2004) 203–207
10. Dawid, A.P.: The Well Calibrated Bayesian. Journal of the American Statistical Association **77** (1982) 605–613
11. Murphy, A.H.: A New Vector Partition of the Probability Score. Journal of Applied Meteorology **12** (1973) 595–600
12. Hand, D.J.: Construction and Assessment of Classification Rules. John Wiley & Sons, New York (1997)
13. Verduijn, M., Peek, N., Voorbraak, F., de Jonge, E., de Mol, B.A.J.M.: Dichotomization of Survival Outcomes based on Model Calibration. Technical Report 2005-01, Department of Medical Informatics, Academic Medical Center – University of Amsterdam (2005)
14. Breiman, L., Friedman, J.H., Olshen, R.A., Stone, C.J.: Classification and Regression Trees. Wadsworth & Brooks, Monterey (1984)
15. Breiman, L.: Bagging Predictors. Machine Learning **26** (1996) 123–140
16. Efron, B., Tibshirani, R.: An Introduction to the Bootstrap. Chapman and Hall, London (1993)
17. Hastie, T., Tibshirani, R., Friedman, J.: The Elements of Statistical Learning. Springer, Berlin (2001)
18. Therneau, T.M., Atkinson, E.J.: An Introduction to Recursive Partitioning using the Rpart Routines. Technical report, Mayo Foundation (1997)
19. Brier, G.W.: Verification of Forecasts Expressed in Terms of Probabilities. Monthly Weather Review **78** (1950) 1–3
20. Metz, C.E.: Basic Principles of ROC Analysis. Seminars in Nuclear Medicine **8** (1978) 283–298
21. Cox, D.R.: Regression Models and Life-Tables. Journal of the Royal Statistical Society B **34** (1972) 187–220
22. Keleş, S., Segal, M.R.: Residual-Based Tree-Structured Survival Analysis. Statistics in Medicine **21** (2002) 313–326
23. Wyatt, J., Altman, D.G.: Prognostic Models: Clinically Useful or Quickly Forgotten? British Medical Journal **311** (1995) 1539–1541
24. Ash, A., Shwartz, M.: R^2: a Useful Measure of Model Performance when Predicting a Dichotomous Outcome. Statistics in Medicine **18** (1999) 375–384

Decision Support Systems

AtherEx: An Expert System for Atherosclerosis Risk Assessment

Petr Berka[1], Vladimír Laš[1], and Marie Tomečková[2]

[1] University of Economic, Prague, Czech Republic
{berka, lasv}@vse.cz
[2] Institute of Computer Science, Academy of Sciences,
Prague, Czech Republic
tomeckova@euromise.cz

Abstract. A number of calculators that compute the risk of atherosclerosis has been developed and made available on the Internet. They all are based on computing weighted sum of risk factors. We propose instead to use more flexible expert systems to estimate the risk. The goal of the AtherEx expert system is to classify patients according to their atherosclerosis risk into four groups. This application is based on the NEST rule–based expert system shell. Knowledge for the AtherEx was obtained (using the machine learning algorithm KEX) from the data concerning a longitudial study of atherosclerosis risk factors and further refined by domain expert. AtherEx is available for consultations on web.

1 Introduction

Atherosclerosis is a slow, complex disease that typically starts in childhood and often progresses when people grow older. In some people it progresses rapidly, even in their third decade. Many scientists think it begins with damage to the innermost layer of the artery. Atherosclerosis involves the slow buildup of deposits of fatty substances, cholesterol, body cellular waste products, calcium, and fibrin (a clotting material in the blood) in the inside lining of an artery. The buildup (referred as a plaque) with the formation of the blood clot (thrombus) on the surface of the plaque can partially or totally block the flow of blood through the artery. If either of these events occurs and blocks the entire artery, a heart attack or stroke or other life-threatening events may result. People with a family history of premature cardiovascular disease (CVD) and with other risk factors of atherosclerosis have an increased risk of the developing of atherosclerosis. Research shows the benefits of reducing the controllable risk factors for atherosclerosis:

- high blood cholesterol (especially LDL or "bad" cholesterol over 100 mg/dL),
- cigarette smoking and exposure to tobacco smoke,
- high blood pressure (blood pressure over 140/90 mm Hg),
- diabetes mellitus,
- obesity (Body Mass Index BMI over 25),
- physical inactivity.

Table 1. Calculators of CVD Risk

system	knowledge source	no. of questions	suitable for	results
NCEP ATP III	ATP III Guidelines	11 + 2	all patients	CVD risk in 10 years
Risk assesment tool	Framingham study	4 + 2	all patients	IM risk in 10 years
Framingham Risk Assessment	Framingham study	5 + 2	all patients	IM risk in 10 years
PROCAM Risk Calculator	PROCAM study	6 + 3	middle-aged men	IM risk in 10 years
PROCAM Risk Score	PROCAM study	7 + 4	middle-aged men	IM risk or death on CVD in 10 years
PROCAM Neural Net	PROCAM study	11 + 5	middle-aged men	IM risk in 10 years
Heart Score	European Society of Cardiology	4 + 2	middle-aged patients	death on CVD in 10 years

Atherosclerosis-related diseases are a leading cause of death and impairment in the United States, affecting over 60 million people. Additionally, 50% of Americans have levels of cholesterol that place them at high risk for developing coronary artery disease. Similar situation can be observed in other countries. So the education of patients about prevention of atherosclerosis is very important.

A number of calculators that compute the risk of atherosclerosis, CVD or myocardial infarction (IM) has been developed and made publicly available on the Internet. These systems usually ask questions about life style (typically about smoking habits) and about results of examination and laboratory tests (typically about blood pressure and cholesterol level) and then compute a risk that given person will suffer from atherosclerosis in 10 years. The computation has a form of weighted sum of used risk factors. The exact formula is based on different knowledge sources: the *NCEP ATP III* system [8] is based on the Adult Treatment Program III guidelines issued by the US National Heart, Lunge and Blood Institute (NHLBI) within the National Cholesterol Education Program (NCEP), the *Risk Assessment Tool* [11] also from NHLBI is based on the data collected within the Framingham Heart Study performed in U.S. - the same study is behind the *Framingham Risk Assessment calculator* [4]. The prospective cardiovascular Münster study (PROCAM) is the background for the *PROCAM Risk calculator* [9] and the *PROCAM Risk score* [10] systems developed in Germany. The *Heart Score* system [7] developed by the European Society of Cardiology is based on data from 12 European cohort studies covering a wide geographic spread of countries at different levels of cardiovascular risks. Tab. 1 summarizes some further information about these systems[1].

---

[1] The column **no. of questions** gives the number of questions on life style (first number) and the number of lab. tests (second number).

The main drawback of using these calculators by an un-experienced user is the necessity to give exact answers to all questions (including questions about values of results of laboratory tests). We believe, that expert systems due to their flexibility and capability to process uncertain or missing information can overcome this obstacle and thus are more suitable for the task of atherosclerosis risk assessment by a non-expert user.

The rest of the paper is organized as follows: section 2 provides a review of the features of NEST with respect to knowledge representation and inference mechanism, section 3 describes the atherosclerosis risk assessment application of NEST (the knowledge acquisition and implementation), and section 4 gives a summary and some future perspectives of the system.

2 Expert System NEST

Expert systems (ES) are typically defined as computer systems that emulate the decision-making ability of a human expert. The power of an ES is derived from presence of a *knowledge base* filled with expert knowledge, mostly in symbolic form. In addition, there is a generic problem-solving mechanism used as *inference engine* [5]. The research in the area of expert systems started in mid-70s, classical examples of early systems that influenced other researchers are MYCIN and PROSPECTOR. The central point of these systems was the *compositional* approach to inference, allowing to compose the contributions of multiple rules (leading to the same conclusion) using a uniform combination function, regardless their mutual dependencies. This approach has later been subject to criticism by most of the uncertainty-processing community. In the design of NEST [3], we attempted to partially overcome the problem that represented the most severe hindrance to compositional system deployment: limited expressiveness of proposition-rule networks for real-world modeling purposes.

2.1 Knowledge Representation

NEST uses attributes and propositions, rules, integrity constraints and contexts to express the task-specific (domain) knowledge.

Four types of attributes can be used in the system: binary, single nominal, multiple nominal, and numeric. According to the type of attribute, the derived propositions correspond to:
- values True and False for a *binary* attribute.
- each value for a *nominal* attribute. The difference between single and multiple nominal attribute is apparent only when answering the question about value of the attribute.
- fuzzy intervals for a *numeric* attribute. Each interval is defined using four points; fuzzy lower bound (FL), crisp lower bound (CL), crisp upper bound (CU), fuzzy upper bound (FU). These values need not to be distinct; this allows to create rectangular, trapezoidal and triangular fuzzy intervals.

Rules are defined in the form

$$condition \Rightarrow conclusion(weight), action$$

where *condition* is disjunctive form (disjunction of conjunctions) of literals (propositions or their negations), *conclusion* is a list of literals and *action* is a list of actions (external programs). We distinguish three types of rules:
- *compositional* - each literal in conclusion has a weight which expresses the uncertainty of the conclusion if the condition holds with certainty. The term compositional denotes the fact, that to evaluate the weight of a proposition, **all** rules with this proposition in the conclusion are evaluated and combined.
- *apriori* - compositional rules without condition; these rules can be used to assign implicit weights to goals or intermediate propositions,
- *logical* - non-compositional rules without weights; only these rules can infer the conclusion with the weight `true` or `false`. **One** activated rule thus fully evaluates the proposition in conclusion.

A list of actions (external programs) can be associated with each rule. These programs are executed if the rule is activated.

As additional knowledge base elements we introduced *integrity constraints* allowing to detect inconsistent patterns of weights and *contexts* that are used to condition the evaluation of attributes or rules.

2.2 Inference Mechanism

During consultation, the system uses rules to compute weights of goals from the weights of questions. This is accomplished by (1) selecting relevant rule during current state of consultation, and (2) applying the selected rule to infer the weight of it's conclusion.

1. The selection of relevant rule can be done using either backward or forward chaining. The actual direction is determined by the user when selecting the consultation mode (see later).
2. For rules with weights (compositional and apriori ones), the system combines contributions of rules using compositional approach described in nest subsection. For rules without weights, the system uses non-compositional approach based on (crisp) modus ponens – to evaluate the weight of a conclusion, and (crisp) disjunction – to evaluate a set of rules with the same conclusion.
   The weights are propagated not only towards the actual goal but by using all rules applicable at given moment.

Uncertainty processing. in NEST is based on the algebraic theory of P. Hájek [6]. This theory generalizes the methods of uncertainty processing used in the early expert systems like MYCIN and PROSPECTOR. Algebraic theory assumes that the knowledge base is created by a set of rules in the form

$$condition \Rightarrow conclusion(weight)$$

where *condition* is a conjunction of literals, *conclusion* is a single proposition and *weight* from the interval $[-1, 1]$ expresses the uncertainty of the rule.

During a consultation, all relevant rules are evaluated by combining their weights with the weights of conditions. Weights of questions are obtained from the user, weights of all other propositions are computed by the inference mechanism. Five combination functions are defined to process the uncertainty in such knowledge base:

1. $NEG(w)$ - to compute the weight of negation of a proposition,
2. $CONJ(w_1, w_2, ..., w_n)$ - to compute the weight of conjunction of literals,
3. $DISJ(w_1, w_2, ..., w_n)$ - to compute the weight of disjunction of literals,
4. $CTR(a, w)$ - to compute the contribution of the rule to the weight of the conclusion (this is computed from the weight of the rule w and the weight of the condition a),
5. $GLOB(w'_1, w'_2, ..., w'_n)$ - to compose the contributions of more rules with the same conclusion.

Algebraic theory defines a set of axioms, the combination functions must fulfill. Different sets of combination functions can thus be implemented. We call these sets "inference mechanisms". The NEST system uses "standard", "logical" and "neural" one. These mechanisms differ in the definition of the functions CTR and $GLOB$ (the respective formulas are shown in Tab. 2).

Standard inference mechanism is based on "classical" approach of MYCIN and PROSPECTOR expert systems. The contribution of a rule is computed Mycin-like, the combination of contributions of rules with the same conclusion is computed Prospector-like.

Logical inference mechanism is based on an application of the completeness theorem for Lukasiewicz many-valued logic. The task of the inference mechanism is to determine the degree in which each goal logically follows from the set of rules (understood as a fuzzy axiomatic theory) and user's answers during consultation [1]. This degree can be obtained by using the *fuzzy modus ponens* inference rule. To combine contributions of more rules, logical inference mechanism uses the *fuzzy disjunction*.

Neural inference mechanism is based on an analogy with active dynamics of neural networks. To obtain results that correspond to the output of a neuron, the contribution of a rule is computed as a weighted input of the neuron and the global effect of all rules with the same conclusion is computed as piecewise linear transformation of the sum of weighted inputs.

The remaining functions are defined in the same way for all three mechanisms: negation of weight w is evaluated as $-w$, conjunction of weights is evaluated as minimum, and disjunction of weights is evaluated as maximum.

Two different notions of "not known" answer are introduced in NEST. First notion, "irrelevant", is expressed by the weight 0; this weight will prevent a rule having either a proposition or it's negation in conditional part from being applied. Second notion, "unknown", is expressed by the weight interval $[-1, 1]$; this weight interval is interpreted as "any weight". Uncertainty processing has thus been extended to work with intervals of weights. The idea behind is to take into account all values from the interval in parallel. Due to the monotonicity of the combination functions, this can be done by taking into account the boundaries of intervals only.

Table 2. Functions CTR and $GLOB$ for different inference mechanisms

inference mechanism	$CTR(a,w)$ for $a > 0$	$GLOB(w'_1, w'_2, ..., w'_n)$
standard	$a \cdot w$	$\frac{w'_1 + w'_2}{1 + w'_1 \cdot w'_2}$
logical	$sign(w) \cdot \max(0, a + |w| - 1)$	$\min(1, \sum_{w'>0} w') - \min(1, \sum_{w'<0} |w'|)$
neural	$a \cdot w$	$\min(1, \max(-1, \sum_{i=1}^{n} w'_i))$

2.3 Consultation with the System

NEST offers several modes of consultation. The *dialogue* mode is the classical question/answer mode when the system selects current question using backward chaining. The *questionnaire* mode allows to fill-in answers in advance; the system then directly infers the goals using forward chaining. In *dialogue/questionnaire* mode the user can input some volunteer information (using questionnaire), during further consultation the system asks questions if needed.

In each of this mode, the user answers the questions concerning the input attributes. According to the type of attribute, the user gives the weight (for binary attributes), the value and its weight (for single nominal attributes), list of values and their weights (for multiple nominal attributes), or the value (for numeric attributes). Questions not answered during consultation get the default answer "unknown" [-1,1] or "irrelevant" [0,0], Answers can be postponed – the user can return to them after finishing the consultation. The result of consultation is shown as a list of goals (resp. all propositions) together with their weights.

3 Building the AtherEx System

3.1 Knowledge Acquisition

The knowledge for the AtherEx system was created in a two-step process. At first a machine learning algorithm has been applied to the data from an epidemiological study of atherosclerosis primary prevention, then, the obtained rule set has been revised and refined by the domain expert.

In the early seventies of the twentieth century, a project of extensive epidemiological study of atherosclerosis primary prevention was developed under the name National Preventive Multifactor Study of Hard Attacks and Strokes in the former Czechoslovakia. The aims of the study were:

1. to identify atherosclerosis risk factors prevalence in a population considered to be the most endangered by possible atherosclerosis complications,
2. to follow the development of these risk factors and their impact on the examined men health, especially with respect to atherosclerotic CVD,

> **KEX algorithm**
>
> **Initialization**
> 1. forall category (attribute-value pair) A add $A \Rightarrow C$ to $OPEN$
> 2. add empty rule to the rule set KB
>
> **Main loop**
> while $OPEN$ is not empty do
> 1. **select** the first implication $Ant \Rightarrow C$ from $OPEN$
> 2. **test** if this implication significantly improves the set of rules KB build so far (we test using the χ^2 test the difference between the rule validity and the result of classification of an example covered by Ant) then add it as a new rule to KB
> 3. for all possible categories A
>   (a) **expand** the implication $Ant \Rightarrow C$ by adding A to Ant
>   (b) **add** $Ant \wedge A \Rightarrow C$ to $OPEN$ so that $OPEN$ remains ordered according to decreasing frequency of the condition of rules
> 4. **remove** $Ant \Rightarrow C$ from $OPEN$

Fig. 1. Simplified sketch of the KEX rule learning algorithm

3. to study the impact of complex risk factors intervention on their development and cardiovascular morbidity and mortality,
4. 10-12 years into the study, to compare risk factors profile and health of the selected men, who originally did not show any atherosclerosis risk factors with a group of men showing risk factors from the beginning of the study.

The data collected within this study thus concern the twenty years lasting longitudinal study of the risk factors of the atherosclerosis in the population of 1 417 middle aged men [2]. To obtain rules from the data we used the algorithm KEX [2]. This algorithm creates decision rules in the form

$$Ant \Rightarrow C(w),$$

where Ant is a conjunction of attribute-value pairs, C is the class attribute, and w is weight of the rule (from the interval [0,1]). During knowledge acquisition, KEX works in an iterative way, in each iteration testing and expanding an implication $Ant \Rightarrow C$. This process starts with default rule weighted with the relative frequency of the class C and stops after testing all implications created according to the user defined criteria. The induction algorithm inserts only such rules into the knowledge base, for which the validity[3] cannot be inferred from the existing rules. The inference (combination of weights of different rules) is based on the pseudobayesian combination function

$$w_1 \oplus w_2 = \frac{w_1 \cdot w_2}{w_1 \cdot w_2 + (1 - w_1) \cdot (1 - w_2)}.$$

---

[2] These data have been used for the ECML/PKDD Discovery Challenge workshops - see http://lisp.vse.cz/challenge for details.
[3] We compute the validity of a rule from the four-fold contingency table as $P(C|Ant)$.

Table 3. Rule bases created from the STULONG data

Rule base	no.rules	overall accuracy	accuracy for non-risk group	accuracy for other groups
1	19	0.87	0.83	0.88
2	39	0.84	0.74	0.87
3	32	0.77	0.63	0.83
4	27	0.73	0.48	0.83

Let us stress, that this function corresponds to the "standard" $GLOB$ function of the system NEST and that the rules created by KEX correspond[4] to the apriori and compositional rules of NEST.

When comparing KEX with divide–and–conquer algorithms (like C4.5) or set covering algorithms (like CN2), we can observe, that:

- KEX creates more rules (because KEX does not remove covered examples),
- the set of rules can obtain both a rule and its sub-rule (the redundancy of rules is evaluated using statistical test),
- examples are assigned to class with uncertainty.

Using KEX we analyzed the data concerning examination of patients when entering the study. These data contain the information about life style, personal history, family history, some laboratory tests and about classification w.r.t atherosclerosis risk (non risk, risky, pathological group). We performed several analyses for different subsets of input attributes:

1. classification based only on already known risk factors (this rule base should confirm the classification of patients in the analyzed data),
2. classification based on attributes concerning life style, personal and family history (but without special laboratory tests),
3. classification based on attributes concerning life style and family history,
4. classification based only on attributes concerning life style.

The classification accuracies (computed using 10 fold cross-validation) of the rule bases resulting from these analyses are summarized in Tab. 3. As a final output from this first (machine learning) step of building the knowledge base, we selected the result of the second type of analyses. The reason for this choice was twofold: the rules have reasonable high classification accuracy and they do not use any "special" attributes concerning laboratory tests.

The set of rules obtained using KEX has been revised by the domain expert who suggested following improvements:

1. add the attribute "total cholesterol" and respective rules,
2. add rules for remaining values of an attribute, if at least one value of this attribute occur in rules obtained from data,

---

[4] We only have to transform the weights of rules from $[0, 1]$ to $[-1, 1]$.

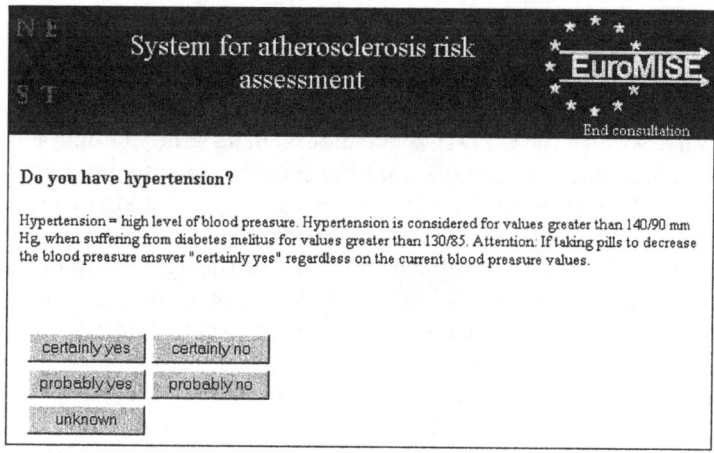

Fig. 2. Screenshot of the system

3. use the goals "no risk", "low risk", "medium risk" and "high risk" instead of original groups taken from data.

3.2 Implementation

We used the client/server version of NEST to implement the AtherEx system. In this version, the server is a web server running under MS Windows and the client is a web browser (like Internet Explorer). Different page layouts can be defined for different knowledge bases. To make AtherEx user-friendly for users who are neither experts in expert systems, nor experts in medicine, we built a front end, that hides the details about inference and uncertainty processing. The system works in dialogue mode, showing one question on a single page. The questions (their number is 22) are grouped into following groups:

- questions concerning personal data (marital status, education, BMI, cholesterol),
- questions concerning life style (smoking, physical activity in job and after job, consumption of alcohol, coffee or tea),
- questions concerning personal history (hypertension, myocardial infarction, diabetes),
- questions concerning family history (hypertension, myocardial infarction, diabetes, angina pectoris or ictus for parents).

The user can answer the questions using predefined values (buttons) "certainly yes", "probably yes", "probably no", "certainly no", or "unknown" (Fig. 2 shows the question about hypertension).

4 Conclusions

The AtherEx expert system described in the paper should help non-expert users to determine their atherosclerosis risk. We see the main advantages of our system (when compared with the CVD risk calculators) in its ability to infer a conclusion from incomplete and/or uncertain input information (the user need not to answer all questions). Our experiments with the machine learning algorithm KEX (see Tab. 3) have shown that the information about life style can be used instead of laboratory tests, that are usually not available for this type of users. AtherEx is now tested by domain expert and other physicians from the EuroMISE center in Prague (http://www.euromise.cz) with similar results. Anyway, the resulting classification does not substitute a diagnosis done by a specialist, it is rather a recommendation that should by consulted with a physician.

AtherEx is available for on-line consultations at http://146.102.170.51. The current version does not consider changes over time. In our future work we plan to include knowledge dealing with the dynamics of the risk factors. As the rules are based on data concerning middle-aged man, we also plan to investigate the applicability of AtherEx to the whole population.

References

1. Berka,P., Ferjenčík,J., Ivánek,J.: Expert system shell SAK based on complete many-valued logic and its application in territorial planning. In: (Novák, et all.) Fuzzy Approach to Reasoning and Decision Making. Academia, Prague and Kluwer, Dodrecht 1992, 67-74.
2. Berka,P., Ivánek,J.: Automated Knowledge Acquisition for PROSPECTOR-like Expert Systems. In: (Bergadano, deRaedt, eds.) Proc. ECML'94, LNAI 784, Springer 1994, 339-342.
3. Berka,P., Laš,V., Svátek,V.: NEST: re-engineering the compositional approach to rule-based inference. Neural Network World, 5/04, 2004, 367-379.
4. Framingham Risk Assessment calculator. Internet, http://chd.uni-muenster.de/framingham.php.
5. Durkin,J.: Expert Systems, Design and Development. Maxmillan Publishing Comp., 1994.
6. Hájek,P.: Combining Functions for Certainty Factors in Consulting Systems. Int. J. Man-Machine Studies 22, 1985.
7. Heart Score. Internet, http://www.escardio.org/knowledge/decision_tools/heartscore.
8. NCEP ATP III system. Internet, http://www.incirculation.net/index.asp?did=23849.
9. PROCAM Risk calculator. Internet, http://www.chd-taskforce.de/calculator/calculator.htm.
10. PROCAM Risk score. Internet, http://www.chd-taskforce.de/risk-english.htm.
11. Risk Assessment Tool. Internet, http://www.nhlbi.nih.gov/guidelines/cholesterol/risk_tbl.htm.

Smooth Integration of Decision Support into an Existing Electronic Patient Record

S. Quaglini[1], S. Panzarasa[2], A. Cavallini[3], G. Micieli[3], C. Pernice[4], and M. Stefanelli[1]

[1] Department of Computer Science and Systems, University of Pavia
[2] CBIM, Pavia
[3] Stroke Unit, IRCCS "C. Mondino", Pavia
[4] TSD Projects, Milan

Abstract. Willingness to use computerised decision support systems is often jeopardised by lack of effective integration into existing user interfaces for electronic patient record. Concepts illustrated in this paper stem from the need of developing a project for the comparison of the physicians' compliance to a clinical practice guideline before and after an electronic version of the guideline was introduced. Before starting the implementation, we performed a deep users' needs analysis. It was accomplished also on the basis of lesson learned on past guideline implementations. The new idea was to classify guideline suggestions on the basis of some attributes, whose values will determine the modality of presentation of the suggestion itself, and on a different management of non compliance advice.

1 Introduction

Despite broad agreement on the necessity to improve quality of care through implementation of clinical guidelines (GLs), and the incredible number of GLs diffused in last years, there is still lack of adherence to them. Since it was soon clear that paper-based GLs, as well as their hypertext representation over the internet, didn't offer adequate decision support in clinical practice, the medical informatics community hypothesised that more formal electronic versions would increase physicians' compliance. Recent reviews are available to compare different GLs representation formalisms [2,5]. However, integrating Gls within a clinical workflow remains a critical issue, and many efforts have been put in developing standard data models for facilitating data sharing among systems. Projects for the Electronic Patient Record (EPR) standardisation are under development [7], but we are still far from a solution. Moreover, in real-world situations a crucial issue is the integration of GLs with existent software and local workflows. If a user is happy with his current information system, the existing human-computer interaction should be preserved and a new system perceived just as a "new release" with some additional functionalities. This paper does not deal with a new formalism for GL representation, nor with standards for EPR, but it describes a users' needs-based approach to challenges posed by the integration of a GL within existing information systems. As a matter of fact, our approach stems from a lesson learned about non compliances with a previous implemented GL [3], and starts analysing the physicians' needs in the various phases of a patient's management. Not only need for GL suggestions, but also communication facilities with colleagues, automatic production and printing of reports in natural language, etc. have been considered. If physicians are not provided with an integrated solution for all these problems, they will not perceive the system as a support, and also GL suggestions will not be taken into the due account. These concepts are currently exploited within a project dealing with the evaluation of compliance to "The Italian guidelines for stroke prevention and management" edited by SPREAD on March 2003 [www.spread.it].

2 The System Analysis

Our goal is to compare the physicians' compliance to GLs before and after the electronic support introduction. Twenty Neurological Units are currently using the same EPR without any decision support (DS). Data will be collected for six months. Then, the same Units will use the GL-supported EPR for additional six months. The EPR has been developed with WINCARE®[1]. The user's interface is based on *Events*, i.e. sections of the clinical chart through which it is possible collecting patient data and generating textual reports. Username and password define the visualization of competent events. In the current version the list of events is not structured at all: it is given in alphabetic order and it is not tailored to the specific patient. As the first step of the study, we performed an analysis of the existing EPR and its user interface in order to (a) find out which additional data needed to be stored, and which data needed to be encoded, in order to verify the compliance with GLs; (b) realise how to integrate the new DS functionalities, within the existing interface, on the "minimal invasiveness" principle. Moreover, we assessed collaboration and agreements with the company providing the EPR in order to (a) allow additional, or different, data input, as derived from point 1; (b) devise a middleware for data sharing between EPR and the GL. As an example for point 1a, the patient's and family's histories were traditionally entered as free text: this was not compatible with the need of interpreting rules such as: "if the patient had a previous myocardial infarction, then ...". "Previous myocardial infarction" of course must be encoded. Thus all the historical information has been encoded through ICD9-CM. This would have been an advantage for the GL engine, but a disadvantage for another aspect of the clinical workflow: in fact, physicians were used to print the histories and attach them to the discharge letter, "as they were": to make ICD9-CM encoding acceptable, a parallel tool has been developed translating the encoded diseases, plus some associated comments, into natural language sentences. The other points are detailed in the next paragraphs.

3 Classification of Guideline Recommendations

We searched for an agreement with neurologists about the best way of communicating GL suggestions; we mean real-time pop-up windows, user's agenda update, use of different colours, special icons, etc. Also non compliances need different management according to suggestions they refer to. Instead of developing ad-hoc solutions, we formulated a general classification of GL recommendations, in which each class could be

---

[1] WINCARE® is a product of TSD-Projects.

associated to a particular GUI modality. This allows building reusable modules for the visualisation of reminds. The key elements of the methodology are that GLs are developed by multidisciplinary groups, they are based on scientific evidence, and recommendations are explicitly linked and graded according to the strength of the supporting evidence[1,6,8]. In the SPREAD GLs, this grade summarizes scientific evidence and applicability. Whichever indicators the GL adopts, users should be aware of how each GL recommendation has been graded.

Our idea has been to build a classification of recommendations taking into account first of all the grading provided by the GL itself, but also other attributes, such as:

1) type of the recommendation: whether it is a diagnostic process, a treatment, a variable monitoring, a message;
2) *sign* of the recommendation: if it is something to do or to rule out;
3) urgency: acute situations must be managed as fast as possible.
4) care provider to whom the recommendation is directed: the communication language could be different for physicians, nurses, technicians, etc.;
5) whether a suggestion addresses a single user, a role (physician, nurse, etc), a group of users or all the care providers involved in a patient treatment.

In agreement with our clinical partners, in order to manage non compliance in a non invasive way, we choose to do it at the patient discharge, in fact preparing the discharge letter requires summarizing the patient hospital stay, and reasoning about. In practice, when physicians fill the DISCHARGE FORM, a set of queries is activated and a sheet is printed with the list of non compliances, that the system can detect automatically starting from the EPR (at that time all data should have been entered).

4 Integration of the Decision Support into the EPR Management

To add the DS functionalities, reengineering of both structure and interface of the EPR was performed. More precisely, we refer to our previous terminology definition given in [4], borrowed from the Workflow Management Coalition. We defined a CfMS as a system that defines, creates and manages the execution of Careflows (Cfs) through the use of software, running under the control of one or more Cfs engines, which are able to interpret the care process definition, interact with Cfs participants and invoke software applications. The Cf model, described on the basis of the SPREAD GL, has been formulated using Oracle Workflow ^{TM}. The CfMS needs patient data in order to fire the GL rules and to generate patient-specific recommendations that, together with messages and alerts, should be communicated to the users (Cf participants) via the end-user application. As already said, our choice is not to create a new specific inter-

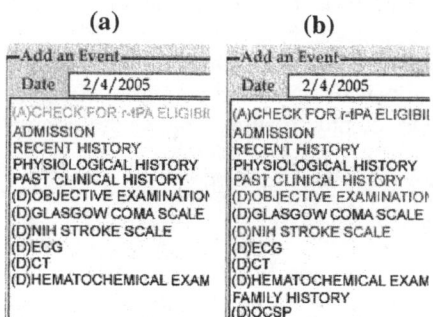

Fig. 1. Changing the list of the tasks as a function of urgency

face for the CfMS, but to integrate all the needed functionalities within the existing system. To this aim, first of all a middleware for data sharing has been developed: whenever there is a new data entry the EPR transfers this data into a support database. On the other hand, when the GL generates a suggestion, or a new list of events, they are put into the same database, and WINCARE can read them and show them through its interface. In the following paragraphs the management of different situations is shown.

Diagnostic and Treatment Processes. In general, GLs suggest a sequence of tasks to be performed according to some routing. Some of these tasks are for all the patients; others are reserved to patients with particular clinical conditions. Concerning scheduling, some tasks are to be done in particular points in time, others have no time constraints. We integrate this information in the events list of WINCARE. In the updated system, the list is no more unstructured: on the contrary it is built taking into account the patient's data and the time spent since the patient's admission. Colours are used to mean that a task has to be done (blue), is being done (orange), it is completed (green) or it has not been executed due to an exception (red). In Fig. 1a, the patient is potentially eligible for the thrombolytic drug r-tPA (information coming from the recent history table). This treatment is both extremely important and delicate: the task list only refers to actions to be done in order to detect possible contraindications. In Fig. 1b, for some reasons, the three-hours temporal window is over, and r-tPA cannot be administered more: "Check for r-tPA eligibility" is red and also less urgent tasks appear in the list.

Grade of Recommendation. It's worth noting that the list of events is not only composed by tasks suggested by the GLs, but also by all the other events useful for the whole patient's management. The GL-related tasks can be recognised by their associated grade (shown as in the textual GL, by letters A-D).

Sign of Recommendation. It's very important to advise also about actions that must not be performed. In fact, if a GL reports such actions, it is very probable that they have been recognised as frequent medical errors. Recommendations with negative sign are represented with crossed text (eg: "I.V. ADMINISTRATION OF STREPTOKINASE IS NOT RECOMMENDED").

Urgency of Recommendations. When there is a tight temporal window for accomplishing a task, the corresponding management form is pop-up window. The window shown in Fig. 2 reports all the contraindications to the r-tPA. The system fills the most crosses as possible, given the available data in the EPR. But the window is popped-up even if the list is not complete, because the decision has to be taken in few tenths of minutes. The remaining crosses will be put by the physician himself. On the other hand, when the suggestion is not urgent, a pop-up window would be boring. In that case, the recommendation is translated into a simple communication, sent to the appropriate

Contraindications	Presence	Absence	Unknown
THERE IS AT LEAST ONE CONTROINDICATION. THROMBOLYYIC THERAPY IS NOT INDICATED			
Suspect of ESA (even with normal CT)			x
Unknown time of the stroke onset		x	
Age > 80 years		x	
Severe patient: stupor or coma		x	
Too mild patient (Scandinavian Stroke Scale score>50 or NIHSS score<6)	x		
Quick improvement before the treatment			x

Fig. 2. Contraindications to thrombolysis. A red sign rules out the treatment

roles, which will be visualised when the users will access their "communication box". A red screen icon on the right top of the screen indicates that the communication box is not empty. An example is shown in Fig. 3: heparin treatment for secondary prevention of deep venous thrombosis may be undertaken in whichever day during the hospital admission.

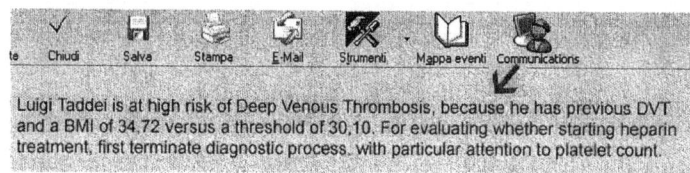

Fig. 3. A communication sent to physicians for evaluating a particular therapy

5 Conclusion

We have illustrated a re-engineering process of a DSS, based on a user needs analysis. The aim was of letting physicians and nurses to exploit system suggestions with the minimum effort and invasiveness with respect to daily routine. To do this, we worked on different levels. At the interface level, we fully integrated the decision support into the EPR interface that neurologists were using since some years. At a cognitive level, we designed modality presentation of both suggestions and non compliances according to a pre-defined classification, based not only on scientific evidence, as in the past, but also on a set of attributes related to the clinical workflow.

References

1. Cook, D.J., Guyatt, G.H., Laupacis, A., Sackett, D.L., Goldberg, R.J.: Clinical recommendations using levels of evidence for antithrombotic agents. Chest **108**(4 Suppl) (1995) 227S-230S
2. de Clercq, P.A., Blom, J.A., Korsten, H.H., Hasman A.: Approaches for creating computer interpretable guidelines that facilitate decision support. Artif Intell Med. **31**(1) (2004) 1-27
3. Micieli, G., Cavallini, A., Quaglini, S.: Guideline Compliance Improves Stroke Outcome-A Preliminary Study in 4 Districts in the Italian Region of Lombardia. Stroke **33** (2002) 1341-1347
4. Panzarasa, S., Bellazzi, R., Larizza, C., Stefanelli, M.: A careflow management system for chronic patients. In: Fieschi, M., Coiera, E., Yu-Chan Jack Li (eds): Medinfo 2004. IOS Press, Amsterdam Berlin Oxford Tokyo Washington DC (2004) 773-777
5. Peleg, M., Tu, S., Ciccarese, P., Kumar, A., Quaglini, S., Stefanelli, M. et al.: Comparing models of decision and action for guideline-based decision support: a case-study approach. JAMIA **1** (10) (2003) 52-68
6. Sackett, D.L.: Rules of evidence and clinical recommendations on use of antithrombotic agents. Chest **89**(2 Suppl.) (1986) 2S-3S
7. Tu, S.W., Campbell, J., Musen, M.A.: The SAGE guideline modeling: motivation and methodology. Stud Health Technol Inform. **101** (2004) 167-171
8. Yusuf, S., Cairns, J.A., Camm, A.J., Fallen, E.L., Gersh, B.J. Evidence-Based Cardiology. 2d edition BMJ Books London (2003)

REPS: A Rehabilitation Expert System for Post-stroke Patients

Douglas D. Dankel II[1] and María Ósk Kristmundsdóttir[2]

[1] University of Florida, C.I.S.E., Box 116120, Gainesville, FL 32611-6120 USA
University of Akureyri, Faculty of Information Tech.,
602 Akureyri, Iceland
ddd@cise.ufl.edu
[2] Selbrekka 1, 200 Kópavogur, Iceland
mok@simnet.is

Abstract. Knowledge-based systems are widely used in many application areas, especially in health care and more recently in rehabilitation. The rehabilitation of cerebrovascular accident (CVA) victims can be a complex and demanding task. This research developed a Rehabilitation Expert System for Post-Stroke Patients (REPS) consisting of an assessment stage and a rehabilitation stage. The assessment is based on internationally validated assessment tools and widely accepted methods of rehabilitation. Both stages are based on the expertise and knowledge of physical therapists at the Fjórðungssjúkrahúsið á Akureyri (FSA) University Hospital in Akureyri, Iceland. This prototype demonstrates the feasibility of knowledge-based systems in the field of physical therapy, in general, and post-stroke rehabilitation, in particular.

1 Introduction

Knowledge-based systems have been developed in many domains with clinical decision support systems and other knowledge-based systems now commonplace in health care [6] [11]. However, most systems are in the fields of medicine and nursing while physical therapy is a relatively untouched domain. One of the most complex and demanding tasks in physical therapy is the assessment and rehabilitation of post-stroke patients. This paper examines REPS, the Rehabilitation Expert System for Post-Stroke Patients.

Two expert systems have been developed for diagnosing and categorizing strokes. Toposcout finds the anatomic location and the corresponding vascular territory of a stroke, based on the clinical signs and symptoms. This system is able to detect typical stroke patterns and was tested for conformity with the final diagnosis of 129 patients in the Hamburg Stroke Data Bank. It was found to have a high level of agreement for hemispheric lesions [3].

Microstroke was designed to categorize and diagnose stroke types based on clinical information. The system's knowledge base includes information from large stroke registries. The system queries the physician for details of the patient's history, the onset of stroke, accompanying symptoms, and pertinent neurological findings. Using these data items, it determines the relevant odds and arrives at the probabilities of different stroke types for a given patient. Stroke type diagnoses by Microstroke, were correct in 72.8% of 250 cases in the Hamburg Stroke Data Bank [4].

According to Myrna Donald [5], three knowledge-based systems have been constructed within the domain of physical therapy. The first, the NIOSH Low Back Atlas prototype, assisted therapists in determining which of three treatment programs was appropriate based on a patient's displayed symptoms. Second is Elexsys, a computer assisted instruction (CAI) prototype that instructs physical therapy students and physical therapists in using interferential therapy. The third system, a prototype developed by Donald [8], attempts to demonstrate the feasibility of knowledge based system applications in the domain of physical therapy. This prototype acts as a clinical decision making aid in the management of post-poliomyelitis cases.

2 Motivation

Fjórðungssjúkrahúsið á Akureyri (FSA) is a university and regional hospital, which serves the town of Akureyri and the surrounding areas in North-Iceland. The hospital was established in 1873 and collaborates with Icelandic universities on the instruction of health classes and resources in health science.

The physical therapy department at FSA consists of 6 physical therapists working mostly in rehabilitation. This involves helping people obtain the best possible physical condition after an operation or an illness. The most complex and demanding task they perform is the rehabilitation of patients who have had a cerebrovascular accident (CVA) or stroke. The repercussions of stroke are very subjective, and it can be very complex and demanding to assess and treat post-stroke patients who often require extensive daily rehabilitation.

CVA is the consequence of a sudden and permanent disturbance of blood flow to regions of the brain caused by vascular disease. This disturbance can be caused by a blockage in a cerebral artery from a blood clot, from an embolism, or because of a hemorrhage into the brain tissue. In each case, the brain cells that are nurtured by the vessel suffer from a lack of oxygen and other nutrients. If these disturbances are short and temporary, the resulting stroke symptoms may appear for only a short time, but, if these disturbances are longer term, a part of the brain dies and the activity of other regions is upset resulting in permanent damage and long-term care. Various diseases may cause CVA and the symptoms that appear are dependant on the location and size of the lesion [12].

A majority of the symptoms can be placed into one of two categories based on which side of the brain is damaged. According to [2], the most common symptoms occurring when the lesion is located in the left hemisphere of the brain are paralysis on the right hand side, aphasia, and an underestimation of ability. The most common symptoms of patients having damage in the right hemisphere are paralysis on the left hand side, an impaired sense of spatial relations, impaired judgment, and neglect. Other symptoms that may appear with CVA patients include motor apraxia, ideational apraxia, and visual field defects.

A doctor treating a CVA patient refers the patient to a physical therapist for rehabilitation. The physical therapist is given the status and medical history of the patient and the location in the brain where the damage occurred. The therapist assesses the patient's condition using two paper forms: the CVA Status sheet and the Modified Motor Assessment Scale (MMAS).

The CVA Status sheet records the assessment of the patient's mobility, which is measured for his/her upper and lower limbs, sitting balance and reflexes, standing balance and reflexes, walking, face and swallowing, and neuropsychological function disorders. This sheet is used in conjunction with the MMAS. The MMAS rates a patient's abilities in turning in bed (supine to side), moving from lying in bed to sitting on edge of bed, sitting, standing up, walking, arm movement, hand movement, and advanced hand movement. Each is rated on a 0-5 scale every time the patient is visited so the patient's progress can be monitored effectively [5]. Based on the results of an assessment, an individualized set of rehabilitation exercises is prescribed [7].

3 Implementation

Analysis of the MMAS and the CVA Status sheet identified that the CVA Status sheet is used to address some of the shortcomings of the MMAS. The MMAS is a standardized sheet that allows no room for personalized and detailed information about the patient. These two assessment tools were combined when implemented in REPS with the categories of the CVA Status sheet used as a skeleton for the knowledge base. Minor modifications resulted in a structure for assessment and treatment that consists of seven categories: upper limb movement, lower limb movement, movement in bed, sitting balance and reactions, standing balance and reactions, walking, and neuropsycological function disorders.

REPS was developed using the C Language Integrated Production System (CLIPS) version 6.2.1 [10] as a rule-based expert system. It contains two sets of facts. The first set, called *initialization facts*, is asserted when the program first starts and drives the assessment process. The second set, the *patient status facts*, is asserted during the assessment process and represents the current status of the assessed patient.

The rules are also divided into two categories. The assessment rules contain patterns that primarily match initialization facts. The rehabilitation rules are driven only by the patient status facts. The rules execute using CLIPS' depth strategy.

4 System Execution

The expected users of REPS are trained physical therapists. While the majority of the users will be accustomed to working with CVA patients, some may have little or no experience in the field and no specific training in computer usage. As a result, the system is designed for easy use and guides the user through the evaluation process.

REPS' functionality consists of consecutive stages. The first involves assessment where the user provides information about the patient. The second is rehabilitation where the system displays advice on rehabilitation based on the assessment.

The assessment stage involves seven phases, which correspond with the seven categories of knowledge derived from the MMAS scales and the CVA status sheet. Each phase asks a series of questions concerning either the patient's rating on a MMAS scale or some specific characteristic of the patient's status.

The system questions the user by displaying the category being evaluated (e.g., *upper limb movement*) and a scale (e.g., set of numbered tasks) for assessing the patient. Finally, the user is asked how many points the patient receives on this scale. The scale is progressive in difficulty with the patient receiving points only to a level where they can complete all of the specified activities.

The *upper limb movement* category has both MMAS scales and some general questions. After the MMAS questions, the user is asked if the patient can actually move the arm. If the answer is "no" then the system does not ask about the arm's spasm and movement patterns. If the answer is "yes," then a more specific question is asked involving the type of movement pattern, either flexion or extension. Finally, two questions are asked regardless of whether or not the patient could move the arm. These questions do not ask about the arm specifically, but rather about weight transference (e.g., the shifting of body weight from the left to right or vice versa) and defense mechanisms in the whole upper body (e.g., the body's reaction of raising arms or moving out of the way when an object is throw at it).

After proceeding through the different phases of assessment, the system provides advice on rehabilitation. This phase is based entirely on the information gathered during the assessment phase and requires no user input. This advice might include a warning if the patient lacks defense mechanisms since the patient is at risk, for example, of falling and not being able to defend himself (e.g., stop the fall by extending his arms to "catch" himself). After displaying the warning, the system provides advice on appropriate exercises to improve the patient's abilities.

5 Conclusion

In summary, assessing and rehabilitating a post-stroke patient is a complex task. The goal of this research was to create a knowledge-based system capturing the knowledge used to determine the appropriate therapy. By doing this, we can make the knowledge permanent, helping the department to maintain the knowledge and the experience that employees have gathered through the years and can make training of new physical therapists easier since the system guides the therapist though the process of assessing and rehabilitating a CVA patient.

REPS was tested for completeness and consistency by searching for eight different types of syntactic errors: redundant rules, conflicting rules, subsumed rules, circular rules, unnecessary IF conditions, dead-end rules, missing rules, and unreachable rules [9]. None of these errors were found. Informal testing was performed to ensure that REPS produces the same output as an expert would when given the same inputs. At meetings with the experts, the system was exercised and viewed. Actual CVA cases were used as test cases to run the system. No major errors where found and any minor problems that were uncovered were fixed.

The current version of REPS is considered a prototype for demonstrating the feasibility of developing a knowledge-based system for assessment and rehabilitation of post-stroke patients. Before this system can be placed in clinical use, it will need to comply with the requirements document for computer systems dealing with medical records, issued by the Ministry of Health and Social Security [1]. Emphasis was placed on creating a complete and comprehensive assessment tool that could be expanded and improved through further research.

Acknowledgements

This research was, in part, supported by a grant from the Fulbright Foundation.

References

1. Almenn kröfulýsing fyrir sjúkraskrárkerfi – Lágmark-skröfur. Heilbrigðis- og tryggingamálaráðuneyti, Reykjavík (2001)
2. Baldursdóttir, B. and Middelink, S.: Almenn fræðsla um heilablóðfall. Fjórðungssjúkrahúsið á Akureyri, Akureyri (2003)
3. Caplan, L.R., Kunze, K., Spizer, K., and Thie, A.: The TOPOSCOUT expert system for stroke localization. Stroke 20(9) (1989) 1195-1201
4. Caplan, L.R., Kunze, K., Spizer, K., and Thie, A.: The Microstroke expert system for stroke type diagnosis. Stroke 20(10) (1989) 1353-1366
5. Carr, J. H., Lynne, D., Nordholm, L., and Shepherd, R. B.: Investigation of a New Motor Assessment Scale for Stroke Patients. Physical Therapy 65(2) (1985) 175-180
6. Coiera, E.: Guide to Health Informatics. Second Edition. Arnold Publishers: London (2003)
7. Davies, P. M.: Steps to Follow: The Comprehensive Treatment of Patients with Hemiplegia. Springer Verlag: New York (1993)
8. Donald, M.: Computer Application for Physiotherapy. M.S. Thesis in Interdisciplinary Studies. University of Manitoba, Winnipeg, Canada (1999)
9. Gonzalez, A. J. and Dankel, D. D.: The Engineering of Knowledge-Based Systems: Theory and Practice. Prentice-Hall: Englewood Cliffs (1993)
10. Riley, G.: What are expert systems? http://www.ghg.net/clips/WhatIsCLIPS.html (2002)
11. Shortliffe, E. H., Perreault, L. E., Weiderhold, G., and Fagan, L. M.: Medical Informatics, Computer Applications in Health Care and Biomedicine. Second Edition. Springer-Verlag: New York (2003)
12. Sigfússon, N., Sveinbjörnsdóttir, S., and Agarsson, U.: Heilablóðfall. Háþrýstingur, hvað er til ráða? http://www.hjarta.is/Qbs/uploads/214.pdf. (2002)

Clinical Guidelines and Protocols

Testing Asbru Guidelines and Protocols for Neonatal Intensive Care

Christian Fuchsberger[1], Jim Hunter[2], and Paul McCue[2]

[1] Innsbruck Biocentre, Division of Medical Biochemistry,
Innsbruck Medical School
info@fuchsberger.it
[2] Department of Computing Science, University of Aberdeen
jhunter@csd.abdn.ac.uk, paul@tiko.demon.co.uk

Abstract. The automatic application of computerized guidelines and protocols in intensive care is not simple, given the high volume of data which must be processed and the need to offer advice on a continuous basis. However most of this data is available automatically and there is therefore the real possibility of improving the quality of care by providing timely advice without placing any additional load on the clinicians. In this paper we describe a prototype system which demonstrates the feasibility of doing this. We then discuss specific issues which arise in applying guidelines for such environments.

1 Introduction

Intensive and high-dependency care is becoming increasingly complex. More physiological parameters (such as heart rate, oxygen and carbon dioxide levels in the blood, body temperatures and blood pressures) are being monitored at higher time resolutions (often one sample per second). Better ventilation, medical and surgical procedures are available. Medical errors in the intensive care unit (ICU) are not uncommon, and although the majority are unimportant and thus might not be classed as 'mistakes', some are significant causing deterioration of the patient and acute anxiety for both relatives and staff. Errors often result from missed symptoms and signs, or a lack of appreciation of their importance. This may be due to staff ignorance, related to inadequate training or experience (most of the time it is relatively junior staff who provide the immediate care). Alternatively it may be related to attentional overload (looking after two or more sick patients or having to handle an emergency in another ward), or to informational overload (so many false alarms occurring that the true situation is not appreciated). Intensive care is an extraordinarily complicated environment and things get forgotten.

Many units have addressed this problem by summarizing the data using complex graphical displays. While this is of significant help to senior clinicians, it has not been shown to improve the performance of the junior staff [1]. One way in which the junior staff might benefit from the collection of this data, would be to deploy automated decision support systems [2].

A parallel development has been the growing interest setting out clear statements of the optimal management for a specific group of patients which, when properly applied, will improve the quality of the care they receive. If these statements can be expressed in a formal language, interpreted by a computer and applied to electronic patient data streams, then the attention of clinical staff could be drawn automatically to the recommendations for the specific patient at the specific time.

Such statements about optimal care are variously referred to as 'guidelines' or 'protocols' [3]. Here, we shall take 'guideline' to refer to the care recommendations which are written down (often by some national committee and usually evidence based) and widely disseminated. We shall take 'protocol' to refer to the recommendations acquired from one clinician (or from a small group of clinicians in the same unit) which represents a more 'local' view. Since most of what we have to say is equally applicable to both guidelines and protocols and since 'guideline' is more commonly used, we shall use it to save repetition (except where we want to refer specifically to a protocol!).

In this paper we describe a prototype system which demonstrates the feasibility of applying computerised guidelines to complex multi-channel data from a (neonatal) ICU. We should emphasise that this was an *off-ward* experiment. Much more development needs to be carried out before we will be in a position to evaluate the application of such guidelines on the ward.

We will look at the various components which need to be in place for the development and application of guidelines within the ICU (section 2). We will then describe the subset of these components which represents our own specific contribution, namely the *test protocol* (section 3), the necessary *data abstractions* and their implementation (section 4), the *test data* (section 5) and the *test infrastructure* used to integrate these components (section 6). We conclude by describing the *test results* (section 7) and discussing some specific problems posed by applying guidelines in the ICU environment (section 8).

2 Application of Computerized Guidelines

In this section we will look at the various elements which need to be in place if we are to implement automated computerized guidelines in a data-rich environment.

Formal Languages for Guidelines and Protocols

In recent years various formal and semi-formal representations of medical guidelines have been introduced. These representations range from workflow representation approaches like Guide, through scenario-based ones, like PRODIGY to sophisticated and complex representations like GLIF, SAGE, ProForma and Asbru; for a review of these languages see [3].

We have chosen to use Asbru, which is a time-oriented, intention-based, skeletal plan-representation language used in the Asgaard Project to represent clinical guidelines [4]. Asbru can be used to express guidelines as skeletal plans that can be instantiated for every patient. Asbru enables the designer to represent both the prescribed actions of a skeletal plan and the knowledge roles required by the various problem-solving methods performing the intertwined supporting subtasks.

Guidelines and Protocols

In adult intensive care there are relatively few existing guidelines and in neonatal intensive care (our area of interest) we are aware only of one [5]. Although this guideline is relevant to our interests, we wanted to concentrate on the particular problem of regulating the levels of oxygen and carbon dioxide in the blood on a continuous basis. We therefore acquired a relatively simple protocol from one of our collaborating clinicians.

Translation and Visualization

The distance between an informal or semi-formalized guideline and its expression in, for example, detailed Asbru XML, is great, and tools are being developed to assist this e.g. [6]. Translated guidelines need to be converted back into some form which can be understood by clinical experts so that the translation can be checked for accuracy, and visual representations constitute one possible modality [7].

Abstraction of the Raw Data

Guidelines will often be expressed using abstractions which are not directly available in the raw data – for example the presence of "multiple bradycardias occurring over several minutes" must be derived from a sequence of real valued measurements of heart rate. These abstractions need to be derived from the data and a variety of signal processing algorithms (both numerical and knowledge-based) must be applied.

One specific problem is that the raw time series data are usually corrupted by artifact from spontaneous patient movement, nursing and medical interventions, etc. Perturbations in the signal do not always reflect changes to the underlying physiology and artifact needs to be removed.

Furthermore, the guidelines may also make reference to physical observations which are not available electronically (e.g. the colour of the patient, degree of spontaneous movement, muscle tone) or to recent actions (e.g. handling, suction, routine care, extubation). However many such aspects of patient state are not captured automatically on a routine basis. Ways need to be found of inferring this information from the data that *is* available electronically or, in extreme and infrequent cases, we must resort to asking the medical staff to input the information themselves.

Execution Engine

This is a program which will apply the formalized guideline to the data stream (or to its abstractions) to generate recommendations for action. We have used the Asbru Run Time Module (AsbruRTM) [8] which executes a clinical guideline written as an Asbru plans. It consists of three core modules: the *data abstraction* unit, the *environment monitoring* unit and the *execution* unit. AsbruRTM has access to the clinical guideline, an interface to the test data set, and a means of exporting the recommendations of the plan.

AsbruRTM is written in Java for platform independence. Asbru plans are written in XML [9] and we need a straightforward transformation of these XML representations to Java classes. We used Castor, an open source data binding framework for Java which generates a Java object model out of an XML Schema.

The *data abstraction* unit connects the incoming data to the *monitoring* unit. In our implementation its name is misleading – although the Asbru language provides a certain amount of computational power, and extensions have been proposed to enhance this [10], we believe that the algorithms required to construct abstractions are better implemented in a more conventional procedural language (in our case, Delphi).

Test Data

Even with good translation and visualization tools, it is unlikely that the completed computerized guideline will work exactly as anticipated and must be tested against sample data. It has been demonstrated that it is very difficult to get experts to make judgments about the correct course of action in a complex situation without a good understanding of the context in which the decision has to be made [11]. For this reason it is desirable that the test data set include as much of that context as possible – in particular which actions had been or were being taken by the staff at and before the time in question. Note that these data may go beyond what is acquired on a routine basis and special measures may need to be taken to acquire them.

Infrastructure

By this we mean the underlying computational and communications system which allows us to access the test data, to apply the abstractions, to deliver the abstractions to the execution engine, and to display both the test data and the recommendations of the guideline.

3 Test Protocol

Consider a neonate who is being artificially ventilated until her lungs are sufficiently mature for her to breathe on her own. Often the immaturity manifests itself in the condition known as respiratory distress syndrome (RDS). The aim of our protocol is to maintain suitable values of the oxygen and carbon dioxide in the blood as measured by a single transcutaneous probe ($PtcO_2$ in kPa and $PtcCO_2$ in kPa). A number of ventilator settings, under the control of the nurse, can be used to provide this regulation (including the peak and end expiratory pressures) but we will consider just two: the fraction of oxygen in the inspired air (FiO_2 as a %). and the respiration rate (*Resp_Rate* in *breaths per minute*). Basically we assume that the nurse uses FiO_2 to control the blood O_2 and *Resp_Rate* to control the blood CO_2.

If *Rec_FiO₂* is the fraction of inspired oxygen recommended by the protocol, then one of our collaborating clinicians provided the following simple rules which were translated by hand into Asbru XML:

IF $PtcO_2$ > O_2-*High* **THEN** $Rec\_FiO_2 = FiO_2 - 5$
IF O_2-*High*> $PtcO_2$ > O_2-*Low* **THEN** $Rec\_FiO_2 = FiO_2$
IF O_2-*Low* > $PtcO_2$ **THEN** $Rec\_FiO_2 = FiO_2 + 10$

In a similar manner if Tgt_PtcCO_2 is the level of CO_2 in the blood that we would like to achieve and *Rec_Resp_Rate* is the respiration rate recommended by the protocol we have:

IF $PtcCO_2 > CO_2\text{-}High$ **THEN** $Rec\_Resp\_Rate =$
$Resp\_Rate * (PtcCO_2 / Tgt\_PtcCO_2)$
WHERE $Tgt\_PtcCO_2 = PtcCO_2 - 2$
IF $CO_2\text{-}High > PtcCO_2 > CO_2\text{-}Low$ **THEN** $Rec\_Resp\_Rate = Resp\_Rate$
IF $CO_2\text{-}Low > PtcO_2$ **THEN** $Rec\_Resp\_Rate =$
$Resp\_Rate * (PtcCO_2 / Tgt\_PtcCO_2)$
WHERE $Tgt\_PtcCO_2 = PtcCO_2 + 5$

O_2-High, O_2-Low, CO_2-High and CO_2-Low are numerical thresholds.

Note that by referring the recommended settings to the actual settings we are basing our recommendations on the state of the world as it is (not as we might like it to be).

4 Data Abstraction

The protocol as presented so far is not explicit about the temporal resolution required. It does not make sense to make recommendations more often than once a minute (at most) – however the raw data is sampled every second.

The first abstraction required is therefore a temporal compression in which the median value of successive blocks of 60 samples is generated (i.e. the effective sampling rate is reduced to 1/minute).

Implicit in the guideline is that the data should be free of artifact – we do not want the guideline to recommend that the FiO_2 be raised simply because the transcutaneous sensor is being repositioned. The artifact detector used is the ArtiDetector devised by Cao [12]. For the $PtcO_2$ and $PtcCO_2$ channels this applies three 'detectors' that, taken together, flag samples as being artifactual or not. The *limit based* detector refers to prior knowledge about the historical distributions of values for the channel and flags up values outside extreme centiles (e.g. 2nd and 98th). The *deviation-based* detector looks at the standard deviation within a moving window and flags values which cause it to exceed a pre-defined limit. The *correlation-based* detector uses the knowledge that, when monitoring multiple data channels, artifacts in one channel can imply artifacts in another. Such artifactual correlation may help identify artifacts missed by less sensitive limit-based or deviation-based detectors. With the combined $PtcO_2/PtcCO_2$ probe, $PtcO_2$ artifacts are usually mirrored by $PtcCO_2$ artifacts and vice versa. If an artifact is detected in the $PtcO_2$ channel (either by its limit-based detector or deviation-based detector), the correlation-based detector is invoked to check if the corresponding $PtcCO_2$ value has a standard deviation greater than a lower threshold. If so, that corresponding value is flagged.

5 Test Data

The test data was collected as a special exercise in a neonatal intensive care unit over a period of about four months [13]. The commercial 'Badger' data collection system which was in operation on the unit, automatically acquired and stored physiological data with a time resolution of one second. The actual variables sampled depended on the monitoring in place but typically included heart rate, transcutaneous O_2 and CO_2, saturation O_2, core and peripheral temperatures, and blood pressures.

In addition a research nurse was employed to observe the activity at the cot and to make as accurate a record as possible; she also recorded other information. The complete data set consisted of:

- the physiological variables;
- the equipment used to monitor, ventilate, etc.;
- the actions taken by the medical staff;
- occasional descriptions of observable state (colour, movement, feeding, etc);
- the alarm limit settings on the monitors;
- the settings on the various items of equipment (including the ventilator);
- the results of blood gas analysis and other laboratory results;
- the drugs administered.

The observational data were entered with a timing accuracy of a few seconds on a laptop computer using a specially written program called 'BabyWatch'. All data (with one or two exceptions) were entered by selecting from pre-compiled lists. In addition the research nurse could enter short free-text comments.

We collected about 407 patient-hours of observations on 31 separate babies consisting of over 32,000 individual data records.

6 Test Infrastructure

The test infrastructure is provided by the Time Series Workbench (TSW) [14]. This provides an expandable range of facilities for viewing, interacting with and analyzing complex multi-channel time series data. Data within the TSW is organized in channels (e.g. heart rate, FiO_2 settings, etc). Channels consist either of a sequence of equi-sampled values (normally real numbers) or a list of timed intervals over which a proposition holds or a variable has a numerical value (e.g. a recommended ventilator setting). Data in channels is manipulated by filters which normally have one or more input channels and one or more output channels. Sources of data are represented by filters which have outputs but no inputs.

The abstractions in our example are performed by two filter types: a windowed median filter (with a window size of 60 samples which is advanced by 60 samples on each application) and a Cao artifact detector (ArtiDetector) which takes in median filtered *$PtcO_2$* and *$PtcCO_2$* and outputs the same channels with the artifacts removed.

More surprisingly perhaps, the TSW treats the AsbruRTM as a filter whose input channels are the outputs of the ArtiDetector and the ventilator settings and whose outputs are recommendations: *Rec_FiO_2* and *Rec_Resp_Rate*. This filter network is illustrated in Figure 1 where OX is short for *$PtcO_2$* and CO for *$PtcCO_2$*.

Given that TSW is written in Borland Delphi and AsbruRTM in Java, we need a communications mechanism; this is provided using CORBA.

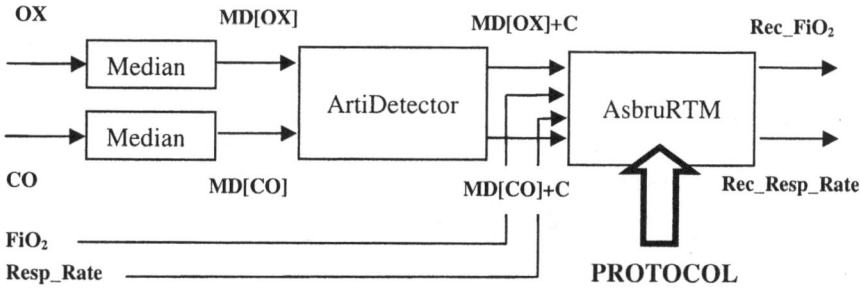

Fig. 1. Filter network

7 Test Results

Figure 2 shows the results of applying the test protocol to a sample of neonatal data. The top two graphs show PtcO$_2$ and PtcCO$_2$ respectively; the faint traces show the raw data and the bold traces the output of the ArtiDetector. The third and fourth graphs show FiO$_2$ and Resp_Rate; the solid traces show the actual values and the dotted traces the recommendations of the protocol. The shaded periods (OP) show the times that the observer (the research nurse) was present. The thresholds used for the protocol were:

O_2-High = 8, O_2-Low = 6, CO_2-High = 10 and CO_2-Low = 5

Of note are the following:

- The protocol recommends increases of the FiO$_2$ at about 09:05, 09:25; and 09:50; the actual FiO$_2$ was changed at the same time or slightly later.
- The protocol did not recommend the increase in FiO$_2$ at 10:15; this is particularly interesting. At this time PtcO$_2$ was already quite high and one wonders why the nurse increased the oxygen. The answer is probably to be found in the bottom trace where short black bars at around 09:34 and 10:20 show the times when the nurse applied suction to the baby in order to clear secretions from the ventilator tube. Suction normally causes distress and a lowering of the PtcO$_2$ levels, and it is routine practice to increase the oxygen before suction. Given that the protocol did not 'know' that suction was about to take place, it had no way of making that recommendation. This demonstrates the value of having collected the information about which actions were performed.
- The protocol tries to correct the increased PtcCO$_2$ values from 09:35 onwards by increasing the respiration rate; the medical staff take no action.

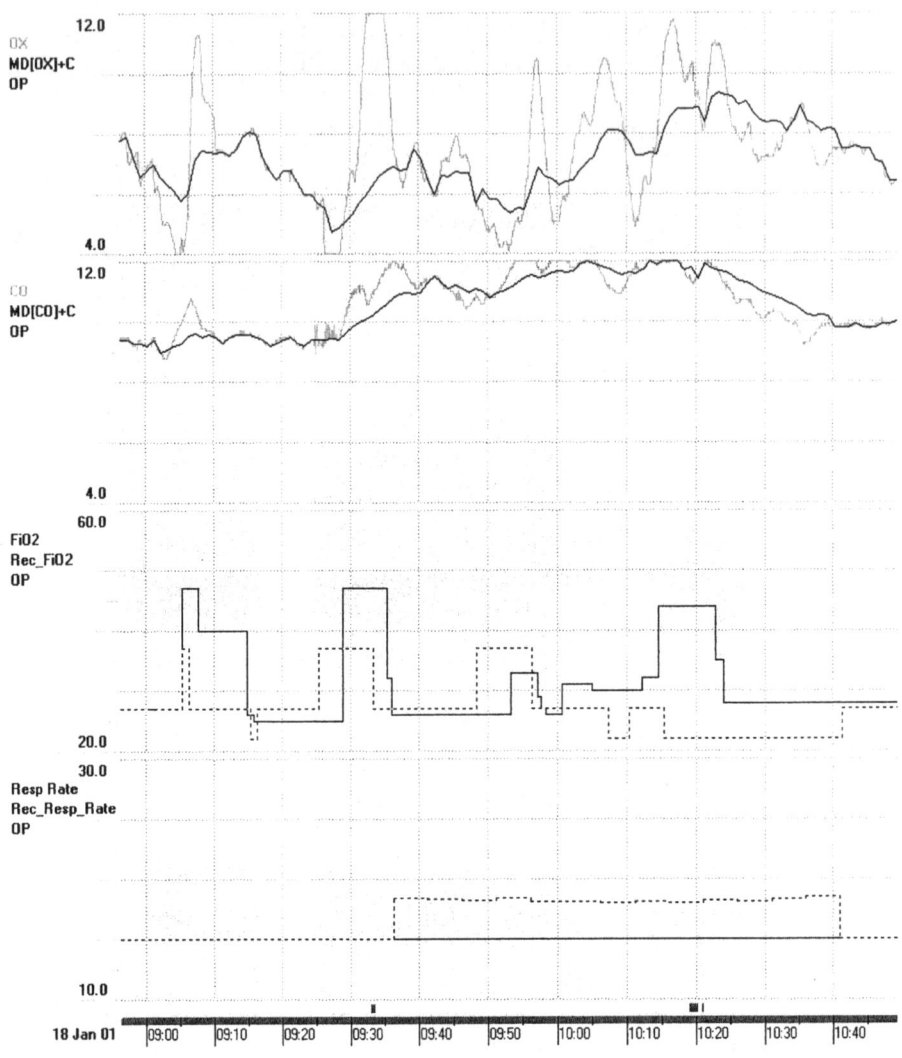

Fig. 2. Test results

8 Conclusions

Most of the individual elements discussed in this paper have been presented elsewhere. However bringing them all together in one coherent system allows us to provide the first realistic test of an Asbru guideline as applied to continuous high-volume data. Up until now, guidelines tend to have been implemented in 'encounter' situations, e.g. an out-patient clinic, where the clinician considers a body of evidence and has to make a decision (or decisions) at a single point in time. The encounter may be repeated, but some time will have elapsed. ICUs are different in a number of ways.

Large volumes of complex multi-channel data are acquired automatically and continuously over time with minimal clinician involvement. This means that we can have the realistic goal of the guideline being applied without any additional clinician input. However the data available to the computer is not as complete as that available to the clinician – the computer lacks the important sensory data that the clinician can see, feel, hear, etc. The challenge is whether we can do without these data, or reconstruct them from what is available. Furthermore, the data is very detailed and noisy; and not expressed in the terms that the guideline requires; a considerable amount of abstraction is required to bridge the gap between the two.

Clinical intervention takes place quasi-continuously, and the guideline needs to deliver advice on a time scale of seconds and minutes. Moreover, it is often possible to detect the actions of the user (e.g. the FiO_2 setting) on a continuous basis and to compare it with the advice proffered by the guideline; we must always remember that the clinical staff are free to ignore the advice. This raises interesting questions as to the appropriate mode for giving advice in such a context. For example, consider a situation where the guideline recommends that the FiO_2 be increased, and where the FiO_2 settings show that the advice has not been heeded. How often should the advice be repeated? One might assume that the frequency of repetition should depend on how far the $PtcO_2$ is below the lower limit. However if it is repeated too often it may come to be viewed as an irritation and ignored. If the staff involved consistently ignore the advice when the $PtcO_2$ is only marginally below the limit, should the guideline 'accept' that the staff have a different view of a marginal situation and adjust its future behaviour accordingly.

Implementing all of the components to generate, implement and test complex guidelines in data-rich environments (as set out in section 2) is probably beyond the resources of one centre. We believe that cooperation between groups is essential – for example sharing test data and agreeing on the best way to implement artifact detection and removal. The current distributed implementation of the TSW infrastructure via CORBA allows this to some extent, in that raw data, the various filters (including AsbruRTM) and the TSW client can all be located on different machines. If it were not for the limitations imposed by firewalls, this technology would be sufficient to allow collaboration over the internet. We are currently developing communications mechanisms based on web-services which will overcome these constraints and allow truly remote collaboration.

All of the above issues, together with the development of more complex guidelines, will be the subject of future research.

Acknowledgements

We gratefully acknowledge the help of our clinical collaborators: Dr Christian Popow, Prof Neil McIntosh and Dr Yvonne Freer. The NEONATE project was supported by the UK PACCIT Programme run jointly by ESRC and EPSRC. Christian Fuchsberger was supported in part by a grant from the Austrian Research Council (FWF), Science Research Center SFB F021.

References

1. McIntosh N, A J Lyon, P Badger, 'Time Trend Monitoring in the Neonatal Intensive Care Unit – Why Doesn't It Make a Difference?', *Pediatrics*, **98**, p 540 (1996).
2. Alberdi E, J-C Becher, KJ Gilhooly, JRW Hunter, RH Logie, A Lyon, N McIntosh and J Reiss, 'Expertise And The Interpretation Of Computerised Physiological Data: Implications for the Design of Computerised Physiological Monitoring in Neonatal Intensive Care', *International Journal of Human Computer Studies*, **55**(3), pp 191-216 (2001).
3. Peleg M, S Tu, J Bury, P Ciccarese, J Fox, R Greenes, R Hall, P Johnson, N Jones, A Kumar, S Miksch, S Quaglini, A Seyfang, E Shortliffe, and M Stefanelli, 'Comparing Computer-Interpretable Guideline Models: A Case-Study Approach', *The Journal of the American Medical Informatics Association (JAMIA)*, **10**(1), pp52–68 (2003).
4. Shahar S, S Miksch and P Johnson, 'The Asgaard Project: A Task-Specific Framework for the Application and Critiquing of Time-Oriented Clinical Guidelines', *Artificial Intelligence in Medicine*, **14**, pp29–51 (1998).
5. Royal College of Paediatrics and Child Health (UK), 'Management of Neonatal Respiratory Distress Syndrome', *http://www.rcpch.ac.uk/publications/clinical_docs/ GGPrespiratory.pdf* (2000).
6. Shahar Y, O Young, E Shalom, A Mayaffit, R Moskovitch, A Hessing and M Galperin, 'DEGEL: A Hybrid Multiple-Ontology Framework for Specification and Retrieval of Clinical Guidelines', *Proceedings of the 9th Conference on Artificial Intelligence in Medicine Europe*, pp 41-45 (2003).
7. Aigner W and S Miksch, Communicating the Logic of a Treatment Plan', *Proceedings of the Symposium on Computer-based Support for Clinical Guidelines and Protocols*, pp 1-16 (2004).
8. Fuchsberger C and S Miksch, 'Asbru's Execution Engine: Utilizing Guidelines for Artificial Ventilation of Newborn Infants', *Workshop on Intelligent Data Analysis in Medicine and Pharmacology and Knowledge-Based Information Management in Anaesthesia and Intensive Care, AIME-03*, pp 119-125 (2003)
9. Seyfang A, R Kosara and S Miksch, 'Asbru 7.3 Reference Manual', *Technical Report Asgaard- TR-2002-1*, Vienna University of Technology, Institute of Software Technology and Interactive Systems (2002).
10. Seyfang A and S Miksch, 'Advanced Temporal Data Abstraction for Guideline Execution', *Proceedings of the Symposium on Computer-based Support for Clinical Guidelines and Protocols*, pp 88-102 (2004).
11. Hunter J, G Ewing, Y Freer, R Logie, P McCue and N McIntosh, 'NEONATE: Decision Support in the Neonatal Intensive Care Unit – A Preliminary Report', *Proceedings of the 9th Conference on Artificial Intelligence in Medicine Europe, AIME-03*, pp 41-45 (2003).
12. Cao CG, IS Kohane, N McIntosh and K Wang, 'Artifact Detection in the PO_2 and PCO_2 Time Series Monitoring Data from Preterm Infants', *Journal of Clinical Monitoring and Computing*, **15**, pp 369-378 (1999).
13. Hunter J, G Ewing, L Ferguson, Y Freer, R Logie, P McCue and N McIntosh. 'The NEONATE Database', *Workshop on Intelligent Data Analysis in Medicine and Pharmacology and Knowledge-Based Information Management in Anaesthesia and Intensive Care, AIME-03*, pp 21-24 (2003).
14. Hunter J, 'Time Series Workbench', *http://www.csd.abdn.ac.uk/~jhunter/research/TSW/* (2003)

EORCA: A Collaborative Activities Representation for Building Guidelines from Field Observations

Liliane Pellegrin[1], Nathalie Bonnardel[2], François Antonini[3], Jacques Albanèse[3], Claude Martin[3], and Hervé Chaudet[1,4]

[1] Equipe "Biomathématiques et Informatique Médicale"
Laboratoire d'Informatique Fondamentale UMR CNRS 6166
Faculté de Médecine, Université de la Méditerranée
27, bd. Jean Moulin 13385 Marseille Cedex 05, France
liliane.pellegrin@medecine.univ-mrs.fr
[2] Centre de Recherche en Psychologie de la Connaissance, du Langage et de l'Emotion,
Département de Psychologie Cognitive et Expériementale, Université de Provence
29, av Robert Schuman, Aix en Provence, Cedex 01, France
nathb@up.univ-mrs.fr
[3] Département d'Anesthésie-Réanimation Hôpital Nord
28, Chemin des Bourelly, 13915 Marseille Cedex 15, France
François.Antonini@ap-hm.fr
[4] Service d'Information Médicale Hôpital Nord
(Assistance Publique des Hôpitaux à Marseille)
28, Chemin des Bourelly, 13915 Marseille Cedex 15, France
lhcp@acm.org

Abstract. In the objective of building care team guidelines from field observations, this paper introduces a representation method for describing the medical collaborative activities during an ICU patient management. An event-centered representation of medical activities is built during a 3-step procedure, successively involving an event-centered observation phase, an action extraction and coding phase, and an event and collaborative representation phase. This method has been used for analyzing the management of 24 cases of neurological and multiple traumas. We have represented the different actions of the medical team members (clinicians, nurses and outside medical consultants), underlining collaborative information management and the strong interaction between information management and medical actions. This method also highlights the difficulty of cases management linked to diagnosis severity, complexity of the situation and time constraints.

Keywords: cognitive modeling, protocols and guidelines, knowledge engineering, collaborative human problem solving, Intensive Care.

1 Introduction

The current use of clinical guidelines and protocols is actually not fully integrated in usual medical activities, though both health organization and physicians widely recognized their usefulness to improve quality of clinical practices. Some proposed solutions to this unwillingness to use clinical guidelines and protocols were firstly, to implement computer-based guidelines to facilitate decision-support [1], secondly, to improve and verify the quality of clinical guidelines programs (as the program AGREE for "Appraisal of Guidelines Research and Evaluation" [2]) and thirdly to explore the existing links between the protocols, the variability of physicians' decision-making and behaviours [3]. In this context, a description of elements of patient medical management observed in real situations that is based upon a formal task analysis should contribute to fill the actual gap between formal medical guidelines and realistic medical activities.

In the project introduced here, our aim was to build a formal method of observation and Event Oriented Representation of Collaborative Activities (EORCA), to describe activities of team members during patient's management in an Intensive Care Unit. The event-centered characteristic of the representation was suggested by the fact that events are the observable parts of medical activities. The most important constraints imposed to this method was to be enough robust and reproducible to allow further qualitative and quantitative analyses of the situations, especially from the objective of improving the quality of patients' care and the reliability of medical decisions associated with the decisions algorithms or guidelines applied in this medical fields [4, 5]. Our method aims at contributing to build and validate protocols in the practice of such specialties in which medical decisions not only result from an isolated physician but also from a group of expert physicians in complex and time-constrained situation [6]. In the future, this method would also allow identifying clinical adverse events, such as potential incidents, dysfunctions and near miss events during patient managements [7].

The goal of this article is to introduce the EORCA main features, its building and the field studies that have been conducted to acquire observation data on the medical cases resolution during 2 years of patients' management observations. This paper is organized as follows. First, we introduce the method we used for analyzing medical team's activities, from observation methodology to the domain ontology that specifies and structures observables, actors and actions. Secondly we present the context of the studies in an ICU service in Marseille (France). In the Results section, we described the application of EORCA model on a set of real data to evaluate its quality as a representation of observed events.

2 EORCA's Approach

Two main rationales have guided the development of EORCA.

Rationale 1: A Standardized Method of Task Observation and Analysis Usable by ICU Team Members

Identifying and formalizing ICU practitioners' actions and decisions during health care from team behavior observation may appear as particularly complex. Human factor approaches can give a complementary view of this problem [8], since some cognitive psychology and ergonomics studies focused on cognitive process involved in anesthesiology, emergency and intensive care tasks [9, 11] and, more recently, on the collective aspects of patient managements [11]. Intensive Care especially requires a coordinating work with a strong collaboration between various specialists such as radiologist, neurologist and nurses. This work situation is also seen as heterogeneous since each actor focused upon a single patient with different activities, motivations and concerns [12]. Our first choice was to base the method upon task observation and representation procedures that would take in account the collaborative dimension of health care as well as the human factors of decision-making in dynamic, complex and critical safety conditions [13]. Stress due to time pressure, specific situation awareness and mental workload, planning and cooperation processes in experts' teams are indeed influent and systematic element of medical decision making that must be considered. Our goal was to develop an accurate and usable task analysis-based tool for observing and representing medical tasks and activities that could be used recurrently by unit staff (doctors or nurses). In addition, the results should be enough stable to allow further qualitative and quantitative analyses of the situations. This method should also allow identifying clinical adverse events, such as potential incidents, dysfunctions and near miss events during patient managements. The resulting descriptive task model would then be the basis for developing the prescriptive task model.

Rationale 2: An Event-Centered Representation of Actions Identified from Observations

Observation methods for studying human actions are, in a general manner, restricted to the level of operations, which are the observable part of a whole, including the operators' underlying cognitive activities. This implies that events involving actors

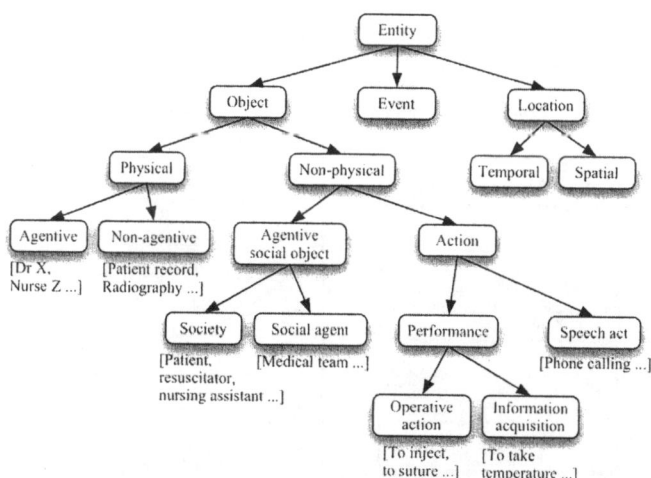

Fig. 1. Top-level categories of the domain-dependant ontology with some examples

are the observable parts of medical activities, hence our choice of an event-centered representation. An event corresponds to the performance or occurrence of an action. If actions are time independent, defining activities that may be conducted by agents for changing world state, events are time and space dependent and may be temporally and spatially connected (i.e. sequential, simultaneous…).A domain-oriented ontology formalizes and organizes every concept involved in observations (Figure 1). This ontology aims at standardizing observation representations. In association with this ontology, an event-oriented language in first order logic (STEEL)[14] derived from Event Calculus, coupled with a graphical representation, allows the formal representation of medical team members' activities.

3 The Method

In accordance with previous rationales, EORCA is based on a three-manual-steps method that allows building the representation of activities from field observations, from patient's admission to his/her transfer or delegation. Figure 2 summarizes the method.

- *Step 1*: This step aims at collecting sequences of events by direct observation, and is ruled by some definite and mandatory instructions that enforce standardization of observation and recording. An "observed event" includes an action with an agentive social object. The action may be a deed or a verbal communication occurring between caregivers as explicit decision-making, requests or questions. Events are recorded in chronological order with non-systematic timestamps. Semi-directive post-task interviews with physicians about the observed cases complete observations. The result of this step is an accurate, constrained and event-oriented written description in natural language of patient's care scenario.

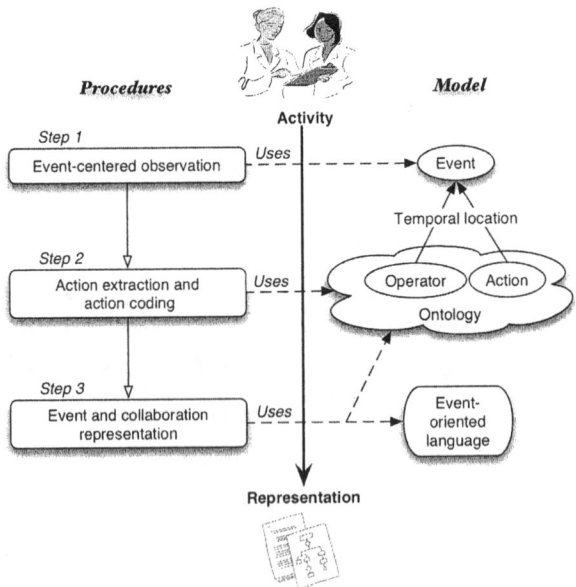

Fig. 2. Overall description of the EORCA's steps, showing correspondences between methods

- *Step 2:* This step analyses the scenario for extracting events' components and sequencing. Actions and agents are identified and coded according to the ontology. The taxonomy of actions included in the ontology is based both upon a yet-existing national codification of medical acts and an analysis of data coming from a first tentative observation campaign. If needed, the lower ontology classes may be completed from observation during this step. The result is a scenario transcription where each event component (i.e. action, agent, time, location) is identified and coded.
- *Step 3*: This last phase consists in rewriting the coded scenario with the event-oriented first-order logic language. Each element of the representation is an event occurrence component, identified during the previous step. A graphical representation of the scenario is directly derived. It allows representing in a single template the main elements of patient's management by medical team members. The result of this step is an event-oriented model of the scenario that may be processed for further analysis

4 Experiment Context

Two studies were successively conducted in the ICU of a public hospital in Marseilles in 2001 and 2003, both of them during 4-5 months. The data we gathered dealt with the management of 24 cases of neurological and multiple traumas occurring during these periods. The data collection was carried out by two ergonomists, for the first study, and by one ergonomist for the second study. Concerning the patient pathologies, multiple traumas and neurological injuries are particularly representative of the kinds of medical problems that are encountered in the ICU, and especially represent the safety-critical characteristics of these problems. Moreover, in this studied unit, these cases constitute a homogeneous and important set of patients. Such pathologies were chosen for two main reasons. The first one is that this department is specialized in neurological traumatisms. Secondly, multiple traumatisms and neurological injuries are particularly representative of the kinds of medical problems that are encountered in the ICU, and especially represent the safety-critical dimension of these problems. The main features of these 24 cases are the various patients' ages (from 19 to 91 years old), and the kind of injuries mainly caused by road accidents.

The data acquisition was manual, directly performed by the observers without videotaped recording [15], computer-based methods using hand-held devices (the FIT technique in the Manser and Whener study [16]) or specific data acquisition tool (such as BabyWatch [17]). Two main reasons are adduced for this restrictive choice. First, the medical team did not accept videotaped recording for legal reasons (the patient cannot give his agreement during the admission). Secondly, we wanted to use the less sophisticated methods of information acquisition and, in the same time, the most opened possible without predefined observable categories. We applied these ecological methods to observe a larger scale of different actions during the patient management by the team members.

5 Results

Assessing the EORCA method implies analyzing its ability to accurately represent the observed events. Based on the data in the final representation, the goal was to identify elements of collaborative information management between the medical team members (clinicians, nurses and outside medical consultants) and interaction between information management and undertaken actions. For this purpose, two kind of analysis have been performed, a quantitative analysis of the observations into classes and sub-classes of actions and a more qualitative analysis of the final graphical representation.

Results About Classes of Observed Actions

Three main classes of observed events were taken in account for analysing the 24 observed patients management:

- *Class of "Speech acts" between the actors*. We define as a speech (verbal or written) act, each information transmission between actors that have been observed and transcribed in the observation sheet. Several sub-classes were identified as for example, the requests for actions from one actor to another one, the explicit decisions for actions upon patient.
- *Class of "operative actions"* gathers actions performed by team members, which were recorded during the patient management as therapeutic deeds linked to major classes of medical acts. Non-strictly medical actions were also identified, essentially collective actions as mutual help, action attempts and actions of time management.
- *Class of "information acquisitions"* includes all actions implying an information acquisition performance as clinical and monitoring examinations, radiology consultations, monitoring and others situation parameters, such as control, observation and verification.

Concerning the repartition of the observations into these 3 main classes, we have hypothesized that information transmissions plays an important role to guide actions, to adjust behaviors when facing to difficulties, to make anticipations and previsions. In the data we gathered, a total amount of 1439 observed actions was obtained (see table 1). Among them, speech acts are the most frequent observations (49.48% of the totality of the identified events). The differences between the study modalities should be not aleatory (Pearson's Chi-squared test, X-squared = 7.9573, df = 2, p-value = 0.01871).

Table 1. Distribution of the recorded observations by year set of management cases and by main categories of action. Percentages are putted into brackets

Cat. of Actions/ Years	Cases 2001	Cases 2003	Total/ Cat.
Speech acts	296 (53.1%)	416 (47.2%)	712 (49.5%)
Operative actions	164 (29.4%)	323 (36.6%)	487 (33.8%)
Information acquisitions	97 (17.4%)	143 (16.2%)	240 (16.7%)
Total/Year	557 (38.7%)	882 (61.3%)	1439

The management of patients by this ICU team should be actually characterized by a majority of information transmissions between the actors of the situation and by care-related actions (operative actions). Events belonging to information acquisitions, essentially clinical examinations and radiological diagnosis are the less observed in these situations. Such activities concern essentially physicians and represent only one part of the overall actions undertaken by all team members, for example the nursing acts. An "Observers/Situations" effect is also observed in the difference between the number of recorded observations in 2001 and 2003. Such results strengthen our positions to build a more efficient observation tool, which would reduce such kind of effect to allow longitudinal studies of patient managements. The analysis of detailed events in the speech acts have highlighted that various kinds of oral communication have been identified as information transmissions per se (transmission of medical information, management of problems and difficulties, phone calling, actions planning), requests for actions or information, explicit decisions expressed to other team members, common discussions between partners.

Application of the Formal Description to a Patient Management Case
Each case has been represented in a final graphical chart using ontology objects. Each chart illustrates explicitly the sequence of different kinds of events and the elements of distributed support for decisions during case resolution. Such distributed decision-making is encountered especially during comments upon radiological results, generally done between resuscitators and radiologists or others specialists. As example, we introduce an observed patient management. This case concerned a patient, age 48, with multiple injuries and neurological traumatisms (with a Glasgow Coma score ≤ 8) transferred to the unit by the fire brigade after a work accident. FA total amount of 12 persons participated to the patient management for total duration of 26 min:

- members of the ICU team (one attending physician, one resident, one anesthetist nurse, two nurses, one medical student were present in the unit)
- external medical consultants (a fire brigade physician, a radiologist, an orthopedist, two anesthetists and a vascular surgeon were required and present at the patient's bedside).

Figure 3 is an excerpt from this example, 10-13 minutes after the beginning, where 9 persons are successively or in parallel participating to this patient management. As quantitative indicators, we have obtained an event density ratio of 1.42 observation/min (37 observations during 26 min of management). 22 speech acts, 8 operative actions and 7 information acquisitions were recorded. It was also possible to provide others indicators extracted from this final event representation such as the amount of 3 overlapping actions, 19 transmission origins (squares), 50 transmission receptions and undertaken actions (ovals) and 8 arrivals or departures. Such kinds of information may be interpreted as an expression of the case management complexity and of global team workload.

Thanks to this representation, it would be possible to describe some features of the caregivers' activity in a situation characterizes as a cognitive cooperation between actors [18]. This activity concerns both a set of individual performances conducted by

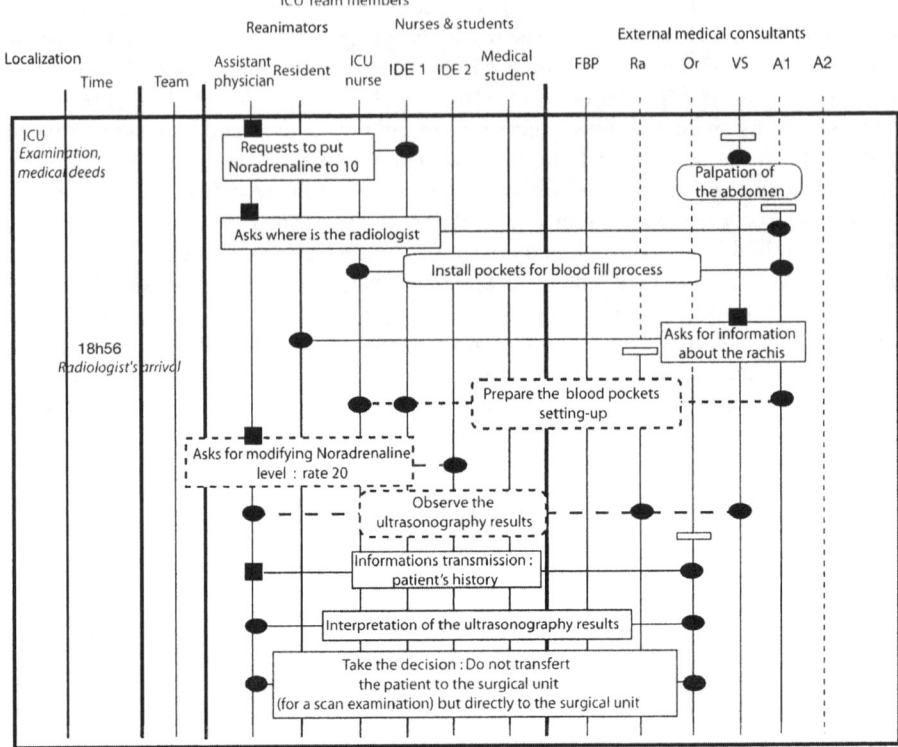

Fig. 3. Excerpt of a patient management by the ICU team. The abbreviations are following: FBP (fire brigade physician), Ra (radiologist), Or (orthopedist surgeon), VS (vascular surgeon), A1 (Anesthesist 1), A2 (Anesthesist 2)

several specialists and a management of all the required tasks by the actors belonging to the team (cooperation in action). The case of cooperative activity observed here could be described as a supervised cooperation implying planning and allocation of the future tasks and actions between staff members (cooperation in planning).

6 Conclusion

EORCA is a method using a representational model associated to a set of procedures for building an event-oriented representation of complex medical situations involving several caregivers. It has been applied upon observations of neurological and multiple traumas managements by an ICU team. The results show that this method is able to report the temporal organization of care management and especially the dynamics of communication and collaboration between actors. All these elements are gathered in a descriptive model of the situation that highlights the difficulties of case management linked to diagnosis severity, the complexity of the situation, and time constraints. It is then adapted to time-constraint and situations at risk where a high level of cooperation and planning is required. In this perspective, we have adopted a task-oriented approach clarifying sequences of actions, goals and decisions during real patients' management. This method should make easier the transcription of a descriptive model of the situation to a prescriptive one in terms of designing or re-designing protocols to adjust them to relevant features of the described situations [19]. But at least two issues remain. The first one is the reproducibility of the method. The set of procedures and the ontology aim at giving this method its reproducibility, but this characteristic remains to be demonstrated. The second is to find the adequate level of abstraction, as for example actions sequences and scenarios, to describe such situations and their specificities with granularity appropriate for guideline writing [20].

Acknowledgements

This project was granted by a national research program Hospital Clinical Research Program (PHRC-2000) from French Heath Department for the years 2000-2003. We whish to thanks Pr. Claude Bastien from the Department of Cognitive and Experimental Psychology (University of Provence) and the students in Cognitive Ergonomics V. Murillo, C. Dobigny, C. Boureau, N. Devictor and also all members of the ICU team of the DAR-Nord for their precious participation in this project.

References

1. De Clerq PA., Blom J., Korsten H., Hasman A: Approaches for creating computer-interpretable guidelines that facilitate decision-support. Artificial Intelligence in Medicine **31** (2004) 1-27.
2. AGREE collaboration: "Appraisal of Guidelines Research and Evaluation" (AGREE) obtained in http://www.agreecollaboration.org/intro/
3. Wang D., Peleg M., Tu SW., Boxwala A., Greenes R., Patel VL., Shortliffe E.: Representation Primitives, Process Models and Patient Data in Computer-Interpretable Clinical Practice Guidelines: A Literature Review of Guideline Representation Models. International Journal of Medical Informatics **68** (2002) 59-70.
4. Bullock, R. & Joint Section on Trauma and Critical Care of the American Association of Neurological Surgeons and the Brain Trauma Foundation. Guidelines for the Management of Severe Head Injury. American Association of Neurological Surgeons, Park Ridge Ill (2000).
5. Albanese J., Arnaud S. Traumatisme crânien chez le polytraumatisé. In Sfar, eds. Conférences d'actualisation. 41ème congrès d'anesthésie et de réanimation. Paris (1999) 737-63.
6. Xiao Y., Milgram P., Doyle DJ. Planning Behavior and Its Functional Role in the Interaction with Complex Systems. IEEE Trans. on Syst., Man, and Cybern., Part A: Systems and Humans **27** (1997) 313-24.
7. Busse, DK., Johnson, CW. Identification and Analysis of Incidents in Complex, Medical Environments. In Johnson CW, eds. First Workshop on Human Error and Clinical Systems, Glasgow (1999) 101-20.
8. Patel VL., Kaufman DR., Arocha JF. Emerging paradigms of cognition in medical decision-making. Journal of Biomedical Informatics. **35** (2002) 52–75.
9. Gaba DM., Howard SK. Situation awareness in Anesthesiology. Human Factors **37** (1995) 20-31.

10. Bricon-Souf N., Renard JM., Beuscart R. Dynamic Workflow Model for complex activity in intensive care unit, International Journal of Medical Informatics. **53** (1999) 143-50.
11. Cicourel AV. The Integration of Distributed Knowledge in Collaborative Medical Diagnosis. In Galegher J., Kraut RE., Egido C., Eds. Intellectual Teamwork. Lawrence Erlbaum Associates, Hillsdale NJ, USA (1990) 221-42.
12. Reddy MC., Dourish P., Pratt W. Coordinating Heterogeneous Work Information and Representation in Medical Care. Prinz W., Jarke M., Rogers Y., Schmidt K., Wulf V., Eds. Proceedings of 7th the European Conference on Computer Supported Cooperative Work-ECSCW'01. Bonn, Germany (2001) 239-258.
13. Blandford A, Wong W. Situation awareness in emergency medical dispatch, Int. J. Human-Computer Studies **61** (2004): 421–52.
14. Chaudet. H. STEEL: A spatio-temporal extended event language for tracking epidemic spread from outbreak reports. In Udo Hahn, ed, Proceedings of KR-MED 2004, First International Workshop on Formal Biomedical Knowledge Representation. Whistler, BC, Canada, (2004), 21-30. Obtained in http:// sunsite.informatik.rwth-aachen.de/Publications/CEUR-WS//Vol-102/chaudet.pdf
15. Xiao Y., Seagull FJ., Mackenzie CF., Klein K. Adaptive leadership in trauma resuscitation teams: a grounded theory approach to video analysis. Cognition, Technology & Work **6** (2004) 158-164.
16. Manser T., Wehner T. Analysing action sequences: Variations in Action Density in the Administration of Anaesthesia. Cognition Technology & Work **4** (2002) 71-81.
17. Ewing G., Ferguson L., Freer Y., Hunter J., McIntosh N. Observational Data Acquired on a Neonatal Intensive Care Unit, University of Aberdeen Computing Science Departmental Technical Report TR 0205 (2002).
18. Hoc JM., Carlier X. Role of common frame of reference in cognitive cooperation: sharing tasks between agents in air traffic control. Cognition, Technology & Work **4** (2002) 37-47.
19. Van Oosterhout EMW., Talmona, J.L. de Clercq P .A. Schouten H.C., Tangea H.J., Hasmana A. Three-Layer Model for the design of a Protocol Support System, International Journal of Medical Informatics **74** (2005) 101—110.
20. Dojat M., Ramaux N., Fontaine D. Scenario recognition for temporal reasoning in medical domains. Artificial Intelligence in Medicine **14** (1998) 139-155.

Design Patterns for Modelling Guidelines[*]

Radu Serban[1], Annette ten Teije[1], Mar Marcos[2], Cristina Polo-Conde[2],
Kitty Rosenbrand[3], Jolanda Wittenberg[3], and Joyce van Croonenborg[3]

[1] Vrije Universiteit Amsterdam, Netherlands
{serbanr, annette}@cs.vu.nl
[2] Universitat Jaume I, Spain
Cristina.Polo@sg.uji.es, Mar.Marcos@icc.uji.es
[3] Dutch Institute for Healthcare improvement CBO, The Netherlands
{k.rosenbrand, j.wittenberg, j.vancroonenborg}@cbo.nl

Abstract. It is by now widely accepted that medical guidelines can help to significantly improve the quality of medical care. Unfortunately, constructing the required medical guidelines is a very labour intensive and costly process. The cost of guideline construction would decrease if guidelines could be built from a set of building blocks that can be reused across guidelines. Such reusable building blocks would also result in more standardised guidelines, facilitating their deployment. The goal of this paper is to identify a collection of patterns that can be used as guideline building blocks. We propose two different methods for finding such patterns We compare the collections of patterns obtained through these two methods, and experimentally validate some of the patterns by checking their usability in the actual modelling of a medical guideline for breastcancer treatment.

1 Introduction

In the last decades a lot of effort has been given to guideline development, since medical guidelines can help to significantly improve the quality of medical care. Currently, the National Guideline Clearinghouse (NGC) contains over 1400 guideline summaries. Recently (2002) the Guidelines International Network (G-I-N) was founded, which seeks to improve the quality of health care by promoting systematic development of clinical practice guidelines and their application into practice. Because modelling guidelines is labour intensive, there is a need for reusable components (patterns), which enables a more systematic development of guidelines.

In this short paper, we describe work in progress. In section 2, we propose two different methods for identifying patterns, that can be used as guideline building blocks, a selection of the patterns that we have obtained by these methods, and some observations about the methods and obtained patterns. In section 3, we

---

[*] This work has been supported by the European Commission's IST program, under contract number IST-FP6-508794 Protocure-II.

report on an experiment of modelling and the use of the identified patterns, and finally, section 4 concludes. The main contribution of this paper is the set of patterns including their categorisation.

2 Methods and Results

In this section we present our results concerning the identification of patterns for constructing guideline models. We present a selection of the identified patterns and present some observations concerning our methods and the identified patterns. First we give a proposal for a categorisation of the obtained patterns.

2.1 Categorisation of Patterns

Following the methods to be discussed in later sections, we found a large number of reusable patterns. Therefore it is necessary to categorise them in such a way that modellers can use them during the modelling activity of a guideline.

We use the following categorisation of patterns. We consider *action patterns*, and patterns concerning with *action ordering*. The action patterns are the primitive building blocks, whereas the action ordering are the complex building blocks, since they can be built up from more simple action patterns. The action patterns are subdivided into action associated with context, action associated with time, action associated with conditions, and action associated with a goal. The action ordering patterns describe different orderings between sets of actions. These patterns are divided into sequence of actions, cyclic (repetitive actions), unspecific-order set (no explicit order is given), trials (try an action and, if it does not succeed, try something else), or selection of actions (concerned with the choice of an action). Most of the patterns found using our two methods fit in this categorisation, as depicted in figure 1.

2.2 Model-Driven Approach

In this approach the patterns have been extracted by knowledge engineers from pre-existing Asbru [1] representations of guidelines, hence the name *(Asbru)*

Categroy of pattern	model-driven	guideline-driven
action/plan	-	1
action associated with conditions	3	9
action associated with goals	2	2
action ordering	-	3
cyclic	2	2
sequence of actions	4	2
unspecific-order set	1	1
trials	2	-
selection of actions	2	3
others	4	9
total	20	32

Fig. 1. Categorisation of patterns obtained with model- and guideline-driven approach

model-driven. The patterns has been identified from the Asbru models of jaundice [2] and diabetes [3] guidelines. Consequently, the patterns are concerned with plans, and have often a high degree of complexity.

The following description serves to illustrate the kind of patterns obtained in this way.

Example of pattern: "Sequence of trials, at least the first action must succeed". Try several actions, in the indicated order and possibly with time delays between some of them; at least the first action must succeed. This pattern can be used whenever a precise sequence of steps must be tried in order to achieve certain target value for a particular parameter.

The Asbru solution makes use of a set of plans (one for each step) grouped into a plan of type `sequentially`, enforcing the described order. Concerning the waiting strategy, the (required) first step is the only one to be included in the `wait-for` option. To prevent the high-level plan to complete after the completion of the first step, the option `wait-for-optional-subplans` must be set to yes.

We have identified 20 patterns with potentials for reuse from the Diabetes and Jaundice Asbru models we analysed. Although these patterns are represented in Asbru, they can be described in general terms and hence they can be exploited independently of this particular target language.

Concerning the nature of the patterns, we can distinguish different types of patterns (see fig. 1). Another important observation is that the patterns obtained from existing Asbru models can be rather complex, because of the design efforts of the modeller. These structures are often not explicit in the original guideline texts.

2.3 Guideline-Driven Approach

In the guideline-driven method we have studied the original text of several guidelines [4, 5, 7] and identified patterns in the guideline text. We looked for general reusable segments of the guideline. After identifying these patterns, we tried to translate them into Asbru patterns The following example is intended as illustration of the kind of patterns obtained with this approach.

Example pattern: "association action-goal" has the following instances:

- Adjuvant hormone therapy for locally advanced breast cancer results in improved survival in the long-term.
- In many patients, radiotherapy achieves good palliation

We found 70 patterns, of which 32 patterns have a counterpart in Asbru, and 38 refer to more general medical aspects that cannot be expressed in Asbru. These patterns are outside the scope of Asbru. For instance, patterns concerning exclusions (ie. "action x should not be part of action y") , rate of success for actions, or support of a hypothesis.

CATEGORY	PATTERN
action/plan	Simple action execution
ass. with conditions	Action along with periodic tests and/or controls
	termination of plan/action
	Monitoring of critical conditions
ass. with goals	Search for treatment, with management of treatment problems
	Management of treatment problems
actions ordering	Ordered action group execution
	Composition of actions
	Actions in parrallel
cyclic	Periodic adjustment of treatment increase of doses of a drug
	Repetitive action with goal specification
sequence	Sequential action composition
	Sequence of actions, none/all of them must succeed necessarily
	Sequence of actions, only applicable ones, any/specific action must succeed
unspecific-order	(Unspecified order) execution of a group of actions
	Unspecified-order set of actions, all of them must succeed
trials	Sequence of two trials
	Series of trials, possibly more than once, a particular action must succeed
	Sequence of trials, at least the first action must succeed
selection	Choice of an action among a list by the user
	Random choice of element from group
	Exclusive alternative branching actions

Fig. 2. Selection of design patterns using the model- and guideline-driven approaches

2.4 Analysis of Approaches

Figure 2 shows a selection of the identified patterns [1]. Although each category contains patterns obtained from both approaches, which may suggest that the patterns they uncover are not very different, there exist differences.

As a general rule, guideline-driven patterns are less specific than model-driven ones, compare, for instance, "action associated with goals" versus "management of treatment problems". As for the level of granularity of the patterns, it differs in general. The guideline-driven patterns cover more generic types of relations, but have a smaller granularity than the relations expressed by the model-driven patterns.

The guideline-driven approach can only expose knowledge which is localized at sentence or paragraph level, while the model-driven approach can capture operational knowledge which is not explicit in the original texts. As result, the patterns obtained through the first approach correspond to complete Asbru fragments and contain medical abstractions, whereas the patterns found with the second one may refer to features broader than Asbru. This makes both approaches complementary to each other.

---

[1] see [6] for the complete collection of patterns.

3 Evaluation of Patterns

The evaluation we have performed, which is limited to the evaluation of the patterns obtained via the model-driven approach, has consisted in modelling in Asbru a part of the CBO[2] breast cancer guideline [7], and subsequently studying the degree of reusability of the different patterns.

The number of plans that we have studied amounts to 52. Only two patterns have been reused in those plans Although the reuse percentage is significant –actual reuse in 12 out of the 38 plans, i.e. 31% of cases– neither the variety nor the complexity of the applied patterns is high. One reason to explain the small number of used patterns might be their specificity with respect to Jaundice and/or Diabetes guidelines. The low complexity of used patterns, could be explained by the fact that the modelling has been restricted to chapters dealing with specific parts of the treatment, which makes the reusability of e.g. high-level coordination patterns less likely. Regardless of the above, the reuse of these patterns for 30% of the plans facilitates the modelling task to a great extent.

4 Conclusions

The main conclusion of this ongoing research is that we were able to identify a large number of patterns, that can be used as guideline building blocks. We have used two different methods for finding such patterns: either by observing regularities in the original text of the guidelines (guideline driven), or analyzing regularities in pre-existing formal guideline models (model-driven). In total we identified 52 design patterns for which we found a counter part in a guideline representation language Asbru. Finally, the lesson from the (limited) evaluation we have performed is that the reuse of patterns can facilitate the modelling task, although in practice only few patterns were reused intensively.

References

1. Y. Shahar, S. Miksch, and P. Johnson. The Asgaard Project: a Task-specific Framework for the Application and Critiquing of Time-oriented Clinical Guidelines. *Artificial Intelligence in Medicine*, 14:29–51, 1998.
2. Protocure I Project IST 2001-33049. Asbru Protocol for the Management of Hyperbilirubinemia in the Healthy Term Newborn, Aug. 2002. www.protocure.org.
3. Protocure I Project IST 2001-33049. Asbru Protocol for the Management of Diabetes Mellitus Type 2, Aug. 2002. www.protocure.org.
4. Scottish Intercollegiate Guidelines Network (SIGN). *Breast Cancer in Women, A National Clinical Guideline, nr. 29.* 1998.
5. Royal College of Radiologists. *Guidelines on the Non-surgical Management of Lung Cancer.* Springer-Verlag, 2001.
6. Deliverable D25: Library of Design Patterns for Guidelines, IST -FP6-508794, 2004. http://www.protocure.org/.
7. Nationaal Borstkanker Overleg Nederland (NABON) Guideline for the Treatment of Breast Carcinoma 2002

---

[2] Dutch Institute for Healthcare Improvement, see http://www.cbo.nl.

Improving Clinical Guideline Implementation Through Prototypical Design Patterns

Monika Moser and Silvia Miksch

Vienna University of Technology, Institute of Software Technology, and
Interactive Systems Favoritenstraße 9-11/E188, A-1040 Vienna, Austria
{moser, silvia}@asgaard.tuwien.ac.at
www.asgaard.tuwien.ac.at

Abstract. Currently, various guideline representation languages are available. However, these languages are too complex and algorithmic to be used by medical staff or guideline developers. Therefore, a big gap is between the information represented in published guidelines by guideline developers and the formal representation of clinical guideline used in an execution model. We try to close this gap by analyzing existing clinical guidelines written in free text, tables, or flow chart notation with the target of detecting prototypical patterns in those guidelines.

1 Introduction

In the last years, clinical guidelines and protocols were introduced in various medical environments. Field and Lohr [1] defined guidelines as "systematically developed statements to assist practitioner and patient decisions about appropriate health care for specific clinical circumstances", and guidelines "are validated policy statements representing best clinical practice, used to support standardized patient care".

The overall objectives of clinical guidelines and protocols convinced various research groups to investigate in the design, the development, and the implementation of such guidelines and protocols. On the one hand, there are the guideline developers who are designing and maintaining guidelines, which are then usually available in free text, tables, or flow chart notation. On the other hand, there are the knowledge engineers and system developers, which aim to represent various guidelines in computer processible format and illustrate that a running system could ease the daily routine of practitioners. Currently, there is a big gap between the guideline developers and the knowledge engineers and system developers – therefore the translation from a guideline in free text to a formal representation (which is used by a guideline execution unit) is a very hard task. This paper illustrates prototypical clinical patterns, which may be used in the authoring of clinical guidelines. Most of these methods are developed within the Asgaard project [2].

2 The Problem

A knowledge engineer usually does not start to develop a guideline from scratch, but uses written guidelines as starting point of the formulation process. Methods are needed to support the marking of different text parts and their corresponding formal counterparts. To support the authoring task our idea is to search for different patterns in already existing clinical guidelines by comparing a specific group of guidelines. The aim of our work is to provide a set of prototypical patterns. The idea of patterns, as they are established in the domain of computer science, is originally conceived of Christopher Alexander in his book "The Pattern Language" [3], where he introduced patterns on the basis of the architectural domain. In computer science, patterns are recognized as a powerful theoretical framework, which can help to solve problems.

3 The Process – Identifying Patterns in Clinical Guidelines

The process of analysing clinical guidelines for prototypical patterns consists of several steps, which can be split up in various tasks:

Definition of criteria – medical and technical – which guidelines have to meet. The basis for guideline selection were the guidelines available in the database of the National Guideline Clearinghouse (NGC, www.guideline.gov). To tackle the huge amount of guidelines provided, several criteria have to be met to receive a representative group for further analysis. We defined *medical* and *technical* criteria.

Pre-selection of guidelines after applying the medical criteria. Restrictions concerning the guideline category, quality, intended user and clinical specialty were defined as important factors. This led to *management* and *treatment* as guideline categories, to *physicians* and *nurses* as intended users, to *Oncology* and *Radiation Oncology* as clinical specialties and to the *evidence-based* quality.

Detailed analysis of guidelines according to the technical criteria. For this purpose the criteria *modularity, structure, temporal dimension* and *intentions* have been defined as technical criteria.

Selecting the group of guidelines for the patterns analysing task. According to the medical criteria, eighteen guidelines have been selected. We selected ten guidelines for further analysis. The selection criteria were availability of the guidelines' text versions at NGC and narrowing the clinical specialties nine guidelines covered different topics of lung cancer and one was about general treatment of cancer patients. These ten clinical guidelines also met the technical criteria and formed the basis for further analysis and the intention of detecting prototypical patterns.

Definition of detected patterns. The core task of our approach was to define the detected patterns. The result consists of a pool of prototypical patterns which can be used for the developing process of new clinical guidelines and provide an overview of the structure and design of existing clinical guidelines.

4 The Details – Developing Prototypical Patterns

The prototypical patterns presented in the following sections – the *Structure Patterns*, the *Temporal Patterns* and the *Element Patterns* – are only valid and significant for the specific text class of clinical guidelines and do not refer to texts in general. For detailed original text examples for all presented patterns and for detailed description of the research work see [4].

Structure Patterns. Structure patterns are the most important one and embody the specific structure of a clinical guideline. Three different types were identified.

The Independent Structure Pattern (Fig. 1). This type represents the simplest type of structure. The textual arrangements of the guidelines are structured in paragraphs. All these parts are clearly separated by content and independent from each other. The XOR structure pattern and the recurring structure pattern represent a further development of the independent structure pattern.

The XOR Structure Pattern (Fig. 2). Guidelines composed in the XOR (exclusive-OR) structure are basically divided in two main parts. Each of these two parts again consists of sub-parts, which are clearly separated by content and independent.

The Recurring Structure Pattern (Fig. 3). The recurring structure consists of clearly separated and independent paragraphs and again, each of these main-paragraphs consists of several sub-paragraphs. These sub-paragraphs exhibit similarity in topic. Due to this similarity in topic the sub-paragraphs are classified as a recurring part in a guideline.

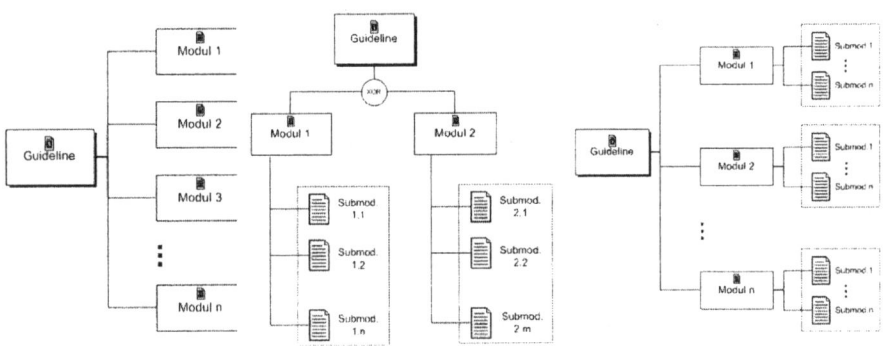

Fig. 1. Indep. Structure   **Fig. 2.** XOR Structure   **Fig. 3.** Recurring Structure

Temporal Patterns. Temporal patterns were found in each guideline. Due to the scientific character of clinical guidelines, they often present clinical trials and statements which include temporal data. Two kinds of temporal patterns were detected. We distinguish between *Single Temporal Statements* (Fig. 4), and temporal statements concerning activities. The latter are either *Simple Temporal Activity* (Fig. 5), which consists of several simple actions arranged in a sequence or *Complex Temporal Activity* (Fig. 6) which consists of a nested structure of several actions.

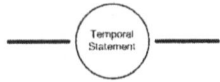

Fig. 4. Single Temporal Statement Pattern

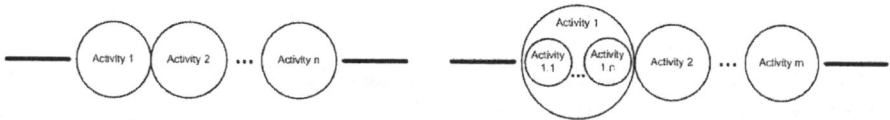

Fig. 5. Simple Temporal Activity Pattern   **Fig. 6.** Complex Temporal Activity Pattern

Element Patterns. The last class of patterns which was detected was the element patterns. These element patterns deduced – headlines, lists and tables and formatted text – refer to frequently used text sequences and text instruments in guidelines with the aim of (i) structuring the text, (ii) presenting facts, scientific results, or achievements; and (iii) using preformatted sequences of text, sentences or words.

A more detailed explanation of the analysis process and the derived patterns is given in *Identifying Pattern in Clinical Guidelines* [4]. It presents the way from patterns to macro – consisting of two steps, the implementation of patterns in the modelling language Asbru and the development of macros in DELT/A (see Section 5).

5 Related Work

Several remarkable methods and tools (Arden, Asbru, EON, GLIF, Guide, Prodigy, ProForma, Glare, and GEM) were developed in the last years – two comparison studies analyzed the benefits and drawbacks of these ([5], [6]). As this paper, Asbru and DELT/A have been developed within the Asgaard Project [2]. Due to this relation and the relevance for the developing process of macros from the detected prototypical patterns as described in [4], Asbru and DELT/A are presented next.

Asbru, a guideline modelling method. Asbru is characterised as a task-specific, intention-based, and time-oriented language for representing skeletal plans [7]. Asbru extends skeletal plans by including temporal dimensions and intentions. Intentions, conditions, and world states are temporal patterns and uncertainty in both temporal scopes and parameters can be flexibly expressed by bounding intervals [8].

DELT/A, a document exploration and linking tool. DELT/A [9] supports the translation task of clinical guidelines into a guideline modelling language such as Asbru. Additionally, DELT/A provides two features – *links* and *macros* – which are supported almost by none of the other modelling tools. In order to work with DELT/A, the operator must have a thorough understanding in clinical guidelines and a guideline modelling language. Therefore, DELT/A is primarily intended for knowledge engineers.

6 Conclusion

We introduced prototypical patterns in clinical guidelines and described the different tasks necessary to achieve the predefined target of this paper – the identification of prototypical patterns in clinical guidelines – and the reduction of the gap between the information represented in clinical guidelines and the formal representation of these clinical guidelines in execution models.

During the analysing process, some remarkable findings have been made. The most important finding have been that clinical guidelines are not as qualified for these analysing tasks as it had been expected beforc. Guidelines are authored at a very high level of abstraction. Furthermore, the evidence-based character of the chosen guidelines had also an impact on the results of the analysis. These two facts were the reason assumed why only few temporal dimensions and intentions have been detected during the analysing process. There were almost no procedural algorithms in clinical guidelines which arose also from the evidence-based character and the level of abstraction. Therefore, the resulting identified patterns are also on a relatively high level of abstraction. Taking these two facts into account, it can be stated, that clinical protocols would provide a more appropriate basis for the research of patterns because of their more detailed and procedural character.

Acknowledgments. This work has been supported by "Fonds zur Förderung der wissenschaftlichen Forschung FWF" (Austrian Science Fund), grant P15467-INF.

References

1. Field, M.J., Lohr, K.N.: Guidelines for Clinical Practice: from Development to Use. Institute of Medicine, Washington, D.C. National Academy Press, 1990.
2. Shahar, Y., Miksch, S., Johnson, P.: The Asgaard Project: A Task-Specific Framework for the Application and Critiquing of Time-Oriented Clinical Guidelines. In: Artificial Intelligence in Medicine, 14, 29-51, 1998.
3. Alexander, Ch., Ishikawa, S., Silverstein, M., Jacobson, M., Fiksdahl-King, I., Angel, S.: A Pattern Language. Oxford University Press, New York, 1977.
4. Moser, M.: Identifying Pattern in Clinical Guidelines. Master's Thesis, Institute of Software Technology and Interactive Systems, Vienna University of Technology, 2004.
5. Peleg, M., Tu, S., Bury, J., Ciccarese, P., Fox, J., Greenes, R., Hall, R., Johnson, P., Jones, N., Kumar, A., Miksch, S., Quaglini, S., Seyfang, A., Shortliffe, E., Stefanelli, M.: Comparing Computer-Interpretable Guideline Models: A Case-Study Approach. Journal of the American Medical Informatics Association 10 (2003) 52–68.
6. de Clercq, P., Blom, J., Korsten, H. and Hasman, A.: Approaches for Creating Computer-Interpretable Guidelines that Facilitate Decision Support, Artificial Intelligence in Medicine 31(1).1-27, 2004.
7. Miksch, S., Shahar, Y., Horn, W., Popow, Ch., Paky, F., Johnson, P.: Time-Oriented Skeletal Plans: Support to Design and Execution. In: S. Steel, R. Alami (eds.), Recent Advances in AI Planning – Fourth European Conference on Planning ECP '97 (EWSP'97), Springer, Lecture Notes in Artificial Intelligence (LNAI), 1997.
8. Miksch, S., Shahar, Y., Johnson, P.: Asbru: A Task-Specific, Intention-Based, and Time-Oriented Language for Representing Skeletal Plans. In: E. Motta, et al. (eds.), 7th Workshop on Knowledge Engineering: Methods & Languages (KEML-97). 1997.
9. Votruba, P., Miksch, S., Kosara; R.: Facilitating Knowledge Maintenance of Clinical Guidelines and Protocols, in 11th World Congress of Medical Informatics (MedInfo 2004).

Automatic Derivation of a Decision Tree to Represent Guideline-Based Therapeutic Strategies for the Management of Chronic Diseases

Brigitte Séroussi, Jacques Bouaud, and Jean-Jacques Vieillot

STIM, DPA/DSI/AP-HP & INSERM, U729, Paris, France
{brigitte.seroussi, jacques.bouaud}@sap.aphp.fr

Abstract. In the management of chronic diseases, therapeutic decisions depend on previously administered therapies as well as patient answers to these prior treatments. To take into account the specific management of chronic diseases, the knowledge base of the guided mode of the system ASTI has been structured as a double level decision tree, a clinical level to characterize the clinical profile of a patient, and a therapeutic level to identify the new recommended treatment when taking into account the patient's therapeutic history. We propose to automatically derive the therapeutic level of the decision tree from the formal expression of guideline-based therapeutic strategies. The method has been developed using Augmented Transition Networks. Preliminary results obtained with additive therapeutic strategies such as $(A, A+B, A+B+C)$ where A, B, and C are therapeutic classes which can be substituted respectively by (A', A''), (B', B''), and (C', C'') are promising. However, the method needs to be extended to take into account more complex patterns.

1 Introduction

In most common chronical conditions (cancer, diabetes, arterial hypertension, etc.), clinical practice guidelines (CPGs) have been developed to formalize care patterns and thus improve the standardization of medical practice. However, if the initial therapy of chronic disease management is actually described, the following steps of the therapeutic strategy are sometimes missing and, when given, proposed as transitions. Nevertheless, it is possible to derive the recommended sequence of treatments $(Tr_1, Tr_2, \ldots, Tr_n)_S$ associated to a specific clinical situation S from the initial therapy and the transitions on the basis of an interpretation framework of the original text [1]. However, although adapted to the clinical situations they are associated with in the CPG, recommended sequences remain theoretical: even when based on "scenarios" [2], they do not take into account the patient-specific therapeutic history, *i.e.* the treatments previously taken by the patient as well as her response, and they are thus never actually "patient-centered".

The guided mode of ASTI[1] [3] has been developed according to the principles of the document-centered approach for medical decision-making support initially proposed

---

[1] The ASTI project has been partially funded by the French Research Ministry. The aim of the project is to design a guideline-based decision support system to be used in primary care.

with OncoDoc [4]. As opposed to "Task Network Models" [5], the knowledge base, built to be browsed by the user clinician, has been represented as a 2-level decision tree, a clinical level to characterize clinical situations, and a therapeutic level to explore recommended therapeutic sequences under the constraint of the patient therapeutic history. However, the building of the decision tree is an expensive manual step. Thus, the aim of the work presented in this paper is to develop a tool allowing to automatically build the therapeutic level of the decision tree from the formalized therapeutic sequences extracted from textual CPGs. The proposed method uses an intermediate step that operationalizes the construction of recommended therapeutic sequences. This step has been implemented with augmented transition networks (ATNs).

2 Method

2.1 Model of a Therapeutic Strategy

The additive sequence is a simple model of therapeutic strategy, nonetheless very frequent. The initial treatment consists in administering drug A. If A is not effective, the next step is to add drug B. Then, if $A + B$ is also ineffective, another drug C is added to reach the level of tritherapy $A + B + C$ (higher levels of drug combination are usually not part of CPGs for general practice). In addition, in case recommended drugs are contraindicated, known drug substitutes may be proposed. If A is contraindicated (*e.g.* allergy) or if A has been previously prescribed and was not tolerated (*e.g.* it had unacceptable side-effects), then A can be replaced by A' in the disease management. Again, if A' is contraindicated or not tolerated, it can be substituted by A''. The formalization of a theoretical therapeutic strategy we used is made of a recommended therapeutic sequence $(A, A + B, A + B + C)$ and the set of the ordered lists of substitutes for every component of the treatment sequence: (A, A', A''), (B, B', B''), and (C, C', C'').

2.2 ATN-Based Operationalization of a Therapeutic Strategy

The operationalization of a therapeutic strategy can be decomposed into several steps. Available therapeutic information about a patient includes her therapeutic history, *i.e.* the list of already prescribed treatments, the effectiveness of these treatments, and a list of contraindicated drugs. In the case of an initial treatment (the therapeutic history is empty), the recommended treatment is the first step of the therapeutic sequence while taking into account patient-specific contraindications. In the case of a patient already treated, it becomes necessary to evaluate the patient's response to the current treatment so that, if ineffective, not tolerated, or both, it could be modified. A new treatment must be proposed constrained by the guideline recommendations and by the patient's therapeutic history. The operationalization of a therapeutic sequence of treatments is implemented using ATNs which can represent recursive procedures.

Choice of the Initial Treatment. The aim is to propose the best non-contraindicated recommended treatment for a given clinical case. The corresponding ATN (figure 1) is decomposed into two subgraphs. The main graph is linear and selects the first treatment A of the recommended sequence (action 1). But this candidate treatment must be tested against potential patient contraindications. This part (action 2 of the main graph) is modeled by the second subgraph (Check_TT_non_CI). If A is contraindicated, its substitutes, given by the list (A, A', A''), are themselves tested. As soon as a substitute is not contraindicated, it is returned to the calling graph and becomes the recommended treatment for the patient.

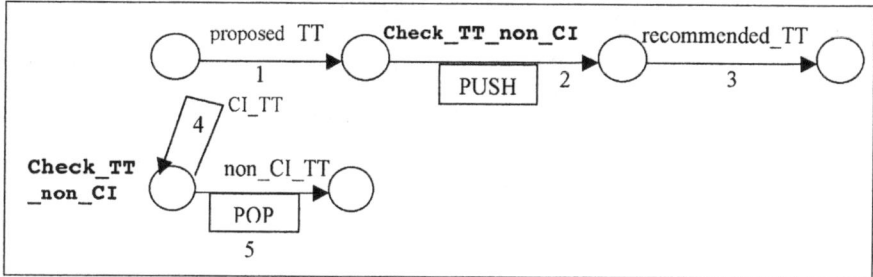

Fig. 1. ATN for prescribing initial therapy

Choice of a Non-initial Treatment. When the patient is currently under treatment, the process of determining the next recommended treatment is more complex since the current treatment has to be evaluated. As a preliminary step, the patient's therapeutic history is updated and the patient's response to the current treatment as to tolerance and effectiveness is recorded. Ineffectiveness of combinations (bi- or tritherapies) is transferred to their components. For instance, if $B + C$ is ineffective while neither B nor C have been prescribed, then B and C are considered ineffective as monotherapies.

The main ATN (figure 2) analyses the patient's response to the current treatment to propose the new appropriate recommended treatment. The first step checks whether the current treatment has been tolerated (action 7). Then, treatment effectiveness is checked. Each of these two checking processes is implemented by a subgraph, respectively Check_TT_tolerated and Check_TT_effective. In any case, when a candidate treatment is proposed, whether it is contraindicated has to be evaluated. This is performed by a call to the Check_TT_non_CI subgraph (figure 1).

If the current treatment is tolerated, the Check_TT_tolerated subgraph yields the same unmodified treatment. Otherwise, each drug component of the current treatment has to be checked with respect to tolerance. Non-tolerated drugs are replaced by their substitutes (action 15), while checking that proposed substitutes are not themselves contraindicated. This subgraph then yields a new treatment which is equivalent in term of level of drug combination (mono-, bi-, or tritherapy).

If the current treatment is ineffective, our therapeutic strategy model consists in successive drug additions to increase the level of drug combination. Action 18 of subgraph Check_TT_effective selects the first recommended drug to be added to the modified current treatment. Then it is checked against contraindications and once a non-contraindicated substitute is identified, it is added to form the final recommended prescription.

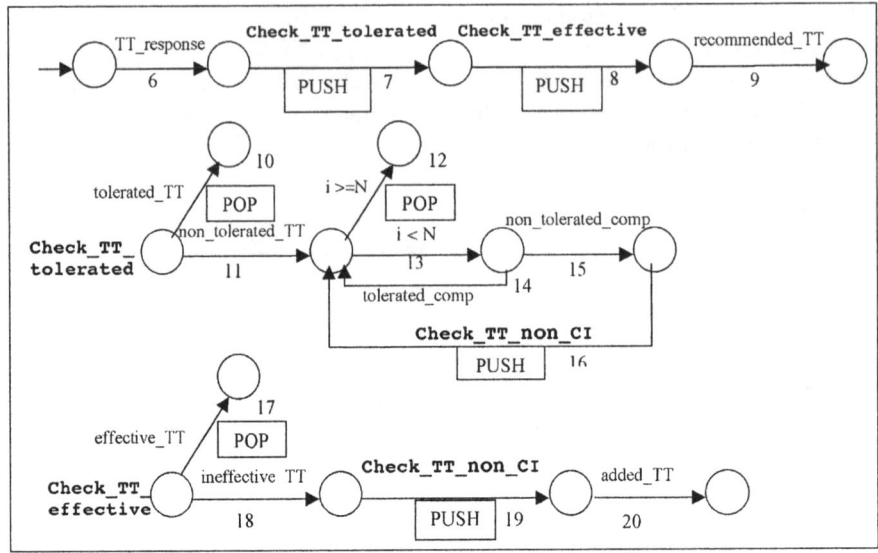

Fig. 2. ATN for current treatment evaluation and revision

2.3 Decision Tree Derivation

In order to generate the knowledge base as a decision tree, we used the previous ATNs while changing the output representation. Instead of computing the recommended treatment for a given patient, ATNs now generate nodes and branches to build the decision tree. Since, all situations must be considered by the decision tree, every transition path in the ATNs has to be traversed in a depth-first search.

The first node of the decision tree consists in determining whether the treatment to prescribe is an initial treatment or not. In the presence of a non-empty therapeutic history, nodes are built to identify the possible levels of drug combination (mono-, bi- and tritherapy) to obtain the relevant part of the theoretical therapeutic sequence. Then, each main ATN is recursively traversed to consider each possible state for each treatment of the recommended sequence taking into account drug substitutes.

3 Results

We compared the decision tree automatically derived from ATNs and the therapeutic level of the decision tree manually built in the ASTI project. We considered the particular, though medically significant, therapeutic sequence $(ACE_i, ACE_i + LD, ACE_i + LD + BB)$ with $(ACE_i, AIIR)$, (LD), and $(BB, DILT)$ as substitution lists. Table 1 displays some quantitative elements of the comparison.

Decision trees generated from ATNs are bigger than those manually built. The automatic derivation is indeed systematic and leads to the production of decision nodes which are not medically relevant although logically valid. These nodes are not created in ASTI when the decision tree is manually built. In addition, there are differences in

Table 1. Comparison between the ASTI decision tree and its equivalent automatically derived from the ATN model

	Manual building	Automatic derivation
Number of nodes	63	131
Number of paths	33	67
Mean value of depth levels	7,03	8,84

the order in which decision parameters are organized. In decision trees derived from ATNs, as the generation is automatic, the order of decision parameters may not follow the medical logics used by the physician in her reasoning process.

4 Conclusion

ATNs are particular graphs that can be used to model recursive problems or, in problem-solving domain, to simplify the resolution of a given complex problem as the resolution of a set of simpler sub-problems. It is this property of ATNs that we used to explore the contraindications of a drug a priori recommended by CPG for a given patient when taking into account her clinical condition, but not actually adapted to the patient because of her specific therapeutic history.

The obtained results are promising in the special case of linear additive strategies such as $(A, A + B, A + B + C)$, even though the procedure can be improved. The approach needs thus to be extended to take into account more complex strategies, e.g. $(A \text{ or } B, A + C \text{ or } B + C, A + B + C)$ or $(A, A + C \text{ or } A + B, A + B + C)$ which include OR choices between therapies that are not substitutes of each other.

References

1. Georg, G., Séroussi, B., Bouaud, J.: Extending the Gem Model to Support Knowledge Extraction from Textual Guidelines. Int J Med Inf **74** (2005) 79–87
2. Johnson, P.D., Tu, S., Booth, N., Sugden, B., Purves, I.N.: Using Scenarios in Chronic Disease Management Guidelines for Primary Care. J Am Med Inform Assoc **7** (2000) 389–393
3. Séroussi, B., Bouaud, J., Chatellier, G.: Guideline-Based Modeling of Therapeutic Strategies in the Special Case of Chronic Diseases. Int J Med Inf **74** (2005) 89–99
4. Séroussi, B., Bouaud, J., Antoine, E.C.: OncoDoc, a Successful Experiment of Computer-Supported Guideline Development and Implementation in the Treatment of Breast Cancer. Artif Intell Med **22** (2001) 43–64
5. Peleg, M., Tu, S.W., Bury, J., Ciccarese, P., Fox, J., Greenes, R.A., Hall, R., Johnson, P.D., Jones, N., Kumar, A., Miksch, S., Quaglini, S., Seyfang, A., Shortliffe, E.H., Stefanelli, M.: Comparing Computer-Interpretable Guideline Models: a Case-Study Approach. J Am Med Inform Assoc **10** (2003) 52–68

Exploiting Decision Theory for Supporting Therapy Selection in Computerized Clinical Guidelines

Stefania Montani, Paolo Terenziani, and Alessio Bottrighi

Dipartimento di Informatica, Università del Piemonte Orientale, Alessandria, Italy
{stefania, terenz, alessio}@mfn.unipmn.it

Abstract. Supporting therapy selection is a fundamental task for a system for the computerized management of clinical guidelines (GL). The goal is particularly critical when no alternative is really better than the others, from a strictly clinical viewpoint. In these cases, decision theory appears to be a very suitable means to provide advice. In this paper, we describe how algorithms for calculating utility, and for evaluating the optimal policy, can be exploited to fit the GL management context.

Clinical guidelines (GL) can be defined as a means for specifying the "best" clinical procedures and for standardizing them. In recent years, the medical community has started to recognize that a computer-based treatment of GL provides relevant advantages, such as automatic connection to the patient databases and, more interestingly, decision making facilities; thus, many different approaches and projects have been developed to this hand (see e.g. [4, 2]).

As a matter of fact, decision making is a central issue in clinical practice. In particular, supporting therapy selection is a critical objective to be achieved. Consider that, when implementing a GL, a physician can be faced with a choice among different therapeutic alternatives, and identifying the most suitable one is often not straightforward. In the clinical practice, various selection parameters (such as the costs and the effectiveness of the different procedures) can be available to physicians when executing a GL. The computer-based GL systems described in the literature offer sophisticated formalizations of these decision criteria. Nevertheless, the available information is often only qualitative in nature, and "local" to the decision at hand. On the other end, a GL represents a *dynamic decision problem*, in which temporally consequent decisions have to be taken with respect to the same patient. The possibility of obtaining a complete scenario of the decision consequences, considering the probability of the different therapy outcomes, the utilities associated to the different health states, and the money, time and resources spent, would therefore be an added value for physicians.Decision theory seems a natural candidate as a methodology for covering this task. To this end, we have recently proposed a systematic analysis of the main GL representation primitives, and of how they can be related to decision theory concepts [5]. In particular, we have observed that in a well-formed GL, each decision is always based on an (explicit or implicit) data collection completed at decision time in order to gather all the needed patient's parameters, and does not depend on the previous history of the patient. We can thus say that the GL describes a discrete-time first-order Markov model. This observation justifies the mapping of GL primitives to the field of decision theory, and in particular allows us to represent a GL as a Markov Decision Process (MDP). The process is also completely observable, since in a GL a decision can be taken only if all the required parameters have been collected: if some needed data are missing, the query action will wait for them and the decision will be delayed. It is then straightforward to define the *state* as the set of patient's parameters that are normally measured for taking decisions and for assessing therapy outcomes. Data collections are the means for observing the state. *State transitions* are produced by all the work (i.e. operative) actions between two consecutive non-trivial therapeutic decisions. Finally, the *utility* of a state can be evaluated in terms of life expectancy, corrected by Quality Adjusted Life Year (QALYs) [3]. Methods for eliciting patient's preferences could be considered as well.

In this paper, we start from such knowledge representation results, to describe how decision theory algorithms (to calculate utility and to obtain the optimal policy) can be exploited, when the goal is the one of supporting therapy selection in a GL management system. We also analyse complex situations which may arise due to the presence of certain types of control flow relations among GL actions, namely iterations and parallel executions. A practical application of this work is represented by the tool which is being implemented in GLARE, a domain-independent system for GL acquisition and execution [7]. The algorithmic choices, and the technical issues discussed in this paper will therefore refer to this specific example. In particular, an earlier version of GLARE already embedded a facility able to calculate costs, time and resources required to complete paths in a GL; the decision theory support can be seen as an extension of that work. The GLARE decision theory facility enables the user: (1) to identify the optimal policy, and (2) to calculate the expected utility along a path. In order to implement these functionalities, we had to take into account the following issues:

Focusing. The possibility of selecting only a sub-part of a given GL is a fundamental issue to be addressed, since it allows one to skip the paths on which decision theory support is not required. In our tool, path selection has been conceived as the first step of the interaction with the user.

Parallel Actions. In case two or more composite actions, each one containing non-trivial decisions, have to be executed in parallel along a selected path, the mapping towards the corresponding Markov model (needed to provide functionality 1 above) is not straightforward. As a matter of fact, in this situation the order of execution of the various actions is not univocally provided. The policy we have chosen to adopt to this end is the one of calculating just one possible order of execution, compatible with the available temporal constraints [9], and to rely on it.

Generating the Markov Model. Once path selection and parallel actions management have been addressed, the next step towards the calculation of the optimal policy (see functionality 1 above) is the mapping of the GL to the corresponding Markov model. In particular, probability values are extracted from the medical literature - when possible; otherwise, in the current implementation, they can be obtained from interviews with expert physicians.

Repeated Actions. On the Markov model, classical algorithms for evaluating the optimal policy can be relied on [1, 8]. When dealing with a finite time horizon, the dynamic programming algorithm can be easily applied. Nevertheless, in the context of clinical GL, it is not infrequent that the number of states, though finite, is not known a priori. This situation may be induced by the presence of iterations to be repeated several times, until a certain exit condition becomes true. The number of repetitions could therefore vary among different executions of the same GL. To handle this problem, the choice made in GLARE is the one of relying on algorithms for calculating the optimal policy on an infinite time horizon (as a matter of fact, "infinite" can be used in the meaning of "unknown a priori"), and in particular on value iteration [8].

Simplifications. Algorithms can be simplified in case the required output is not the optimal policy, but the expected utility of all the different paths selected by the user (see functionality 2 above). Note that following a path corresponds to apply a specific policy, i.e. to make the hypothesis of knowing what is the decision to be taken at any decision node. In case of a finite time horizon, since the policy is known, we can calculate the utility by applying the dynamic programming algorithm, avoiding to maximize the expected value of the cumulative utility function wrt the different actions. On the other hand, when iterations with an exit condition have to be tackled, we can ask the user physician the minimum and maximum number of times that the action has to be repeated, given the specific patient's characteristics. Then, we can generate the paths corresponding to these two extreme situations, thus reducing to a finite time horizon, on which it is possible to calculate utility and costs as described above. In the case of utility, however, we can also keep working on an infinite time horizon, not having to rely on the physician's estimate of the number of iterations, and resort to value iteration. Again, since the policy is fixed, the algorithm can be simplified by avoiding maximization wrt the different actions. This second strategy is clearly not applicable to costs, which are additive. It is up to the user physician to select the preferred output in these cases.

As an example, we present an application of the GLARE decision theory tool to a GL for asthma treatment. Figure 1 shows part of the GL. Patients affected by mild persistent asthma (see upper branch in the figure) may be treated by four different therapies (as indicated by the four edges exiting the T1 node): inhaled beta-2-agonists (A), oral beta-2-agonists (OA), inhaled anticholinergics (IA) or theophylline (TH). Each therapy implementation consists of a daily dose. Basically, the four drugs for mild asthma are clinically equivalent; therefore, indications about implications of each alternative could be useful in deciding. If the therapy does not work, the patient could worsen to moderate asthma. In this case, another therapeutic decision has to be taken (action T2), in order to

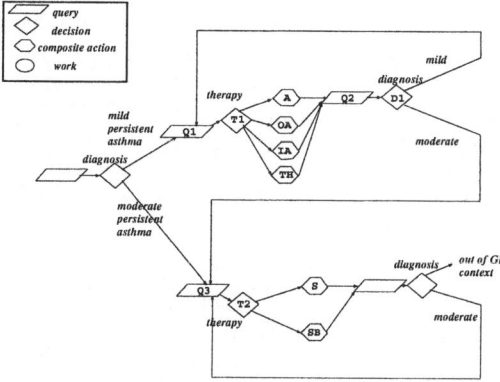

Fig. 1. Part of the asthma treatment guideline. Node types legend is provided as well

Table 1. Probabilities of transition between states

Therapy	From	To	Probability
A	Mild asthma	Mild asthma	0.9
A	Mild asthma	Moderate asthma	0.1
OA	Mild asthma	Mild asthma	0.85
OA	Mild asthma	Moderate asthma	0.15
IA	Mild asthma	Mild asthma	0.6
IA	Mild asthma	Moderate asthma	0.4
TH	Mild asthma	Mild asthma	0.5
TH	Mild asthma	Moderate asthma	0.5
S	Moderate asthma	Moderate asthma	0.85
S	Moderate asthma	Severe asthma (out of GL)	0.15
SB	Moderate asthma	Moderate asthma	0.95
SB	Moderate asthma	Severe asthma (out of GL)	0.05

implement a more effective treatment. It is possible to select between inhaled steroids (S) and inhaled steroids plus bronchodilators (SB). Again, these drugs have to be provided daily. Periodically (e.g. weekly), the patient's state is reassessed, and the therapeutic decision has to be repeated in a loop, until this guideline becomes not applicable for the patient at hand (because asthma is now severe, and a different guideline has to be referred to, or because asthma improves: this case is not explicitly represented in figure 1).

In the GLARE formalism, the treatment of mild asthma has to be represented as an iterated plan with an exit condition, that corresponds to the onset of moderate asthma. Analogous considerations hold for the treatment of moderate asthma. The utility of the mild persistent asthma state is 86, while the utility of moderate asthma is 82, and the utility of severe asthma is 78 [6]. Table 1 lists the probabilities of transition, that were provided by medical experts. Since the GL includes two cycles, which are repeated a number of times not known a priori, in this example the optimal policy has been calculated using the value iteration algorithm, which has identified A as the optimal therapy in case of

Table 2. Utilities of the asthma GL states having fixed the various policies (i.e. paths). Numbers have been normalized wrt the maximum value

Policy	Utility Mild asthma	Utility Moderate asthma
A-S	0.57590	0.24231
A-SB	1	0.66641
OA-S	0.46470	0.24231
OA-SB	0.88879	0.66640
IA-S	0.32570	0.24230
IA-SB	0.74979	0.66639
TH-S	0.30902	0.24230
TH-SB	0.73311	0.66639

mild asthma, and SB as the optimal therapy in case of moderate asthma. We have applied (simplified) value iteration also for calculating the utility of all the possible paths in the GL; the corresponding values are reported in table 2.

In conclusion, a decision theory facility would be an added value for a computerized system for GL management. In this paper we have underlined what integrations and specific choices are required to deal with non trivial GL control flow constructs, namely iterations and parallel executions.

References

1. R. Bellman. *Dynamic programming*. Princeton University Press, 1957.
2. D.B. Fridsma (Guest Ed.). Special issue on workflow management and clinical guidelines. *Journal of the American Medical Informatics Association*, 1.
3. M.R. Gold, J. E. Siegel, L. B. Russell, and M. C. Weinstein. *Cost-Effectiveness in Health and Medicine*. Oxford University Press, New York, 1996.
4. C. Gordon and editors. J.P. Christensen. *Health Telematics for Clinical Guidelines and Protocols*. IOS Press, Amsterdam, 1995.
5. S. Montani and P. Terenziani. Decision theory issues for supporting therapy selection in computerized guidelines. In B. Bouchon-Meunier, G. Coletti, and R.R. Yager, editors, *Proc. Information Processing and Managing of Uncertainty in Knowledge-based Systems (IPMU) 2004*, pages 591–598. Casa Editrice Università la Sapienza, Roma, 2004.
6. M.L. Moy, E. Israel, S.T. Weiss, E.F. Juniper, L. Dube, and J.M. Drazen. Clinical predictors of health-related quality of life depend on asthma severity. *Am. J. Respir. Crit. Care Med.*, 163(4):924–929, 2001.
7. P. Terenziani, S. Montani, A. Bottrighi, M. Torchio, and G. Molino. Supporting physicians in taking decisions in clinical guidelines: the glare "what-if" facility. In *Journal of the American Medical Informatics Association (JAMIA) Symposium supplement*, pages 772–776, 2002.
8. H.C. Tijms. *Stochastic modelling and analysis: a computational approach*. Wiley and Sons, 1986.
9. L. Vila. A survey on temporal reasoning in artificial intelligence. *AI Communications*, 1(7):4–28, 1994.

Helping Physicians to Organize Guidelines Within Conceptual Hierarchies

Diego Sona[1], Paolo Avesani[1], and Robert Moskovitch[2]

[1] ITC/irst - Trento, Italy
[2] Ben Gurion University - Beer Sheva, Israel

Abstract. Clinical Practice Guidelines (CPGs) are increasingly common in clinical medicine for prescribing a set of rules that a physician should follow. Recent interest is in accurate retrieval of CPGs at the point of care. Examples are the CPGs digital libraries National Guideline Clearinghouse (NGC) or Vaidurya, which are organized along predefined concept hierarchies. In this case, both browsing and concept-based search can be applied. However, mandatory step in enabling both ways to CPGs retrieval is manual classification of CPGs along the concepts hierarchy, which is extremely time consuming. Supervised learning approaches are usually not satisfying, since commonly too few or no CPGs are provided as training set for each class.

In this paper we apply *TaxSOM* for multiple classification. *TaxSOM* is an unsupervised model that supports the physician in the classification of CPGs along the concepts hierarchy, even when no labeled examples are available. This model exploits lexical and topological information on the hierarchy to elaborate a classification hypothesis for any given CPG. We argue that such a kind of unsupervised classification can support a physician to classify CPGs by recommending the most probable classes. An experimental evaluation on various concept hierarchies with hundreds of CPGs and categories provides the empirical evidence of the proposed technique.

1 Introduction

Clinical practice guidelines (CPGs) are an increasingly common and important format in clinical medicine for prescribing a set of rules and policies that a physician should follow. It would be best if automated support could be offered to guideline-based care at the point of care. It is often important to be able to quickly retrieve a set of guidelines most appropriate for a particular patient or task. Correctly classifying the guidelines, along as many semantic categories as relevant (e.g., therapy modes, disorder types, sighs and symptoms), supports easier and more accurate retrieval of the relevant guidelines using concept based search.

Traditional text retrieval systems use the *vector-space-model*, in which retrieval is based on the terms appearance in the text. Concept based search extends this approach, in which documents and queries are mapped into concepts taxonomy based on their contents. Such an approach is implemented in

Vaidurya - a concept based and context sensitive search engine for clinical guidelines [1]. Electronic CPGs repository, such as the National Guideline Clearinghouse (NGC) provide a hierarchical access to electronic CPGs in a free-text or semi-structured format (see <http://www.ngc.org>). However, to implement an accurate concept based search, manual classification of CPGs should be applied by an expert. This task is extremely time consuming, therefore, an automatic process that classifies CPGs along the concepts hierarchy is crucial, while very challenging.

The main aim of this paper is to provide a tool that assists the domain expert (physician), who classifies the CPGs, suggesting the most probable classes for each CPG, even when concept hierarchies is built from scratch, and no examples of labeled CPGs are provided for each class. In this case there is no premise for a successful training of any existing supervised classifier, therefore, recommendations can be given only using an unsupervised model, a task known as the *bootstrapping* problem [2]. Then, once the physician is provided with the set of recommended classes for each CPG she can select the most appropriate ones.

The interesting part of this approach is that while the physician manufactures the concept hierarchy she also inserts some prior knowledge on the desired organization of data. Thus, each concept is described by some keywords and has several descendants sub-concepts, which are more specific. This prior knowledge is exploited by the proposed model in order to perform a preliminary classification of CPGs according to their contents and the desired organization within the hierarchy.

An evaluation of the proposed approach was made on the NGC dataset with encouraging results. Section 2 gives a description of the addressed task with some references to related works. Section 3 introduces the model used to test the proposed solution. Section 4 describes the experimental setup and gives some results. Finally, Section 5 draw some conclusions.

2   Task Definition

A concept hierarchy (taxonomy) is a hierarchy of categories (classes), represented in a *tree-like* structure. Each node is described in terms of both linguistic keywords, ideally denoting their "semantic meaning", and relationships with other categories. The leaves of the tree represent the most specific concepts while nodes near the root represent more general concepts. In our particular task, each node of the hierarchy, also intermediate, can contain CPGs and, in general, each CPG can belong to more than one category (multiple classification).

A typical task in text categorization is to identify a set of categories that best describe the content of a new unclassified CPG. A wide range of statistical and machine learning techniques have been applied to text categorization [3, 4, 5, 6, 7, 8, 9]. However, these techniques are all based on having some initial labeled examples, which are used to train a (semi)-supervised model.

These problems are partially solved within the setup we use in the *TaxSOM* model [10]. The model uses the prior knowledge to drive a clustering process and, as a result, it organizes the CPGs on a given concept hierarchy without any supervised training stage. Basically, the model bootstraps the given taxonomy with a preliminary classification of CPGs that afterward need to be reviewed by the taxonomy editor. The basic idea of the *bootstrapping* process is to support and alleviate the manual labeling of a set of unlabeled examples, providing the user with an automatically determined preliminary hypothesis of classification. Specifically, the goal here is to recommend the user with a list of the most probable k classes for each CPG.

3 Classification Models

A simple strategy to classify documents only using prior knowledge is to build a reference vector for each category, through the encoding of all keywords in the current node and in all its ancestors, i.e., all keywords of the nodes in the path from the root to the current node. In this way the codebooks contain both the lexical and the topological information. The documents are then associated to the category having the nearest reference vector. This is a standard prototype based minimum error classifier that in the following will be referred to as *baseline* approach.

The above idea has been further extended in the *TaxSOM* model [10]. Specifically, a *TaxSOM* is a collection of computational units connected so as to form a graph having the shape isomorphic to the given taxonomy. Such computational units, namely codebooks, are initialized only using local lexical information. Then an unsupervised training algorithm (similar to Self Organizing Maps training) adapts these codebooks considering both the documents similarity and the constraints determined by the node keywords and the relationships between units.

Once a *TaxSOM* has been properly trained the final configuration of the codebooks describes a clustered organization of documents that tailors the desired relationships between concepts. The learning procedure of a *TaxSOM* is designed as an iterative process, which can be divided into two main steps: a competitive step and a cooperative step. During the *competitive* step the codebook most similar to the current input vector (a document) is chosen as the *winner* unit. In the *cooperative* stage all codebooks are moved closer to the input vector, with a learning rate proportional to the inverse of their topological distance from the winner unit. The iterations of the two steps are interleaved with an additional phase where the codebooks are constrained by the prior lexical knowledge localized on the nodes (refers to [10] for a detailed description).

4 Experimental Evaluation

We used the NGC CPGs collection to evaluate the suggested approach. The CPGs in the NGC repository are classified along two hierarchical concept trees (*Disorders* and *Therapies*) having each roughly 1,000 unique concepts, where in some regions the concepts trees are 10 levels deep, but the mean is 4 to 6 levels.

Table 1. Results of *baseline* and *TaxSOM k-coverage* with two different values for k

	\multicolumn{4}{c}{k-coverage}			
	baseline		TaxSOM	
taxonomies	$k=10$	$k=20$	$k=10$	$k=20$
diagnosis	11.3	23.3	32.9	46.8
neoplasms	38.2	46.2	47.2	63.7
organic chemicals	60.7	71.0	73.1	80.0
pathol. sympt. cond. signs	42.8	55.4	64.2	76.5
surgical operative proced.	44.1	70.4	68.8	76.9
system diseases nervous	26.1	38.9	53.5	71.2
therapeutics	23.9	39.2	52.5	69.0
virus diseases	27.5	48.9	58.0	72.5
disease condition	8.0	14.0	21.6	34.7
treatment intervention	3.9	5.9	11.2	20.0

There are 1136 CPGs, each CPG may have multiple classifications at different nodes. CPGs have a mean of 10 classifications, not necessarily on the leaves. To evaluate the model with a plurality of taxonomies, we have split the two original trees into eight smaller and different datasets. The variability of the hierarchies structure (number of concepts and CPGs) enabled us to evaluate the model without any biases caused by any prior knowledge of the taxonomy.

The depth of the eight trees ranges from 5 to 9, where the number of concepts ranges from 124 to 326, and the mean ratio of documents per concept is 2.6. The content of documents and the category keywords were cleaned removing stop–words, stemming, and reducing the resulting vocabulary to 500 important words plus the keywords. This selection was done separately for each taxonomy using the notion of Shannon Entropy[1]. Finally, CPG contents were encoded with a *set–of–words* representation (i.e., binary vectors).

As previously outlined, since to our knowledge there are not models devised to solve the proposed bootstrapping problem, we compared *TaxSOM* with the *baseline* approach. The model was tested on each taxonomy performing an hypothesis of classification for all CPGs, and the results were then compared with the original labeling. Actually, the addressed task requires the multi-classification of CPGs, therefore, given a CPG, both models generate a membership value for each class. These membership values are then used to rank the classes, and this ranking is then used to select the best classes to recommend to the user.

For the evaluation we devised a specific measure – the *multi-classification k-coverage precision*. This measure allows a comparison of models rather than an objective evaluation. The measure counts the percentage of CPGs "correctly" classified with respect to the total number of CPGs. The definition of *k-coverage* is strongly related to the definition of "precise classification". A document is correctly classified when all the first k recommended classes include the real

---

[1] Entropy is a standard information theoretic approach used to evaluate the amount of information provided by the presence of a word in the dataset.

classes. Thus, a model having *k-coverage* equal to 60% for $k = 10$ means that for 60% of the documents all the corresponding correct classes appear in the first ten ranked classes.

The results in Table 1 are shown for two settings of k. Based on the results it seems that for all taxonomies *TaxSOM* outperforms the *baseline* approach. The table also provides the results of the same type of analysis done for the original two NGC hierarchies, indicating the same magnitude but with lower performance caused by the lower rate of documents per concepts.

5 Conclusions and Future Work

In the paper we presented an approach for helping physicians to organize CPGs within hierarchies of concepts. The challenge was twofold: to avoid the need of labeled documents in advance and to exploit relational knowledge encoded by a taxonomy. Preliminary evaluation on a collection of CPGs is encouraging. We are in the process of evaluating the system based on other settings of k.

References

1. Moskovitch, R., Hessing, A., Shahar, Y.: Vaidurya - a concept-based, context-sensitive search engine for clinical guidelines. In: Proc. of the joint conf. of AMIA04 and Medinfo-2004, San Francisco, CA, US (2004)
2. Adami, G., Avesani, P., Sona, D.: Bootstrapping for hierarchical document classification. In: Proc. of CIKM-03, 12th ACM Int. Conf. on Information and Knowledge Management, ACM Press, New York, US (2003) 295–302
3. Ceci, M., Malerba, D.: Hierarchical classification of html documents with WebClassII. In: Proc. of the 25th European Conf. on Information Retrieval (ECIR'03). Volume 2633 of Lecture Notes in Computer Science. (2003) 57–72
4. Cheng, C., Tang, J., Fu, A., King, I.: Hierarchical classification of documents with error control. In: PAKDD 2001 - Proc. of 5th Pacific-Asia Conf. on Knowledge Discovery and Data Mining. Volume 2035 of Lecture Notes in Computer Science. (2001) 433–443
5. Doan, H., Domingos, P., Halevy, A.: Learning to match the schemas of data sources: A multistrategy approach. Machine Learning **50** (2003) 279–301
6. Dumais, S., Chen, H.: Hierarchical classification of web document. In: Proc. of the 23rd ACM Int. Conf. on Research and Development in Information Retrieval (SIGIR'00). (2000)
7. Moskovitch, R., Cohen-Kashi, S., Dror, U., amd A. Maimon, I.L., Shahar, Y.: Multiple hierarchical classification of free-text clinical guidelines. In: Intelligent Data Analysis In Medicine And Pharmacology (IDAMAP-04) Stanford University CA. (2004)
8. Ruiz, M., Srinivasan, P.: Hierarchical text categorization using neural networks. Information Retrieval **5** (2002) 87–118
9. Sun, A., Lim, E.: Hierarchical text classification and evaluation. In Cercone, N., Lin, T., Wu, X., eds.: ICDM 2001 - Proc. of the 2001 IEEE Int. Conf. on Data Mining, IEEE Computer Society (2001) 521–528
10. Adami, G., Avesani, P., Sona, D.: Clustering documents in a web directory. In: Proc. of WIDM-03, 5th ACM Int. Workshop on Web Information and Data Management, ACM Press, New York, US (2003) 66–73

MHB – A Many-Headed Bridge Between Informal and Formal Guideline Representations[*]

Andreas Seyfang[1], Silvia Miksch[1], Cristina Polo-Conde[2], Jolanda Wittenberg[3], Mar Marcos[2], and Kitty Rosenbrand[3]

[1] Vienna University of Technology, Austria
[2] Universitat Jaume I, Spain
[3] Dutch Institute for Healthcare Improvement, The Netherlands

Abstract. Clinical guidelines are becoming more and more important as a means to improve the quality of care by supporting medical staff. Modelling guidelines in a computer-processable form is a prerequisite for various computer applications, to improve the quality of guidelines and to support their application. However, transforming the original text into a formal guideline representation is a difficult task requiring both the skills of a computer scientist and medical knowledge.

To bridge this gap, we have designed an intermediate representation called the MHB. It is a *Many-Headed Bridge* between informal representations such as free text and tables and more formal representations such as Asbru, GLIF, or PROforma. Obtaining an MHB representation from free text should be easier than modelling in a more formal representation because the vague expressions found in the guideline do not need to be replaced by precise information immediately.

1 Introduction

Clinical guidelines are "systematically developed statements to assist practitioner and patient decisions about appropriate health care for specific clinical circumstances" [1]. A guideline describes the optimal care for patients and therefore, when properly applied, it is assumed that they will improve the quality of care. Evidence-based guidelines are becoming an important and indispensable part of quality health care.

There are several formal guideline representations. Asbru, EON, GLIF, Guide, Prodigy and PROForma have been compared by [2]. Further representations are Glare [3] and GEM [4]. Although the degree of formalization varies between these approaches, the majority of them represent the guideline in a format which is precise enough to execute it (semi-)automatically.

While it is desirable to produce a formal model of a guideline, it is difficult and expensive. If a guideline is revised, the modelling effort is lost and it is not easy to detect which changes in the formal model are required by the changes in the original text. The main reason for this is that there is a large gap between natural language and the currently available formal representations. To close the above described gap in a versatile manner we designed an *intermediate representation* called MHB.

---

[*] This work has been supported by the European Commission's IST program, under contract number IST-FP6-508794 Protocure-II.

2 The Many-Headed Bridge MHB

As the name suggests, the MHB is not designed as a unidirectional bridge from a one type of natural language guideline to one formal representation. Instead, it is designed as a versatile device to improve guideline quality.

The overall structure of an MHB file is a series of *chunks*. Each chunk corresponds to a certain bit of information in the natural language guideline text, e.g., a sentence, part of a sentence, or more than one sentence. The information in a chunk is structured in various *dimensions*, e.g. control flow, data flow. Dimensions consist of optional *aspects* which contain attributes. The aspects of different dimensions are independent, i.e. a chunk can have any combination of aspects (i.e. several dimensions).

All aspects contain link elements which store the connection between each part of the MHB file and the original guideline text. Most aspects contain an attribute degree-of-certainty to explicitly show the confidence the original guideline authors expressed in this statement (e.g., *should, seems advisable*), independent of the formal grade of evidence which is derived from the quality of the studies this statement is based on. Chunks can also contain a refer-to element used to refer to other chunks placed elsewhere within the file to make the reuse of chunks possible.

The subsections below describe the representation of each of these dimensions. Due to space limitations, we only show the main features of this language. The full specification can be found in [5] at www.protocure.org.

2.1 Dimension Control Flow

One of the most prominent aspects of a guideline is: *when* to do *what*. MHB offers the following means to express this.

Decisions. In MHB the basic structure of a single decision is if-then. It consists of a condition, a condition-modifier, a result, a result-modifier. The condition-modifier supports various categories of choices, such as negative recommendations and strong and weak arguments pro and contra a certain option. The result designates the recommended action. In MHB the element option-group is used to group several if-then elements. The options can exclude each other or not as specified by the attribute selection-type.

Decomposition. A task can be decomposed into subtasks. The MHB element decomposition names a task as an attribute and the names of its subtasks. Often one task is performed more then once – either for a certain number of times or at certain times during another task. In these cases, repetition specifies a task ("envelope task") which continues during all the repetitions and a subtask ("repeated task") which is performed repeatedly.

Figure 1 shows an example for a contra-indication. The corresponding text in the guideline is

> *Absolute contra-indications for BCT: multicentricity (two or more tumors in different quadrants of the breast); ...*

CHUNK-10041			
control	if-then	condition	multicentricity
		condition-modifier	strong rule-out
		result	BCT
data	usage	name	multicentricity
	definition	name	multicentricity
		description	two or more tumors in different quadrants of the breast
structure		status	recommendations

Fig. 1. Model of an absolute contra-indication

2.2 Dimension Data Flow

Interwoven with control flow is the description of the data processing involved in the diagnosis and treatment of the patient. In MHB, we distinguish the following (compare Figure 1): The definition of a data item; The usage of a data item is made explicit to varying degrees in actions described in the guideline and calculation of other values. The input of a data item is sometimes explicitly described in the description of the patient interview or diagnosis. abstraction-rules describe the calculation or abstraction of one data item based on others.

2.3 Dimension Temporal Aspects

Both data and control flow may have temporal aspects which can be qualitative or quantitative. MHB covers the complexity of Asbru (which has the most complex means of modelling the temporal dimension) in modelling temporal aspects, but adds more standard concepts such as average or precise duration. For each of start, end, and duration, the minimum, maximum, estimate, and precise value can be given. The precise value excludes others, but the other three values can be combined. The difference between estimate and precise value lies in the semantics given in the guideline. If start or end are given relative to a certain starting point and it is not obviously the start of the plan described, then reference point must be noted together with the offset in the respective attribute.

In addition to the above, the temporal dimension also models qualitative temporal relations such as "A is started after the end of B". While this could be implemented using the above elements, we provide a distinct element for qualitative relations to improve the comprehensibility of the model.

2.4 Dimension Evidence

An evidence-based guideline builds a bridge from carefully examined pieces of evidence which are obtained for the problem to generally applicable recommendations. Evidence for a statement can appear in various forms:

For so called summary statements of the evidence (also called scientific conclusion), a grade is given to show the overall strength of the evidence supporting this conclusion. In addition, every single literature reference that this statement is built on is graded by a `level` of evidence. This level depends on the quality of the study and the study design. Statements in the guideline can have a `literature-reference`.

2.5 Dimension Background Information

Background information describes various aspects of the topic. This may refer to a particular statement or group of statements or may only be loosely coupled to particular statements or recommendations. Also the potential for formal encoding can vary.

Intentions. of the described actions or recommendations inform and motivate the reader about the reasons for certain steps. *Effects* are relations between data or phenomena and other phenomena which are not seen as events or actions. *Relations* are similar to effects, but do not postulate that one of the two named entities is the cause of the other. Other *educational information* and *explanations* give further information on details of the disease not directly related to guideline execution. *Indicators* are measurable elements of health care that give an indication about the quality.

2.6 Other Dimensions

Resources. Each action consumes resources of various nature: *Personal* resources such as the working time of clinical staff; *Devices* such as treatment facilities; and *Financial cost*.

Patient Related Aspects. While the resources dimension mostly represents the view of the care provider, there are several other general issues mentioned in a guideline which see treatment from the patient perspective: *Risk, patient discomfort,* and *health prospective* related a certain treatment option or diagnostic action.

3 Evaluation

Our evaluation of the MHB was performed both on a theoretical and on a practical level. On the *theoretical level*, the mapping between MHB and various formal representations for clinical guidelines and protocols was discussed and documented [5].

In a *practical evaluation* we modelled a significant part of the Dutch Guideline for the Treatment of Breast Carcinoma [6] in MHB. Our experience has shown that MHB is appropriate to model the statements found in the significant guideline parts. MHB not only provides constructs to express the essential knowledge we intended to model, but also allowed for a modelling with the degree of detail necessary for our purposes. An initial problem was the variation observed across the MHB models obtained initially. To solve this, we elaborated a series of basic MHB modelling recommendations. Thanks to these recommendations, the degree of variation was greatly decreased, regardless of the different background of the modellers.

Currently, we are translating the MHB model to Asbru. Although this is still work in progress, our initial experience shows that the MHB model together with the original guideline text forms a better basis for guideline formalization than the original guideline text alone. Already at this stage of modelling, various analyses have been performed, e.g. to detect the unintended use of synonyms and missing knowledge.

4 Conclusions

Our experiences in the Protocure [7] project led to the following conclusions. MHB is easier to understand than Asbru by those without computer background. However, a significant effort in training was necessary.

It is easier to create an MHB model from the original guideline text than an Asbru model. The main reason for this is that MHB does not demand complete information. Also, MHB can be structured like the guideline, while formal representations such as Asbru and others model a guideline as a hierarchy of plans or tasks which is not easy to detect in the original guideline text.

It is easier to create an Asbru model based on MHB than based on the original text alone. While missing knowledge and vague information in the guideline text still cause modelling problems, they are more efficiently handled since they are already displayed in the MHB model.

The major drawback of MHB compared to other, more strict representations such as Asbru or GLIF lies in the fact that the syntax of MHB does not impose strict rules for the usage of each attribute (or aspect). The usage is only described in a guidelines [5] and it is the author's responsibility to follow them. While this is an advantage in the early modelling phase, it takes considerable effort to arrive at a uniform naming scheme for the tasks and data items in the guideline. However, this is a known problem shared by all formal guideline representations.

Weighing the advantages and limitations of MHB, we conclude that MHB is a suitable solution for bridging the gap between the original guideline text and formal representations such as Asbru.

References

1. Field, M.J., Lohr, K.H.: Clinical Practice Guidelines: Directions for a New Program. National Academy Press (1990)
2. Peleg, M., Tu, S., Bury, J., Ciccarese, P., Fox, J., Greenes, R., Hall, R., Johnson, P., Jones, N., Kumar, A., Miksch, S., Quaglini, S., Seyfang, A., Shortliffe, E., Stefanelli, M.: Comparing computer-interpretable guideline models: A case-study approach. Journal of the American Medical Informatics Association **10** (2003) 52–68
3. Terenziani, P., Molino, G., Torchio, M.: A modular approach for representing and execution clinical guidelines. Artificial Intelligence in Medicine **23** (2001) 249–276
4. Shiffman, R.N., Karras, B.T., Agrawal, A., Chen, R., Marenco, L., Math, S.: GEM: A proposal for a more comprehensive guideline document model using XML. Journal of the American Medical Informatics Association **7** (2000) 488–498
5. Seyfang, A., Miksch, S., Votruba, P., Rosenbrand, K., Wittenberg, J., von Croonenborg, J., Reif, W., Balser, M., Schmitt, J., van der Weide, T., Lucas, P., Homersom, A.: Specification of Formats of Intermediate, Asbru and KIV Representations. EU Project Protocure (2004)
6. Nationaal Borstkanker Overleg Nederland (NABON): Guideline for the Treatment of Breast Cancinoma. Van Zuiden Communications B.V. (2002)
7. Balser, M., Coltell, O., van Croonenborg, J., Duelli, C., van Harmelen, F., Jovell, A., Lucas, P., Marcos, M., Miksch, S., Reif, W., Rosenbrand, K., Seyfang, A., ten Teije, A.: Protocure: Supporting the development of medical protocols through formal methods. In Kaiser, K., Miksch, S., Tu, S., eds.: Computer-based Support for Clinical Guidelines and Protocols, IOS Press (2004) 103 – 107

Clinical Guidelines Adaptation: Managing Authoring and Versioning Issues

Paolo Terenziani[1], Stefania Montani[1], Alessio Bottrighi[1],
Gianpaolo Molino[2], and Mauro Torchio[2]

[1] DI, Univ. Piemonte Orientale, Via Bellini 25, Alessandria, Italy
{terenz, stefania, alessio}@mfn.unipmn.it
[2] Lab. Informatica Clinica, Az. Ospedaliera S. G. Battista, C.so Bramante 88, Torino, Italy
{mtorchio, gmolino}@molinette.piemonte.it

Abstract. One of the biggest issues in guideline dissemination nowadays is the need of adapting guidelines themselves to the application contexts, and to keep them up to date. In this paper, we propose a computer-based approach to facilitate the adaptation task. In particular, we focus on the management of two different levels of authors (users and supervisors), and of the history of the guideline versions.

1 Introduction

Clinical guidelines can be roughly defined as frameworks for specifying the "best" clinical procedures and for standardizing them. Many authors have shown the advantages of adopting computer-based guidelines as a support for improving physician's work and/or optimizing hospital activities, and several computer systems have been developed (consider, e.g., [5], [3]).

Usually, clinical guidelines are developed/revised by committees of expert physicians, and all the existing alternatives are deliberately described in order to make the guidelines as general as possible. Despite this valuable effort, however, a guideline may include no alternatives which can be really put in practice in a given hospital. As a matter of fact, one of the most relevant obstacles to guideline use and dissemination is the need of *adapting* them to *local constraints* (see also [2]) in local settings (e.g., hospital resources availability, available practitioners' skills). Moreover, a basic issue is what we call *upgrade adaptation*, i.e., the fact that, periodically, guidelines have to be updated in order to include relevant novelties in the clinical field (e.g., new therapies) and, possibly, to remove obsolete ones. We proposed our approach to resource adaptation in [11]. In this paper, we extend our work to deal with upgrade adaptation.

2 Functionalities

In principle, periodical updates to guidelines could be provided by general practitioners (GPs); a team of supervisors will have to accept (i.e. validate) them before modifying the original version. Of course, one might want to record the identity of the author(s) of the proposals and of the acceptances. Moreover, also maintaining the "history" of the guideline *versions* is very important. For instance, a physician might be called to justify her/his actions on a given patient P in the time span T on the basis of her institution's guidelines, but only considering the guidelines that were valid at time T (e.g., further upgrades cannot be considered, since they were not available at the time the physician had to operate). To summarize, we think that the following functionalities should be provided to support *upgrade* updates to guidelines:

(i) management of authors (distinguishing between GPs and supervisors);
(ii) management of the status of any piece of knowledge in the guideline (distinguishing between proposed and accepted knowledge);
(iii) management of the history of knowledge (considering proposal vs acceptance times);
(iv) facilities for selecting the parts of a guideline to be changed/updated;
(v) facilities for modifying (part of) a guideline;
(vi) facilities for formulating queries and for visualising the updates.

In order to devise a modular, general, and system independent approach to face the above issues, we propose a three-layered architecture, consisting of:

(1) a data model layer, defining the data model and providing the basic operations;
(2) a query language layer, supporting an SQL-like high-level manipulation and query language, based on layer (1);
(3) an interface layer, based on the previous ones, that provides users with high-level functionalities, accessed through a user-friendly graphical interface.

For the sake of brevity, only the first layer is discussed in this paper.

3 A Data Model Supporting Updates

In the following, we rely on an general and abstract model of guideline knowledge, in which guidelines are represented as actions, each one described by a set of <property – value> pairs (for the sake of brevity, we do not cope with multi-valued properties). Actions may be organized in a *composed-by* hierarchy. In order to devise a general and system-independent approach providing the above functionalities (i)-(vi), the standard guideline data model has to be enriched with the possibility of representing, for each unit of information (action, property or value; henceforth *IU*)

(1) the time t_P and the author A_P of the proposal;
(2) (if accepted) the time t_A and the author (supervisor) A_A of the acceptance.

Since in many cases IU are described in terms of their components, the treatment of *composite* IU deserves specific attention. Suppose, for instance, that an action A in a guideline G has been described (at the time t_0 when the guideline has been originally entered) as the sequence of two sub-actions A_1 and A_2, and that, at time t_1, an update has been made in the properties of A_2. In such a case, we would like to propagate along the *composed-by* chain the update, stating that also the super-action A has been updated at time t_1. This bottom-up propagation needs to be applied recursively along the whole chain to all the super-actions of A, and has been made explicit in our approach for the sake of clarity.

In order to support the history of IU, we associate two temporally ordered lists of pairs <t,A> to each IU: the *TP* list for the proposals and the *TA* list for the acceptances. Rejected proposals are physically deleted. Such an extended model is paired with the definition of two primitive functions, *insert* and *update* (we model *delete* operations as updates where no new value is substituted to the old one), which properly operate on the data model, by inserting/modifying the IU, updating their TP and TA lists, and, if necessary, propagating the update to the TP and TA lists of the upper IU in the *composed-by* chain.

In the following, we exemplify our approach via the abstract example in figure 1, in which the history of the sample guideline records the changes below:

(0) The *initial* situation is modelled by the bold part of figure 1. We suppose we have a (part of a) guideline which, at the time t_0 of acquisition, is composed by an action A, which has a property P with value v, and is composed by A1 (with property P1 with value v1) and A2 (with property P2 having value v2). Let $S=\{S1\}$ the set of supervisors, and $U=\{U1,U2,U3\}$ the set of practitioners. In particular, notice that, by default, in the initial situation, proposal and acceptance times exactly correspond

(1) At time t_1, practitioner U1 proposes to change the value of property P1 to v1'. This results in: (i) adding the $<t_1,U_1>$ pair to the TP list of P1; (ii) inserting the new IU P1=v1', with TP equal to $<t_1,U_1>$; (iii) propagating the proposal of update to A1 and A, so that the $<t_1,U_1>$ is also appended to the TP lists of A and of A1.

(2) At time t_2, the supervisor S1 accepts the above update. This results in adding the $<t_2,S_1>$ pair to the TA list of P1, A1 and A.

(3) At time t_3, practitioner U2 proposes to insert a new property P3 to A2, with value v3. This results in adding the IU P3=v3 in A2 and appending $<t_3,U_2>$ at the end of the TP lists of P3, A2 and A.

(4) Finally, the acceptance at time t_4 of the proposal in t_3 leads to the final situation shown in figure 1.

A   {TP: **<t$_0$,S1>**,<t$_1$,U1>,<t$_3$,U2> # TA: **<t$_0$,S1>**,<t$_2$,S1>,<t$_4$,S1>}
P=v   {TP: **<t$_0$,S1> # TA : <t$_0$,S1>**}

     A1   {TP: **<t$_0$,S1>**,<t$_1$,U1> # TA: **<t$_0$,S1>**,<t$_2$,S1>}
     P1=v1   {TP: **<t$_0$,S1>**,<t$_1$,U1> # TA: **<t$_0$,S1>**}
     P1=v1'   {TP: <t$_1$,U1>; <TA : < t$_2$,S1>}

     A2   {TP: **<t$_0$,S1>**,<t$_3$,U2> # TA: **<t$_0$,S1>**,<t$_4$,S1>}
     P2=v2   {TP: **<t$_0$,S1> # TA: <t$_0$,S1>**}
     P3=v3   {TP: <t$_3$,U2>#TA : <t$_4$,S1>}

Fig. 1. Internal representation of the history of a (simplified) guideline. Boldface text describes the initial situation (at time t_0)

Notice that our data model proposal is deliberately a general one, so that it can be implemented both in a relational and in an object-oriented DB.

On the basis of the above data model, different types of information can be extracted about the guideline history, considering (i) the *status* of the IUs (proposed vs accepted), (ii) the *authors* of the proposals/acceptances, and (iii) their *time*. These three dimensions are mostly independent, so that the different combinations of their values provide a powerful and extended three-dimensional space of possible types of queries. In the following, we propose some examples, considering the IU in Figure 1.

Q1: Give me the current description of A2.
STATUS={accepted}; AUTHOR={any Supervisor}; TIME=NOW;
      A2.P2=v2   A2.P3=v3

Q2: Give me the description of A2 at time t_0.
STATUS={accepted}; AUTHOR={any Supervisor}; TIME= t_0;
      A2.P2=v2

Q3: Give me the update proposals regarding A made by U1 or U2 in the period $[t_0,t_2]$
STATUS={proposed}; AUTHOR={U1,U2}; TIME=$[t_0,t_2]$;
      A1 part-of A; A1.P1=v1 ➔ A1.P1=v1'
Note. The updates to A1 are taken into account since A1 is part of A.

Q4: Give me the history of (acceptances regarding) A
  STATUS={accepted}; AUTHOR={ any Supervisor}; TIME= "all-time"
      At time t_0:   A.P=v A1 part-of A; A1.P1=v1 A2 part-of A; A2.P2=v2
      At time t_2:   A1 part-of A; A1.P1=v1 ➔ A1.P1=v1'
      At time t_4:   A2 part-of A; added A2.P3=v3

4 Comparisons, and Future Work

In this paper, we have proposed a system-independent approach to guideline upgrade adaptation, considering authoring and versioning issues.

Several approaches in the literature have focused on clinical guideline adaptation.
As concerns the adaptation based on resources availability, Shahar et al. [8] have proposed to manage a high level description of the guideline's intentions, in order to ensure the adaptability of the procedure to different contexts still preserving the guideline's intentional objectives. Such an approach has been followed in CAMINO (see [4]). [1] suggested an approach in which the dependencies between actions in a guideline can be explicitly described, and where users' modifications to a general guideline must respect these dependencies. [6] proposes a versioning approach that records the reasons for changes and uses queries to summarize changes by grouping them by concept or relationship type. To the best of our knowledge, however, none of the approaches in the computer guideline literature take into account the distinction between different levels of authors (general practitioners vs supervisors), and manages in a general an principled way the "history" of guideline updates, which are the core of our contribution.

Our approach is also innovative with respect to the area of Temporal Databases (TDB). In particular, although the distinction between time of *proposal* and time of *acceptance* resemble TDB's distinction between *transaction* and *valid* time [9], and many approaches to DB schema versioning have been proposed [7], there seems to be no counterpart of our two-level treatment of authoring and of our management of proposal/acceptance times in the TDB literature.

In the future, we are planning to extend GLARE (Guideline Acquisition, Representation and Execution), a computer-based manager of clinical guidelines [10], [11] in order to offer the facilities described in this paper.

References

[1] Boxwala, A.A., Applying axiomatic design methodology to create guidelines that are locally adaptable. Proc. AMIA 2002 (2002)
[2] Cabana, M.D. , Rand, C.S.N.R. Powe, C.S., Wu, A.W., Wilson, M.H., Abboud, P.C., Rubin, H.R.: Why don't physicians follow clinical practice guidelines? A framework for improvement. JAMA 282(15) (1999) 1458-1465
[3] Fridsma, D.B. (Guest ed.): Special Issue on Workflow Management and Clinical Guidelines. AIM Journal, 22(1) (2001) 1-80
[4] Fridsma, D.B., Gennari, J.H., Musen, M.A.: Making generic guidelines site-specific. Proc. AMIA 1996 (1996) 597-601
[5] Gordon, C., Christensen, J.P.: Health Telematics for Clinical Guidelines and Protocols, IOS Press (1995)
[6] Peleg, M., Kantor, R.: Approaches for Guideline Versioning using GLIF, Proc. AMIA 2003 (2003) 509-513
[7] Roddik, J.F.: A survey of Schema Versioning Issues for Database Systems. Information and Software Technology 37(7) (1995) 383-393
[8] Shahar, Y., Miksch, S., Johnson, P.: An intention-based language for representing clinical guidelines. Proc AMIA 1996 (1996) 592-596
[9] Snodgrass, R.T., Ahn, I.: "Temporal Databases", IEEE Computer 19(9) (1986) 35-42
[10] Terenziani, P., Molino, G., Torchio, M.: A Modular Approach for Representing and Executing Clinical Guidelines. Artificial Intelligence in Medicine 23 (2001) 249-276
[11] P. Terenziani, S. Montani, A. Bottrighi, M. Torchio, G. Molino, G. Correndo, A context-adaptable approach to clinical guidelines. Proc. MEDINFO'04, M. Fieschi et al. (eds), Amsterdam, IOS Press (2004) 169-173

Open-Source Publishing of Medical Knowledge for Creation of Computer-Interpretable Guidelines

Mor Peleg[1], Rory Steele[2], Richard Thomson[2,3], Vivek Patkar[2], Tony Rose[2], and John Fox[2,3]

[1] Department of Management Information Systems, University of Haifa, 31905, Israel
morpeleg@mis.hevra.haifa.ac.il
[2] Advanced Computation Laboratory, Cancer Research UK,
Lincoln Inn fields, London,
WC2A 3PX, UK
{rs, vp, tr, jf}@acl.icnet.uk
[3] OpenClinical
rt@openclinical.org
www.openclinical.org

Abstract. Guidelines, care pathways, and other representations of high quality clinical practice can now be formalized and distributed in executable form. It is widely recognized that the ability to apply knowledge at the point of care creates an opportunity to influence clinicians' behavior, encouraging compliance with evidence-based standards and improving care quality. The ability to share formal knowledge may also enable the medical community to build on work done by others and reduce content development costs. We propose a Medical Knowledge Repository and content model that supports assembly of components into new applications. Some types of resources that may be included in such a repository are defined, and a frame-based representation for indexing and structuring the components is described. The domain of breast cancer is used as a case study for demonstrating the feasibility of the approach.

1 Introduction

A number of studies of computer applications that can deliver patient-specific clinical knowledge to the point of care during patient encounters have shown positive impacts on clinicians behavior [1]. Since developing such resources requires much effort, we would like to be able to share them, enabling the community of clinical guideline developers, publishers, and users to work collaboratively, leveraging prior work.

There are several potential ways for sharing medical knowledge that is in a computer-interpretable format. One way is to permit multiple formalisms to exist and to translate between different representation formalisms, as required. This appears to be infeasible based on the experience of the InterMed project [2].

A second option is to adopt a single standard. The HL7 Clinical Guidelines Special Interest Group (CGSIG) is engaged in a process of developing and standardizing components of a standard computer-interpretable guideline (CIG) model. Standardizing CIG components would enable sharing of significant parts of encoded guidelines across different CIG modeling methods. The selection of CGSIG components was influenced by the results of a study that compared CIG formalisms in terms of components that capture the structure of CIGs [3].

A third way to facilitate sharing of computer-interpretable (CI) components of medical knowledge is to create a library of resources that could be used as components for developing executable guidelines. Guideline developers can use this Medical Knowledge Repository (MedKR) to assemble guidelines from CI knowledge components. The idea is similar to Common Object Request Broker Architecture (CORBA) [4], an open, vendor-independent architecture and infrastructure that computer applications use to work together over networks. Similar architectures, which address interoperability of components defined by different standards, security and administration challenges, include Web Services Architecture (WSA) [5] and Semantic Web Services Framework (SWSF) [6]. The knowledge components would be units of operational software that deliver specific functionality (and may include data relevant to the function being delivered). The components will share a common interface for specifying the operation that is performed and its arguments. In this way, a client object could request an operation to be performed on a server, with appropriate parameters, which would perform the operation and return the results to the client.

2 Executable Medical Resources That Could Be Shared

Many types of medical resources could be published and later used to assemble executable CIGs. A few examples include:

1. Medical calculators (e.g., http://www.medalreg.com/; http://www-users.med.cornell.edu/~spon/picu/calc/)
2. Risk-assessment tools (e.g., http://www.yourdiseaserisk.harvard.edu/),
3. Drug databases (http://www.medscape.com/druginfo),
4. Controlled terminologies (e.g., SNOMED-CT http://www.snomed.org/),
5. Authoring, validation, and execution tools for CIGs [7]

How might we create a CIG, care pathway, or other application by bringing subsets of such a wide variety of resources together in a single application?

Components may exhibit different granularities. For example, medical calculators may be shared by linking them as nodes within a CIG's task network. In this way, any CIG formalism that conforms to the task network model [3], such as Asbru, EON, GLIF3, GUIDE, PRODIGY, or PRO*forma* may call upon predefined components. On the other hand, components may be shared at finer granularity. For example, different CIG formalisms might use the same expression language to express decision and eligibility criteria, and may refer to the same patient data model, which may be different than the expression language and patient model that their CIG formalism uses.

Figure 1 shows an example of our proposed component definition for sharability and interoperability. It includes input and output types, which can be conventional data types or semantic types that are defined in an external ontology. The definitions of CORBA components and Web services descriptions have been extended by developing a frame-based representation that includes, in addition to the above-mentioned attributes, attributes by which the resources could be indexed and organized in a repository. One of these is the component's *goal* — a semantic type based on an ontology originally developed for the breast cancer domain [8], which includes about 20 general classes of goals, broadly categorized as knowledge goals and action goals. Currently, most of these semantic types contain only a "goal sentence", which is free text, but some semantic types also have additional slots. Work is under way to structure the goal sentence [9], and to suggest a restricted vocabulary for coding.

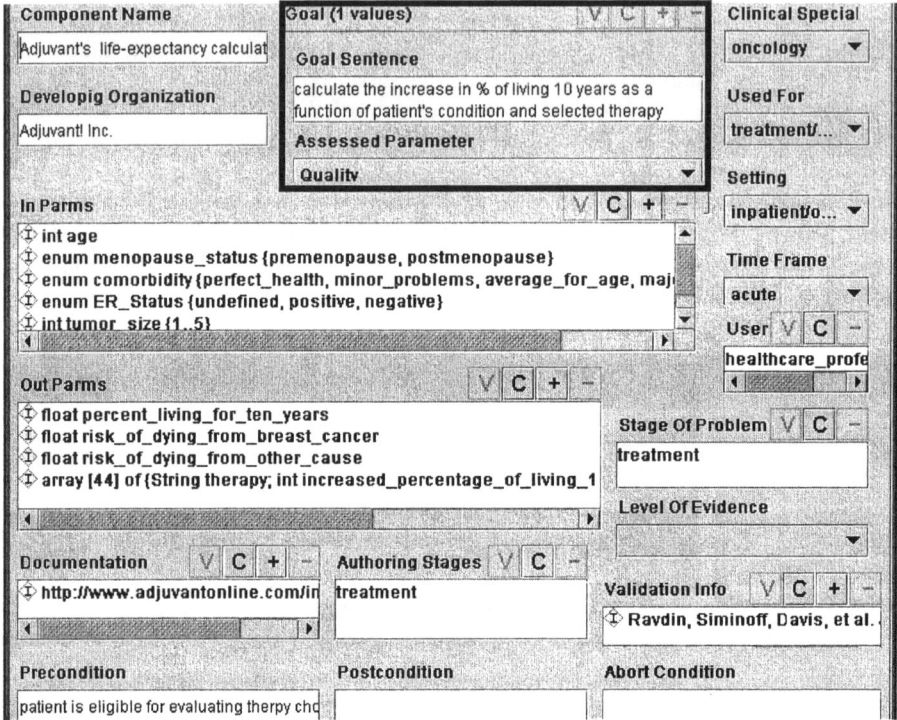

Fig. 1. The interface of Adjuvant's life-expectancy calculator specified as a frame using the Protégé-2000 knowledge modeling tool. Input and output parameters are specified as instances of the well-defined Parameter_Definition class hierarchy, which consists of classes for simple and complex parameters and for enumerated types. In the figure, only the short names for the parameters are shown

The goal shown in Fig. 1 is of type Assessment and has a slot called "assessed_parameter" which can hold the following symbols: urgency, need, risk, quality. Additional attributes describe the clinical sub-domain that the component addresses. They are taken from a schema for indexing CIGs that was developed by Bernstam and colleagues [10] and is an extension of the classification scheme used by the National Guideline Clearinghouse. Additional attributes include pre- and post- and abort-conditions for using the component, the authoring stage at which the component could be used, information about the component's developers, version, pointers to documentation, the level of evidence supporting the component, and information on how the component has been validated, including pointers to test cases.

Components can be indexed and searched based on their attributes. Especially useful are attributes that specify the clinical sub-domain, the relevant authoring stages, and goals.

Components could be assembled into CIGs by specifying the guideline's skeleton into which components can be integrated. When a CIG engine that enacts the skeletal CIG formalism calls a component, it passes control to a broker that acts as an interface between the engine and the MedKR, passing parameter values and returning results. The broker will have services for converting vocabulary terms, measurement units, and data-type casting.

3 Case Study Example

We have chosen guidelines in the domain of breast cancer to test the applicability of these proposals. This is a good area because knowledge in the domain is abundant, evidence-based, and structured. Figure 2 shows an example of a PRO*forma* CIG that call external components: Adjuvant's life expectancy calculator, which calculates the density of breast masses from radiographs (www.adjuvantonline. com), and Gail's breast cancer risk assessment module (http://www2.swmed.edu/breastcarisk/).

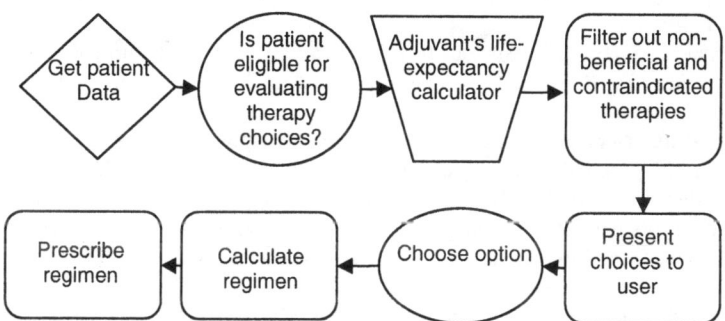

Fig. 2. A PRO*forma* CIG that provides advice on regimens for treating breast cancer. The CIG includes an external *component* (trapezoid), whose interface definition is given in Fig. 1. Different types of native PRO*forma* tasks are shown: *enquiry* (diamond), *decision* (circle), and *plan* (round-cornered square)

4 Discussion

A repository of executable medical knowledge components that would be published on the Web would enable guideline developers to piece together CIGs from components that have been independently developed and tested. In this paper, we suggested a framework for specifying the interface of executable components so that they could be searched for and integrated within a CIG specification. Unlike publets, which are encoded solely in the PRO*forma* formalism, our approach permits a CIG to be encoded in any CIG formalism, integrating components written in different formalisms. We hope that the notion of creating a repository of tested knowledge components and

CIGs would be appealing to the community of content developers, and developers of CIG formalisms. We hope developers and researchers will contribute components and tested CIGs to the MedKR. We are currently working on implementing a simple guideline using our approach

References

1. Shea S, DuMouchel W, Bahamonde L. A Meta-analysis of 16 Randomized Controlled Trials to Evaluate Computer-based Clinical Reminder Systems for Preventative Care in the Ambulatory Setting. J Am Med Inform Assoc 1996;3(6):399-409.
2. Peleg M, Boxwala AA, Tu S, Zeng Q, Ogunyemi O, Wang D, et al. The InterMed Approach to Sharable Computer-interpretable Guidelines: A Review. J Am Med Inform Assoc 2004;11(1):1-10.
3. Peleg M, Tu SW, Bury J, Ciccarese P, Fox J, Greenes RA, et al. Comparing Computer-Interpretable Guideline Models: A Case-Study Approach. J Am Med Inform Assoc 2003;10(1):52-68.
4. Siegel J. CORBA 3 Fundamentals and Programming, 2nd Edition: John Wiley & Sons; 2000.
5. W3C. Web Services Architecture. Champion M, Ferris C, Newcomer E, Orchard D, editors. 14 November 2002 ed: W3C; 2002.http://www.w3.org/TR/2002/WD-ws-arch-20021114/
6. Domingue J, Cabral L, Hakimpour F, Sell D, Motta E. -III: A Platform and Infrastructure for Creating WSMO-based Semantic Web Services. Proc Workshop on WSMO Implementations 2004.
7. Clercq PAd, Blom JA, Korsten HH, Hasman A. Approaches for creating computer-interpretable guidelines that facilitate decision support. Artif Intell Med 2004;31(1):1-27.
8. Fox J, Alabassi A, Black E, Hurt C, Rose T. Modelling Clinical Goals: a Corpus of Example and a Tentative Ontology. Proc Symp Comput Guidelines and Protocols 2004: 31-45.
9. Fox J, Alabassi A, Patkar V, Rose T, Black E. An ontological approach to modelling tasks and goals. Comput in Biol & Med, in press 2004.
10. Bernstam E, Ash N, Peleg M, Tu S, Boxwala AA, Mork P, et al. Guideline classification to assist modeling, authoring, implementation and retrieval. Proc AMIA Symp. 2000: 66-70.

A History-Based Algebra for Quality-Checking Medical Guidelines*

Arjen Hommersom, Peter Lucas, Patrick van Bommel, and Theo van der Weide

Department of Information and Knowledge Systems,
Nijmegen Institute for Computing and Information Sciences,
Radboud University Nijmegen

Abstract. In this paper, we propose a formal theory to describe the development of medical guideline text in detail, but at a sufficiently high level abstraction, in such way that essential elements of the guidelines are highlighted. We argue that because of the fragmentary nature of medical guidelines, an approach where details in guideline text are omitted is justified. The different aspects of a guideline are illustrated and discussed by a number of examples from the Dutch breast cancer guideline. Furthermore, we discuss how the theory can be used to detect flaws in the guideline text at an early stage in the guideline development process and consequently can be used to improve the quality of medical guidelines.

1 Introduction

In order to control and improve the quality of medical care, organisations of medical professionals, such as medical specialists and nursing staff, are increasingly making use of evidence-based medical guidelines [8]. The goal of our work is to develop a representation of a guideline in detail, but at a sufficiently high level abstraction, in such way that essential elements of the guidelines are highlighted. As the ultimate aim is to verify properties and to study the quality of medical guidelines, the theory is necessarily formal in nature.

A major problem in achieving the ends mentioned above is that guidelines are fragmentary, which renders it hard to formalise them, as one way or the other, the gaps have to be filled in, or the modelling language should allow omitting detail. The former approach is often used in guideline modelling languages such as Asbru [6] and GLIF [5] which represents a guideline as a program-like structure. In that case, program verification techniques can be used to investigate properties of the original guideline. In this article, we take the latter approach, which is the main reason why we have decided to abstract from the details of a guideline text. Other, more logical oriented approaches such as PRO*forma* [2], which also allow fragmentary formalisation of guidelines are different in the sense that we concentrate on the medical knowledge concerning patient-groups and ultimately on the composition of a guideline rather than the decision making. This results in different design choices.

---

* This work has been partially supported by the European Commission's IST program, under contract number IST-FP6-508794 PROTOCURE II.

2 Framework for Modelling Medical Guidelines

2.1 Basic Elements

Time. Time is used in a guideline to model the changes in situation of the patient and its environment. Research has shown that an imprecise time axis is sufficient in most cases. However, sometimes guidelines are more specific and actually give reasonably precise time frames, but only in a limited number of cases medical science is as precise as physics. Hence, a formalisation of time should allow for an extension of the cause-consequence relationship. Consequently, we assume there is a set Time and a relation $\preceq$: Time × Time such that $\preceq$ is reflexive and transitive, i.e., $\preceq$ is a pre-order. Note that $\preceq$ is not anti-symmetric in general, because there can very well be different descriptions of the same points in time. Moreover, we do not assume that this ordering is known, but in general there are known constraints with respect to this order.

State. A state can provide a description of the actual situation of a patient given all known facts and more general situations of individual patients. The traditional technique to abstract from a certain situation (a model) is by providing a logical language that refers to one or more situations without fixing all the details. Typical elements in the state of a patient are symptoms, signs and other *measurable* elements. Because many of these elements are unknown and often irrelevant we have chosen to define the state space as a many-sorted first order logic State including equality, but excluding any free variables. Let there be a structure $\mathcal{A}$ consisting of a domain for every sort σ and an interpretation I of every constant of a given sort to the domain of this sort such that $I(c_i^\sigma) \neq I(c_j^{\sigma'})$ where $i \neq j$ or $\sigma \neq \sigma'$, i.e., we assume unique names. Let State be a language built up inductively consisting of terms and propositional connectives in the traditional manner (see for example [3]) such that elements of State can be interpreted on the structure. For example, typically temperature = 37 ∨ systolic-blood-presure = 120 is an element of State. Note that in the upcoming sections we will leave the different sorts implicit.

Intervention. Interventions include medical actions that influence the condition or the environment of a patient. The domain of interventions is formalised as a countable set Interventions. The interpretation of a subset of the Interventions is a treatment where each intervention is applied, either in sequence or in parallel. Furthermore, we have a closed-world assumption for each set of interventions I which says that if $i \notin I$, then intervention i is not applied.

2.2 Histories

A medical guideline contains descriptions of processes concerning the disease, medical management and recommendations. Static descriptions of the different aspects of patient groups as we have described above are captured in a history.

Let $\wp(X)$ denote the powerset of X and let $[V \to W]$ denote the function space of functions $f : V \to (W \cup \{\epsilon\})$, where ϵ will have the interpretation 'undefined'. Let a time constraint be of the form $t \preceq t'$ or $t \not\preceq t'$. A model of a set of constraints is a total pre-order. A history is defined as an element of the set History such that History = [Time → (State × $\wp$(Intervention))] in combination with a set of time constraints $\mathcal{C}$.

The examples we present here were extracted from a medical guideline regarding breast cancer by CBO [1], an institute that has supported the development of most of the guidelines developed so far by the Dutch medical specialists.

Example 1. After a mastectomy or breast-conserving treatment, there is an increased risk of movement problems, impaired sensation, pain, and lymphoedema. Adjuvant radiotherapy increases the risk of limited movement of the shoulder and of lymphoedema. Physiotherapeutic intervention can have a positive effect on the recovery of mobility and functionality of the shoulder joint. Early initiation of intensive remedial therapy (in other words, during the first postoperative week) has an unfavourable effect on the wound drainage volume and duration.

There are several possible ways to formalize this excerpt depending on the focus of the modeller. One possibility is to pick some patient-group, for example the patient-group which receives physiotherapy too early after the mastectomy. We can denote this history h algebraically as follows.

$h = \{(t_0, \text{breast cancer}, \varnothing), (t_1, \text{breast cancer}, \{\text{mastectomy}\}), (t_2, \text{lymphoedema},$
$\varnothing), (t_3, \text{lymphoedema}, \{\text{physiotherapy}\}), (t_4, \text{high drainage}, \varnothing)\}$

Note that these elements of Time do not express anything about the *distance* between the time points. So the distance between t_0 and t_1 is not necessarily the same distance as the distance between t_1 and t_2. In addition to being imprecise about certain patients it also allows us to 'instantiate' patients of a certain patient-group by adding patient-specific information to this history.

2.3 Expectations

When dealing with guidelines, we are concerned with the dynamic aspect, for example, the description of how a history is *expected* to continue. As a consequence, this means that the history is extended with new information. A typical example is an expectation of a treatment, i.e., the expected history that a certain treatment yields. We formalise this notion below.

Given a history h and h' then h' is an extension of h iff $dom(h) \subseteq dom(h')$ and for all $t \in$ Time: $h(t) \neq \epsilon$ implies $h(t) = h'(t)$. The projection of a history h to two elements $i, j \in$ Time, denoted as $\langle h \rangle_{(i,j)}$, is defined as the history h' such that: (1) $dom(h') \subseteq dom(h)$, (2) for all $t \in$ Time: $h(t) \neq \epsilon$ implies $h(t) = h'(t)$ and, (3) $t \in dom(h') \Rightarrow i \preceq t \preceq j$. Obviously, a history is always an extension of a projection on itself. The expected continuation of a given history is the function space E = [History → $\wp$(History)] such that for each $e \in$ E and $h \in$ History the following hold: (1) $e(h) \neq \{h\}$ (the expectation introduces new information), (2) $h' \in e(h) \Rightarrow h'$ is an extension of h (no information is lost) and, (3) let $m \in min(dom(h)), M \in max(dom(h)), i \geq M$: $e(h) \supseteq \bigcup_{h' \in e(h)} e(\langle h' \rangle_{m,i})$ (the expectation function is consistent with respect to its own expectations). For example, consider a patient with breast cancer p where $p = \{(t_1, \text{breast cancer}, \{\text{chemo-therapy}\})\}$. The use of chemo-therapy can cause an infection, which we can describe as an expectation $e(p) = \{h\}$ where $h = \{(t_1, \text{breast cancer}, \{\text{chemo-therapy}\}), (t_2, \text{infection}, \varnothing)\}$. Note that this is of course a rather naive example, because in this case we can, by definition of an expectation function, deduce that $e(e(p)) = e(p)$. In a more realistic setting, more alternatives would be listed, such that this simple relation does not hold.

3 Application to Fragments of Medical Guidelines

As an application to check the quality of a guideline we consider its consistency. Because of the commitment of guideline developers to produce high quality guidelines, we do not expect to find blatant inconsistencies within a guideline. Nonetheless, it is expected that during the process of developing guidelines different views on how the patient should be treated are considered. Clearly, in many cases these views will be inconsistent and it is therefore of great use to detect these inconsistencies.

Every country typically develops their own version of a guideline about similar subjects. Therefore, we have the possibility to simulate the process as described above by comparing recommendations of different guidelines. We have chosen to compare the Dutch CBO guideline with the Scottish SIGN guideline for breast cancer [7]. Consider chapter 13.2 of this guideline concerning local recurrence in the axilla after mastectomy.

Example 2. nodule(s)/nodes should be excised (...) and if not previously irradiated, locoregional radiotherapy should be given.

Thus, the following patient-group is consistent, and it can be argued this is implied by a closed world assumption that is taken to hold in many medical applications, with the SIGN guideline:

$h = \{(t_0, \text{breast cancer}, \{\text{mastectomy}\}), (t_1, \text{breast cancer}, \{\text{radiotherapy}\}),$
$\quad (t_2, \neg\text{breast cancer}, \varnothing), (t_3, \text{breast cancer}, I)\}$

such that $t_0 \prec t_1 \prec t_2 \prec t_3$ and radiotherapy $\notin I$. The more recent CBO guideline discusses the local treatment of local recurrence following modified radical mastectomy.

Example 3. If an isolated local recurrence occurs in a previously irradiated area, high-dose radiotherapy is not an option. In that case, low-dose re-radiation with hyperthermia is the treatment of choice.

Hence, in this case we find that there are patient-groups which are treated taking this guideline into account described by:

$h' = \{(t_0, \text{breast cancer}, \{\text{mastectomy}\}), (t_1, \text{breast cancer}, \{\text{radiotherapy}\}),$
$\quad (t_2, \neg\text{breast cancer}, \varnothing), (t_3, \text{breast cancer}, \{\text{radiotherapy}, \text{hyperthermia}\})\}$

such that $t_0 \prec t_1 \prec t_2 \prec t_3$. Hence, we find by definition that h and h' are inconsistent. In particular, we find that these fragments are inconsistent with respect to their interventions.

4 Discussion

We have presented a framework for quality-checking of medical guidelines. Use was made of algebraic theory and insights that we have gained during formalisation of a part of the Dutch breast cancer guideline. In our previous work [4], a method was presented for verifying parts of a medical guideline using temporal logic and abduction in the context of theorem proving. The framework presented here allows for more realistic and elaborate modelling of the guideline, while preserving the advantages of a formal model such as the possibility to use abduction and automated theorem proving for its verification.

Like in many other guideline description languages, time has a central role in our approach. There are important differences however. One of the main differences is that time is inherently less precise than in other languages. For example, in PRO*forma* or Asbru, to refer to imprecise time points, one must use time intervals. However, these intervals are defined by exact time points and while this is imperative to create a task hierarchy or even to schedule the tasks in a consistent manner, we argue it is not imperative to have this information to check many of the quality criteria of a medical guideline.

In our future work we will extend the theory in a number of ways. Firstly, more high-level methods are being developed that allow the characterization of a history, either by embedding histories in a logical language or by defining certain patterns in histories, e.g., a history with a monotonically increasing parameter. Secondly, we will work towards establishing a formal relation between histories, or expectations that people have of treatment and processes that occur within a patient on one hand and recommendations on the other, i.e., the construction of a guideline.

References

1. CBO. *Richtlijn Behandeling van het mammacarcinoom.* van Zuiden, 2002.
2. J. Fox and S. Das. *Safe and Sound - Artificial Intelligence in Hazardous Applications.* The MIT Press, 2000.
3. W. Hodges. Elementary predicate logic. In Gabbay D.M. and Guenthner F., editors, *Handbook of philosophical logic*, volume 1, pages 1–129. Kluwer Academic Publishers, 2nd edition, 2001.
4. A.J. Hommersom, P.J.F. Lucas, and M. Balser. Meta-level verification of the quality of medical guidelines using interactive theorem proving. In J. J. Alferes and J. Leite, editors, *Logics in Artificial Intelligence, JELIA'04*, volume 3225 of *LNAI*, pages 654–666, Heidelberg, 2004. Springer-Verlag.
5. L. Ohno-Machado, J. Gennari, and S. Murphy. Guideline interchange format: a model for representing guidelines. *Journal of the American Medical Informatics Association*, 5(4):357–372, 1998.
6. Y. Shahar, S. Miksch, and P. Johnson. The asgaard project: a task-specific framework for the application and critiquing of time-oriented clinical guidelines. *Artificial Intelligence in Medicine*, 14:29–51, 1998.
7. SIGN. *Breast Cancer in Women.* SIGN, 1998.
8. S.H. Woolf. Evidence-based medicine and practice guidelines: an overview. *Cancer Control*, 7(4):362–367, 2000.

The Spock System: Developing a Runtime Application Engine for Hybrid-Asbru Guidelines

Ohad Young and Yuval Shahar

Medical Informatics Research Center,
Department of Information Systems Engineering,
Ben Gurion University, Beer Sheva84105, Israel
{ohadyn, yshahar}@bgumail.bgu.ac.il
http://medinfo.ise.bgu.ac.il/medlab/

Abstract. Clinical Guidelines are a major tool for improving the quality of medical care. A major current research direction is automating the application of guidelines at the point of care. To support that automation, several requirements must be fulfilled, such as specification in a machine-interpretable format, and connection to an electronic patent record. We propose an innovative approach to guideline application, which capitalizes on our *Digital electronic Guidelines Library (DeGeL)*. The DeGeL framework includes a new hybrid model for incremental specification of free-text guidelines, using several intermediate representations. The new approach was implemented, in the case of the Asbru guideline ontology, as the *Spock* system. Spock's hybrid application engine supports the application of guidelines represented at an intermediate format. Spock uses the IDAN mediator for answering complex queries referred to heterogeneous clinical data repositories. Spock was evaluated in a preliminary fashion by applying several guidelines to sample patient data.

1 Introduction

Clinical practice guidelines are a powerful method for standardized improvement of medical care quality, and sometimes even the survival of patients [1]. Clinical guidelines are most useful at the point of care [2]. However, care-providers, overloaded with information rarely have the time, nor the computational means, to assist them in utilizing the valuable knowledge of free-text guidelines, during treatment. Therefore, there is a pressing need to facilitate the automation of guideline-based care.

During the past 20 years, there have been several efforts to support complex guideline-based care over time in automated fashion. An excellent comparative review of most current approaches to the support of complex guideline-based care is provided by Peleg et al.'s [3] and de Clercq et al.'s [4] comprehensive paper

An effective framework for support of automated application of clinical guidelines must address several key requirements [2] such as: (1) formal specification of guidelines, to enable interpretation by computers; (2) reuse of encoded guidelines achieved through the sue of standard terms originating from controlled medical vocabularies; (3) access of patient data electronically, to apply a formal guideline to a particular patient in an automated fashion; (4) smooth integration with the local clinical host systems; (5) ability to store the runtime application state, to support episodic guideline application over extended periods, and various documentation and legal needs.

1.1 The DeGeL Guideline-Automation Framework

Typically guideline-application systems require as input a guideline in a formal format. However, most guidelines are in free text, and their conversion to a formal format is a highly complex and time consuming task [2].

To gradually convert clinical guidelines to formal representations we have developed a *hybrid* (i.e., one that has multiple representation formats co-existing simultaneously), multifaceted representation, and an accompanying distributed computational architecture, the *Digital electronic Guideline Library* (*DeGeL*) [5]. The conversion process intertwines the expertise of both the expert physician and knowledge engineer to gracefully convert guidelines from free-text through semi-structured and semi-formal (i.e., intermediate representations) to a formal representation format. Thus, the output of the guideline conversion process is a *hybrid representation* which contains, for each guideline, or even for different knowledge roles within the same guideline, a mixture of the above formats and a pointer to the original textual source.

In addition, the DeGeL specification tools are linked to a set of controlled medical vocabularies, which, in conjunction with a search and retrieval vocabulary engine, enable the author of the guideline to embed in it standard terms originating from international medical-terminology standards (e.g., SNOMED).

1.2 The Hybrid Asbru Guideline-Specification Language

The default ontology for guideline specification in DeGeL is the Asbru ontology [6]. Hence, a hybrid version of it, *Hybrid-Asbru,* was defined according to the structure of DeGeL's hybrid-guideline model. The Hybrid-Asbru guideline ontology includes all of Asbru's knowledge-roles. Each semantically meaningful knowledge role (e.g., *Intentions*) contains a slot for the semi-structured content. In addition, more complex structures, which adhere to formal Asbru, were created to store the content of the semi-formal format. For example, *temporal-patterns,* the building blocks of a guideline in Asbru, are expressed using combinations of text, logical operators (e.g., AND, OR) and time-annotations.

2 The Spock Hybrid Runtime Guideline Application System

We propose a new approach for supporting application of clinical guidelines in an automated fashion, which capitalizes on our work in the DeGeL project. We introduce the *Spock* system, an architecture aimed to assist a care provider in application of guidelines, specified using Hybrid-Asbru ontology, over long time periods at the point of care. It is designed to support the application process to some extent, regardless of the guideline's representation level. It is also designed to conduct a practical dialog with the care-provider, regardless of whether an Electronic Patient Record (EPR) exists. Naturally, the services offered by Spock improve as the level of sophistication of the knowledge and data representation increases. The application model of Spock is *hybrid* in two senses: (1) The guideline representation level – due to DeGeL's hybrid representation model, a candidate guideline for application can be in a variety of representation levels; (2) The availability of an EPR– unfortunately, the patient data required for guideline application is not always available electronically.

The two dimensions of the hybrid application model imply four possible scenarios for applying guidelines. Although application of guidelines in a fully-automated fashion is feasible only when the guideline is in a formal format, automated support to some extent can be provided to guidelines in any of the intermediate representation levels, especially when an EPR is not available. Although most of the decision making is carried out by a human agent rather than by a computerized one, the overall workload on the care-provider is significantly diminished, since the care-provider is not required to consult the original textual guideline. Since we expect most guidelines to be in intermediate representations within the near future, the current version of Spock focuses mainly on the scenarios of having an intermediate represented guideline with or without an EPR available.

The Spock client-server architecture relies on external resources for its operation such as: (1) a service for retrieving hybrid guidelines content from the DeGeL framework, (2) a service that can access heterogeneous clinical data repositories, available via the IDAN [7] architecture; and (3) a patient-data visualization and exploration tool, KNAVE-II [8].

2.1 The Spock Guideline Application Engine

For answering desideratum four, integration local clinical host systems, the guideline application engine was developed according to the *Model-View-Control (MVC)* design pattern, which enables the decoupling of the logic layer (i.e., Model), applying a Hybrid-Asbru guideline, from all other layers (e.g., data access and the presentation layers). For example, a customizable user interface (i.e., View), can be developed to meet specific demands at potential deployment sites without the need to recode the logic layer again. Albeit, the Spock system includes a default user interface (figure 1) developed mainly for testing purposes. Thus, the Spock guideline application engine consists of: (1) namespace of classes and interfaces encapsulating the semantics of how to apply a hybrid-Asbru guideline, for example a *ParallelPlanBody* class which handles the application of plan steps in parallel; (2) a parser for interpreting the content of a Hybrid-Asbru guideline which is in XML format; (3) a specialized module, the Controller, which synchronizes the communication between the system layers and external services (e.g., DeGeL).

For each application of a guideline, an *application-instance* is created. As the application proceeds, a *plan-instance* is created for every recommended subguideline (or plan) that is activated. The application process of each plan-instance follows the semantics of the Hybrid-Asbru ontology, for example Asbru's state transition model.

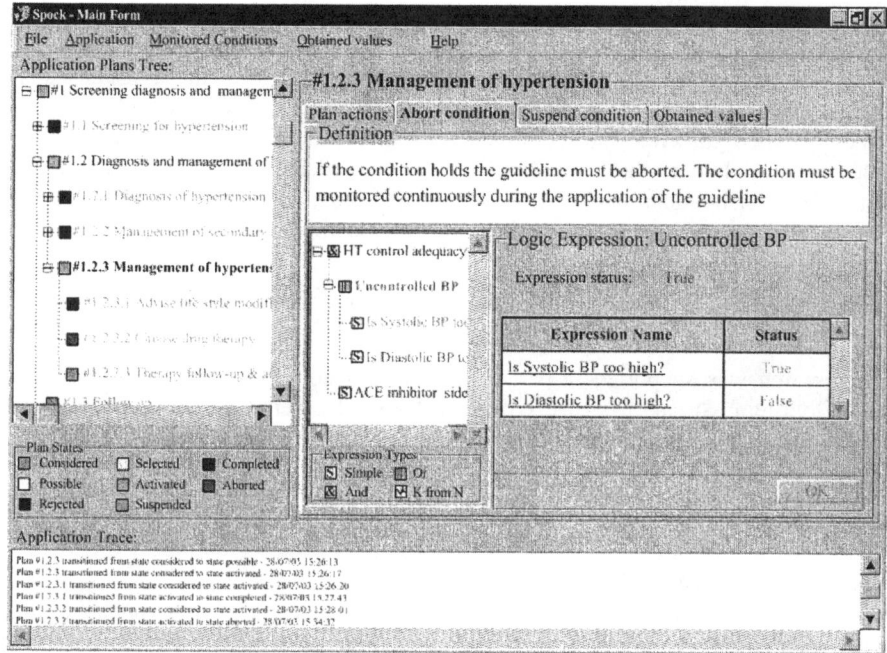

Fig. 1. The default graphical user interface (GUI) of the Spock system

2.2 Guideline Application Log

For answering desideratum five, storing the runtime application state, essential to the Spock system since its process of applying a guideline is a process spanning long time periods performed in an episodic fashion during patient's visits. The guideline application log contains several data structures for each application-instance such as: (1) state transitions of a plan-instance (e.g., *selected* → *activated* → *completed*), (2) list of all recommended plan-steps issued during application (e.g., order a certain lab test), and (3) list of obtained-values relevant for each plan-instance.

Thus, when resuming an application-instance which had been started previously, the history of its previous application sessions is retrieved in order to continue from the point last stopped at. Furthermore, other modules can benefit from the historical information, for example a retrospective quality-assessment module. Finally, the application log is stored on a centralized repository located on a remote server, accessible to any Spock client operated from a computer anywhere in the local network.

3 Preliminary Results

We have recently finished specifying several guidelines in various clinical domains (e.g., Endocrinology, Pulmonology and Gynecology) using the Hybrid-Asbru ontology, with medical collaborators from several medical centers associated with *Stanford University*, California, USA, and the *Ben-Gurion University*, Beer-Sheva, Israel. In addition, sample patient records, covering various options, for all specified guideline were prepared as well. The focus of the evaluation was to test the feasibility of applying guidelines represented in intermediate formats. Thus, with the assistance of a medical expert, a list of expected recommendations was prepared for each combination of specified guideline and set of patient simulated records. Meanwhile, the Spock system was applied to the same guidelines and simulated patient records. The expected recommendations list is then compared to Spock's output. The initial results were encouraging and we are currently in the process of a more formal evaluation.

Acknowledgments

This research was supported in part by NIH award no. LM-06806. We thank Drs. Mary Goldstein, Susana Martins, Lawrence Basso, Herbert Kaizer, Eitan Lunenfel, and Guy Bar, who were extremely helpful in assessing the various DeGeL tools.

References

1. Micieli, G., Cavallini, A., and Qauglini, S., *Guideline Compliance Improves Stroke Outcome - A Preliminary Study in 4 Districts in the Italian Region of Lombardia.* Stroke, 2002. **33**: p. 1341-7.
2. Zielstorff, R., *Online Practice Guidelines: Issues, Obstacles and Future Prospects.* Journal of the American Medical Informatics Association, 1998. **5**(3): p. 227-36.
3. Peleg, M., Tu, S., Bury, J., et al., *Comparing Computer-Interpretable Guideline Models: A Case-Study Approach.* Journal of the American Medical Informatics Association, 2003. **10**(1): p. 52-68.
4. de Clercq, P., Blom, J., Korsten, H., et al., *Approaches for creating computer-interpretable guidelines that facilitate decision support.* Artificial Intelligence in Medicine, 2004. **31**(1): p. 1-27.
5. Shahar, Y., Young, O., Shalom, E., et al., *A Framework for a Distributed, Hybrid, Multiple-Ontology Clinical-Guideline Library and Automated Guideline-Support Tools.* Journal of Biomedical Informatics, 2004. **37**(5): p. 325-44.
6. Miksch, S., Shahar, Y., and Johnson, P. *Asbru: A Task-Specific, Intention-Based, and Time-Oriented Language for Representing Skeletal Plans.* in *Proceedings of the 7th Workshop on Knowledge Engineering: Methods & Languages.* 1997: The Open University, Milton Keynes, UK.
7. Boaz, D. and Shahar, Y. *Idan: A distributed temporal-abstraction mediator for medical databases.* in *Proceedings of the 9th Conference on Artificial Intelligence in Medicine-Europe (AIME).* 2003.
8. Martins, S., Shahar, Y., Galperin, M., et al., *Evaluation of KNAVE-II: A tool for intelligent query and exploration of patient data.* Proceedings of Medinfo 2004, the 11th World Congress on Medical Informatics, 2004.

AI Planning Technology as a Component of Computerised Clinical Practice Guidelines

Kirsty Bradbrook[1], Graham Winstanley[1], David Glasspool[2], John Fox[2], and Richard Griffiths[1]

[1] School of Computing, Mathematical and Information Sciences, University of Brighton
[2] Advanced Computing Laboratory, Cancer Research UK

Abstract. The UK National Health Service (NHS) is currently undergoing an intensive review into the way patient care is designed, delivered and recorded. One important element of this is the development of care pathways (clinical guidelines) that provide a reasoned plan of care for each patient journey, based on locally-agreed, evidence-based best practice. The ability to generate, critique, and continually evaluate and modify plans of patient care is considered important and challenging, but in the case of computerised systems, the possibilities are exciting. In this paper we outline the case for incorporating AI Planning technology in the generation, evaluation and manipulation of care plans. We demonstrate that an integrative approach to its adoption in the clinical guideline domain is called for. The PRO*forma* Clinical Guideline Modelling Language is used to demonstrate the issues involved.

1 Introduction

AI techniques have been employed for many years in the medical domain to assist in decision support. However, one of the most heavily researched areas of AI – planning technology – has not seen widespread application in medical informatics. It is our contention that AI planning technology is eminently suitable for incorporation into medical IT systems that are intended to provide support to medical staff in generating, evaluating and manipulating standardised care plans, and for tailoring care plans for individual patients and health care settings.

One of the central problems that computerised clinical practice guidelines (CPGs) address is the ever-increasing amount of clinical knowledge required in diagnosis and treatment, and the need to continually update this knowledge to conform to the principle of evidence-based best practice exacerbates the problem. The availability of standard care pathways for particular medical conditions opens the possibility of uniform and consistently high standards of care, regardless of a clinician's specialist knowledge. Unambiguous documentation is also important [1], [2]. Indeed, current initiatives in the UK NHS have ambitions to generate a database of methodologies indicating the ideal route that any patient in a particular circumstance should follow [3]. However, the effective deployment and maintenance of CPGs requires a great deal more than simply translating a "paper" guideline to machine-readable form [4], [5]. For example in [3] a "patient journey" is designed within a multi-disciplinary, patient-centric environment in which variation from the 'ideal' is both recorded and later evaluated. We start in section 2 by identifying the main processes in the entire "lifecycle" of a computerised guideline, with an eye to the requirements these may impose on the technology. In section 3 we discuss the possibility that many of these requirements will be well served by a combination of techniques well-known in the AI planning literature. Section 4 supports this claim by demonstrating that a typical CPG modelling language, PRO*forma*, is comparable with existing AI planning standards.

2 Elements of Effective Guideline Representation

The "life-cycle" of a practical computerised clinical guideline includes many steps. The first step is to select, analyse and specify the guideline to be implemented, a difficult process in itself [4]. Once an unambiguous requirements specification has been produced, we can identify the following steps in producing and using a computerised guideline. For each step we identify the possible support computerised techniques can provide and the requirements these imply for effective guideline modelling.

a) Guideline authoring: To support the process of authoring an electronic guideline a representation format is required that allows guideline process logic to be clearly and efficiently represented. Experience shows that a representation must support both instantaneous and durative actions, allow states of actions to be represented during execution (relevant, established, requested, accepted, cancelled), and allow libraries of useful actions and action sequences to be established. An effective representation should allow guideline flow – both sequencing and scheduling of actions – to be defined. This might include sequential, parallel and cyclical execution, definition of constraints between actions, and should in principle allow strict linear plan ordering and resource allocation to be delayed until execution (i.e. elements of least commitment planning).

b) Tailoring plans to an individual setting and an individual patient: A standard guideline, disseminated in electronic form either regionally or nationally, is unlikely to be directly appropriate to a particular patient or a particular local setting [5]. However support may be provided within the representation for manually fine-tuning a guideline. This might include representation of constraints on, and effects of, actions (so that harmful interactions can be recognised), and hierarchical decomposition of plans allowing a high-level action to be implemented in alternative ways to suit both local conditions and patient preferences.

c) Critiquing and justifying plans: It is necessary to be able to evaluate the plan looking for inconsistencies, unwanted interactions, etc. The syntax and semantics of the representation should be amenable to automatic validation. With appropriate representations it may be possible to factor financial or resource optimality, and risk assessment based on patient records, into guidelines at development time (e.g. [6]).

d) Plan integration: It is common for patients to be simultaneously treated on a number of clinical guidelines. For example a diabetic patient might simultaneously be treated under diabetes, cardio-vascular and stroke prevention guidelines. Computer-based CPGs provide the potential to integrate multiple guidelines, perhaps using critiquing methods to help identify possible interactions or side-effects caused by the application of multiple treatment regimes.

e) Guideline delivery: The guideline representation should be executable, possibly with alternative modes of delivery (e.g. reminder-based or on-demand [7]). Fully automated care is not realistic, but mixed-initiative planning techniques can allow an appropriate mix of clinician/computer-based intervention. Effective decision support during guideline delivery requires representation of decision alternatives, procedures for ranking decision options, and the information to provide explanations for decisions to a user. It should be possible to represent patient and clinician preferences, potentially including the visualisation of several different plan refinements for evaluation prior to enactment.

f) Monitoring and repairing guidelines: The effective monitoring of a patient's journey along a prescribed care pathway is essential. An automated comparison of expected against actual progress could lead to the generation of alerts. These could be used to suggest the suspension or abortion of a plan which is failing, or the removal of plan steps that are no longer necessary. Effective monitoring requires some degree of modelling of expected and actual patient states (perhaps including desirable and undesirable states), and of execution states of guideline components (e.g. plans might be suspended or aborted, restarted, completed successfully etc). The automatic or semi-automatic repair of a plan following a failed action is an exciting possibility. If clinical goals and intentions are modelled effectively, alternative means might be sought to achieve a goal if one procedure fails. Hierarchical organisation of plans facilitates this, offering alternative low-level implementations for high-level goals, and stored in libraries. Representation of the medical facts and reasoning underlying the recommendations of the guideline will be required for effective automatic repair.

g) Guideline maintenance: Continuing maintenance of a guideline is essential to its effective operation clinically. This extends beyond timely updating of the medical content to reflect current best practice. Computerised variance tracking and monitoring methods promise to provide a means of automatically identifying incomplete, inconsistent or outdated documentation, or errors in clinical practice and documentation. The specification of a guideline in a non-ambiguous and standard format also opens the possibility of widespread dissemination and peer-review of guidelines, a further, and possibly very effective, form of guideline maintenance.

3 AI Planning Techniques and Their Relevance to CPGs

In this section we discuss the range of established AI planning techniques which may address the requirements listed above. Planning can be seen as the process of searching for and deciding on a set of actions that can be temporally sequenced and executed in such a way to achieve a set of desired outcomes, or goals. 'Classical' (AI) planning is considered to be a substantial subset of currently available paradigms, and can be described as the transformation of a set of initial, to a set of final logical (goal) states. A very simplistic view of the classical planning process has as its heart: An initial world description I; a goal state description G; and a set of possible actions known to the planner, called the domain theory α. A valid plan is (naively) said to exist when $A_{(s0)} \vDash G_{(s\infty)}$ ($I \neq G$ in most cases), Where A is an ordered set of non-conflicting deterministic actions applied in I, $A \subseteq \alpha$, (s0) is the initial state and (s∞) is the end state in the temporal order of plan execution expressed in the Situation Calculus. Actions in the classical sense are composed of three basic components:

- preconditions that must be satisfied in order for the action to be selected and executed
- effects that define the changes made to the world state after the action's execution
- an action body that provides a vehicle for establishing parameters, constraints, etc, and can be seen as the procedural element of the action

These components match some of the basic requirements of guideline representation (elements a and b of section 2). We, and others [9], [10], have identified a clear link between the needs of a computerised clinical guideline system and the facilities offered by AI planning technologies.

Early planning algorithms, mostly based on state-space search, produced plans as totally ordered sequences of ground actions, i.e. strict linear sequences of actions leading to the goal state. This places a significant burden on the planner to make early decisions about the inclusion of every primitive action, and furthermore the process must take place in a strict chronological order. However, in most realistic problem domains, it is desirable and even sometimes necessary, to delay decisions on strict ordering until a later time, concentrating on 'important decisions' first (element a).

The ability of a planner to generate actions that are not (all) linearised is intuitively termed Partial Order Planning (POP) [11], and by delaying the processing and allocation of resources, a least commitment strategy ensues. This introduces the importance of constraints, and indeed partial plans have been defined as "any set of constraints that together delineate which action sequences belong to the plan's candidate set, and which do not" [12] (c.f. section 2 elements a and b). Figure 1 is an example of an action taken from a guideline for treating weight loss [13]. It has an unbound variable ?x, one precondition and one effect.

```
(:action GI_treatments                   ;; name of action
  :parameters (?x – patient)             ;; variable ?x of type "patient"
  :precondition (diagnosis ?x peptic_ulcer) ;; precondition that ?x has a peptic ulcer
  :effect (weightloss ?x treated) )      ;; effect that ?x's weightloss is treated
```

Fig. 1. Action for treating weight loss expressed as a potential plan step

Formally, a partial-order planning problem can be expressed as a three-tuple [11] <A, O, L>, where: A is a set of deterministic actions (the domain theory), O is a set of (partial) ordering constraints over actions, and L is a set of constraints that provide protection to precedence relationships. These have been termed 'Causal Links' [11] and record explicitly the causal dependencies between actions.

Contemporary approaches [12] go further by expanding on the concept of constraints beyond causal link protection. By defining multiple constraint types, such as codesignation, non-codesignation and 'auxiliary' constraints that further control ordering and bindings, plus the facility for constraint propagation, the means exists to control not only strict dependencies between actions, but also which states must be temporally 'preserved' between actions. This power and flexibility is important in care pathway planning, and it highlights the importance of constraint satisfaction. Graph-based [14] and satisfiability approaches [15] have also seen success in terms of the complexity of problems solved and the time taken to plan.

Partial order planners operate by successively performing 'refinements' to the existing plan, either by adding new actions to the plan set, or by re-ordering existing plan steps. This process proceeds by nondeterministically repairing 'flaws' in the existing plan, e.g. a precondition not satisfied either in the initial state or by the effects of a preceding step, a causal link between two plan steps that is threatened by an intervening step, or the violation of auxiliary constraints. Such threats are readily detected in POP systems, and remedial actions can be either automatically applied or suggestions made via constraint satisfaction techniques.

Partial order planning allows for concurrent tasks to be represented in the same manner as they are currently represented in many of the current computerised guideline representations, and the ability to represent and process various types of constraints holds the potential, not only for a clear and logically sound representation, but the programmatic means to generate and validate plans in a logical and legible way. The generic nature of POP, in representation and reasoning, also leads to the inherent capability of merging plans, i.e. of merging multiple treatment regimes (element d of section 2).

Conditional, or contingency planning techniques, allow for alternatives to be declared at given choice points (see elements b and f). This is appropriate in situations in which safety is paramount, and in procedural terms minimises the need for later replanning. However it would be difficult and error-prone to produce contingencies for every conceivable choice point. One potential solution, to interleave planning and execution [16], caters for unbounded indeterminacy by monitoring the world state during the execution of the plan to ensure that the plan remains valid until its completion. This provides an opportunity to re-plan in any new or unexpected situations should they appear. For example if a patient's status changed unexpectedly (element f). It may also be wise to predefine intervals at which checks are made (perhaps suggested by the healthcare worker responsible for the plan) to ensure safety standards. This method of plan revision could be of great use when dealing with volatile and unpredictable situations.

Hierarchical planning involves refinement in the space of partial plans expressed hierarchically. Planning can be seen as a decomposition process which links successively less abstract actions and action sequences, from an initial high-level set of goals to a set of actions expressed at whatever level is deemed satisfactory (see elements b and f). Thus a network of actions is produced, linking each decomposed action to a higher level in the hierarchy. Such planners have been intuitively termed Hierarchical Task Network (HTN) Planners, and in addition to the refinement methods used in POP, such systems rely heavily on what has been called 'task reduction methods' that search for, select, and merge plans at increasing more specific levels.

The domain theory in this area consists of a library of plans, sub-plans and/ or atomic actions that collectively describe CPGs or components of them.

Task reduction (decomposition) proceeds by non-deterministically choosing an action a ∈ A, selecting a task reduction method R to decompose a, and then merging the new action into the developing plan A. This is not a trivial problem. Constraint satisfaction must take place in order to remove any conflict that may have been introduced, ordering constraints that previously (might have) existed between actions one level up the abstraction hierarchy must now be updated to reflect the new ordering constraints introduced at the lower level, and the same considerations must be given to the causal links and any auxiliary binding constraints there may be.

Representing CPGs hierarchically as shown in Figure 2 provides the means to share common guidelines at one level of abstraction while delegating institution and patient-specific tasks and processes to lower levels to be instantiated in individual situations. This has implications both for the design and delivery of CPGs (especially elements b and f).

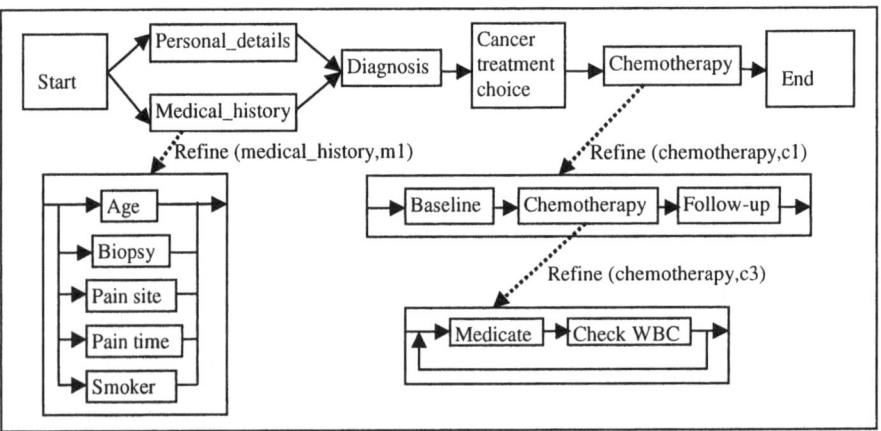

Fig. 2. An example of a hierarchical task network which shows the simplified cancer guideline. There may be several different refinements for each abstract action (medical_history for example)

One important issue is the need to specify the interface between higher and lower levels in the hierarchy, which is typically done by defining goals which lower-level actions should achieve. Unambiguous specification of medical goals is a non-trivial task; however some progress has been made [17].

Case-based reasoning (CBR) uses past experience in an attempt to match similar cases and solve new planning problems [18], and can offer many advantages, including improved facilities for developing and maintaining guidelines. Case-based approaches require that information on cases be recorded, leading to an inherent ability to provide for the important tasks of variance tracking and best practice review (section 2 element g). Plans produced via HTN and POP techniques, supported by contingency and execution monitoring approaches, provide the potential for the storage of completed plans along with a reasoned history of plan suspension, abortion, modifications, etc. (element a). It is important to note that CBR is not proposed as simply an organised data store and quality assessment tool, but would also provide an effective means to facilitate knowledge management. However, issues relating to case similarity, effective and efficient indexing and the free-form nature of existing variance documentation remain.

Mixed-initiative planning involves human interaction, which is essential in any computer system responsible for defining and guiding patient care (element e). Safety is a primary concern, but also the integration of clinician and patient preferences must be accommodated. One of the central tenets of our work is that computerised guidelines should perform as informed assistants or "knowledge levers." One major element of the UK government's IT strategy is that patients should have some level of control over their treatment [3], and to facilitate this, healthcare workers require the ability to manipulate plans while they are being generated and throughout the patient journey. The cycle of task selection, task reduction, plan merging, critiquing (constraint satisfaction), and manipulation, that is inherent in HTN planners employing POP techniques, is amenable to human interaction at whatever level of detail is required. During the various stages in the cycle, human involvement may be readily facilitated, i.e. conforming to the principle of reminder-based or on-demand modes of delivery. One interesting approach is the 'argumentation' method developed for the PRO*forma* CPG modelling language to provide assistance in the decision-making processes, based on a knowledge base of evidential and theory-based research. This is an important research direction currently being taken at Cancer Research UK [8]. It may also be possible to define preference levels for action options, showing their proximity to the "ideal" guideline, and which could be used to assist the planner in keeping as closely as possible to the model patient journey when re-planning after variances.

We conclude from this survey that, while no single AI planning technique discussed above can match all the requirements established in section 2, a combination of technologies has the potential to make a significant contribution to every one of the seven "elements". An appropriate combination would incorporate a least commitment and partially ordered hierarchical element (for plan generation and repair), with a reactive facility provided by execution monitoring and replanning. Case-based planning methods (to deal with plan maintenance during execution, variance tracking and guideline maintenance) provide the potential for variance tracking and management.

4 Standards in Representation: PRO*forma* and PDDL

We have suggested that AI planning techniques may make a substantial contribution to computerised care plan representation and execution. It is instructive to compare the style of representation which has evolved in the AI planning community with that developed in medical informatics. The Planning Domain Definition Language (PDDL), is a domain and problem specification language originally created for use in the biennial planning competition held in conjunction with the international AI planning conference [19], but which has been widely accepted as an evolving standard. PRO*forma* is a formal knowledge representation language capable of capturing the structure and content of a clinical guideline in a form that can be interpreted by a computer. The language forms the basis of a method and a technology for developing and publishing executable clinical guidelines [8]. It has been developed over a number of years by the Advanced Computing Laboratory at Cancer Research UK and there are currently many clinical applications of PRO*forma* both in use and in development over a range of different medical domains. A detailed description of the PRO*forma* language can be found in [20]. There is clear similarity between PRO*forma* and PDDL, both in syntax and semantics, and the neutrality of PDDL provides the opportunity to review and experiment with existing planning technology. One element of PDDL that maps well onto the medical domain is the level of separation between the domain (which includes generic CPGs) and the problem (the specific situation).

```
PROforma
plan :: 'plan1';
    caption ::"Surgery";
    description ::"Care pathway for surgery";        action :: 'action1';
    precondition :: result_of( decision2) = Surgery;     caption ::"Refer to surgeon";
    component :: 'action1';                          procedure ::'Refer to surgeon';
        number_of_cycles ::1;                        end action.
        ltwh :: 39,121,35,35;
    end plan.

PDDL
(:action plan1_surgery
    :parameters (?x – patient)
    :precondition (and (^^ (decision2 ?x completed) (goal-type: achievable) )
                       (^^ (result_of decision2_cancer_treatment ?x surgery) (goal-type: filter)))
    :effect (and (^^ (refer_to_surgeon ?x) :primary-effect)
                 (^^ (plan1_surgery ?x completed) :side-effect)
                 (^^ (weightloss ?x treated) :primary-effect)) )
```

Fig. 3. Comparing the PRO*forma* and PDDL methods of representing plan steps

Figure 3 compares the simplified plan step 'surgery', represented in the PRO*forma* and PDDL syntax. It should be noted from this very simple example, that there is a distinct syntax and structure to PDDL, and that the classical notions of pre and postconditions are catered for. The '^^' notation permits some qualification. Semantically, '(^^(precondition literal),(X))' provides the means to add meta-level 'advice' (X) to the planner. For example the '(decision2 ?x completed)' precondition must be *achieved* before the plan step can be executed, but the second precondition '(result_of decision2_cancer_treatment ?x surgery)' is specified as a 'filter' condition, i.e. the plan step 'surgery' is *only applicable* when the decision is surgery.

In the version of PRO*forma* currently under development a structure exists, called a "keystone." The idea is that it could be used as an "intervention" or marker which would be inserted into a plan when no details about the task to be performed at that point were known. This is similar to partial order and HTN planning techniques, requiring the planning algorithm to search the library of actions to replace the unspecified keystones with a network of actions that fulfil the guideline requirements. Incorporation of the argumentation process would be useful in assisting clinicians with the generation of possible reasons surrounding variances which may occur during execution, allowing for more accurate or appropriate resolutions and plan repairs to be found.

5 Conclusions

While much progress is being made in the area of computerised CPGs, there remain challenging problems associated with care plan generation, evaluation, manipulation and standardisation. It has been shown in this paper that AI planning techniques have the potential to facilitate many of the requirements identified, although it would appear that each technique addresses only part of the overall problem. Our thesis is that a hybrid combination of AI planning technologies, incorporating a least commitment and partially ordered hierarchical element with a reactive facility provided by execution monitoring and replanning is the way forward. Contemporary approaches are seen to provide much of the functionality required for merged treatment regimes, and the technology's advanced use of constraint manipulation techniques leads to an inherently knowledge-rich reasoning capability. Case-based planning methods may form an interesting basis for variance tracking and management, and ultimately to effective and efficient maintenance of the CPGs themselves. Formalised representational standards have evolved in the CPG and AI Planning communities, and their respective similarities and common aims leads to the possibility of seamless integration.

Acknowledgements

This work was supported in part by award L328253015 from the UK Economic and Social Research Council and Engineering and Physical Sciences Research Council.

References

1. NHS Information Authority: Care Pathways Know-How Zone. URL http://www.nelh.nhs.uk/carepathways/icp_about.asp (2003).
2. NHS Information Authority: Care Pathways Know-How. URL http://www.nelh.nhs.uk/carepathways/icp_benefits.asp (2003).
3. The NHS Confederation: *Briefing 88: The national strategy for IT in the NHS*. London: NHS Confederation Publications Sales (2003).
4. Shiffman, R. & Greenes R.: Improving clinical guidelines with logic and decision-table techniques. *Medical Decision Making.* **14**(3) p.247-343, (1994)
5. Waitman, L. R. & Miller, R. A.: Pragmatics of implementing guidelines on the front lines. *l American Medical Informatics* Assoc. **11**(5), p.436-438. (2004)
6. Glasspool, D. W., Fox, J., Castillo, F. C. and Monaghan, V. E. L.: Interactive Decision Support for Medical Planning. In M. Dojat, E. Keravnou and P. Barahona (Eds.) *Proc. 9th Conference on AI in Medicine in Europe, AIME 2003*. Berlin: Springer-Verlag. p. 335-339, (2003).
7. Bouaud J. & Séroussi B.: Reminder-based or on-demand guideline-based decision support systems. From CPG2004. URL http://www.openclinical.org/cgp2004.html (2004)

8. Fox, J. & Dunlop, R.: *Guideline modelling methods: PROforma.* London: OpenClinical. URL: http://www.openclinical.org/gmm_proforma.html (2004)
9. Veloso, M., et. al.: Integrating planning and learning: The prodigy architecture. *Journal of Experimental and Theoretical AI* 7(1) p.81-120, (1995)
10. Miksch, S.: Plan Management in the Medical Domain. *AI Communications* 12 p.209-235, (1999)
11. Penberthy, J. S. & Weld, D.: UCPOP: A sound, complete, partial order planner for ADL. *Proc 3rd Int Conf Principles of KR and R.* p.103-114. URL http://www.cs.washington.edu/homes/weld/papers/ucpop-kr92.pdf (1992)
12. Kambhampati, S.: Refinement planning as a unifying framework for plan synthesis. *AI Magazine.* 18(2) p.48, (1997)
13. Fox, J. & Das, S.: *Safe and Sound: Artificial intelligence in Hazardous Applications.* London: MIT Press, (2000)
14. Blum, A. & Furst, M.: Fast planning through planning graph analysis. Proc 14th IJCAI p.1636-1642. Morgan Kaufmann, (1995)
15. Kautz, H.A. and Selman, B.: Pushing the envelope: Planning, propositional logic, and stochastic search. *Proc 13th National Conf on AI.* AAAI Press, (1996)
16. Pryor, L. and Collins, G.: Planning for contingencies: a decision-based approach. JAIR **4**, p 287-339, (1996)
17. Fox, J., Alabassi, A., Black, E., Patkar, V. & Rose, A.: An ontological approach to modelling tasks and goals. *Computers in Biology and Medicine*, in press (2005).
18. Watson, I. & Marir, F.: Case-Based Reasoning: A Review. *Knowledge Engineering Review.* 9(4) p.355-381, (1994)
19. McDermott, D.: The 1998 AI Planning Systems Competition. *AI Magazine* **21**(2) Summer (2000)
20. Sutton, D. & Fox, J.: The Syntax and Semantics of the PRO*forma* guideline modelling language. *JAMIA.* **10**(5) p.433-443, (2003)

Gaining Process Information from Clinical Practice Guidelines Using Information Extraction

Katharina Kaiser, Cem Akkaya, and Silvia Miksch

Institute of Software Technology & Interactive Systems,
Vienna University of Technology, Vienna, Austria
{kaiser, silvia}@asgaard.tuwien.ac.at
http://ieg.ifs.tuwien.ac.at

Abstract. Formalizing Clinical Practice Guidelines for subsequent computer-supported processing is a cumbersome, challenging, and time-consuming task. But currently available tools and methods do not satisfactorily support this task.

We propose a new multi-step approach using Information Extraction and Transformation. This paper addresses the Information Extraction task. We have developed several heuristics, which do not take Natural Language Understanding into account. We implemented our heuristics in a framework to apply them to several guidelines from the specialty of otolaryngology. Our evaluation shows that a heuristic-based approach can achieve good results, especially for guidelines with a major portion of semi-structured text.

1 Introduction

Computer-supported guideline execution is an important instrument for improving the quality of health care. To execute Clinical Guidelines and Protocols (CGPs) in a computer-supported way, the information in the guideline, which is in plain textual form, in tables, or represented in flow charts, has to be formalized. That means that a formal representation is required in order to make the information computable. Thus, several so called *guideline representation languages* have been developed to support the structuring and representation of various guidelines and protocols and to make possible different kinds of application.

Many researchers have proposed frameworks for modelling CGPs in a computer-interpretable and -executable format (a comprehensible overview can be found in [1] and [2]). Each of these frameworks provides specific guideline representation languages. Most of these languages are sufficiently complex that the manual formalization of CGPs is a challenging project. Thus, research has to be directed in such a way that tools and methods are developed for supporting the formalization process. Currently, using these tools and methods the human guideline developer needs not only knowledge about the formal methods, but also about the medical domain. This results in a very challenging, time-consuming, and cumbersome formalization task.

Thus we will look for new approaches that can facilitate the formalization process, and support the developer by providing these kinds of knowledge, as well as intelligent methods for a simplified guideline modelling processing.

2 Related Work

In this Section, we present a short discussion of some relevant work describing guideline formalization tools as well as some examples of Information Extraction (IE) systems.

2.1 Guideline Formalization Tools

For formalizing clinical guidelines into a guideline representation language various methods and tools exist, ranging from simple editors to sophisticated graphical applications and multistep methodologies.

Several markup-based tools exist, like *Stepper* [3], the *GEM Cutter* [4], the *Document Exploration and Linking Tool/Addons (DELT/A)*, formerly known as *Guideline Markup Tool (GMT)* [5], and *Uruz*, part of the *DEGEL* [6] framework. There are also graphical tools that assist formalization. For instance, *AsbruView* [7] uses graphical metaphors to represent Asbru [1, 2] plans. *AREZZO* and *TALLIS* [8] support translation into PROforma by means of graphical symbols representing the task types of the language. *Protégé* [9] is a knowledge-acquisition tool, where parts of the formalization process can be achieved with predefined graphical symbols. In addition, methodologies (e.g., *SAGE* [10]) have been developed that should help by making the formalization traceable and concise by using a multi-step approach.

But still, in all of the above mentioned cases, the modelling process is complex and labour intensive. Therefore, methods are needed that can be applied to automate a part of the this task.

2.2 Information Extraction Systems

Information Extraction systems have been developed for various domains. For example, the BADGER system [11] is a text analysis system, which summarizes medical patient records by extracting diagnoses, symptoms, physical findings, test results, and therapeutic treatments based on linguistic concepts. At the University of Sheffield extensive research in Natural Language Processing, and especially IE, has been devoted (e.g., the AMBIT system [12] to extracting information from biomedical texts). In the legal domain, Holowczak and Adam developed a system that supports the automatic classification of legal documents [13].

Besides these domain specific systems, there are also other systems using Machine Learning techniques, which can be applied in various domains. WHISK [14], for example, learns rules for extraction from a wide range of text styles; its performance varies with the difficulty of the extraction task. RAPIER [15] uses pairs of sample documents and filled templates to induce pattern–match rules that directly extract fillers for the slots in the template.

Finally, different kinds of wrappers have been developed to transform an HTML document into an XML document (e.g., XWRAP [16] or LiXto, which provides a visual wrapper [17]). These methods and tools are very useful in the case of highly structured HTML documents or if simple XML files need to be extracted. However, CGPs are more complex and more structured XML/DTD files are needed in order to represent them.

3 Our Approach: A Multi-step Transformation Process Based on Heuristic Methods

Most guideline representation languages are very powerful and thus very complex. They can contain many different types of information and data. We therefore decided to apply a multi-step transformation process (cf. Fig. 1). It facilitates the formalization process by using various intermediate representations that are obtained by stepwise procedures.

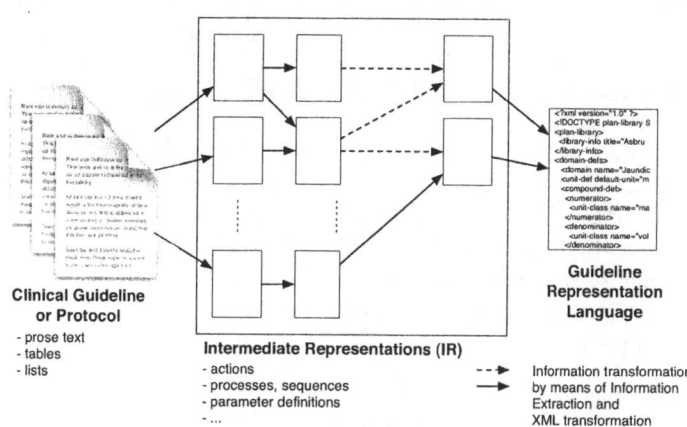

Fig. 1. Guideline transformation process. A multi-step process using intermediate representations to transform clinical guidelines and protocols (CGPs) into a formal representation language

The benefits of the intermediate representations are:

- Concise formalization process
- Different formats for various kinds of information
- Separate views and procedures for various kinds of information
- Application of specific heuristics for each particular kind of information
- Simpler and more concise evaluation and tracing of each process step

To process as large a class as possible of documents and information we need specific heuristics. These are applied to a specific form of information, for instance:

- **Different kinds of information**
  Each kind of information (e.g., processes, parameters) needs specific methods for processing. By presenting only one kind of information the application of the associated method is simpler and easier to trace.
- **Different representations of information**
  We have to take into account various ways in which the information might be represented (i.e., structured, semi-structured, or free text).
- **Different kinds of guidelines**
  CGPs exist for various diseases, various user-groups, various purposes, various organizations, and so on, and have been developed by various guideline developers'

organizations. Therefore, we can speak about different classes of CGPs that may contain similar guidelines.

To transform information by applying Information Extraction (IE) methods, we generated specific templates that can present the desired information. Heuristic methods detect relevant information, which is filled into the templates' slots for subsequent processing. In the next section we present a method that extracts process information from clinical guidelines for otolaryngology using heuristic algorithms. The output of this method is a unified format, which can be transformed into the final representation.

4 Process Extraction of Clinical Guidelines and Protocols

CGPs present effective treatment processes. One challenge when authoring CGPs is the detection of individual processes and their relations and dependencies. We try to detect these by means of IE. CGPs consist of semi-structured and free text. The resulting output can subsequently be processed to yield refined representations, leading ultimately to the representation in the guideline representation language.

By analyzing treatment processes of otolaryngology contained in the guidelines we detected the following processes:

- Sequential processes
- Processes without temporal dependencies
- Processes which exclude each other (i.e., one process has to be selected from several)
- Processes containing subprocesses
- Recurring processes

We have therefore developed heuristics in order to acquire treatment processes from the CGPs, where a process is described by at least one sentence. This means that a sentence, for instance, *'Take acetaminophen or ibuprofen.'*, presents only one process and not a selection of two processes. The heuristics are categorized into three groups: (1) heuristics for detecting the relevant sentences, (2) heuristics for detecting whether the sentence is the description of a process, an annotation, or a negative action, and (3) heuristics for detecting relations between processes (for the latter two groups an outline is shown in Fig. 2). The heuristics are developed for XHTML-conforming documents. Before going into the details of our heuristics we describe our dictionary that they use.

4.1 Dictionary for Extracting Processes: CGPs of Otolaryngology

The dictionary we use for this purpose includes various classes, such as

- *Medical* terms (i.e. drug agents, surgical procedures, and diagnostic terms)
- *Action* terms (mainly verbs; e.g., 'activate', 'perform', 'prescribe', 'treat', 'receive')
- *Condition* terms (i.e. regular expressions, such as 'if [Ê, : \.]+', 'in case(s)? [ˆ,: \.]+', 'for .*<diagnosis-term>')
- *Dose unit* terms (e.g. '(m|d|c)?(l|g)(/kg/day)?', 'drop(s)?', 'teaspoon(s)?', 'tsp')
- *Time unit* terms (e.g. '(m(illi)?)?sec(ond)?(s)?', 'min(ute)?(s)?')

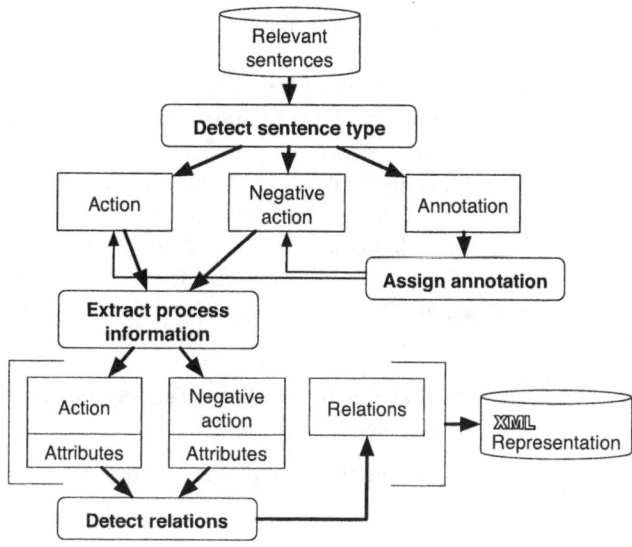

Fig. 2. Processing the relevant sentences to obtain a representation of processes and their relations

- *Relation* terms (e.g. 'after', 'before', 'during', 'while')
- *Negative action* terms (i.e. expressions describing actions that should not be performed; e.g. 'no .*(benefit|advantage)', 'not to perform', 'not be (used|treated)')

The medical terms are based on a subset of the Medical Subject Headings (MeSH)[1] of the United States National Library of Medicine. We adapted them according for missing terms, different wordings, acronyms, and varying categorization.

4.2 Task 1: Detecting Relevant Sentences

Detecting relevant sentences is a challenging task, which we undertake in two steps: (1) detecting irrelevant sentences to exclude them from further processing and (2) detecting relevant sentences.

In both steps we use special keywords to detect whether a sentence is irrelevant or relevant. Keywords describing irrelevant sentences are 'history', 'diagnosis', 'criteria', 'symptom', 'clinical assessment', 'risk factor', 'complicating factor', 'etiology', and so on. These terms point out that the following paragraph does not describe treatment processes, but that it describes symptoms, demonstration of diagnoses, and so on. If such a term appears within a caption the corresponding section is removed.

Detecting relevant sentences is not a trivial task. First, we parse the entire document and split it into sentences. Then we process every sentence with regard to its context within the document and its group affiliation. Thereby, the context is obtained by captions (e.g. *'Acute Pharyngitis Algorithm Annotations | Treatment | Recommendations:'*) and a group contains sentences from the same paragraph or the same list, if there are

---
[1] http://www.nlm.nih.gov/mesh/

no sublists. Besides, we mark explicitly described annotations (i.e., sentences or paragraphs starting with *'Note'* or *'Notice'*).

Each sentence is now checked for relevance. Relevant sentences are identified by the occurrence of an agent term or surgical procedure or their context contains specific terms. These terms (i.e., 'measure', 'remedies', 'medication', 'treatment') are important, because they specify actions that may not contain agent terms or surgical procedures (e.g. *'Maintain adequate hydration (drink 6 to 10 glasses of liquid a day to thin mucus)'*). Furthermore, we assign a therapy list to each sentence, which contains all agent terms and surgical procedures contained in the sentence.

Now that we have collected the relevant sentences from the guideline, we can proceed with the next step.

4.3 Task 2a: Detecting Whether a Sentence Is the Description of a Process, an Annotation, or Describes a Negative Action

First, we check, whether a sentence describes an action or a negative action (cf. Algorithm 1).

Algorithm 1. *Checking whether each sentence describes an action or a negative action*

```
1. for each Sentence s do {
2.      if s.listEntry is true
3.          s is relevant
4.      split s.content in subclauses
5.      for each SubClause sc do {
6.          if sc contains a negative-action-term and
             an (agent term or surgical procedure) {
7.              if the negative-action-term contains 'not '
8.                  set s.notAction to true
9.              else {
10.                 remove all agents or surgical procedures
                    in sc from the therapy-list
11.         }   }
12.         if s.listEntry is false
13.             if sc contains an (agent term or surgical
                procedure) and an action term {
14.                 s is relevant
15.                 mark sc as mainClause
16. }   }   }
17. store relevant sentences
```

Negative actions are instructions that an action should not be performed, often under specific conditions (e.g. *'Do not use aspirin with children and teenagers because it may increase the risk of Reyes syndrome.'*). Most guideline representation languages will handle such actions by inverting the condition. But languages may exist which will handle these in other ways. Therefore we will provide a representation for such actions that can be used in a general way.

Detecting explicitly described annotations has already been described in subsection 4.2. To detect implicitly described annotations we have developed a special heuristic.

This is done by checking whether the agent terms or surgical procedures in a sentence also appear in processes belonging to the same group appearing above this sentence in the text. If this happens, the sentence is added as an annotation to all these processes.

Explicitly mentioned annotation sentences are added to each process of the same group appearing before the annotation sentence. If there are no sentences in front of the annotation, the annotation sentences are added to each process of the parent group.

If the sentence is not an annotation, it is added as a new process and augmented by additional information. The additional information contains conditions, the duration and iterative aspects of the process, as well as the dosage in case of a drug administration. The information obtained is presented as single-slot values. As we decided to one sentence as one process, a multi-slot system is not necessary at this time. If there are processes with multiple filled slots, the processes can be refined in subsequent steps, if this is wanted.

4.4 Task 2b: Detecting Relations Between Processes

The default relationship between processes is that there is no synchronization in their execution. But as we determined when we analyzed the guidelines, there are more kinds of relations (see Section 4).

To group processes in a *selection* they must fulfill the following requirements: (1) the processes have to belong to the same group and (2) agents or surgical procedures have to be associated to the same category. For instance, processes describing the administration of *Erythromycin*, *Cephalexin*, and *Clindamycin* within one group are combined in a *selection*, as all these agents are antibiotics. If processes are grouped in a selection, one of these processes has to be selected to be executed.

Furthermore, we try to detect relations between processes that are explicitly mentioned within the text, as well as relations that are implicitly given by the document structure. The former is very difficult to detect, as we often cannot detect the reference of the relation within the CGP (e.g., *'After 10 to 14 days of failure of the first line antibiotic ...'*). Nevertheless, we found heuristics that arrange processes or process groups if the reference is unambiguously extractable from the text.

The latter we detect by patterns in the document structure (e.g. *'Further Treatment'* appears after *'Treatment'* or *'Treatment'* appears before *'Follow-Up'*). Thereby, we developed structure patterns that are used to determine the relations between several groups.

5 Evaluation

To evaluate our heuristics we developed a framework and used several guidelines from otolaryngology. We obtained 18 CGPs from the National Guideline Clearinghouse (NGC)[2] that describe the treatment and management of various diseases of otolaryngology. The CGPs were developed from eight different organizations in North America and Europe. We split the CGPs into two groups: (1) six guidelines for developing and

---

[2] http://www.guidelines.gov/

improving the heuristics and (2) twelve guidelines for testing our heuristics. To select the CGPs for the two groups was not trivial. Organizations that develop guidelines dont always use the same hierarchical structure. Therefore, we were unable to select the CGPs according to the organization that developed them. However we used the complexity of the hierarchical structures as selection criteria and distributed them evenly to each group.

Before applying our heuristics we have to carry out some pre-processing. This consists of making the documents XHTML-conform and applying additional structuring elements. The latter is done by converting paragraphs and their corresponding headings to list elements. In this way, we obtained a unique document format containing lists and sublists as well as paragraphs.

We then detected relevant sentences in Task 1 as explained in Section 4.2. Task 2 summarizes the detection of the type of sentence, additional information, and the relations between processes as explained in Sections 4.3 and 4.4. We evaluated our heuristics using Recall and Precision measures. The *Recall* score measures the ratio of correct information extracted from the texts against all the available information present in the text. The *Precision* score measures the ratio of correct information that was extracted against all the information that was extracted [18].

Task 1 produced promising results, although the lower recall score implies that detecting relevant sentences has to be improved. The high precision score shows that irrelevant sentences are barely categorized as relevant.

The input to Task 2 consists of the sentences detected in Task 1. The task's recall score is very high, which means that only a few slots were spuriously not detected. The precision score implies there are some incorrect slot fillers. These arise from not always detecting the correct type of sentence and especially assigning annotations to their particular actions, which has to be improved. Overall evaluation results are presented in Table 1. Detailed evaluation results are presented in [19].

Thus, refining and enhancing our heuristics, especially for documents with a minor portion of semi-structured text, will be one of our next steps in order to provide a good basis for subsequent transformation steps.

Table 1. Evaluation measures of Task 1 and Task 2

	COR	POS	ACT	Recall	Precision
Task 1	379	497	392	**0.76**	**0.97**
Task 2	847	898	1011	**0.94**	**0.84**

Scoring Key:
COR – Number of correctly identified slots by the system
POS – Number of slots according to the key target template
ACT – Number of slots identified by the system
Recall – Ratio of COR slot fillers to POS slot fillers
Precision – Ratio of COR slot fillers to ACT slot fillers

6 Conclusion and Future Work

We have shown that it is possible to extract process information from CGPs applying heuristics. Our heuristics use patterns in the structure of the document as well as of specific expressions. Thus, we do not need to use Natural Language Understanding.

We have applied a framework in order to evaluate our heuristics that can cope with both semi-structured and free text documents. The resulting information is filled in single-slot templates, which can represent processes and their relations. The information extracted can then be used in further transformations to finally generate a representation in a guideline representation language.

Our next step is to improve our heuristics and to enhance them for guidelines which contain processes of higher complexity. Furthermore, we want to support the modelling process by giving the plan modeler the ability to evaluate and intervene after each step, making the process traceable. We will therefore implement *links* that connect the origin of the information and the extracted or transformed information, thereby making it possible to evaluate the individual steps by means of DELT/A [5], which can visualize these links.

Acknowledgments. We would like to thank Jim Hunter for his useful comments. This work has been supported by "Fonds zur Förderung der wissenschaftlichen Forschung FWF" (Austrian Science Fund), grant P15467-INF.

References

1. Peleg, M., Tu, S.W., Bury, J., Ciccarese, P., Fox, J., Greenes, R.A., Hall, R., Johnson, P.D., Jones, N., Kumar, A., Miksch, S., Quaglini, S., Seyfang, A., Shortliffe, E.H., Stefanelli, M.: Comparing Computer-Interpretable Guideline Models: A Case-Study Approach. Journal of the American Medical Informatics Association (JAMIA) **10** (2003) 52–68
2. de Clercq, P.A., Blom, J.A., Korsten, H.H.M., Hasman, A.: Approaches for creating computer-interpretable guidelines that facilitate decision support. Artificial Intelligence in Medicine **31** (2004) 1–27
3. Růžička, M., Svátek, V.: Mark-up Based Analysis of Narrative Guidelines with the Stepper Tool. In Kaiser, K., Miksch, S., Tu, S.W., eds.: Computer-based Support for Clinical Guidelines and Protocols. Proceedings of the Symposium on Computerized Guidelines and Protocols (CGP 2004). Volume 101: Studies in Health Technology and Informatics., Prague, Czech Republic, IOS Press (2004) 132–136
4. Polvani, K.A., Agrawal, A., Karras, B., Deshpande, A., Shiffman, R.: GEM Cutter Manual. Yale Center for Medical Informatics. (2000)
5. Votruba, P., Miksch, S., Kosara, R.: Facilitating knowledge maintenance of clinical guidelines and protocols. In Fieschi, M., Coiera, E., Li, Y.C.J., eds.: Proc. from the Medinfo 2004 World Congress on Medical Informatics, IOS Press (2004) 57–61
6. Shahar, Y., Young, O., Shalom, E., Mayaffit, A., Moskovitch, R., Hessing, A., Galperin, M.: DEGEL: A hybrid, multiple-ontology framework for specification and retrieval of clinical guidelines. In Dojat, M., Keravnou, E., Barahona, P., eds.: Artificial Intelligence in Medicine: 9th Conference on Artificial Intelligence, in Medicine in Europe, AIME 2003, LNAI 2780, Protaras, Cyprus, Springer-Verlag (2003) 122–131

7. Kosara, R., Miksch, S.: Metaphors of Movement: A Visualization and User Interface for Time-Oriented, Skeletal Plans. Artificial Intelligence in Medicine, Special Issue: Information Visualization in Medicine **22** (2001) 111–131
8. Steele, R., Fox, J.: Tallis PROforma Primer – Introduction to PROforma Language and Software with Worked Examples. Technical report, Advanced Computation Laboratory, Cancer Research, London, UK (2002)
9. Gennari, J.H., Musen, M.A., Fergerson, R.W., Grosso, W.E., Crubézy, M., Eriksson, H., Noy, N.F., Tu, S.W.: The Evolution of Protégé: An Environment for Knowledge-based Systems Development. International Journal of Human Computer Studies **58** (2003) 89–123
10. Tu, S.W., Musen, M.A., Shankar, R., Campbell, J., Hrabak, K., McClay, J., Huff, S.M., McClure, R., Parker, C., Rocha, R., Abarbanel, R., Beard, N., Glasgow, J., Mansfield, G., Ram, P., Ye, Q., Mays, E., Weida, T., Chute, C.G., McDonald, K., Mohr, D., Nyman, M.A., Scheital, S., Solbrig, H., Zill, D.A., Goldstein, M.K.: Modeling guidelines for integration into clinical workflow. In Fieschi, M., Coiera, E., Li, Y.C.J., eds.: Proc. from the Medinfo 2004 World Congress on Medical Informatics, IOS Press (2004) 174–178
11. Soderland, S., Aronow, D., Fisher, D., Aseltine, J., Lehnert, W.: Machine Learning of Text Analysis Rules for Clinical Records. Technical report, University of Massachusetts, Amherst, MA (1995)
12. Gaizauskas, R., Hepple, M., Davis, N., Guo, Y., Harkema, H., Roberts, A., Roberts, I.: AMBIT: Acquiring medical and biological information from text. In Cox, S.J., ed.: Proceedings of the UK e-Science All Hands Meeting, Nottingham, UK (2003)
13. Holowczak, R.D., Adam, N.R.: Information Extraction based Multiple-Category Document Classification for the Global Legal Network. In: Proc. of the 9th Conference on Innovative Applications of Artificial Intelligence, AAAI Press/MIT Press (1997) 992–999
14. Soderland, S.: Learning Information Extraction Rules for Semi-Structured and Free Text. Machine Learning **34** (1999) 233–272
15. Califf, M.E., Mooney, R.J.: Relational Learning of Pattern-Match Rules for Information Extraction. In: Proceedings of the Sixteenth National Conference on Artificial Intelligence (AAAI-99), Orlando, FL (1999) 328–334
16. Liu, L., Pu, C., Han, W.: XWRAP: An XML-enabled Wrapper Construction System for Web Information Sources. In: Intern. Conference on Data Engineering (ICDE). (2000) 611–621
17. Baumgartner, R., Flesca, S., Gottlob, G.: Visual Web Information Extraction with Lixto. In: Proceedings of the Conference on Very Large Databases (VLDB). (2001)
18. Lehnert, W., Cardie, C., Fisher, D., McCarthy, J., Riloff, E., Soderland, S.: Evaluating an Information Extraction system. Journal of Integrated Computer-Aided Engineering **1** (1994)
19. Kaiser, K., Akkaya, C., Miksch, S.: Gaining process information of clinical practice guidelines using information extraction. Technical Report Asgaard-TR-2005-04, Institute of Software Technology & Interactive Systems, Vienna University of Technology (2005) (extended version).

Ontology-Driven Extraction of Linguistic Patterns for Modelling Clinical Guidelines*

Radu Serban[1], Annette ten Teije[1], Frank van Harmelen[1], Mar Marcos[2], and Cristina Polo-Conde[2]

[1] AI Department, Vrije Universiteit, The Netherlands
{serbanr, annette, frankh}@few.vu.nl
[2] Departament d´ Enginyeria i Ciéncia dels Computadors,
Universitat Jaume I, Castellón, Spain
Mar.Marcos@icc.uji.es, Cristina.Polo@sg.uji.es

Abstract. Evidence-based clinical guidelines require frequent updates due to research and technology advances. The quality of guideline updates can be improved if the knowledge underlying the guideline text is explicitly modelled using the so-called **guideline patterns (GPs)**, mappings between a text fragment and a formal representation of its corresponding medical knowledge.

Ontology-driven extraction of linguistic patterns is a method to automatically reconstruct the control knowledge captured in guidelines, which facilitates a more effective modelling and authoring of clinical guidelines. We illustrate by examples the use of a method for generating and searching for linguistic guideline patterns in the text of a guideline for treatment of breast cancer, and provide a general evaluation of usefulness of these patterns in the modelling of the guideline analyzed.

1 Introduction

Authoring and maintenance of medical guidelines is recognized as an important factor for improving the quality of healthcare, but also a costly process.

Medical guidelines change frequently due to research and technology improvements, but only parts of the guideline need updates. Guideline formalization makes explicit a modular organization of medical knowledge and produces an executable model from the guideline recommendations, therefore facilitating a more effective update of the guideline knowledge and verification of guideline properties. To avoid repeating guideline formalization from scratch each time a guideline is updated, recent research ([3, 13]) suggests to split the formalization into several steps, isolating procedural, medical, organizational knowledge and defining the so-called **guideline patterns (GPs)**, which represent mappings between text fragments and a more formal representation of its underlying knowledge.

---

* This work has been supported by the European Commission's IST program, under contract number IST-FP6-508794 Protocure-II.

A few linguistic constructs are frequently recurring in the text of clinical guidelines, regardless of the domain addressed by the guideline. For instance, conclusions and recommendations typically have a modular structure, easy to recognize and useful in modelling the guideline.

If linguistic regularities such as these:

In the event of [*MedContext*], *the treatment of choice is* [*Treatment*]. or
In the event of [*MedContext*], [*Treatment*] *is recommended*.

can be given a formal representation, it seems natural to define knowledge templates that are instantiated by these statements, which can be reused when making new guidelines or changing a particular type of knowledge. These so-called linguistic pattern templates help us in establishing a set of modular components for modelling guidelines in the form of: (1) a shared vocabulary and (2) a language to describe linguistic regularities conveying a specific type of knowledge. This mapping between text and the knowledge underlying it makes validation of this knowledge straightforward and eases the modelling task. Authoring and updating of guidelines can also benefit from these modular components, as only the parts concerned with a changing piece of knowledge need updated.

In this paper we focus on knowledge templates that describe control (procedural) knowledge, and investigate their role in improving modularization and formalization of clinical guidelines. We propose a method that uses linguistic regularities in the text of a guideline, and an ontology of the medical domain, to generate a list of linguistic templates, which is explained in section 2 and summarized in figure 1. In section 3 we discuss our algorithm for searching instances of linguistic patterns and their use in the guideline formalization. In section 4

Algorithm 1.1
GUIDELINE–FORMALIZATION(TF,PT)
▷ *TF:text fragment; PT:set of patt.templates*

1. build an ontology from a corpus of guideline texts;
2. semantically tag the guideline text using the ontology: replace terms in the text with their corresponding ontological categories;
3. generate control templates using the ontological categories identified;
4. select a set of core templates, by eliminating templates covered by or made of other templates;
5. establish a formal translation for the core templates;
6. find instances of core templates in the guideline;
7. translate pattern instances into their formal equivalent using the translation pattern of their corresponding template;
8. select the linguistic templates instantiated in more than one guideline text, as guideline building blocks.

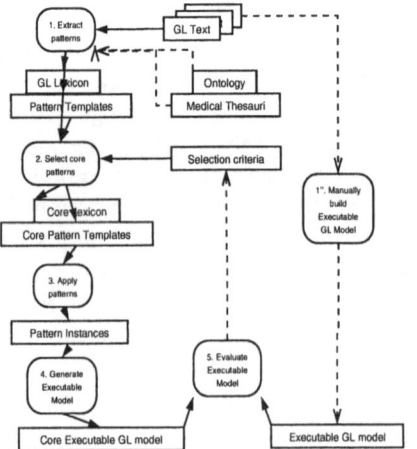

Fig. 1. Guideline formalization using patterns

Fig. 2. Steps for extracting and evaluating linguistic patterns

we evaluate the effectiveness of pattern detection in generating an executable model of a breast-cancer guideline. Section 5 presents related work and section 6 summarizes the paper contribution, emphasizing the benefits of using linguistic patterns as support for guideline formalization. Figure 2 depicts the steps for building a set of core linguistic templates. Activities are marked as rounded rectangles, the objects produced by them are shown as plain rectangles.

2 A Text-Driven Approach to Pattern Extraction

Starting from a practical experiment in guideline formalization using the Stepper tool ([13]), we propose the use of patterns in guideline formalization, as depicted by the algorithm in figure 1.

Linguistic patterns can be extracted from the textual representation of the guideline through abstraction, using medical knowledge such as the one depicted in figure 3. This ontology contains "*is_a*" hierarchical relations between medical concepts, "*instance_of*" relations between medical concepts and medical terms, and labeled semantic relations between medical concepts. The ontology can be built from an existing ontology (WordNet) or medical thesauri such as MeSH [1], UMLS [4], or NCIOncology [2].

Generating Pattern Templates. We aim at generating control templates such as action sequencing, decomposition or condition-action, to capture the procedural aspect of a guideline. Initially, simple templates are generated, such as a medical action, followed by a control operator and an additional medical category (e.g., medical action or goal). Then more specific and complex templates could be generated by (1) adjusting the level of abstraction of the concepts in the pattern, (2) replacing them with specific ones, (3) replacing by operators the semantic relations among several concepts from the ontology, or (4) merging two instances of simpler templates (e.g., if they share a word).

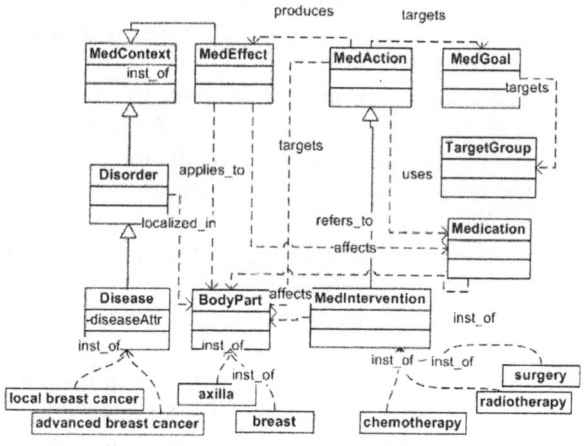

Fig. 3. Relations between medical terms and concepts in the medical ontology

(1) *Recommendation:* Patients with locoregionally advanced breast cancer should receive multidisciplinary treatment with curative intent.
  ⇓ refined_as
(2) {*Recommendation*}: {*Patients with*} [disease] {*should receive*} [treatment] {*with*} [med_goal].
  ⇓ refined_as
(3) {*Recommendation*}: [Target_group] [recommendation_op] {*receive*} [treatment] {*with*} [med_goal].
  ⇓ refined_as
(4) {*Recommendation*}: [med_context] [recommendation_op] [complex_treatment].

Fig. 4. Abstraction steps for extracting a pattern template

Guideline developers use the implicit knowledge captured by these semantic relations when producing the guideline. Guideline formalization can benefit from reverse engineering of the domain addressed by the guideline, since a part of the formal representation of the guideline is represented by these relations.

The example in figure 4 illustrates how pattern templates can be extracted from the text of a recommendation taken from the 2002 **CBO guideline for treatment of breast cancer** ([5]). If we replace instances present in the recommendation text (1) with their categories in the ontology, we obtain a skeletal representation of the sentence. This intermediate representation of a pattern template contains concepts from an ontology and terms from a non-medical lexicon (2). If we apply the categorization rules in the ontology (which contains relations such the ones depicted in figure 3), to represent the sentence skeleton at a higher level of abstraction, the recommendation is rewritten as expression (3). Finally, if we ignore the linking words (of the lexicon) and consider only the categories present in the ontology, we obtain a more compact template of the recommendation, as depicted in expression (4).

The recommendation contains an instance of *med_context* ("Patients with locoregionally advanced breast cancer") followed by a *recommendation_op* ("should") and an instance of *med_action* ("receive multidisciplinary treatment with curative intent"); the latter can be further refined as a sequence of: *treatment* ("multidisciplinary treatment") followed by *med_goal* ("with curative intent"). The advantage of having such a conceptual sketch of the linguistic construct "med_recommendation" is that the template of any recommendation will include one of the following ordered lists of medical categories, obtained by refining parts of the linguistic component:
(med_context, recommendation_op, med_action)
(target_group, recommendation_op, treatment, med_goal), and so on.

The goal of finding linguistic templates in the text requires us to find n-grams with elements belonging to either a medical category, such as *target_group* or *med_goal*, or to a lexical category such as *ctx_op*, *recommendation_op*, which links medical terms. Disambiguation of some of the terms is required, nonetheless the use of a terminology system when authoring the guidelines would reduce the importance of this task. By filtering the detected n-grams using the relevant semantic relations provided by the ontology, a grammar for defining linguistic pattern templates can be derived. Even though pattern templates can be generated and instantiated automatically using this method, producing meaningful linguistic pattern templates cannot be fully automated.

3   Detection of Pattern Instances in the Guideline Text

For identifying instantiations of existing pattern templates in the guideline text we use our custom built ontology of the medical domain, summarized in section 2. Figure 3 contains a few examples of concepts from this ontology:

1. **medical specific categories**: disease, medication, body_part, med_effect, med_action;
2. **operator categories** - lexical terms corresponding to semantic relations between medical categories in the ontology: relational operators (assoc_rel_op, temp_rel_op, causal_rel_op) or action operators (decomp_op, act_op)

We built an application that generates templates as sequences of medical concepts that are connected using control relations in the ontology, for instance:
$template([med\_action, effect\_op, med\_effect])$ **covers**
   $ontology\_fragment(MedAction\ produces\ MedEffect)$
We define a set of control relations relevant for the operational model of the guideline: causal relationships between actions, ordering and decomposition of actions, correlations condition-action, action-intention, action-effect, etc. We transform them into pattern templates and look up their instances in the guideline.

Implementation. The guideline text is split into sentences and further into word-level chunks. A *guideline chunk* is a pair $\langle TF, Ann \rangle$, where TF represents a text fragment potentially relevant for the pattern detection, and Ann is a list of semantic annotations for TF. Initially, the chunk is set at the word level, but during semantic annotation, it can group together several words and even sentences, depending on the level of granularity at which patterns are recognized.

A pattern template is the abstraction of a text fragment as a list of concepts from two sources: a medical ontology and a non-medical lexicon containing frequent link words. We define patterns at different levels of granularity: (1) patterns at word-level are in fact semantically tagged medical terms in the guideline text; (2) pattern at sentence level define concepts from different semantic categories which correspond to well-defined formal constructs.

For instance, the sentence "*Treatment1 consists of axillary surgery followed by radiotherapy.*" consists of two basic (core) patterns:
$action_1\ consists\_of\ action_2, action\_3$, a hierarchical decomposition, and
$action_2\ followed\_by\ action\_3$, an action sequencing.

Initially, the sentence is split into word-level chunks, and the list of annotations of each word contains only the relative position of the term in the guideline text. At each processing of the sentence, in search for patterns, the annotations

```
i1(axillary_surgery, following, excision))
i2(biopsy, following, excision))
i3(breast_reconstruction, following, mastectomy))
```
⇓ instance_of
p1(med_action, act_op, med_action)

Fig. 5. Pattern template extracted from several instances

can be expanded as follows: when the term of the chunk is an instance of a medical term, its semantic categories are added to the annotation list; when a pattern is recognized, of which the chunk can be a part, it is added as annotation of that chunk, etc. When medical terms are recognized in the sentence, several chunks corresponding to the component words are merged into one chunk, together with their annotations. In the next step the analysis focuses on sentence-level chunks. Sentence-level chunks are sequences of word-level chunks, annotated with possibly overlapping pattern instances found in that sentence.

Results of Pattern Detection. The parameters of pattern detection are: (1) the medical ontology; and (2) a set of target pattern templates sought in the text. After applying the algorithm described above for the reference guideline ([5]), and reviewing the instances found, the most frequent operational patterns were:
$p_{1.1}(A : med\_action, \{following\} : seq\_act\_op, B : med\_action)$ and
$p_{1.2}(A : med\_action, \{after\} : act\_op, B : med\_action)$.
They are subclasses of a more abstract pattern - sequence of two medical actions, denoted: $p1(med\_action, seq\_act\_op, med\_action)$. In figure 5 we have depicted the template $p1$ corresponding to three pattern instances $i1, i2, i3$. Pattern $p1$ says that a frequent template consists of an ordered list of slots, of which the first and the third one can be filled with instances of medical actions, and the middle one can be filled with any instance of an action operator, describing relations between actions. For instance, in chapter 3, 134 out of 179 sentences were deemed relevant for analysis, and 226 such pattern instances (including overlappings) were identified.

By grouping together pattern instances that instantiate same templates or share common words, the most frequent linguistic constructs can be retrieved and reused in guideline authoring and formalization. For instantiations of control patterns, an equivalent executable representation can be generated automatically, based on the translation of the underlying pattern template into actions.

Selection of Core Patterns. The process of pattern detection produces a list of pattern templates and a core lexicon of link words that connect medical terms in the pattern instances detected. For the guideline analyzed ([5]), the lexicon contains link words such as:

conditional_op : if, in_the_case_of, in_the_event_of
effect_op : results_in, improves, is_expected_to
sequential_op : after, following, followed_by, before, initially
causal_op : since, because, due_to
recommendation_op : should, is_recommended, advisable_to

The list contains relational operators grouped according to the type of semantic relation they describe: ordering of actions, quantification of action effects, etc.

Relations Between Linguistic Templates. After the instances of medically-relevant pattern templates have been looked up in the guideline text, we choose as basic pattern templates those which have the highest support and are more abstract than other templates.

A semantic annotation $SemAnn : T_{GL} \rightarrow Cat$ of the guideline text T_{GL} produces a list of semantic categories from the set Cat. Medical background knowledge expected in the guideline is represented as a set of facts BK about elements in Cat. A schema is a collection of primitive items in Cat connected by relations between items or sets of items. The set of all schemas produced by Cat is denoted S_{Cat}. A schema $S \in S_{Cat}$ is called maximal if it is not a subschema of any other schema $S_1 \in S_{Cat}$. Pattern templates with a high level of abstraction represent maximal schemas. For selecting the core templates, we define relations between linguistic patterns $PT_1 = [C_{11}, C_{12}, \ldots, C_{1n}]$ and $PT_2 = [C_{21}, C_{22}, \ldots C_{2n}]$, using the hierarchical relations in the ontology:

is-more-specific(PT_1, PT_2) iff for all $i = \overline{1,n}$: is_a(C_{1i}, C_{2i});
contains(PT_1, PT_2) iff $\{C_{21}, C_{22}, \ldots C_{2n}\} \subset \{C_{11}, C_{12}, \ldots, C_{1n}\}$.

The list of core pattern templates with high coverage among the instances identified is depicted in table 1, with frequencies for three guideline chapters used in the evaluation in section 4.

Table 1. Coverage of core pattern templates in the chapters analyzed

Template	Translation	Ch.2-4
Association action-goal : $[med\_action, assoc\_rel\_op, disorder]$ $[surgery, to\_reduce, tumour\_load]$	action-goal	10
Action decomposition : $[med\_action, decomp\_op, med\_action, med\_action]$ $[current\_treatment, consists\_of, surgery, radiotherapy]$	decomp.	3
Association condition-action : $[med\_context, med\_action]$ $[multidisciplinary\_treatment, chemotherapy]$	if-then	12
Action sequencing : $[med\_action, act\_op, med\_action]$ $[radiotherapy, following, neoadjuvant\_chemotherapy]$	sequencing	29
Associations action-effect : $[disorder, temp\_rel\_op, med\_action]$ $[tumour\_recurrence, following, radiotherapy]$	action-effect	2
Preference for actions : $[treatment, assoc\_rel\_op, med\_action]$ $[treatment\_of\_choice, is, neoadjuvant\_chemotherapy]$	preferences	19

4 Evaluating the Use of Patterns in Guideline Formalization

Guideline formalization is a transformation that takes as input a guideline GL and a set of formalization rules RF, and produces an executable representation E of the procedural part of the guideline. Formalization involves the following

Table 2. Evaluation: linguistic patterns vs. manual annotation in modelling guidelines

	(autom.) processed sentences	(manual.) modelled sentences	modelled sentences processed	modelled sentences with patterns
chapter 2	130	41	30 (73%)	8 (19.5%)
chapter 3	134	20	16 (80%)	7 (35%)
chapter 4	91	25	18 (72%)	7 (28%)

steps: [1.] select a set of control relations relevant for the target model, then generate templates corresponding to these relations; [2.] detect instances of the control templates in the guideline text; [3.] transform these instances into their formal equivalent. The text-driven approach to formalization consists of deriving a set of constraints RF by reverse-engineering, using a domain-specific lexicon, of the mappings between text fragments and medical knowledge, and using the representation of that knowledge in the guideline representation language to obtain E. To evaluate how close two executable models are, in this paper we make a simplifying assumption: an executable representation of a guideline consists of the actions and the control relations referenced in the guideline.

Evaluation Results. We have compared the results of modelling chapters 2, 3 and 4 of the **CBO guideline for treatment of breast cancer** ([5]) in the medical language MHB [14], using two methods: one which generates a guideline model from pattern instances found automatically as described in this paper, and one which employs a human knowledge engineer (KE) to build the model manually. To estimate the usefulness of applying patterns in guideline formalization, the executable model produced using the linguistic patterns identified automatically is evaluated against and expected to be aligned with the "golden standard" model produced by the human modeller.

We used only instances of templates denoting control relations: action sequencing and decomposition, which were deemed relevant for a medical executable model. To assess if these patterns are suitable to be used for knowledge acquisition in the beginning of guideline formalization, we evaluated whether it is possible to build a coherent fragment of an executable MHB model from the pattern instances detected. The evaluation consisted of: (1) a rough comparison (quantitative) of the amount of knowledge (automatically) identified by using patterns with respect to the knowledge modelled by (manual) knowledge acquisition; for this, we compared the amount of sentences in which the pattern search application has found patterns with respect to the sentences modelled by the KE as procedural knowledge. (2) an analysis (qualitative) of the utility of the pattern instances identified in specific fragments of the guideline; we studied whether a significant piece of a medical executable model can be directly obtained from the pattern instances. This gives an indication of the potential of the pattern detection process for knowledge acquisition.

We have evaluated the coverage of the detection process with respect to the procedural parts modelled by the KE by calculating the percentage of sentences where patterns were detected. Table 2 shows the numbers obtained for the different chapters modelled. Column 1 shows the number of sentences processed by the application and considered relevant for the guideline topic, using a keyword list as criteria for relevance. Columns 2 and 3 give respectively the number of sentences actually modelled by the KE (i.e. the sentences considered relevant from the KE's viewpoint) and, among them, the amount of sentences processed by the application (both the number and the percentage with respect to the modelled sentences). Finally, the last column shows the amount of sentences modelled by the KE and also processed by the application where some patterns have been found. The amount of sentences considered relevant by the application exceeds the modelled knowledge, but covers it to a significant extent, between 70% and 80%. The relatively low coverage of the executable model is explained by the low granularity of the automatically detected patterns, and the absence of some semantic relations from the ontology. Other obstacles in automatic detection were the use of tables and references to non-medical actions and terms absent from the ontology, that could not be extracted from tables. Better coverage heavily depends on having a complete classification of medical terms, particularly actions. Using a richer thesaurus for generating the skeleton executable model from patterns would prove helpful in supporting formalization.

5 Related Work

Guideline patterns reflect modelling decisions when medical guidelines are transformed into an executable form. The task of extracting structure and semantics from annotated and unannotated text, for supporting querying and natural language understanding, has been addressed by recent research in text and data mining (see, for instance, the MedLEE system and related work [7]). The main trend has been extraction of vocabularies or simple syntactic constructs from untagged text ([6, 10, 11, 12]), in some cases guided by the use of a dictionary, thesaurus, or positive examples ([8]). Assigning domain-specific categories to text is done using background knowledge in the form of conceptual graphs ([15, 16]) or simpler mappings between concepts in an ontology and terms in the target domain of the textual description. Statistical and probabilistic models ([6]) were used to increase the performance when ambiguous textual constructions are present. Our work has similarities with concept and relation extraction, but focuses on the use of an ontology to generate, not only validate, pattern candidates for a category of texts with rather strict formatting rules.

6 Conclusions

Searching linguistic patterns is motivated by the need for reusable guideline blocks in guideline formalization and authoring, and by the high overlap between the medical vocabularies used by the oncology guidelines analyzed. The pattern search process is guided by the mappings between medical terms and concepts in a medical ontology, which help us to: 1. extract control knowledge from text, in the form of pattern templates; 2. select a set of core pattern templates, using pattern relationships; 3. identify pattern instances for existing pattern templates. The process takes as input the text of an existing guideline, and an ontology, and attempts to reverse engineer the recurring linguistic pattern templates containing those terms from the ontology that were used to produce the text.

Linguistic patterns are basic building blocks from which semantically-richer fragments can be built, facilitating modularization, validation and reuse of the background knowledge covered by guidelines. The use of patterns produces a lexicon and a skeleton of the formal model covered by the procedural part of the guideline, automatically. The method proposed can be extended to non-procedural knowledge, therefore authoring and formalization of clinical guidelines can benefit from the use of the ontology-driven approach to obtaining linguistic patterns.

References

1. Mesh (Medical Subject Headings). URL: http://www.nlm.nih.gov/mesh/meshhome.html.
2. Natl. Cancer Institute Ontology. URL: http://www.mindswap.org/2003/CancerOntology
3. Protocure 2 Project. URL:www.protocure.org
4. Unified Medical Language System. URL: http://www.nlm.nih.gov/research/umls/
5. CBO. *Guideline for the Treatment of Breast Carcinoma*. 2002. PMID: 12474555.
6. E. Frank; G.W. Paynter; I.H. Witten, C. Gutwin and C. Nevill-Manning. Domain-Specific Keyphrase Extraction. In *Procs. Int. Joint Conf. on AI*, pages pp.668–673. Morgan Kaufmann Publishers, San Francisco, CA, 1999.
7. C. Friedman and G. Hripcsak. Evaluating Natural Language Processors in the Clinical Domain. In *Procs. Conf. on Natural Language and Medical Concept Representation*, pages 41–52. IMIA WG6, 1997.
8. Scott B. Huffman. Learning Information Extraction Patterns from Examples. In *Learning for Natural Language Processing*, pages 246–260, 1995.
9. S. Miksch; Y. Shahar and P. Johnson. Asbru: A Task-Specific, Intention-Based, and Time-Oriented Language for Representing Skeletal Plans. In *Procs. 7th W-shop on Knowledge Engineering: Methods and Languages (KEML-97)*, 1997.
10. A. Moreno and C. Perez. From Text to Ontology: Extraction and Representation of Conceptual Information. In *Procs. Conference on TIA*, May 2001.
11. E. Riloff. Automatically Generating Extraction Patterns from Untagged Text. In *Procs. 13th Nat. Conf. on AI (AAAI-96)*, pages 1044–1049, 1996.
12. E. Riloff and J. Shoen. Automatically Acquiring Conceptual Patterns without an Annotated Corpus. In *Procs. 3rd W-shop on Very Large Corpora*, pages 148–161, New Jersey, 1995. Assoc. for Computational Linguistics.
13. V. Svatek and M. Ruzicka. Mark-up Based Analysis of Narrative Guidelines with the Stepper Tool. In *Procs. Symposium on Computerized Guidelines and Protocols (CGP-04)*. IOS Press, 2004.
14. A. Seyfang, S. Miksch, and P. Votruba. Specification of Formats of Intermediate, Asbru and Kiv Representations. TR-D2.2a, Protocure-II, June 2004.
15. I. Witten. Adaptive Text Mining: Inferring Structure from Sequences. *J. of Discrete Algorithms*, 2000.
16. J. Zhong; H. Zhu; J. Li and Yong Yu. Conceptual Graph Matching for Semantic Search. In *ICCS*, pages 92–196, 2002.

Formalising Medical Quality Indicators to Improve Guidelines*

Marjolein van Gendt, Annette ten Teije, Radu Serban,
and Frank van Harmelen

Vrije Universiteit Amsterdam, Dept. of Artificial Intelligence,
De Boelelaan 1081a, 1081HV Amsterdam, Netherlands
{mtvgendt, annette, serbanr, frank.van.harmelen}@cs.vu.nl

Abstract. Medical guidelines can significantly improve quality of medical care and reduce costs. But how do we get sound and well-structured guidelines? This paper investigates the use of quality indicators that are formulated by medical institutions to evaluate medical care. The main research questions are (i) whether it is possible to *formalise* those indicators in a specific knowledge representation language for medical guidelines, and (ii) whether it is possible to *verify* whether such guidelines do indeed satisfy these indicators. In a case study on two real-life guidelines (Diabetes and Jaundice) we have studied 35 indicators, that were developped independently from these guidelines. Of these 25 (71%!) suggested anomalies in one of the guidelines in our case study.

1 Introduction

Medical guideline are accepted as an instrument for contributing to a higher quality of care. It is evident that high quality of guidelines is important. [7, 2] present formalisation as a technique for guideline quality improvement. Such formalisation points out anomalies. Analysing these anomalies can result in improvement of a guideline. Given a formalisation, verifying the guidelines against particular properties could improve the guideline even further. The question is then *which* properties are useful to verify.

This paper evaluates the use of medical quality indicators as properties to verify. Medical guidelines prescribe the actions medical practitioners should undertake. The medical quality indicators are designed to judge the execution or performance of the care. These quality indicators are systematically engineered by medical experts and therefore give us new insights into what properties the medical care and thus the medical guidelines should satisfy. The motivation for the research question is that the guideline prescribes the care beforehand, whereas the indicators judge the care afterwards, so one would expect these two to correspond (also suggested in e.g. [3]).

Earlier work. [7] already used an indicator to formally verify a medical guideline, but the formalisation of the indicator was done in an ad hoc fashion. In this

---

* This work has been partially supported by the European Commission's IST program, under contract number IST-FP6-508794 Protocure-II.

paper, we study the systematic formalisation of such indicators, and their use in guideline improvement. In this research we build that bridge by interpreting indicators as properties or requirements of the medical guidelines.

Our main research question therefore is: *Can medical guidelines be improved using medical quality indicators?* This leads to the two sub-questions: (i)whether the medical quality indicators can be *formalised*, and (ii) whether they can be used for *verification*.

Structure of this paper. Section 2 describes the general approach of using medical indicators for quality improvement of guidelines. Section 3 describes the results of modelling the indicators and thus answers the *formalisation* question. Section 4 studies the *verification* question. Section 5 shows the overall conclusions from the preceding two sections. This section also shows related and future work.

2 Approach

This research consists of a number of steps. At first the indicators from the relevant medical areas are selected. These indicators must be formalised in the same language as the guidelines, in order to be able to verify their satisfaction by the guideline. During this formalisation anomalies can surface, for instance that an indicator describes a medical action which is not present in the guideline. In such a case the indicator cannot be formalised. The indicators that can be formalised are used for a manual verification against the appropriate guideline. During this verification it might turn out the guideline does not comply with the indicator. Both these types of anomalies point at possible improvements of the guidelines. This section explains these steps in more detail.

Choice of representation language. We have chosen Asbru as modelling language [14]. It is a modelling language constructed specifically for guidelines. Asbru is a task-specific, intention-based and time-oriented language for representing skeletal plans. Its main characteristics are the hierarchy of plans, the possibility to define timing aspects and to define dependencies between plans in a rich control structure. Another important characteristic of Asbru are the constructs for modelling intentions of a plan. In this research these intention constructs are used for the formalisation of the indicators. When a guideline and indicator are modelled in the same language a check on similarities or discrepancies can be performed.

Choice of guidelines. We have used two medical guidelines that were already formalised by the Protocure project[1]. These guidelines concerned Diabetes [13] and Jaundice [1] and this prior work determined the case studies chosen for this research. The original Jaundice guideline is 10 pages of text and is modelled in an Asbru model containing 40 plans (18 pages of Asbru, [9]) while the original Diabetes guideline is 4 pages of text and is modelled in an Asbru model containing 68 plans (58 pages of Asbru, [10]).

---

[1] www.protocure.org

Choice of indicators. For Jaundice the MAJIC indicators are used [6] and for Diabetes the CBO quality indicators [15]. A strong point of our case study is that these indicators are developed independently from the respective guidelines, by different organizations. This avoids the possibility that the guidelines will trivially satisfy the indicators because are both based on the knowledge and experience from the same experts. The results of this research are not limited to only the MAJIC and the CBO diabetes indicators, because a small search revealed many other indicators for both diabetes [12, 4, 8] and for other diseases [11] which were similar to the indicators studied here.

Translating indicators as goals. Indicators usually are measurements of the number of people for which the care has been performed as it should have been. In order to regard indicators as goals or intentions of a care-performance, we need to rephrase the indicators. For instance if an indicator states *"Percentage of people with diabetes suffering retinopathy"*, the corresponding goal becomes *"minimize the number of people with diabetes with retinopathy"*. In other words the indicators must first be translated into goals to be achieved during guideline execution to be useful for verification purposes.

Modelling the indicators. For the actual modelling of the indicators in Asbru a step-wise translation is used. The natural language indicators are first divided into parts that map onto concepts used in Asbru (such as the time annotation). The second step involves the actual formal translation. The results from the formalisation are described in section 3.

Verifying the indicators. After the modelling, the formalised indicators can be used for verification. The verification has to be done manually, because no automated techniques are available yet. This manual verification is quite labour intensive, but produces good results, as can be seen in section 4. Manual verification consists of a walk through the plans in a guideline during which conditions are checked as to whether a required action will be performed under the required circumstances.

3 Modelling

In this section, we discuss the modelling of the indicators and the problems that we encountered. We illustrate them by a concrete example. Furthermore we give an overview of the anomalies that we found during this phase.

Categories of indicators. During modelling, we divided the indicators in a number of categories, due to their differing characteristics.

1. Result vs. process indicators
2. Maximizing vs. minimizing the number of people the indicator applies to
3. Time-related vs. time-unrelated indicators
4. Quantitative vs. qualitative indicators

During the modelling it turned out that the first dimension is the most important. Result indicators refer to *situations or states* that should be true or avoided, whereas process indicators refer to *actions* that should be undertaken or avoided.

How to model indicators in Asbru. Intentions would seem to be the most appropriate Asbru-construction to model indicators. That is because indicators are seen as the goals that must be obtained during or after guideline execution. Plans are the central and essential part of Asbru. Their structure captures the sequence of and the relationship between all the actions. An Asbru intention defines the rationale of a plan i.e. it indicates what purpose a plan has. Intentions are attached to a specific plan and consist of three components. The first component is a Verb. This can be Achieve, Maintain or Avoid. Second there is the indication whether the statement should hold at some time during (Intermediate) or at the successful completion (Overall) of the plan's life cycle. The third building block indicates whether the intention concerns a State (parameter evaluation) or an Action (execution of a plan). In addition to these building blocks an intention consists of a temporal pattern and optionally a time annotation. The time annotation specifies the time period when the parameter proposition used in the intention should hold or be tested. The temporal pattern is the core of every intention, because it describes the situation or action the intention aims for. Within the temporal pattern it is also possible to define a context for an intention. The intention will only be evaluated if the parameter values match the values specified in the context description.

It is interesting to note that the ontology for medical goals as proposed in [5] is very close to the notion of intentions from Asbru. The proposal in [5] consists of the following five components: context, intention verb, target function, temporal constraint, and priority of the goal. This proposal maps rather well to the components of Asbru's intentions, suggesting some concensus among researchers on the elements required for goal modelling.

Example of an indicator in Asbru. Figure 1 shows an example of an indicator that is modelled in Asbru. The example should apply to people with diabetes, so the context for the formalised indicator is a glucose-evaluation of DMT2 (Diabetes Mellitus Type 2). The expressions occuring in the indicator are restricted to those concepts that already occur in the guideline. In this example, both the glucose-evaluation parameter and the diastolic blood pressure already were present in the formalised guideline, so could be used to express the indicator.

The type of the indicator in terms of the four categories mentioned at the beginning of this section, has consequences for the formalisation. The result

Example result indicator (Diabetes)	
original	Percentage of people with diabetes with a diastolic blood pressure smaller than or equal to 90 mmHG
intermediate	maximise (people with diabetes with (a diastolic blood pressure smaller than or equal to 90 mmHG))
formal	Intermediate-state (Achieve (context glucose-evaluation = DMT2) lower-blood-pressure $\leq$ 90)

Fig. 1. An example indicator modelled in Asbru

indicators usually map onto state-intentions, whereas the process indicators map onto action-intentions. If the indicator must be maximized, the verb used is either Maintain or Achieve. For minimization the Avoid-verb is appropriate. If an indicator is time-related a time-annotation is needed and otherwise this can be ignored. The fourth category has no effects on formalisation.

Different types of anomalies. The potential anomalies in the guideline or in the indicator, can be divided in the following groups:

1. Type mismatch: Parameters in the guideline have a value that is of different type or has a range mismatch to the value mentioned in the indicator. For instance, one CBO indicator mentioned *"Percentage of people with diabetes and microalbumin > 30 mg/hr or blood pressure above 150/85 mmHg who get anti-hypertensive medication"*. However, the microalbumin parameter in the guideline ('microalbuminuria') did not match the 'microalbumin' from the indicator, since the one in the guideline is a Boolean value, whereas the one in the indicator is measured in mg/hr.
2. Missing Parameter: The parameter referred to in the indicator is not used at all in the guideline. An example is the following indicator: *"Percentage of people with diabetes who have had a laboratory test for HbA1c during the last 12 months"*, while the parameter HbA1c does not occur in the diabetes guideline.
3. Missing Action: The action required by the indicator is not covered by the guideline. An example is the following indicator: *"Percentage of people with diabetes with just diagnosed or worsening proliferating retinopathy who have undergone vitrectomy or laser coagulation during the last 3 months"*. The indicator presumes much more detail regarding this than the guideline contains, since the actions vitrectomy and laser coagulation are not mentioned in the guideline.
4. Missing medical knowledge: An example from Diabetes is the following indicator: *"Percentage of people with diabetes and angina pectoris who get anti-angina medication"*. The phrase "anti-angina medication" does not occur in the guideline. If it is clear what this medication exactly is, it might be possible to still model the indicator. In that case one could search for other parameters indicating the same substances. This problem can be overcome by consulting a medical expert. In this case there turned out to be no parameters matching 'anti-angina medication' present in the guideline.

Empirical results. Figure 2 summarizes our modelling results[2]. For Diabetes we investigated 21 indicators, of which 12 process indicators and 9 result indicators. We found 10 anomalies in total, which are mainly incompleteness anomalies. The remaining 11 indicators were successfully modelled in Asbru's intentions,

---

[2] In the table the numbers sometimes do not add up for two reasons. The failure to formalise an indicator can have multiple causes and in one case an indicator is formalised in two parts ('achieve intermediate action' as well as 'achieve intermediate state').

Diabetes					
# indicators	21	# anomalies	10	# modelled	11
process	12	Incomplete	8	avoid intermediate state	2
result	9	- missing parameter	5	achieve intermediate state	5
		- missing action	3	maintain intermediate state	3
		Type mismatch	3	achieve intermediate action	2
		Missing medical knowledge	1		

Fig. 2. Indicators and anomalies obtained from the modelling phase

for which we used 4 different intention patterns (notice that in principal 12 different intention patterns are possible in Asbru). For Jaundice, we modelled 14 indicators (all of which were process indicators), which resulted in 3 anomalies, and 11 succesfully modelled indicators. Again only a few (namely 4) intention patterns were needed for modelling 11 process indicators.

In total for the two guidelines, we studied 35 indicators, of which no fewer than 13 (37%) gave rise to potential anomalies.

Especially the indicators that resulted in an "incompleteness" anomaly are of use for guideline improvement. These modelling failures show differences between the guideline and the indicator content, suggesting that either of these would have to be changed.

The above shows that the formalisation of indicators by itself is already a useful contribution to guideline improvement. In the next section we will check whether the modelled intentions do actually hold for the given Asbru models.

4 Verification

The formalisation of the indicators allows us in principle to formally verify whether a guideline complies with the indicator. Such a verification is preferably done automatically. In our case study we perform this verification process manually, for lack of suitable software tools. We have performed this verification for both the Diabetes and the Jaundice guidelines and their corresponding indicators. Our verification is limited to process indicators, and excludes result indicators, because we do not have access to patient data (ie. the outcomes of actions).

Two types of indicators for verification. We distinguish two types of indicators which require different approaches to the verification process: achievement indicators that intend to maintain or achieve an action, and avoidance indicators that intend to avoid an action. The only two conditions that can make a plan stop are the abort and complete conditions. Thus, when an action must be avoided, the abort and complete conditions of the plans must be checked, because if those conditions are met the plan stops and thus the action-leaf will not be reached. If an indicator-action must be achieved or maintained, all conditions and the control structure must match the situation sketched in the indicator.

Achievement indicator (Diabetes)	
original	Percentage of people with diabetes with a known albumin value measured during the last 12 months
intermediate	maximize [people with diabetes] with [a known albumin value] measured [during the last 12 months]

formal	Intermediate-state Achieve
	(or ((context glucose-evaluation = DMT2)
	    albumin-in-urine = known [[0,_][_,1Y][_,_],*now*])
	((context glucose-evaluation = DMT2)
	    albumin-creatinin-ratio-in-urine = known [[0,_][_,1Y][_,_],*now*])))

Fig. 3. Original text, intermediate and formal version of an achievement indicator for the Diabetes guideline

The verification of this type of indicator requires much more work than the avoidance indicators.

4.1 Example Verification

We give an example of the verification of an achievement indicator. Figure 4 shows the relevant part of the Asbru plan hierarchy for the Diabetes guideline; figure 3 shows the original text, the intermediate version and the formal version of an achievement indicator for the Diabetes guideline.

We start with the main plan Diabetes-Mellitus-Type-2. This plan contains two sub-plans, Diagnostics and Policy. Due to the continuation-specification[3] only one of the two sub-plans must necessarily be performed. The wait-for-optional-subplans condition specifies that although only one of the sub-plans must be performed, both of them will be tried and executed if the conditions are met.

Of these two, we first investigate the Diagnostics plan. Again, its wait-for-optional-subplans value dictates that all of its sub-plans must be tried, one of which is the Risk-inventory plan[4]. The filter-precondition of Risk-inventory says: glucose-evaluation = known and glucose-evaluation = DMT2, implying that the plan only applies to people with diabetes. This is indeed also the case for the indicator (figure 3), yielding our first (positive) verification result.

Continuing with the recursive descent down the plan-hierarchy, we arrive at (among others) the Albumin-test subplan of Risk-inventory. The Albumin-test plan has two optional sub-plans: Albumin-test-manual and Albumin-creatinin-ratio-in-urine. These plans aim to obtain just the two values needed in the formal version of the indicator from figure 3: albumin-in-urine and albumin-creatin-ratio-in-urine. Because the values occur in an OR-statement, at least one of these two subplan must be executed. However, neither of these subplans is decorated with a time-annotation that guarantees the requirement stated in the indicator that these two values must date from within the last year. As a result, this aspect of the indicator is not fulfilled by this branch of the diabetes guideline.

Another option for the fulfilment of this indicator is via the Annual-control-plan, reachable from the top-plan via a recursive descent not discussed here (see

---

[3] The detailed conditions of these plans are not shown in figure 4 for space reasons.
[4] In the full verification the other subplans of Diagnostics are also traced, but we skip these here for space reasons

fig. 4). This plan does indeed guarantee the required 1-year period from the indicator, because it is repeated every 46-50 weeks[5]. Unfortunately, the body of Annual-control-plan only calls the required Albumin-test-plan under the condition if age < 50. Consequently, this path of the overall plan also does not verify the indicator in all cases.

Concluding, there is no single path through the Diabetes-Mellitus-Type-2-plan which completely fulfills all the conditions imposed by the indicator from figure 3. In summary, one branch of the plans misses the time-annotations needed to ensure the required timeless of some parameter-readings, while another branch, while ensuring the required timeless of the parameter-readings, only applies to a subset of all patients. This discrepancy can be caused by a mistake either in the guideline or in the indicator. When consulted, a medical expert from CBO, the institution that produced the diabetes indicators, clarified that in this case the indicator was not precise enough, and should have been refined to limit its applicability to patients under 50 (exactly as stated in the guideline).

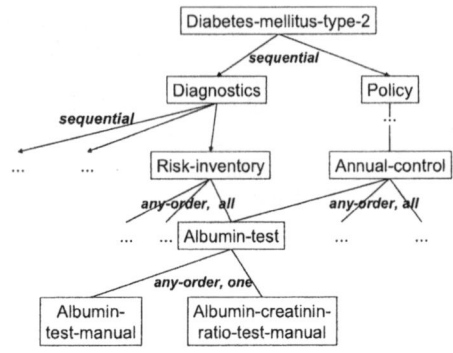

Fig. 4. Part of Asbru plan for Diabetes guideline

Indicators	Diabetes	Jaundice	percentage
Total Attempted	11	11	100%
Succesfully Verified	4	0	18%
Not Succesfully Verified	3	9	55%
- provably untrue	3	6	
- additional assumptions needed	0	3	
Unverifiable	4	2	27%
- need patient data	4	0	
- too complicated for manual effort	0	2	

Fig. 5. Total verification results for both guidelines

4.2 Overall Verification Results

Figure 5 summarizes our verification results for both guidelines. In total we verified 11 indicators for each guideline, namely exactly the indicators that were indicated as succesfully modelled in figure 2. Only a surprisingly small number of the indicators could be successfully verified (a mere 18%). Of the 12 indicators (3+9, 55%) that could not be successfully verified, 3 could be verified, but

---

[5] Again, body of the plan not shown

only under additional assumptions which should be discussed with a medical expert. This leaves a signficant number of 9 indicators (6+3) that were provably incompatible with the guideline. For a remaining category of 6 indicators (27%) we were not able to perform a verification, because either they would require patient data (the result indicators discussed in section 3), or because the verification proof was too complicated to complete by hand.

Especially the category of "not succesfully verified" indicators (12 indicators, 55%) can be of use for improving the guideline, because they point at differences of opinion between the creators of the guidelines and of the indicators.

5 Conclusion and Future Work

Medical quality indicators can be used to improve medical guidelines and thus medical care. The guideline and the indicator must be formalised to do this. In this case study we have used Asbru as a modelling language to formalise guidelines and indicators in the Diabetes and Jaundice domains. Our main findings are as follows:

- A translation of the indicators into a formal guideline modelling language is possible. This translation already reveals a number of potential anomalies, which can be divided into 4 different groups (type mismatch, missing parameter, missing action and missing medical knowledge).
- The formal modelling of the indicators for Diabetes and Jaundice resulted in a significant number of potential anomalies. For the Diabetes guidelines almost 50% of the indicators suggested some kind of anomaly in the guideline. For Jaundice, this percentage was much lower (20%), but still significant.
- The formalisation of indicators enabled the verification of compliance between guidelines and indicators. Only a disappointing 18% of the indicators could be succesfully verified. For a suprisingly high number of indicators (55%) the verification revealed non-compliance of the guideline with the indicator. For the remaining 27% the result remains undecided for a variety of practical reasons.
- Overall, we have started with 35 independently developped indicators for two guidelines. Of these, 13 suggested a possible anomaly during the modelling phase. Of the remaining 22, a further 12 suggested anomalies during the verification phase. In other words 25 out of 35 indicators, a staggering 71%, suggested anomalies in one of the guidelines in our case study.

Future work.
- An obvious next step in this research is the validation of our results with medical experts, to evaluate which changes should be incorporated into the guidelines.
- Another issue is the enhancement of the formalisation process. The manual verification should be replaced by automatic verification and the process must become more formal, for example by using an interactive theorem prover [7].
- Verification of the result indicators should be done on the basis of patient data, which was unavailable at the time of our case study.
- A possible resolution of the mismatch-anomalies could be to use an ontology for semi-automatically bridging the mismatches between guideline and indicator.

References

1. American Academy of Pediatrics, Provisional Committee for Quality Improvement and Subcommittee on Hyperbilirubinemia. Practice parameter: management of hyperbilirubinemia in the healthy term newborn. *Pediatrics*, 94:558–565, 1994.
2. M. Balser, O. Coltell, J. van Croonenborg, C. Duelli, F. van Harmelen, A. Jovell, P. Lucas, M. Marcos, S. Miksch, W. Reif, K. Rosenbrand, A. Seyfang, and A. ten Teije. Protocure: Supporting the Development of Medical Protocols through Formal Methods. *Proceedings of the Symposium on Computerized Guidelines and Protocols (CGP 2004)*, number 101 in Studies in health technology and informatics, pages 103–108, IOS press, 2004.
3. A. Casparie, et al. *Ontwikkeling van Indicatoren op Basis van Evidence-based richtlijnen*. Van Zuiden Communications, Alphen aan den Rijn, 2002.
4. B. Fleming, S. Greenfield, M. Engelgau, L. Pogach, S. Clauser, M. Parrott. Diabetes care. *The Diabetes Quality Improvement Project*, 24:1815–1820, 2001.
5. J. Fox, A. Alabassi, E. Black, C. Hurt, and T. Rose. Modelling Clinical Goals: a Corpus of Examples and a Tentatove Ontology. In *SCGP-04, Proceedings of the Symposium on Computerized Guidelines and Protocols*, pages 31–45. IOS Press, 2004.
6. MAJIC. MAJIC Steering Committee Meets. *MAJIC Newsletter*, 1(2), 1998.
7. M. Marcos, M. Balser, A. ten Teije, F. van Harmelen, and C. Duelli. Experiences in the Formalisation and Verification of Medical Protocols. In *AIME-2003*, pgs 132–141. Springer, 2003.
8. L. Nyberg and M. Lawrence. Overall Quality Indicators in Health Care and Medical Services, 2001.
9. Protocure I Project. Asbru Protocol for the Management of Hyperbilirubinemia in the Healthy Term Newborn, August 2002. Technical Report, URL: http://www.protocure.org.
10. Protocure I Project. Asbru Protocol for the Management of Diabetes Mellitus Type 2, August 2002. Technical Report, URL: http://www.protocure.org.
11. T. C. of State, t. A. o. S. Territorial Epidemiologists (CSTE), T. C. D. P. D. (ASTCDPD), the National Center for Chronic Disease Prevention, H. P. C. for Disease Control, and Prevention. Indicators for chronic disease surveillance, 2001. http://cdi.hmc.psu.edu/pathways/ breastcancer.html.
12. Rockville. AHRQ Quality Indicators - Guide to Prevention Quality Indicators: Hospital Admission for Ambulatory Care Sensitive Conditions. *Agency for Healthcare Research and Quality*, AHRQ Pub, no. 02-R0203, 2004. revision 3.
13. G. Rutten, S. Verhoeven, R. Heine, W. de Grauw, P. Cromme, K. Reenders, E. van Ballegooie, and T. Wiersma. NHG-Standaard Diabetes Mellitus Type 2 (eerste herziening). *Huisarts en Wetenschap*, 42(2):67–84, 1999. First revision.
14. Y. Shahar, S. Miksch, and P. Johnson. The Asgaard Project: a Task-specific Framework for the Application and Critiquing of Time-oriented Clinical Guidelines. *AIM*, 14:29–51, 1998.
15. G. Storms, P. ten Have, and R. Dijkstra. *Indicatoren voor Verbetering van de Diabeteszorg*. Van Zuiden Communications, Alphen aan den Rijn, 2002.

Ontology and Terminology

Oncology Ontology in the NCI Thesaurus

Anand Kumar[1] and Barry Smith[1,2]

[1] IFOMIS, University of Saarland, Saarbruecken, Germany
[2] Department of Philosophy, SUNY at Buffalo, NY, USA
akumar@ifomis.uni-saarland.de, phismith@buffalo.edu

Abstract. The National Cancer Institute's Thesaurus (NCIT) has been created with the goal of providing a controlled vocabulary which can be used by specialists in the various sub-domains of oncology. It is intended to be used for purposes of annotation in ways designed to ensure the integration of data and information deriving from these various sub-domains, and thus to support more powerful cross-domain inferences. In order to evaluate its suitability for this purpose, we examined the NCIT's treatment of the kinds of entities which are fundamental to an ontology of colon carcinoma. We here describe the problems we uncovered concerning classification, synonymy, relations and definitions, and we draw conclusions for the work needed to establish the NCIT as a reference ontology for the cancer domain in the future.

Keywords: Ontology, Oncology, NCI Thesaurus, Clinical Bioinformatics.

1 Introduction

The NCI Thesaurus (NCIT)[1] is a public domain Description Logic-based terminology produced by the National Cancer Institute's Center for Bioinformatics as a component of its caCORE distribution.[2] NCIT was initially conceived as a terminology server to be used within the various NCI departments. However, it has slowly gained acceptance also outside the NCI as a source for carcinoma terminology. The Thesaurus spans clinical and biological domains. It is one of the earliest terminologies to operationally federate with another ontology system (the MGE Ontology) and to embrace the goal of harmonizing with external ontology modeling practices. The NCIT is thus to be welcomed because it covers an unusually large domain with limited resources. This means also however that it is marked by certain inaccuracies, which are currently managed in an ad hoc way via updates on the basis of criticisms received. The NCIT's impressively broad coverage makes it a good dictionary or lexicon. As argued in [Ceusters et al 2004], however, if the NCIT is to conform to the best practices of ontology building, then it needs to do more than resolve reported inaccuracies in an ad hoc fashion. It should rather be rebuilt on the basis of a sound ontology and its constituent terms should be evaluated in light of this ontology. Such an exercise will guarantee that it has the sort of robust organization that can support

---

[1] http://nciterms.nci.nih.gov/NCIBrowser/Startup.do
[2] http://ncicb.nci.nih.gov/core

the drawing of inferences involving the different sub-domains of oncology in a maximally efficient and reliable way.

In a series of earlier papers we have drawn attention to certain characteristic families of errors in biomedical terminologies and ontologies such as SNOMED-CT,[3] the UMLS Semantic Network[4] and the Gene Ontology[5] [Kumar & Smith 2004a, Kumar & Smith 2004b, Ceusters et al 2004, Kumar et al 2004, Kumar & Smith 2003], pointing especially to problems with is_a and part_of relations and to logical errors in the formulation of definitions. [Ceusters et al 2004] continues this work in relation to the NCIT. Here we concentrate on one particular aspect of the Thesaurus: its representation of the entities involved in colon carcinoma. To this end we draw on our previous work in collaboration with the Swiss Institute of Bioinformatics [Kumar et al 2005], which uses SNOMED-CT and Gene Ontology annotations, the Swissprot mutant protein database and the Foundational Model of Anatomy to construct an onco-ontology within the Protégé 2000 ontology editing environment, supplementing these digital information resources with deVita's text book [deVita 2004 CD].

Our strategy was to assess the degree to which the NCIT lives up to its goal of serving as a reference ontology for the cancer domain, by attempting to represent within it the entities belonging to our onco-ontology for colon carcinoma. As concerns the salient anatomical entities we also compared the NCIT with the Foundational Model of Anatomy[6] (FMA).

2 The Colon and Adjacent Anatomical Structures

We begin with the normal anatomy and physiology of the colon. The NCIT incorporates the UMLS Semantic Network (SN), meaning that it provides for each class the SN semantic type provided within the UMLS Metathesaurus. Problems arise because SN sometimes conflicts with the subsumption relations provided by the Thesaurus itself and also with the assertions derivable from its incorporation of relational expressions (such as 'Anatomic_Structure_is_Physical_Part_of') in which the types of the relata are explicitly stated.

The ontology of *colon carcinoma* revolves around the *colon*, the anatomical structure which bears the carcinoma and upon whose existence the carcinoma depends. NCIT has:

colon is_a *gastrointestinal system part*

gastrointestinal system part is_a *body part, organ or organ component*

The NCIT does not provide definitions of 'is_a' or of its other relational expressions. For present purposes, however, we can define 'is_a' (meaning: is a subkind of / is a subtype of) as follows:

$$A \text{ is\_a } B =_{def} \forall x \, (Ax \rightarrow Bx)$$

---

[3] http://www.snomed.org/
[4] http://www.nlm.nih.gov/research/umls/
[5] http://www.geneontology.org/
[6] http://sig.biostr.washington.edu/projects/fm/AboutFM.html

Here 'Ax' abbreviates 'individual x is an instance of kind A.' '$\forall$' is the standard universal quantifier of first-order logic (signifying 'for all values of') and '$\rightarrow$' is the logical connective 'if ... then'. In a full version of the ontology we would need to take account of time for continuant entities and write 'Axt' for 'x is an instance of A at t'. We could then assert for example an axiom to the effect that

$$A \text{ is\_a } B \rightarrow \exists xt(Axt \text{ \& } Bxt),$$

which means that is_a statements imply also the existence of corresponding instances. (Here '$\exists$' is the standard existential quantifier, signifying 'for some value of'.)

The NCIT has:

colon is_a *body part, organ or organ component*

Here the use of the disjunctive class name '*body part, organ or organ component*' does not reflect good ontology authoring practices [Ceusters et al 2005]. Moreover its use means that, unlike the FMA, NCIT does not define what an *organ* is and makes no statement from which we can infer that *colon* is in fact an *organ*. *Organs* have specific properties and belong to a specific level of granularity, which is different from that of both *organ systems* and *organ parts*.

3 Large Intestine

NCIT also has:

colon Anatomic_Structure_is_Physical_Part_of *large intestine*

We presume that the oddly named relation: Anatomic_Structure_is_Physical_Part_of comes close to the part_of relation for anatomical structures as defined within the FMA. We could then reformulate the above as:

colon part_of *large intestine*

where A part_of B is defined as: for every instance x of A there is some instance y of B which is such that x **part_of** y. In symbols:

$$A \text{ part\_of } B =_{def} \forall x (Ax \rightarrow \exists y (By \text{ \& } x \textbf{ part\_of } y))$$

(Here **part_of** is the instance-level parthood relation obtaining between individuals, illustrated for example by Mary's_colon **part_of** Mary.)

Unfortunately, NCIT also has:

colon synonym *large intestine*

This is problematic first of all because synonymy relations (unlike part relations) hold not between classes or kinds, but rather between the corresponding *names*. Thus we should more properly write:

'colon' synonym 'large intestine'

though even this (as any dictionary will verify) is an error.

Such mistakes have adverse implications when for example we attempt to use a resource like Swissprot to derive information pertaining to those mutant proteins which are involved in colon carcinoma specifically and not in carcinomas of both the colon and the rectum, or to draw on the information in Swissprot pertaining to the markers present within rectum carcinomas of the *squamous* and of the *adenocarcinoma* type.

4 Colorectal Carcinoma

'Colorectal carcinoma' is a term used in some contexts to represent a carcinoma which affects both the colon and the rectum, and in others to represent a kind of carcinoma which is sometimes present in the colon, sometimes in the rectum, and sometimes in both. Unfortunately NCIT, which should have provided some regimentation in the use of this term, has not only:

colon carcinoma is_a *colorectal carcinoma*

but also assertions to the effect that the colorectal carcinoma is located both within the colon and the rectum and within the small intestines.

5 Colon Epithelium

Colon epithelium in the FMA is an *organ part* which is asserted to stand also in a parthood relation to *colon*. The NCIT, in contrast, has

epithelium is_a *tissue*

tissue is_a *other anatomic concept*

other anatomic concept is_a *anatomic structure, system or substance*

The classification of *tissue* as *other anatomic concept* reflects a characteristic confusion, found still today in many terminologies, between concepts and entities in the world. This represents a departure from the principles of good ontology not least because it blocks inferences on the basis of the physical characteristics of the entities at issue [Smith et al 2005b]. Thus it blocks such inferences regarding *adenomatous polyposis coli*, one of the prime predisposing factors for *colon carcinoma*, for which we have:

adinomatous polyposis coli Disease_Has_Normal_Tissue_Origin *epithelium*

We find analogous mistakes with respect to specific organ parts, e.g. in:

large intestinal muscularis mucosa is_a *large intestinal mucosa*

which, because the muscularis mucosa is not a type of but rather a part of the mucosa, confuses mereology with subsumption.

Consider also:

large intestinal muscularis mucosa is_a *large intestinal wall tissue*

large intestinal wall tissue is_a *normal tissue*

normal tissue is_a *microanatomy*

which involves a confusion between a kind of entity and a branch of science.

6 Is_a Overloading

The *is_a* relation can reflect different types of partition of reality. For example in a partition on the basis of pathology we have:

colon carcinoma is_a *disease of colon*

The former is a specification of the latter reflecting the added factor of (carcinomatous) *pathology*. In a partition on the basis of location, in contrast, we have

colon carcinoma is_a *carcinoma*

the specification here deriving from the factor: *location within the colon*. The specification is in each case a child (type) of the relevant partitioning entity. Thus, carcinomatous pathology is a type of pathology and colon location is a type of location. Where distinct specification factors are combined within a single tree errors often result. Thus in the NCIT we find:

mutagen is_a *chemical modifier*

chemical modifier semantic_type *chemical viewed functionally*

drugs and chemicals, functional classification semantic_type *classification*

drugs and chemicals, functional classification is_a *drugs and chemicals*

so that *functional classification* is classified as a subtype of *drugs and chemicals*.

DNA damage, which plays an important role within the pathogenesis of colon carcinomas, is asserted to belong to the *semantic type: Cellular or Molecular Dysfunction*. In:

DNA damage Biological_Process_Has_Associated_Location *chromosome structure*

DNA damage Biological_Process_Has_Initiator_Chemical_or_Drug *mutagen*

however, NCIT asserts also that *DNA damage* is a *process*. The problem here is that functions and processes belong to ontologically distinct top-level categories. The former are continuants, the latter occurrents.[7] Functions are powers or potentials which can be realized in corresponding processes. That function and process cannot be identified follows also from the fact that many functions are never realized.

Even if *DNA damage* were a biological process (which we doubt), then one would still not need to represent this fact twice, once by means of an explicit assertion of an is_a relation, and again by making it explicit within the assertion of relationships in which *DNA damage* enters as a term. The NCIT's complex relational expressions bring not only redundancy (and occasional contradiction) but also serve as an obstacle to the goal of integration with other ontologies, for which it is important that relations be both clearly defined and maximally general in scope. [Smith et al 2005]

---

[7] http://ontology.buffalo.edu/bfo/BFO.htm

7 Predisposing Factors

Alcohol consumption is one of the predisposing factors for colon carcinoma. There are both physical and behavioral aspects of such consumption, and NCIT mixes the two together by taking over definitions of 'alcohol consumption' from two distinct sources, defining it both as: 'consumption of liquids containing ethanol; includes the behavior of drinking the alcohol (CSP2003)' and as: 'behaviors associated with the ingesting of alcoholic beverages, including social drinking (MeSH2001)'. The Thesaurus thus asserts that *alcohol consumption* is:

a. *physical consumption* (from the definitions)
b. *individual behavior* (from SN)
c. (on some occasions) *social behavior* (from MeSH)

This is a good example of the mistakes which result when term-to-term matching is used to create an "ontology of ontologies" on the basis of component parts which are of varying quality and without careful consideration of the meanings associated with the terms in the different sources.

The Thesaurus assigns to *physical activity* the semantic type: *Daily or Recreational Activity* (!). At the same time it asserts:

physical activity is_a *health behavior*

Each case of physical activity, then, is a case of health behavior (!).

The confusion between physical activity and behavior is extended in the case of *obesity* which is on the one hand assigned the semantic type *Sign or Symptom* and is on the other hand classified as follows:

obesity is_a *symptom*

symptom is_a *other finding*

Here the physical parameters are not considered at all. Rather *obesity* is classified as a *finding*, an extremely broad class (analogous to *concept*), which is applied on the basis of how the corresponding knowledge is gained by healthcare professionals. Such jumps from one partition to another leave gaps which cannot be spanned by inference.

For *old population* we have:

old population is_a *population group*

population group is_a *social concept*

A population group, then, is a certain kind of concept.

Confusions also arise with relations which are not well defined. For example, *APC gene* is asserted to stand in the following relations

APC gene Gene_is_Element_in_Pathway *TGF beta signaling pathway*

APC gene Gene_is_Element_in_Pathway *WNT signaling pathway*

APC gene Gene_Plays_Role_in_Process *cell adhesion*

APC gene Gene_Plays_Role_in_Process *cytoskeletal modeling*

Pathways are built out of multiple subprocesses, here called 'Elements'. Yet the processes of *cell adhesion* and *cytoskeletal modeling* mentioned in the above relations are also composed of many subprocesses and thus do not differ in their ontology from those classes here called 'Pathways'. It therefore makes little sense to represent a gene as an Element of the one and as a Role Player in the other. We do not really understand what the Thesaurus means by 'Element' but we surmise that it is meant to represent the fact that there are other subprocesses in which the particular gene at issue is not involved. This is also true, however, for cell adhesion and for cytoskeletal modeling, and thus the relations involved should be identical in all of the four cases.

8 Clinical Manifestations

The inaccuracies related to the representation of the clinical management of colon carcinoma are very similar to those already mentioned above. For example, *obstruction* and *perforation* are assigned the semantic type: *Finding*. *Rectal hemorrhage* is classified as *other finding*.

There are situations where the Thesaurus puts *neoplasm*, a continuant and *neoplastic process*, an occurrent, together under a single heading. This *mucinous neoplasm*, one of the most aggressive kinds of colon carcinoma, is classified as follows:

mucinous neoplasm is_a *neoplasm by morphology*

neoplasm by morphology is_a *neoplasm*

mucinous neoplasm semantic type *neoplastic process*

This is rather as if one were to identify fracturing process with the fracture itself, the result of such a process. On the therapeutic side, there are many cases where an agent used within a therapy is classified together with the therapy itself. *BCG therapy*, which involves the use of an immunomodulator, is assigned three distinct semantic types – *bacterium*, *immunologic factor* and *pharmacologic substance*, none of which represent it as a therapy.

On the other hand there are cases where a drug combination itself is represented as a therapy even if it mentions only the names of the involved drugs. Thus *Capecitabine/DJ-027* is assigned the semantic type *Therapeutic or Preventive Procedure* and is classified as follows:

Capecitabine/DJ-027 is_a *chemotherapeutic regimen*

9 Conclusion

In adhering to its legacy in the UMLS Semantic Network, the NCI Thesaurus has increased the number of its inaccuracies. But there are also mistakes which are the responsibility of the Thesaurus itself. If the Thesaurus were to be used for representing entities involved in the location, pathogenesis or management of carcinomas, then it needs to be thoroughly restructured, and this is all the more the case if Electronic Health Records are to use the Thesaurus as the source of terms for the entities involved in carcinomas.

The NCIT does provide a rich terminology for carcinomas, which makes it a good starting point for ontology work in the cancer domain. Moreover, the problems which are present within the Thesaurus are, as we have seen, not new. One of the reasons why current Electronic Health Record standards restrict the use of standard terminologies and ontologies as code providers is to ensure that employing a particular code would convey a single corresponding term. And when one attempts to go further than that on the basis of current approaches, in order to use the structures of terminologies and ontologies in a way that supports the drawing of inferences, then experience has shown that one is confronted by formidable obstacles. If the necessary integration is to be accomplished, then the structure found within those terminologies and ontologies must be aligned with each other and with those found within Electronic Health Records on the basis of robust formal principles. We established in a controlled comparison that FMA, though its representation is restricted to the domain of (non-pathological) anatomy, does far better in this respect. We therefore recommend a thorough audit of the NCI Thesaurus on the basis of the principles followed by the FMA.

Acknowledgements. Work on this paper was carried out under the auspices of the Wolfgang Paul Program of the Humboldt Foundation and also of the EU Network of Excellence in Semantic Datamining and the project "Forms of Life" sponsored by the Volkswagen Foundation.

References

1. Ceusters W, Smith B, Goldberg L. A terminological and ontological analysis of the NCI Thesaurus. Methods of Information in Medicine.(2005). In press
2. Ceusters W, Smith B, Kumar A, Dhaen C. Ontology-Based Error Detection in SNOMED-CT® Medinfo. 2004 (2004) 482-6.
3. Devita VT, Hellman S, Rosenberg SA. Principles and Practices of Oncology. Chapter 33. Cancers of the Gastrointestinal Tract. 33.7 Cancer of the Colon. 6th edition. CD
4. Kumar A, Yip L, Smith B, Grenon P. Bridging the Gap between Medical and Bioinformatics Using Formal Ontological Principles. Computers in Biology and Medicine. 2005. In press
5. Kumar A, Smith B. On Controlled Vocabularies in Bioinformatics: A Case Study in Gene Ontology. Drug Discovery Today: BIOSILICO, 2, (2004) 246-252 [2004a]
6. Kumar A, Smith B. Towards a Proteomics Metaclassification. IEEE Fourth Symposium on Bioinformatics and Bioengineering, Taichung, Taiwan. IEEE Press. (2004) 419-427 [2004b]
7. Kumar A, Smith B, Borgelt C. Dependence Relationships between Gene Ontology Terms based on TIGR Gene Product Annotations. CompuTerm Aug 29, 2004: 3rd International Workshop on Computational Terminology: 31-38.
8. Kumar A, Smith B. The Universal Medical Language System and the Gene Ontology: Some Critical Reflections. Lecture Notes in Computer Science. (2003) Sep; 2821/2003: 135 – 148.
9. Smith B, Ceusters W, Koehler J, Klagges B, Kumar A, Lomax J, Mungall C, Neuhaus F, Rector A, Rosse C. Relations in Biomedical Ontologies Genome Biology. 2005;6:R46. 2005a
10. Smith B, Ceusters W, Temmerman R. Wuesteria. MIE 2005. (2005) in press. 2005b

Ontology-Mediated Distributed Decision Support for Breast Cancer

S. Dasmahapatra, D. Dupplaw, B. Hu, P. Lewis, and N. Shadbolt

IAM, School of Electronics and Computer Science (ECS),
University of Southampton Southampton, SO17 1BJ, UK

Abstract. We have developed a prototype system to support decision making in Breast Cancer, wherein the varied nature of expertise is modelled by multiple ontologies that provide domain-specific grounding to concepts and relationships used. While the different medical experts need to be co-present at a meeting, our system employs a distributed architecture for handling data and invoking services appropriate for the requirements of this decision-making process. This distributed system is built upon Semantic Web technology, which enables the possibility of Web-based tele-medicine.

1 Introduction

The increasing necessity of incorporating specialist knowledge in critical medical domains has introduced a rearrangement of the sites of patient-doctor engagement. Thus, the patient's condition is described by different specialists, offering complementary views which determine the course of intervention or treatment. In the domain of breast cancer, this multiplicity of views is the norm, so a decision support environment for this domain needs to incorporate the distribution of sources and type of knowledge, and provide methods to collate the case-specific information based on the concepts used in the various specialist domains. In particular, the domains of interest that are relevant involve radiology, X-ray, magnetic resonance images (MRI) and ultrasound images are routinely used; pathology, histopathologists and cytopathologists produce microscopic slides from cells and tissues extracted from the patient; and clinicians, oncologists and surgeons also deliberate on possible interventions they can suggest based on prognostic factors implied by the interpretations of these images.

The integration of heterogeneous types and formats of information sources for the purpose of retrieval is one of the envisaged positive outcomes of Semantic Web technology [1]. In this paper, we describe a prototype system for providing decision support which used Semantic Web technology—domain ontologies for describing the relevant specialist information as indicated, a declarative (ontological) characterisation of the methods and services that are invoked in order to enable relevant information flows within a Web-based distributed environment. This provides a flexible open-ended architecture for the integration of services which can be described at the knowledge level, and hence possibly chained together in order the requirements of the users' decision-making deliberations. The application building process is also made more flexible with distributed service implementers having control over their methods which are called through a mediating task registry. This is crucial in a medical application such as ours, as institutional control over data is critical as ethical issues create an independent channel regulating the flow of information within the system.

2 Domain Ontologies for Breast Cancer

The medical domains represented by ontologies in this project are X-ray mammography, MRI, ultrasound imaging and histopathology. These were developed independently of each other using a variety of sources and implemented in the Web Ontology Language (OWL-DL). For X-ray, MRI and ultrasound, we could make use of lexicons developed in standardising efforts of the American College of Radiologists, called BI-RADS[3]. The histopathology ontology was created from UK National Health Service guidelines for reporting [2] in breast cancer cases as well as from papers in medical journals. The National Cancer Informatics (NCI) ontology [4] is a very useful resource, but its sheer size (38MB) and breadth of coverage meant having to throw out most of the terminological concepts that were not relevant to breast cancer. Moreover, the terms that we required in order to provide terminological support for the cases that we were provided by our medical partners were not completely covered in the NCI ontology. In addition to these medical specialist terminological coverage, we also have an ontology to describe basic patient information like age, a description of the procedures that she may have undergone and so on. Within each class in each of the ontologies, sub-concepts are usually introduced not just with expressive names borrowed from the lexicon, but as refinements with respect to values in the range of some discriminatory relation, such as morphological features taking particular descriptive names as values.

The principal role these ontologies play in our system is to provide a framework within which relevant information pertaining to a case can be retrieved and related information reached by navigation. To that end, we have a mechanism of exposing aspects of the web of conceptual terms to the user should it be necessary or desirable (as illustrated in Figure 1).

3 Distributed Decision Support

In this section, we give an overview of the system architecture which allows the inclusion of different knowledge-based services. The system design is a declarative specification based on information flow within the system, which is driven by the demands for the relevant knowledge by the medical users of the system. Access to information is contrained by legal and ethical concerns, and we have assumed local storage under institutional custodianship. Any algorithms or clients that are instantiated through the system retrieve the patient information, such as x-ray images directly from these distributed sources.

As with the domain ontology where the interactions between the different sources of knowledge about a case was organised into the separation of different groups of concepts, here too we develop an "service composition ontology (SCO)" that organises the different services that are invoked and trigger information transfers around the system, so that the client can invoke the available distributed services described. Apart from the client and the server, a general task invocation framework allows remotely developed and appropriately packaged modules to be called upon, should they be relevant to the knowledge handling requirements for use. This too is described in SCO and is run on a remote server.

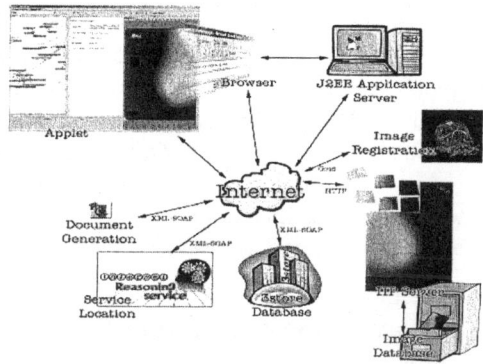

Fig. 1. The System Architecture

Declarative Specifications and Applications

The task invocation sub-system uses a number of different mappings to provide task-level invocation of functionality on disparate systems. The idea in the task invocation sub-system is first and foremost to protect the client application from changes in the remote web-resources. Secondly, it provides a clean interface for the execution of web-resources that are accessed through different interfaces. The flexibility provided by the system also provides a good base for application deployment.

In the task invocation framework, a Task Registry plays the analogous role, but here it is the inputs and outputs of the services that have to remain uncorrupted, not the internal workings of the modules. The Task Registry is a dictionary-like structure that maps tasks on to task implementations. The task's identification (its name and other parameters) is represented by a Task Description. A specific task implementation may be used in more than one task description, although new instances of that implementation are used in each task. Both task descriptions and task implementations can have default arguments and both can have mappings applied to any argument names. This also ensures flexibility between the task descriptions and the task implementations.

Knowledge Services

Our system provides a generic platform to compose various medically relevant services designed particularly for Breast Cancer Domain. A number of such services are provided by some of our partners in the project from other universities and they have been and are being written up elsewhere. These include MRI diagnostic classification tasks, natural language generation from case annotations against our domain ontologies, image registration, and so on. Here, we report on some of the knowledge rich diagnostic support services we have implemented. The architecture accommodates, among other methods, classification services based on features automatically extracted from images or its hand-drawn segments. In addition, in the multi-disciplinary meeting for patient management, the cases already come with expert labels attached—shape features for masses seen in X-rays, for example. We have also built classifiers which take BI-RADS descriptors and other ontological metadata labels for X-ray images as input and classify cases according to their likelihood of being benign or malignant. We have packaged a few classifiers – trained on 1500 cases from the Digital Database for Screening Mammography (DDSM) of the University of South Florida [5] – to run as services that can be accessed remotely via task invocation methods. Also, with the descriptive framework for task invocation in place, the future availability of semantic web service description standards could then be used to advertise such capabilities in appropriate semantic web service repositories.

4 Related Work and Looking Ahead

While there are several aspects of the system we have not described here, we would like to indicate some future directions we would like to go in. As indicated in Figure 1 one of the service modules delivers image feature vectors from X-ray images—these are grayscale histograms, shape, perimeter and area measures on hand-annotated closed curves on the image indicating regions of interest, wavelet features, and so on. Association of features of an image or region of interest with the concepts in the ontology may be manually or semi-automatically generated, or retrieved from legacy data. Association of a feature to concepts defined in the ontology is provided by a simple point and click mechanism. The user highlights the feature which they are going to associate with a concept, and finds the relevant concept in one of the concept browsers to right click and link. The feature vector is stored in a feature database, which provides indexed, feature-dependent retrieval of features, and the unique ID of the feature vector is inserted as an instance of the given concept. This image feature extraction algorithms are provided to the client mainly through the web-service interface. This API provides functionality for storing, retrieving, and comparing feature vectors from images, and automatically provides feature modules with the relevant regions from the source media. There is another use to which we can put these classifiers. As different hospital practices and radiologists use slight variations in ontological terms and relations in describing x-ray images, the collation of information for statistical analysis becomes difficult. We will use these image to concept label classifiers to assist the ontology mapping process, where the system will enable the remote exchange of images.

Recent work in feature extraction for diagnosis is featured in [6], which framework would be amenable to the word-picture matching problem[7]. As for the system presented, a quite similar architecture was described in [8]. The content-based soft annotation (CBSA) tool [10] uses Bayesian classifiers to commute semantic labels between image sets, providing content based semantic labeling. Marques and Barman [9] use feature clustering and ontological labeling to provide semi-automatic image annotation. They map the image into feature space (based on automatically extracted colour, shape and texture features) and retrieve the ontological concepts that been associated with the nearest cluster.

Future work on this system and the requirements of the domain will initially be drawn from the ideas presented above. As a proof of concept of a prototype for this domain, the system succeeds in pulling together web services and Grid based image registration services through an ontologically indexed architecture. While we have had substantial clinical input, we are currently trying to use this framework in a limited clinical setting.

References

1. T Berners-Lee, J Hendler, O Lassila. "The Semantic Web." *Scientific American*, 2001.
2. R Wilson, D Asbury, J Cooke, M Michell and J Patnick (eds.). Clinical Guidelines for Breast Cancer Screening Assessment. NHSBSP Publication No 49, April 2001.
3. American College of Radiology. Breast Imaging Reporting and Data System: BI-RADS.
4. The National Cancer Informatics Thesaurus and Ontology. Available from http://www.mindswap.org/2003/CancerOntology/nciOncology.owl.gz
5. M. Heath, K.W. Bowyer, D. Kopans et al. Current Status of the Digital Database for Screening Mammography. *Digital Mammography*, p 457-460, Kluwer Academic Publishers, 1998.
6. P Sajda, C Spence and L Parra. A multi-scale probabilistic network model for detection, synthesis and compression in mammographic image analysis *Medical Image Analysis* 7 (2003) 187204.
7. K Barnard, P Duygulu, N de Freitas, D Forsyth, D Blei and M I Jordan. Matching Words and Pictures. *Journal of Machine Learning Research*, 3, pp 1107-1135, 2003.
8. M Addis, M Boniface, S Goodall, P Grimwood, S Kim, P Lewis, K Martinez, A Stevenson. SCULPTEUR: Towards a new paradigm for multimedia museum information handling. *International Semantic Web Conference (ISWC)* 2003, October 20-23, 2003, FL.
9. O. Marques, and N. Barman. Semi-automatic semantic annotation of images using machine learning techniques. *International Semantic Web Conference (ISWC)* 2003, October 20-23, 2003, FL.
10. E. Chang, K. Goh, G. Sychay, and G. Wu. CBSA: Content-Based Soft Annotation for Multimodal Image Retrieval Using Bayes Point Machines. *IEEE Transactions of Circuits and Systems for Video Technology*, 13(1):26-38, January 2003.

Multimedia Data Management to Assist Tissue Microarrays Design

Julie Bourbeillon, Catherine Garbay, Joëlle Simony-Lafontaine,
and Françoise Giroud

Laboratoire TIMC-IMAG, IN3S, Faculté de Médecine,
38706 La Tronche cedex, France
{Firstname.Name}@imag.fr

Abstract. In oncology research, Tissue Microarray (TMA) technology allows for the mass treatment of hundreds of tissue samples and rapid visualisation of molecular targets. Since this technique is relatively new, there are very few dedicated information systems and little formalised knowledge about the technique is available. We therefore intend to set up an integrated system around TMA technology that is accessible from the Internet. In particular we intend to set up a multimedia document generation system to assist with TMA design.

1 Introduction

Tissue Microarray (TMA) technology [1] is a new technique used in oncology research. It allows for quick *in situ* visualisation of molecular targets in thousands of tissue samples. In this technique patients are selected according to the study to be conducted. A pathologist analyses a histological slide for each patient biopsy block and marks areas of interest. Tissue cores are extracted from each biopsy paraffin block (donor block) and inserted in a new paraffin block (receiver or TMA block) in which slides are cut and treated as conventional slides would be. Images for TMA slides are acquired annotated and submitted to image analysis treatments.

Compared to classical studies, those using TMA technology economise on reactants and biological material. Moreover, mass treatment brings a statistical dimension to the pathologist's work. Both advantages can be increased by using the virtual TMA slide concept: spot images can be reorganised according to a new study without constructing a new real block. However TMA technology suffers from a lack of formalised knowledge and automation of TMA design and data analysis.

A major step in the computerisation of TMA technology has been the definition of the TMA Data Exchange Specification [2]. But most tools focus on data management [3], and an increasing need for assistance in data mining is being noticed [4]. We therefore intend to set up an integrated web-based system providing assistance in real TMA block design and TMA data mining through the generation of virtual representations of future TMA blocks or virtual TMA slides. The system will have to generate these representations "on the fly", according to a user query. These will have to be a complex mix of heterogeneous data adapted to users' needs.

In this paper we present preliminary work to formalise this adaptation process.

2 Related Works

User-adaptive software systems and especially adaptive hypermedia and adaptive web [5] compute the layout and contents of web pages according to a user model. Beyond this simple personalisation according to preferences, some systems such as e-Learning or on-line newspapers [6] aim at representing a narrative coherence through a spatial organisation. Compared to such approaches the envisioned system intends to reach a representative thematic organisation according to a query which is analytic by nature. This implies that we also focus on task adaptation.

Indeed, as with all information retrieval systems the goal is to provide some relevant information according to a user query. In our case however, as with web page summarising [7] or news tracking systems (such as News-map [8]), the returned data must be seen as an organised collection of documents. In the pictured system, the collected data is even meant to support data mining operations. As a consequence, the retrieved data has to be selected and organised to present an overview of the complete collection through a representative set which keeps the variety present in the original collection and allows for statistical analysis.

To achieve these adaptations, it is necessary to acquire and represent some knowledge about the adaptation task and the application domain. Using ontologies [9] will facilitate the modelling and knowledge sharing amongst human and software agents.

3 TMA Design: Problem Overview

Given a request the document to be designed may be thought of as an arrangement of objects, each being characterised by information extracted from a data repository. Therefore virtual representations of real TMA blocks and virtual TMA slides can be described as collections of multimedia documents that are generated according to a user request. They consist of a user query defining the study that the biologist or the physician wants to conduct (for instance comparing two patients groups...) and a TMA grid (the assembly of spot images selected and spatially arranged according to the user query). Each spot can be linked with data regarding the corresponding patient (clinical data...), image annotation and analysis (staining quantification...).

Starting from available data and knowledge, the tool we intend to build has to generate the TMA multimedia document on the fly. This is a complex problem which can be split into three sub-problems:

- **Selection:** Building a TMA can be thought of as looking at a list of elements (biopsy areas or spots) for a collection (the list for pertinent patients or spots) which fits the demand (the user query) and complies with some general rules.
- **Spatial organisation:** These objects (cores or spots) have to be placed on a grid.
- **Presentation:** The previously generated set has to be displayed to the user in the most user-friendly way while still allowing for varying user preferences.

The complexity of the problem is first of all linked to the heterogeneity of the data to handle. Some elements are purely computer data (virtual objects such as the numeric representation of the slides) and others are references to real objects such as the slides themselves. Some, such as staining intensity, are quantitative, whereas others such as patient gender are qualitative. The difficulty is increased due to the associated combinatorics.

Moreover the query is more than just inclusion/exclusion criteria since the aim is to obtain a spatially organised collection of documents which will be used for data mining. As a consequence, it appears necessary to acquire some knowledge about the TMA technology domain and the adaptation process at hand. This will be achieved using ontologies.

4 TMA Design: Ontologies

Building a TMA design ontology first of all requires modelling the pathology field. Currently available medical ontologies are either too general for our purpose or do not include abnormal tissue structures [10]. As a consequence, a colon carcinoma ontology has been put forward by Dr. Joëlle Simony-Lafontaine (a pathologist from the Centre Régional de Lutte Contre le Cancer in Montpellier, France). We also need to represent the objects and concepts associated with the technology. All these notions are integrated in a TMA domain ontology.

Along this domain ontology a task ontology needs to be modelled. An example of a query made by a pathologist expressed in natural language might be: 'Study of colon cancer evolution among men with a virtual TMA slide and using the Ki67 marker.' Such a query can be decomposed into several elements. The Goals of the Study guide the way to arrange the objects into the TMA grid. Inclusion Criteria define the list of patients or spots to take into account to build the grid. The Samples are a list of interesting areas in the biopsies where samples should be taken. The Document Logical Model is the TMA document type to build. The Lab protocols list specific protocols to build the TMA. This decomposition led us to construct a query ontology which guided the formalisation presented in Table 1.

The generation of a TMA document is a process of selection, spatial organisation on a grid, and presentation of this grid to the user. This is a process of adaptation of the final document to a query which is directed by a set of criteria. Some of these criteria can be influenced by user preferences expressed in the query or in a profile.

Table 1. Example for a formalised query where the elements are referenced according to the query ontology

Query Element	Problem Element	Formalism ([Father Element]...) [Element] (= [Value])
Goal of the Study	Organisation	[Goal] [Patient] [Diagnostic] [pTNM grade]
Inclusion Criteria	Selection	[Inclusion Criteria] [Patient] [Sex] = [Male]
Samples	Selection	[Sample] [Area] = [Colon] [All]
Document Logical Model	Selection / Organisation	[Document Logical Model] = [Virtual]
Lab Protocols	Selection / Organisation	[Lab Protocol] [Grid Size] = [Default] [Lab Protocol] [Nail diameter] = [Default] [Lab Protocol] [Marker] = [Ki67]

5 Adaptation Process

Given the collection of criteria introduced in the previous section the TMA design issue consists of selecting and ordering a group of relevant criteria, and categorising them according to the query and user preferences in order to propose an **adaptation plan**. The manipulation of such a criteria collection is a complex problem because of its size and possible contradictions. However the studies that can be conducted can be classified into families of similar studies. We can also build an **adaptation model** for each of these families. An adaptation model consists of a more specialised subset of constraints and rules extracted from the whole collection according to the specifics of the corresponding study family.

To achieve the adaptation of the final TMA document to the task those adaptation models have to be instantiated with data extracted from the query. As a consequence adaptation models constitute a representation layer depending on the goal of the study which plays an intermediate role between the domain and query layers.

Three specialisation layers have then been defined. The **Domain Layer** includes the complete collection of criteria for the considered application domain. The **Goal Layer** includes a subset of the previous collection, selected, ordered and parametrised according to the goal of the corresponding query family. The **Query Layer** includes an adaptation model specialisation according to the current query and user preferences.

Following these three specialisation layers, three composition levels corresponding to the three sub-problems to solve can be defined. The **Factual Level** deals with the selection stage where data or facts are analysed in order to present a pertinent element list. The **Logical Level** deals with the spatial organisation step where a thematic

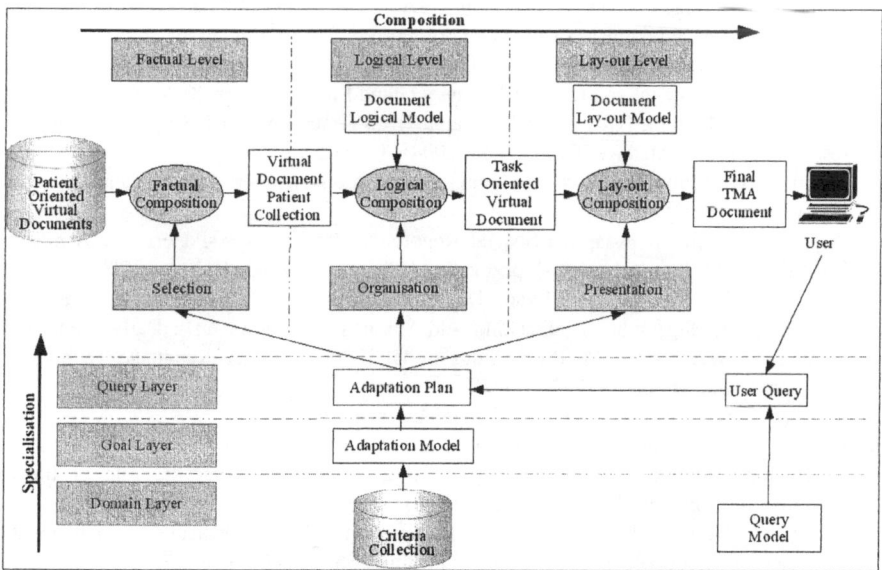

Fig. 1. Adaptation Engine Architecture

ordering of the previous list is achieved. The **Lay-out Level** deals with the presentation stage where the the previous document is prepared to be displayed while taking into account some user preferences.

A TMA document generation is a two-stage process which is achieved by the adaptation engine presented Figure 1. The adaptation engine goes through the three specialisation layers to generate the Adaptation Plan. The application of the adaptation plan to the three composition levels allows to create the final TMA document.

6 Conclusion

In this paper we have proposed an architecture for an adaptation engine which for now, is dedicated to TMA design assistance. The proposed architecture relies on an adaptation engine operating along two axes. The multi-layer Specialisation consists of a progressive refinement of the adaptation procedure towards a particular case. It facilitates knowledge representation and acquisition and allows for flexible query formulation. The multi-level Composition consists of a progressive refinement of the adaptation process through successive steps. It allows for task decomposition and it eases the formalisation of expertise.

The next step would be to go further into the conception and build a prototype.

References

1. Kallioniemi, OP., Wagner, U., Kononen, J., Sauter, G.: Tissue microarray technology for high-throughput molecular profiling of cancer. Hum Mol Genet. 10(7) (2001) 657-662
2. Berman, JJ., Edgerton, ME., Friedman, BA.: The tissue microarray data exchange specification: a community-based, open source tool for sharing tissue microarray data. BMC Med Inform Decis Mak. 3(1) (2003) 5
3. Henshall, S.: Tissue microarrays. J Mammary Gland Biol Neoplasia. 8(3) (2003) 347-358
4. Shergill, IS., Shergill, NK., Arya, M., Patel, HR.: Tissue microarrays: a current medical research tool. Curr Med Res Opin. 20(5) (2004) 707-712
5. Brusilovsky P.: From Adaptive Hypermedia to the Adaptive Web. Communications of the ACM. 45(2) (2002) 31-33
6. Iksal, S., Garlatti, S.: Adaptive Special Reports for On-line NewsPapers. In: Workshop Electronic Publishing,Adaptive Hypermedia (AH) 2002. Malaga, Espagne. (2002)
7. McKeown, K., Barzilay, R., Evan, D., Hatzivassiloglou, V., Klavans, J., Sable, C., Schiffman, B., Sigelman, S.: Tracking and Summarizing News on a Daily Basis with Columbia's Newsblaster. In: Proceedings of HLT 2002: Human Language Technology Conference. San Diego. USA (2002)
8. http://www.marumushi.com/apps/newsmap/newsmap.cfm
9. Gruber, TR.: Toward principles for the design of ontologies used for knowledge sharing. International Journal of Human-Computer Studies. Special issue: the role of formal ontology in the information technology 43(5-6) (1995) 907-928
10. Rosse, C., Mejino, JL. Jr.: A reference ontology for biomedical informatics: the Foundational Model of Anatomy. J Biomed Inform. 36(6) (2003) 478-500

Building Medical Ontologies Based on Terminology Extraction from Texts: Methodological Propositions

Audrey Baneyx[1], Jean Charlet[1,2], and Marie-Christine Jaulent[1]

[1] INSERM, U729, Paris, F-75006 France
15 rue de l'Ecole de Médecine, 75006 Paris, France
[2] STIM - DSI/AP-HP
{Audrey.Baneyx, Jean.Charlet, Marie-Christine.Jaulent}@spim.jussieu.fr

Abstract. In the medical field, it is now established that the maintenance of unambiguous thesauri is accomplished by the building of ontologies. Our task in the PERTOMed project is to help pneumologists code acts and diagnoses with a software that represents medical knowledge by an ontology of the concerned specialty. We apply natural language processing tools to corpora to develop the resources needed to build this ontology. In this paper, our objective is to develop a methodology for the knowledge engineer to build various types of medical ontologies based on terminology extraction from texts according to the differential semantics theory. Our main research hypothesis concerns the joint use of two methods: distributional analysis and recognition of semantic relationships by lexico-syntactic patterns. The expected result is the building of an ontology of pneumology.

1 Introduction

For about ten years, French hospitals have had to communicate information about their medical activities. For each patient, information is gathered as patient discharge summary, using the international classification of diseases CIM-10 [1] for the diagnoses codification and CCAM[2] for the acts. The French PMSI[3] coding process is usually done manually by physicians using medical specialty thesauri based on common terminologies. However it has become obvious that wording of thesauri is ambiguous and non-exhaustive. We think that the automation of the coding task requires a conceptual modelling (an ontology non-contextual and unambiguous) of medical items whose meaning would be written inside the model's structure itself [1] [2]. The main difficulty is to identify and classify the concepts of a given domain. Since classification criteria depend on purposes and are not universal, we do not seek to build a universal ontology, but merely a specific ontology of pneumology [3] [4]. This work is part of the PERTOMed [4] research

---

[1] The French version of the International classification of diseases.
[2] Common classification of medical acts.
[3] Program of medicalization of information systems.
[4] http://www.spim.jussieu.fr/Pertomed

project whose objective is to develop methods and tools to produce and use terminological and ontological resources in the medical field. We build our specific ontology by applying natural language processing (NLP) tools to analyse textual corpora. We hypothosize that this kind of ressource is the best source to characterize notions useful for the ontological modelling and the semantic content that is associated with them. In this paper, we discribe an experimentation that combines two methods in order to build an ontology according to the differential semantics principles [4]. A differential ontology is a hierarchy of concepts and relationships organized according to the similarities and differencies between them. We expect to extract from this experimentation a methodology for the knowledge engineer to be applied to building medical ontologies.

Section 2 presents the material and tools used and section 3 details the different steps of the methodology. Section 4 presents the results we obtained and last, in section 5, we conclude this paper by discussing perspectives expected from this work.

2 Material

In order to cover the whole area of pneumology, we have gathered 1 038 patient discharge summaries (corpus named [PDS]) from six hospitals in Paris. We added a teaching book (corpus named [BOOK]) to that first corpus. The [PDS] corpus has about 417 000 words and the [BOOK] corpus has about 823 000 words. We use SYNTEX-UPERY as an NLP tool. SYNTEX is a syntax analyser module based on the hypothesis of similar dependencies between terms which have a close meaning. Thus, this module allows us to identify relationships of syntactic dependencies between terms or syntagma (noun vs noun phrase, verbs vs verbal syntagma ...). At the end of the process, we have a network of syntactic dependencies – or a terminological network – whose elements are the candidate terms that will be used to build the ontology. Then, the UPERY module proceeds to the distributional analysis [5]: it computes distributional proximities between candidate terms on the basis of shared syntactical contexts and exploits all the network data to cluster terms. We obtain a network of candidate terms, their contextual associations, and their links to the corpus. The results of the analysis can be viewed with TERMONTO, the data access and data process software interface. The editor DOE[5] allows us to build our ontology according to the differential semantics. This software also permits us to complete the ontology with the addition of the English translation of concepts and relationships, and their encyclopaedic definitions. Finally, the ontology is exported into OWL, a knowledge representation language recommended by the W3C Consortium.

3 Method

The Bachimont's methodology used to design differential ontologies allows us to describe variations of the words' meaning in context and stresses the importance

---

[5] The Differential Ontology Editor, http://opales.ina.fr/public

of the textual corpus [4]. There are four successive steps in this methodology: 1) the constitution of the corpus of knowledge and its analysis by NLP tools, 2) the semantic normalization of the set of terms through the application of differential principles, 3) the ontological engagement to formalize defined concepts, 4) the finalization of the process in a language based on description logic and understandable to the computer. Our research in pneumology brings both precision and adapts the first two steps of the methodology to the knowledge engineer. This experimentation combines two methods to enrich the ontology building : a) the building of terminological resources by distributional analysis applied to the [PDS] corpus [6], and b) the semantic relationship recognition through the observation of corpus sequences, illustrating the desired relationship applied to the [BOOK] corpus [7].

The two [PDS] and [BOOK] corpora resources are processed to obtain an anonymous [PDS] corpus and a [BOOK] corpus both in XML format. Next, the [PDS] corpus is processed by SYNTEX-UPERY. The results of the analysis allow us to build the basic elements – i.e. primitives – of the ontology. The second [BOOK] corpus is analysed to identify semantic relationships (hyperonymy, synonymy...) between candidate terms, using the previously defined lexico-syntactic patterns [7]. These links help us to control and enrich the hierarchy. Candidate terms[6] (CT) representative of pneumology are chosen within the results provided by SYNTEX-UPERY from the [PDS] corpus in two steps:

- We select the noun phrases (NP) provided by the syntactical analysis that appear in the [PDS] corpus more than 12 times (2% of the corpus). Four conceptual axes are distinguished: symptoms, pathologies, treatments and examinations. The CT are linked with one of these axes. In this way, 35% of the CT classified are used in the second step.

- The distributional analysis connects terms sharing the same contexts (descendants in head and descendants in expansion). It also connects the contexts according to the terms they share (neighbours in head and neighbours in expansion). For instance, *effusion* is the head of the NP *effusion of pleura* and *of pleura* is its expansion. Descendants in head yield information on what could be child-concepts or defined concepts. Descendants in expansion provide information about the concept's position in the hierarchy. Neighbours in head and in expansion allow us to constitute the groupings of CT semantically close to the one under study, *effusion of pleura*. Groupings are a great help for the development of the hierarchical structure of the ontology, for the both horizontal and vertical axes. The example below shows a first possible connection: we can link group A {*effusion, lesion, infection, uncompensation*} with {*symptoms*}. For this example, our first hypothesis will be to consider CT of group A as sibling-concepts (sharing the same semantical context) and *symptoms* as the parent-concept of the group.

---

[6] A candidate term is a noun phrase composed by a head and an expansion. For instance, in the NP *Opacity in the left lung*, the term *Opacity* is the head and *in the left lung* is its expansion.

In order to work the hierarchy out, the CT are organised by refining the differential principles that define them. We have to express in natural language the similarities and differences of each concept with respect to its parent-concept and its sibling-concepts. The meaning of a node is given by the gathering of all similarities and differences defined for each concept between the node target and the root. The four axes are refined in that way. In addition, we use the results of the processing of the [BOOK] corpus to help us in applying the differential principles according to the method described in [3]. The analysis based on lexico-syntactic pattern recognition yields clues on how to apply the differential principles. The lexico-syntactic patterns are representative of specific semantic relationships [8]. These patterns are built around a marker which is the lexical relationship indice, such as *kind of*, for hyperonymy relationships. To build differential ontologies, we apply this method to look for definition statements in the corpus (for instance: *Dry cough is a symptom for bronchitis and it is also a pathology*). The patterns used were developed by Malaisé et al. [7]. The extracted lexical units are manually confirmed. At the end of this stage, we have a semantic normalization of the set of terms of the specialty and we have represented the hierarchy of primitive concepts and relationships with DOE.

4 Current Results

After using SYNTEX process, the [PDS] corpus gives 36 881 NP and the [BOOK] corpus gives 17 666 NP. Using the lexico-syntactic patterns for the definition recognition, 799 lexical units were extracted. 15% are confirmed. This study gives precision and help us to order the hierarchy. Our ontology includes today 600 primitive concepts stemming from the first analysis of the CT. Given that the building stages 1 and 2 are iterative, we will rapidly increase the hierarchy by examining the CT which appear less than 12 times in the [PDS] corpus. The ontology is to be evaluated in terms of both quality and coverage. The conceptual hierarchy must be corrected and validated by pneumologists from the French Pneumology Society with whom we collaborate.

5 Discussion and Conclusion

The purpose of this work is to show that our methodology allows a knowledge engineer, non-specialist of the medical field, to build an ontology based on texts using NLP tools. The initial results of our research coupled with a recent work on surgical intensive care gives us reasons to think we are moving in the right direction [6]. This work of knowledge processing shows that it is necessary to use jointly NLP tools (SYNTEX-UPERY) and modelling tools (DOE). The physicians we are working with are interested in formal representations of knowledge based on patients records to be able to perform epidemiological studies from patient data. To do that, an ontological representation is essential. We develop specific ontologies, connected to existing thesauri of the domain. From that point of view, our work is closer to the GALEN's terminological server[7] [9] than to the SNOMED-CT approach playing both the role of thesaurus and ontology. The evaluation will also test the completeness of the ontology compared to the specialty thesauri. To estimate that completeness, we will check the possibility of building a conceptual representation of medical knowledge by combining the primitive concepts and the relationships in the ontology. It is important to notice that the last validation stage of the ontology will be to use it in concrete applications available in the framework of the PERTOMed terminological plateform. To conclude we have presented a range of methodological principles for the building of differential medical ontologies based on texts. We plan to complete this ontology by connecting it to the head (conceptual high level) of the MENELAS project ontology[8] [10]. This allows us to verify whether there exists, in part, a common high level in the medical field that can be used in other contexts.

References

1. Rector, A.: Thesauri and formal classifications: Terminologies for people and machines. Methods of Information in Medicine **37** (1998) 501–509
2. Staab, S., Studer, R.: Handbook on Ontologies. 1 edn. Springer, Germany (2003)
3. Charlet, J., Bachimont, B., Jaulent, M.: Building medical ontologies by terminology extraction from texts: An experiment for the intensive care units. Computer in Biology and Medicine (2005) *To appear*.
4. Bachimont, B., Isaac, A., Troncy, R.: Semantic commitment for designing ontologies: A proposal. In: Proceedings of EKAW, Sigenza, Espagne, Springer (2002) 114–121
5. Harris, Z.: Mathematical Structures of Language. John Wiley and Sons, New-York, USA (1968)
6. Le Moigno, S., Charlet, J., Bourigault, D., Degoulet, P., Jaulent, M.: Terminology extraction from text to build an ontology in surgical intensive care. In: Proceedings of the AMIA Annual Symposium 2002, San Antonio, Texas (2002) 430–435
7. Malais, V., Zweigenbaum, P., Bachimont, B.: Mining defining contexts to help structuring differential ontologies. In Ibekwe-San, J., Condamines, A., Cabr, T., eds.: Application-Driven Terminology Engineering, Termonology. John Benjamins (2005) 21–53
8. Hearst, M.: Automatic acquisition of hyponyms from large text corpora. In Zampolli, A., ed.: Proceedings of the 14 th COLING, Nantes, France (1992) 539–545
9. Trombert-Paviot, B., Rodrigues, J., Rogers, J., Baud, R., van der Haring, E., Rassinoux, A., Abrial, V., Clavel, L., Idir, H.: Galen: a third generation terminology tool to support a multipurpose national coding system for surgical procedures. International Journal of Medical Informatics **58-59** (2000) 71–85
10. Zweigenbaum, P., Bouaud, J., Bachimont, B., Charlet, J., Sroussi, B., Boisvieux, J.F.: From text to knowledge: a unifying document-oriented view of analyzed medical language. Methods of Information in Medicine **37** (1998) 384–393

---

[7] http://www.openclinical.org/prj_galen.html
[8] http://www.biomath.jussieu.fr/Menelas/Ontologie

Translating Biomedical Terms by Inferring Transducers

Vincent Claveau[1] and Pierre Zweigenbaum[2]

[1] OLST - University of Montreal, Montreal QC, H3T 1N8, Canada
Vincent.Claveau@umontreal.ca
http://olst.ling.umontreal.ca/~vincent
[2] AP-HP, STIM/DSI; INSERM, U729; INALCO, TIM, Paris, France
pz@biomath.jussieu.fr
http://www-new.biomath.jussieu.fr/~pz

Abstract. This paper presents a method to automatically translate a large class of terms in the biomedical domain from one language to another; it is evaluated on translations between French and English. It relies on a machine-learning technique that infers transducers from examples of bilingual word pairs; no additional resource or knowledge is needed. Then, these transducers, making the most of the high regularity of translation discovered in the examples, can be used to translate unseen French terms into English or vice versa. We report evaluations that show that this technique achieves high precision, reaching up to 85% of correct translations for both French to English and English to French tasks.

1 Introduction

In the biomedical domain, the international research framework and fast knowledge update make producing, managing and updating multilingual resources an important issue. Within this context, this paper presents and evaluates an original method to automatically translate a large class of biomedical simple terms (*i.e.*, composed of one word) from one language to another; it is tested on translations from French into English and English into French.

Our approach relies on two major hypotheses: (*i*) a large class of French and English terms are morphologically related; (*ii*) differences between French and English terms are regular enough to be automatically learned. These two hypotheses make the most of the fact that biomedical terms often share a common Greek or Latin basis, and that their morphological derivations are very regular (*e.g. ophtalmorragie/ophthalmorrhagia, leucorragie/leukorrhagia*...). Our technique relies on a supervised machine-learning algorithm, called OSTIA[1] (Oncina, 1991), that infers transducers (*cf.* next section) from examples of bilingual term pairs. Such transducers, when given a new term in English (respectively French), must propose the corresponding French (resp. English) term.

Only few researches aim at directly translating terms from one language to another (Schulz *et al.*, 2004). Nonetheless, closely related problems are often

---

[1] The authors wish to thank J. Oncina for giving them access to the code of OSTIA.

addressed in the domain of automatic corpus translation (cognate detection or statistical word alignment in bitexts (Véronis, 2000)). These approaches heavily rely on bitexts, which are not always available, and they look for an existing translation in a text (*i.e.* a relational problem) while we are willing to produce the translation of a term without other information (a generation problem).

In the next section, we present the machine-learning technique we use to infer transducers. In Section 3, we describe the methodology and the data used in our experiments. Section 4 details the results obtained for both French to English and English to French translation tasks. Last, some perspectives for this work are given in Section 5.

2 Inferring Transducers

2.1 Sub-sequential Transducers

The transducers inferred with OSTIA and used here to translate biomedical terms are an extension of the classical transducers called sub-sequential transducers. We give readers a basic background of these sub-sequential transducers; for formal definitions, please refer to (Oncina *et al.*, 1993).

Transducers are finite-state machines that can be seen as graphs in which an input symbol and an output string are associated to each edge and having one initial state I and one or more final states. An input sequence E is said to be *accepted* if there exists a path of edges from I to a final state such that the concatenation of the input symbols of these edges gives E. The *transduction*, or *translation* of an input sequence E corresponds to the concatenation of the output strings associated to the edges used to accept E. A sub-sequential transducer is a deterministic transducer (two edges with the same input symbol cannot emerge from the same state) in which all the states are final, and having an output string associated to each state. This string is produced when the input sequence to be accepted by the transducer ends on the state it is associated with.

Figure 1 presents a simple sub-sequential transducer with the usual notations of the automata. It represents the transduction function that translates ϵ (the empty word) into D, $a(bc)^n$ into $A(BC)^n E$ and $a(bc)^n b$ into $A(BC)^n BF$. A word like *abca* is not accepted and thus not translated by this transducer.

2.2 The OSTIA Algorithm

OSTIA is the machine learning technique used to infer sub-sequential transducers from examples of French/English pairs of biomedical terms. OSTIA is formally presented by J. Oncina (1991); here, we only give an outline of its principles. It is illustrated with an example: we want to learn the transducer presented above

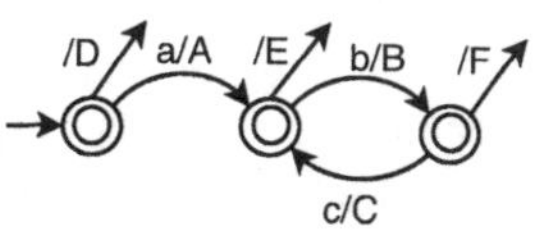

Fig. 1. A simple sub-sequential transducer

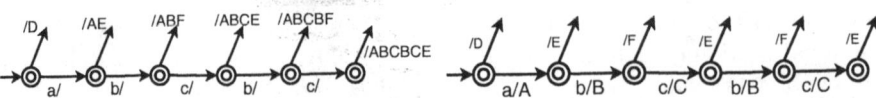

Fig. 2. Transducer at the end of step 1   Fig. 3. Transducer at the end of step 2

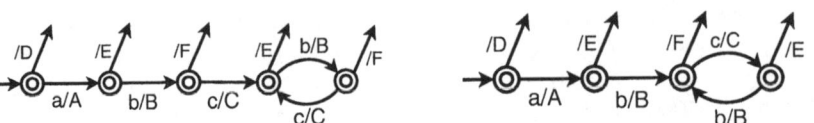

Fig. 4. Transducer after one merge   Fig. 5. Transducer after two merges

in Figure 1 from the training set T containing the 6 following input/output examples: $\{\epsilon/D, a/AE, ab/ABF, abc/ABCE, abcb/ABCBF, abcbc/ABCBCE\}$. OSTIA works in three steps (Oncina, 1998):

1. a prefix tree of every input sequence in T is built up. Empty output strings are associated to each internal state and edge of the tree and the complete output strings are associated at the leaves of the branch accepting the corresponding input sequence (*cf.* Figure 2).
2. every common prefix of the output sequences is moved up from the leaves towards the root of the tree (Figure 3).
3. last, starting from the root, every possible pair of states of the transducer is considered and is merged if the resulting transducer does not contradict the training data (Figures 4 and 5). When no further merge can be done, the algorithm ends.

3 Experiments

3.1 Learning Data and Evaluation Set

The data we use to train and test this translation technique are taken from an on-line French medical dictionary (Dictionnaire Médical Masson) in which some of the entries contain English equivalent terms. We selected those entries that were simple terms both in French and English, avoiding proper nouns and acronyms. About 12,000 bilingual term pairs were collected this way.

In order to focus on morphologically related pairs, a formal similarity was computed for each pair through the string edit distance. Pairs were then ordered in a list according to their scores in descending order.

3.2 Methodology

It is important to provide OSTIA only with training pairs that are actually morphologically related (*i.e.* from the top part of the list presented above). In contrast, the data used to evaluate our technique can be taken from any part of this list, even though obviously no automatic system can provide good translations of terms at the end of the list. To take this point into account and provide a fair and complete evaluation, we run two experiments:

exp. 1. training pairs and testing pairs are taken from the first half of the list;
exp. 2. training pairs are taken from the first half of the list and testing pairs from the whole list.

For each experiment, we test our approach for the translation of terms from French to English and from English to French. The inference process is repeated 10 times: the initial set is divided in 10 folds and OSTIA uses 9 of these folds; the tenth fold is different each time. Thus, ten transducers are inferred; this allows us to average their results (see Section 4). Each test set comprises 2000 pairs (of course different from the training pairs).

Since ten transducers are inferred each time, it is possible to compare the translations they propose for each term in the testing set. The more frequently a translation is proposed, the more likely it is to be the correct one. Thus, we also implement a simple voting process: for each testing term, we keep the translation that was proposed most often by the ten transducers. In case of a tie between several translations, one of them is chosen at random.

4 Results

In order to evaluate the performances of the inferred transducers, the only measure we use is the precision of the produced translations. It is the rate of correctly translated terms from the source language into the target language. If a term is not accepted by the transducer, it is considered as incorrectly translated. This precision rate is computed for both experiments with respect to the number of training examples used by OSTIA. Figures 6 and 7 present the resulting graphs for experiment 1 and 2, for translation from English to French; similar graphs, not reported here, are obtained for French to English. We report the average precision of the 10 transducers inferred for each number of examples, as well as the precision obtained through the vote of the 10 transducers as described above. As a baseline, we compute the precision that would be obtained by a system systematically proposing the source term as its own translation.

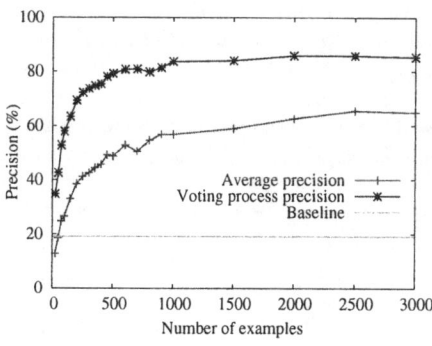

Fig. 6. Exp. 1 precision with respect to training set size En to Fr

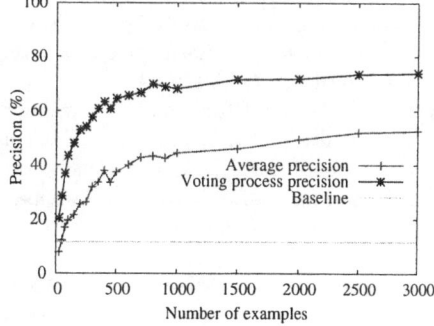

Fig. 7. Exp. 2 precision with respect to training set size En to Fr

The average precision is quite good and much better than the baselines: with 3,000 examples, about 64% of the terms are correctly translated in Experiment 1, and about 52% in Experiment 2. The precision obtained with the voting process is even better: in Experiment 1 it reaches about 85% of correct translations and 75% for Experiment 2. The good results for Experiment 2 are particularly interesting since it represents the performance of our technique on any term, even those with a non-morphologically related translation.

5 Perspectives

Many perspectives are foreseen for this work. From a technical point of view, future work is planned to improve the voting process between the inferred transducer. Indeed, the correct translation of a term is proposed by at least one of the 10 inferred transducers 93% of the time for Exp. 1 and 85% for Exp. 2. Thus, these figures represent the upper limits an optimal voting method could reach. Secondly, considering the terms as sequences of morphs instead of sequences of letters (*e.g. broncho⊕pleuro⊕pneumo⊕nia*) could yield better results. Morphological analysis systems for French biomedical terms exist (Namer & Zweigenbaum, 2004) and could be used with OSTIA. Another possible extension concerns translation of complex terms (with several words). If we are able to translate word by word a complex term, it may be possible to produce a translation of the term as a whole, provided we are able to handle terminological variations (*virus de la variole/virus variolique, variola virus/variolic virus*) (Jacquemin, 2001).

References

Jacquemin C. *Spotting and Discovering Terms through NLP*. Cambridge: MIT Press (2001).

Namer F. & Zweigenbaum P. Acquiring Meaning for French Medical Terminology: Contribution of Morpho-Semantics. In *Proceedings of MEDINFO 2004*, San-Francisco, CA, USA (2004).

Oncina J. *Aprendizaje de Lenguajes Regulares y Transducciones Subsecuenciales*. PhD thesis, Universidad Politécnica de Valencia, Valencia, Spain (1991).

Oncina J. The Data Driven Approach Applied to the OSTIA Algorithm. In *Proceedings of the Fourth International Colloquium on Grammatical Inference, ICGI'98*, p. 50–56, Ames, IA, USA (1998).

Oncina J., García P. & Vidal E. Learning Subsequential Transducers for Pattern Recognition Interpretation Tasks. *IEEE Transactions on Pattern Analysis and Machine Intelligence*, 15(5), 448–458 (1993).

Schulz S., Markó K., Sbrissia E., Nohama P. & Hahn U. Cognate Mapping - A Heuristic Strategy for the Semi-Supervised Acquisition of a Spanish Lexicon from a Portuguese Seed Lexicon. In *Proceedings of the 20th International Conference on Computational Linguistics, COLING'04*, p. 813–819, Geneva, Switzerland (2004).

J. Véronis, Ed. *Parallel Text Processing*. Dordrecht: Kluwer Academic Publishers (2000).

Using Lexical and Logical Methods for the Alignment of Medical Terminologies

Michel Klein[1] and Zharko Aleksovski[1,2]

[1] Vrije Universiteit Amsterdam, department of Artificial Intelligence
michel.klein@cs.vu.nl
[2] Philips Research Eindhoven
zharko@few.vu.nl

Abstract. Standardized medical terminologies are often used for the registration of patient data. In several situations there is a need to align these terminologies to other terminologies. Even when the terminologies cover the same domain, this is often a non-trivial task. The task is even more complicated when the terminology does not contain much structure. In this paper we describe the initial results of a procedure for mapping a terminology with little or no structure to a structure-rich terminology. This procedure uses the knowledge of the structure-rich terminology and a method for semantic explicitation of concept descriptions. The first results shows that, when compared to approaches based on syntactic analysis only, the recall can be greatly improved without sacrificing much of the precision.

1 Terminology Alignment for Non-structured Lists

The use of standardized terminologies for the registration of patient data is a very common practice in modern health-care. There can be many reasons to link (part of) the patient data to other data sources, e.g. for registration purposes, to find relevant literature references, to compare hospitals, and so on. These tasks often involve the alignment of the used terminology with another terminology.

There already exist several techniques for ontology[1] alignment [2, 3, 4, 5]. However, the existing techniques are most effective when the ontology contains structure. In practice there are quite some terminologies in use that have no or only minor structure (e.g. a controlled list of terms). This often implies that the alignment has to be based on lexical techniques only. In this paper, we report on a method for aligning a flat list of terms with a structure-rich ontology. In this method, we use the knowledge in the ontology as background knowledge. The results of the method are suggestions for mapping candidates to users that perform an ontology alignment task.

In the next section, we briefly describe the two terminologies that are used in our procedure. In Section 3, we describe the alignment procedure itself and we explain our choices. Section 4 presents the first results, and in the last section we discuss our approach and look forward.

---

[1] In this paper we do not make a distinction between a structured terminology system and an ontology and use the terms intermixed. See [1] for a more detailed positioning of both.

2 Description of Terminologies

There are two terminologies used in the experiments. The first terminology is a list of "problems" related to patients at an intensive care unit (ICU), developed in a local hospital. This list is partly based on the ICD-9-cm[2]. During its use in the past three years the list has been extended with additional descriptions of medical conditions of patients at the ICU. The resulting list is a mixture of problem descriptions at several levels of abstraction with minor redundancy. The list is mainly in Dutch but also contains some English terms. In the remainder of this paper we will refer to this terminology as the *local hospital list*. This list contains 1399 problem descriptions consisting of maximal 7 words. 95% of the descriptions consists of three words or less.

The second terminology is a structured ICU ontology, developed at the Academic Medical Center in Amsterdam [6]. The ontology defines around 1460 'reasons for admission' at the ICU. These concepts are defined via five axes, i.e. 'tractus', 'abnormality', 'activity', 'anatomical location' and 'aetiology'. The concepts in the ontology are related to at least one term and often to more. This ontology can be seen as a combination of two distinct parts: the taxonomy of 'reasons for admission' itself and an ontology with background knowledge about anatomy, abnormalities etc.

3 Alignment Approach

The goal of the approach is to map the unstructured descriptions in the local hospital list to concepts that are defined in 'reason for admission' subtree in the ontology.

1. Apply lexical mapping techniques to match terms in the problem descriptions to terms from the five defining axes in the ontology (i.e. the background knowledge).
2. Translate problem descriptions from the local hospital list into logical formulas.
3. Create logical formulas for ontology concepts using both its term and the terms from the five defining axes.
4. Classify formulas from the local hospital list in the ontology.

The first step results in an annotated version of the local hospital list, in which each term in the descriptions is labelled with the name of the axis in the ontology in which the term or a synonym of it is found. For example, the description colon carcinoom is not directly found in the ontology. However, the term colon is found in the 'anatomical location' subtree, while a synonym of the term 'carcinoom' is found the 'abnormality' subtree. The resulting annotation is colon^{location} carcinoom^{abnormality}. Not all terms can be found in the ontology, so there will also be unlabelled terms.

For the classification, we apply an approximate matching method that is described in [7]. The idea behind this method is to transform the concepts from two ontologies into propositional formulas and then to discover matchings by finding equivalence or subsumption relations between the formulas of the different ontologies. The transformation of the concepts into formulas consists of two parts: transforming the natural language descriptions into logical formulas—*semantic explicitation*, and using the relations among the concepts in the ontologies—*contextualization*.

---

[2] http://www.cdc.gov/nchs/about/otheract/icd9/abticd9.htm

The *semantic explicitation* is intended to capture the meaning of the natural language descriptions into logic formulas. In some cases, certain word combinations will make no sense and should be discarded. The idea behind the *contextualization* is to make the knowledge that is encoded in the structure of the ontology explicit. For example, a concept can be represented as a disjunction of its preferred term and all its synonyms; or it can be represented in conjunction with its superconcepts, since superconcepts are naturally assumed to have broader meaning.

In our experiment, the logical formulas for the descriptions in the local hospital list are formed by creating a disjunction of all possible interpretations of the word combinations that are likely to make sense. For example, the term abdominal aneurysm aorta is translated into the following formula:

(abdominal ∩ aneurysm ∩ aorta) ∪ (abdominal_aneurysm ∩ aorta) ∪
(abdominal ∩ aneurysm_aorta) ∪ (abdominal_aneurysm_aorta)

This encodes all different interpretation of the description in which subsequent terms can form one composite term or separate terms.

The 'reasons for admission' concepts in the ontology (only these concepts, *not* the terms from the five defining axes) are translated by taking the disjunction of all terms and the conjunction of the values of the attributes that are defined on them. For example, the concept Pneumonia with synonym longontsteking, abnormality infection and location lungs will be translated into:

(pneumonia ∪ longontsteking) ∪ (infection ∩ lungs).

The intuition behind this translation is that the meaning of the concept is either completely captured in one of it terms, or in the combination of its defining attributes. If preferred terms or synonyms consist of several words, they are translated in a similar way as the descriptions in the local hospital list, encoding all possible different interpretations.

Subsumption and equivalence is now decided by comparing the formulas from both terminologies. This is possible because they partly use the same terms, i.e. the terms from the five defining axes (the background knowledge). The ontology concepts were directly defined using these terms, while the local hospital list is mapped to the (synonyms of the) terms in the background knowledge.

4 Experiment

In the lexical comparison step, we first compared the complete problem descriptions from the local hospital list with the terms and synonyms used in the 'reason for admission' subtree in the ontology. This step is necessary to find all descriptions that have direct syntactic equivalents in the ontology. Then, we compared each individual term in the local hospital list one-by-one with the terms in the five 'axes' of the ontology.

Many terms in the local hospital list are composite terms and therefore not matched to terms in the ontology. This is a consequence of the Dutch language, in which it is under certain conditions allowed to concatenate nouns. Terms like aortaklepvervanging (aorta-valve replacement) and coloncarcinoom are not directly matched, although the component terms are known in the ontology. To solve, this, we also look for "partial" matches of terms (substrings of at least 3 characters at the beginning or the end of a string).

Table 1. Number of matches for different categories in the ontology

category	exact	partial	total
reason-for-admission concept (complete)	171	31	202
activity	49	41	90
abnormality	182	99	281
anatomical location	87	95	182
aetiology	25	9	34
tractus	2	0	2
named-values	70	13	83
reason-for-admission term	125	50	175

4.1 Results of Lexical Comparison with Background Knowledge

The procedure resulted in 1123 exact matches and 702 partial matches, which gives a total of 1835 matches. The complete local hospital list contains 1399 descriptions consisting of 2558 terms. This means that when we require 100 % precision (i.e. only exact matches) we find a match for almost 49 % of the terms in the hospital list. Table 1 shows the distribution of the matches over the different categories in the ontology.

The table shows that only 202 of the 1399 problem descriptions in the local hospital list (14%) have direct syntactic equivalents in the ontology. Using the comparison to the background knowledge, we find *some* match for 800 descriptions, i.e. 57 %. The other 599 descriptions did not match to anything in the ontology.

4.2 Results of Classification

We performed the classification in two directions: 1) we determined which formulas from the local hospital list are contained in formulas from the ontology, and 2) we determined which formulas from the 'reasons for admission' are contained in formulas from the local hospital list. In the first direction, 308 statements were derived, while the second direction resulted in 965 statements. In total, 1273 subclass statements were derived for 800 concepts.

Our first analysis of the results give the impression that around 85% of the suggestions make sense. Around 50% of the suggested subclass relations are trivial suggestions based on the containment of the set of words, e.g. "Epstein-Barr virus hepatitis subClassOf Hepatitis" or "Exploratieve laparotomie subClassOf Laparotomie". Some others are less trivial and could only be found using background knowledge, e.g. "Hypernatraemische encephalopathie subClassOf Coma" or "Maligne melanoom subClassOf Tumor"

There are also some statements that are clearly incorrect, e.g. "Excision of atrial thrombus subClassOf Thrombus". Many incorrect statements are surgical procedures (like 'excision', 'biopsy' etc.) that are classified as subclass of their object. Others are more subtle, like the Infected placenta, which is classified as subclass of Pregnancy.

Another observation is that some descriptions are considered as subclasses of fairly general concepts in the ontology, e.g. tumor. Although this is correct, it might be that there are more specific concepts in the ontology to which could be mapped. However, because we see the results as suggestions to a human that performs the alignment, this is still a useful result: the number of choices is drastically reduced.

5 Discussion and Outlook

A direct matching approach with linguistic techniques between the descriptions from the local hospital list and the 'reason for admission' subtree in the ontology falls short because not all descriptions are syntactically similar to the the ontology concepts. Using the background knowledge from the ontology looks as a promising approach because much more terms from the descriptions can be found, seemingly without many errors being introduced.

Although in our experiments we use the background knowledge from the ontology itself, we think that this is not required. The two main requirements for our approach are a structured ontology with definitional knowledge of concepts and a shared vocabulary for the individual terms. We expect that background knowledge could also be provided by (combinations of) other ontologies, for example semi-standards like the Foundational Model of Anatomy[3] or UMLS sources.

This paper presents initial results which show that the approach seems to be worthwhile. There are several improvements to the method described that can be made. For example, better natural language techniques might help to improve the number of matches found in the lexical analysis phase. Using other classification techniques, e.g. classification based on Description Logic, is another line of research.

Acknowledgements

This research was partly supported by the Netherlands Organisation for Scientific Research (NWO) under project number 634.000.020.

References

1. de Keizer, N.F., Abu-Hanna, A., Zwetsloot-Schonk, J.: Understanding Terminological Systems I: Terminology and Typology. Methods of Information in Medicine **39** (2000) 16–21
2. Rahm, E., Bernstein, P.A.: A Survey of Approaches to Automatic Schema Matching. VLDB Journal **10** (2001)
3. Doan, A., Madhavan, J., Domingos, P., Halevy, A.: Learning to Map Between Ontologies on the Semantic Web. In: WWW '02: Proceedings of the Eleventh International Conference on World Wide Web, ACM Press (2002) 662–673
4. Noy, N.F., Musen, M.A.: PROMPT: Algorithm and Tool for Automated Ontology Merging and Alignment. In: Proceedings of the Seventeenth National Conference on Artificial Intelligence (AAAI-2000), Austin, TX, AAAI/MIT Press (2000)
5. McGuinness, D.L., Fikes, R., Rice, J., Wilder, S.: The Chimaera Ontology Environment. In: Proceedings of the Seventeenth National Conference on Artificial Intelligence and Twelfth Conference on Innovative Applications of Artificial Intelligence, AAAI Press / The MIT Press (2000) 1123–1124
6. de Keizer, N.F., Abu-Hanna, A., Cornet, R., Zwetsloot-Schonk, J., Stoutenbeek, C.: Design of an Intensive Care Diagnostic Classification. Methods of Information in Medicine **38** (1999) 102–112
7. Aleksovski, Z., ten Kate, W., van Harmelen, F.: Semantic Coordination: a New Approximation Method. In: Proceedings of the Workshop Meaning Coordination and Negotiation, ISWC 2004, Hiroshima, Japan (2004)

---

[3] See http://sig.biostr.washington.edu/projects/fm/.

Latent Argumentative Pruning for Compact MEDLINE Indexing

Patrick Ruch, Robert Baud, Johann Marty,
Antoine Geissbühler, Imad Tbahriti, and Anne-Lise Veuthey

University Hospital of Geneva and Swiss Institute of Bioinformatics,
Medical Informatics Service and Swiss-Prot Group, 1205 Geneva, Switzerland
patrick.ruch@sim.hcuge.ch

Abstract. PURPOSE: We evaluate how argumentation in scientific articles can be used to propose an original index pruning strategy, which significantly reduce the size of the engine's indexes but having a limited impact on retrieval effectiveness. METHODS: A Bayesian classifier trained on explicitly structured MEDLINE abstracts generates these argumentative categories. The categories are used to generate four different argumentative indexes. A fifth index contains the complete abstract, together with the title and the list of Medical Subject Headings (MeSH) terms. This last index is used as baseline to compare results obtained when only a specific argumentative index is retrieved. RESULTS and CONCLUSION: When titles and medical subject headings are also stored in the respective indexes, querying PURPOSE and CONCLUSION indexes can respectively achieves 78.4% and 74.3% of the baseline, while the size if the index is divided by two. It is concluded that argumentation can be a powerful index pruning strategy in complement to more traditionnal approaches.

1 Introduction and Background

Fast and precise text search engines are widely used to search biomedical litteratures [1] as well as clinical records [2] through Web and desktop applications [3]. Efficient query evaluation is attained in these search engines by use of an inverted file, which provides an association between textual entities used as indexing units (words, stems, terms...) and documents in the collection. Indexing a large collection of documents might result in huge index files that are hard to maintain. Therefore, it is important to utilize efficient compression methods for index files. The importance of index compression is fostered by the emergence of hand-held devices [4]. Equipping these devices with advanced index-based search capabilities is desirable, for quick reference and browsing purposes, but storage on hand-held devices is still sufficiently limited that indices need to be very compact. There are two complementary approaches in the field of index compression: lossless compression and lossy compression. Lossless approaches do not lose any information; instead, they use more efficient data structures. Thus, under lossless approaches, posting lists have a very compact representation [5]. On the other hand, under lossy approaches, certain information is discarded. The two approaches are complementary. That is, after selected document postings have been pruned using lossy methods, the index can be further compressed in a lossless manner. Thereby, a smaller index size can be attained than is possible by either one of the methods separately. Examples of the lossy approach include stopword omission, posting pruning [6], field-driven indexing [7] or vocabulary-driven indexing [8]. Another separation concerns the type of the knowledge needed for applying these approaches. Posting pruning are based on statistical profiling, whereas stopwords removal, field-driven and vocabulary-driven indexing rely on some domain expertize to reduce the size of the inverted file. Thus, field-driven indexing is used in Web engines to separate between highly relevant and less content bearing web contents by exploiting topological HTML markup, such as headings or anchor texts found in the context of hyperlinks. Our approach relies on the argumentation as found in biomedical articles to reduce the size of the indexes. The basic idea is that some argumentative contents are more relevant than others for information retrieval. So, following the above proposed typology for pruning systems, our approach relates to field-driven approaches, because it relies on some topological specificities, but like LSI it uses statistical distributions to make explicit the latent argumentative structure of the abstract. In contrast to vocabulary-driven methods, which are highly domain-dependent, our approach is only genre-specific: we only assume that the indexed documents contains some logical underlying moves.

Experimental research is often described as a problem solving activity. In full text scientific articles, as well an in short abstracts, this problem-solution structure has been crystallized in a fixed presentation known as *Introduction, Methods, Results* and *Conclusion*. This structure is often presented in a much-compacted version in the abstract and it has been clearly demonstrated by Schuemie et al. 2004 [9] that abstracts contain a higher information density than full text. Correspondingly, the 4-move problem-solving structure (standardized according to ISO/ANSI guidelines) has been found quite stable in scientific reports [10]. The argumentative structure of an article is rarely explicitly labeled: less than 5% of MEDLINE abstracts contain such markers. To find the most relevant argumentative status that describes the content of the article, we employed a classification method to separate the content dense sentences of the abstracts into the argumentative moves. An evaluation of the argumentative categorizer can be found in [11], where the tool has been used for information extraction tasks in genomics and proteomics, such as the identification of gene functions in the LocusLink database. The average recall and precision score (F-score) is in the range of 85%, when evaluated on a large sample of MEDLINE abstracts.

2 Methods

The performance of the engine on the pruning-free index will provide a baseline measure, that is the maximal effectiveness that can be theoretically achieved on a given benchmark. In information retrieval, benchmarks are developed from three resources: a document collection, a query collection and a set of relevance rankings, which relates each query to the set of documents. Once a good baseline is established, following experiments attempt to reduce the number of stems in the inverted file with minimal negative effects on the retrieval effectiveness.

Document sets, query sets and relevance judgements were obtained from the *Cystic Fibrosis* (CF) collection [12]. Measures are based on the Mean Average Precision (MAP), which is the standard metric for assessing retrieval effectiveness. For indexing, we used the easyIR system, which implements standard vector space IR schemes (following SMART [13]). Every experiment is conducted with Porter's conflation and using a list of 544 English stopwords. We also evaluate the use of a large thesaurus (400 000 items), extracted from the Unified Medical Language System (UMLS). The term-weighting schema, composed of combinations of term frequency, inverse document frequency and length normalization is varied to determine the most relevant output ranking. To establish a strong baseline, we tested different weighting schema: standart *tf.idf* as well as more advanced ones, such as *pivoted normalization* [14] and *deviation from randomness* [15]. A formal description of the different weighting schema, following the SMART standard representation used in the following, can be found in [16]. For *tf.idf* schema the first letter triplet applies to the document, the second letter triplet applies to the query (cf. [17] for a short introduction).

The classifier segments the abstracts into 4 argumentative moves: PURPOSE, METHODS, RESULTS, and CONCLUSION. The basic segment is the sentence; therefore the abstract is splitted into a set of sentences before being processed by the argumentative classifier. In this setting only one argumentative category is attributed to each sentence, which makes the decision model binary. The classification unit is the sentence which means that abstracts are preprocessed using an ad hoc sentence splitter. To determine the value of each argumentative move for index pruning, the argumentative categorizer first parses each abstract, generating four groups each representing a unique argumentative class. Each argumentative index contains sentences classified in one of four argumentative classes. Because argumentative classes are equidistributed in MEDLINE abstracts, each index contains approximately a quarter of the complete CF collection. Separately, we also evaluate the effect of adding titles and MeSH keywords in the argumentative indexes.

3 Results

To obtain the baseline measure, we tested different weighting schema (including atn.ntn, ltc.lnn), with and without the thesaurus. The lnu.ltn weighting schema in combination with the thesaurus produced the best results (0.2502), therefore these settings are used as baseline for all subsequent experiments and comparisons. Table 1 gives the compression ratio obtained by each type of index. The compression ratio (CR) is measured by counting the number of stems, used as indexing units in each index) divided by the number of indexing units in the full collection. In the same table, we also provide the results achieved by each of the four argumentative indexes. For each index, the table indicates the perfor-

Table 1. Mean average precision (MAP) and compression ratio (CR) results for querying the collection using different argumentative index

Indexes	MAP	Ratio (%)	# stem	CR (%)
CF collection	0.2502	100	8047	100
PURPOSE	0.2293	**64.6**	1734	21.5
METHODS	0.2307	17.4	1651	20.5
RESULTS	0.2344	18.7	1466	18.2
CONCLUSION	0.2389	**58.0**	1625	20.2
PURPOSE + Title + MeSH	0.2293	**78.4**	3709	46.1
METHODS + Title + MeSH	0.2307	37.2	3631	45.0
RESULTS + Title + MeSH	0.2344	37.9	3443	42.8
CONCLUSION + Title + MeSH	0.2389	**74.3**	3602	44.8

mance of the engine, when titles and MeSH are also added in the index. Adding MeSH and title' contents in each argumentative index implies that we trade compactness for retrieval effectiveness.

Table 1 shows the sentences classified as PURPOSE provide the most useful content to retrieve relevant documents. An average precision of 64.6% is achieved when using only this section of the abstract. The CONCLUSION move is the second most valuable, achieving 58.0% of the baseline average precision, while the compression ratio is about 20% (one indexing unit out of five in the full collection is stored in the index). The METHODS and RESULTS sections appear less content bearing for retrieving relevant documents, 16.4% and 17.6%, respectively, of the baseline. Each argumentative set represents roughly a quarter of the textual content of the original abstract. Querying with the PURPOSE section, (25% of the available textual material) realizes almost 2/3 of the average precision and for the CONCLUSION section, it is more than 50% of the baseline precision.

4 Conclusion

We have reported on the construction of an original index pruning strategy, which select indexing units based on their argumentative classes. Our results show that querying the PURPOSE index, which reduces the inverted file by a factor five, is sufficient to achieve about two-third (65.8%) of the baseline precision, while querying exclusively the CONCLUSION index achieves 54.2% of the baseline. When titles and medical subject headings are also stored in the respective indexes, querying PURPOSE and CONCLUSION indexes can respectively achieves 78.4% and 74.3% of the baseline, while the size if the index is divided by two (respectively 46.1% and 44.8%). Roughly, these results suggests that indexing between 20% and half of the argumentative content is sufficient to achieved between two third and 80% of the retrieval effectiveness. It is concluded that argumentation can be a powerful index pruning strategy in complement to more traditionnal approaches.

Acknowledgements

The study is supported the Swiss National Foundation (EAGL project, 3252BO-105755 - http://www.genisis.ch/natlang/eagl/).

References

1. Aronson, A., Mork, J., Gay, C., Humphrey, S., Rogers, W.: The NLM Indexing Initiative's Medical Text Indexer. MedInfo'89 Proceedings (2004)
2. Ruch, P., Baud, R.: valuating and Reducing the Effect of Data Corruption when Applying Bag of Words Approaches to Medical Records. Int J Med Inf **67 (1-3)** (2002) 75–83
3. Névéol, A., Soualmia, L., Douyère, M., Rogozan, A., Thirion, B., Darmoni, S.: Using cismef mesh "encapsulated" terminology and a categorization algorithm for health resources. Int J Med Inf **73(1)** (2004) 57–64
4. Tschopp, M., Lovis, C., Geissbühler, A.: Understanding usage patterns of handheld computers in clinical practice. Proc AMIA Symp (2000) 806–9
5. Witten, I., Moffat, A., Bell, T.: Managing Gigabytes. Morgan Kaufman, San Francisco (1999)
6. Carmel, D., Cohen, D., Fagin, R., Farchi, E., Herscovici, M., Maarek, Y., Soffer, A.: Static index pruning for information retrieval systems. Proc of ACM-SIGIR (2001) 43–50
7. Craswell, N., Hawking, D., Wilkinson, R., Wu, M.: Overview of the trec 2003 web track. In: TREC. (2003) 78–92
8. Aronson, A., Bodenreider, O., Chang, H., Humphrey, S., Mork, J., Nelson, S., Rindflesch, T., Wilbur, W.: The indexing initiative. A report to the board of scientific counselors of the lister hill national center for biomedical communications. Technical report, NLM (1999)
9. Schuemie, M., Weeber, M., Schijvenaars, B., van Mulligen, E., van der Eijk, C., Jeliert, R., Mons, B., Kors, J.: Distribution of information in biomedical abstracts and full text publications. Bioinformatics (2004)
10. Orasan., C.: Patterns in Scientific Abstracts. (In: Proceedings of Corpus Linguistics) 433–445
11. Ruch, P., Chichester, C., Cohen, G., Coray, G., Ehrler, F., Ghorbel, H., Müller, H., Pallotta, V.: Report on the TREC 2003 Experiment: Genomic Track. In: TREC-12. (2004)
12. Shaw, W., Wood, J., Wood, R., Tibbo, H.: The cystic fibrosis database: Content and research opportunities. LSIR **13** (1991) 347–366
13. Salton, G., Fox, E., Wu, H.: Communications of the acm. Journal of the American Society for Information Science **26 (11)** (1983) 1022–1036
14. Singhal, A., Buckley, C., Mitra, M.: Pivoted document length normalization. ACM-SIGIR (1996) 21–29
15. Amati, G., van Rijsbergen, C.: Probabilistic models of information retrieval based on measuring the divergence from randomness. ACM Transactions on Information Systems (TOIS) **20 (4)** (2002) 357–389
16. Savoy, J.: Report on clef-2003 monolingual tracks: Fusion of probabilistic models for effective monolingual retrieval. CLEF 2003 (2003)
17. Ruch, P.: Using contextual spelling correction to improve retrieval effectiveness in degraded text collections. COLING 2002 (2002)

A Benchmark Evaluation of the French MeSH Indexers

Aurélie Névéol[1,2], Vincent Mary[3], Arnaud Gaudinat[4], Célia Boyer[4], Alexandrina Rogozan[1], and Stéfan J. Darmoni[1,2]

[1] PSI Laboratory, Rouen, France
{aneveol, arogozan}@insa-rouen.fr
[2] CISMeF & CGIS, Rouen, France
stefan.darmoni@chu-rouen.fr
[3] Rennes Medical School, France
vincent.mary@univ-rennes1.fr
[4] HON Foundation, Geneva, Switzerland
Firstname.Lastname@healthonthenet.org

Abstract. The increasing demand on both practitioners and librarians to encode medical documents with controlled vocabularies calls for automatic tools and methods to help them perform this task efficiently. This paper presents the Benchmark evaluation of the French MeSH indexing systems carried out under the umbrella of the VUMeF consortium. The CISMeF, NOMINDEX and HONMeSHMapper systems are introduced, and evaluated on a set of 82 resources randomly taken from the CISMeF catalogue. The automatic MeSH indexing produced by each system was compared to the manual gold standard provided by the CISMeF medical librarian team. The automatic systems achieve at best a precision close to 50% at rank 1 (HONMeSHMapper, CISMeF) and HONMeSHMapper achieves the best overall F-measure. A qualitative evaluation of the indexing provided indicates that all systems tend to misevaluate the specificity of the terms to retrieve.

1 Introduction

The internet has become a very prosperous source of information in numerous fields, including health and molecular biology. Several projects have been initiated in order to meet the users' information needs related to these fields. Among them, the Health On the Net foundation (HON[1]) aims at guiding both lay and specialist audiences to trustworthy medical information. HON has developed automatic search engines to crawl and index the web, and an accreditation system based on their HONcode principles. Some 4,600 websites are currently accredited and annually reviewed. The Nomindex project[2] aims at organising health information for a more efficient retrieval. CISMeF[3] (French acronym of Catalogue and Index of Medical On-Line Resources) describes and indexes more than 14,000 resources of institutional health information in French. Indexing is a decisive step for the efficiency of information

---

[1] http://www.hon.ch/ (accessed on February 1st, 2005)
[2] http://www.med.univ-rennes1.fr/nomindex/ (accessed on February 1st, 2005)
[3] http://www.cismef.org (accessed on February 1st, 2005)

retrieval within these systems, and if performed manually, it is a highly time consuming task. Automatic tools have been developed for MeSH indexing in English as early as the 80s [1]. More recently, such tools have also been available for French. This paper presents the results of the Benchmark evaluation of the French MeSH indexing systems which was carried out in 2004 under the umbrella of the VUMeF [2] consortium. The aim of this evaluation is twofold: first, it provides a comparison of the systems. Secondly, through the analysis of the results, the strengths and weaknesses of each system may be identified. If appropriate, the complementarity of the systems – or of the resources they use, may be exploited.

2 Material and Methods

2.1 The French MeSH Indexing Systems

CISMeF - Natural Language Processing Approach (NLP)
This approach (detailed in [3]) is built on the three-step manual indexing procedure: analysis of the resource to be indexed, translation of the emerging concepts into the appropriate controlled vocabulary (here, the MeSH) and revision of the resulting index. First, a MeSH dictionary is used to extract medical concepts. The variants of the concepts (inflected forms, synonyms, etc.) are taken into account to compute the frequency of each concept. The dictionary contains the necessary information to translate the concepts into MeSH terms. A tf*idf normalization is then used to compute relevance scores for each MeSH term. The hierarchical information drawn from the MeSH is used to select and promote the most precise terms. Moreover, recurring check tags are promoted at the top of the candidate list to ensure their selection. Eventually, indexing rules are applied in order to revise the candidate list before the final index selection using a breakage function [3]. Although this system is able to retrieve isolated keywords, it was conceived to retrieve keyword/qualifier pairs.

NOMINDEX
Nomindex [4] was developped in order to identify medical concepts in natural language sentences. Then, these concepts are stored in a database which may be used for information retrieval. Nomindex uses a lexicon derrived from the ADM [5] (Assisted Medical Diagnosis) knowledge base which contains 130.000 terms, including associated words, compound words, prefixes and suffixes. First, document words are mapped to ADM terms and reduced to reference words (for instance, "cephalalgia" is mapped to "headache"). Then, ADM terms are mapped to the equivalent French MeSH terms, and also to their UMLS Concept Unique Identifier. Finally, every reference word of the document is then attributed its corresponding UMLS CUI. A relevance score (tf*idf) computed for each concept found in the document, is used in various tools : keyword identification, document similarity and automatic document synthesis.

HONMeSHMapper
HONMeSHMapper was developed in 1997 for the automatic categorization and retrieval of online medical documents. It is encapsulated in a more generic term

extractor which uses generic terminological resources such as the UMLS. Initially developed for HONselect and enhanced through the years, HONMeSHMapper has become a major component of the WRAPIN project [6] for MeSH keyword extraction and mapping. Initially, it was a lexical mapper [7] based on Cooper's assumptions [8] that (1) "the medically meaningful content in free-text clinical records would be contained within noun phrases" and (2) "all the important medical words worth recognizing in free-text noun phrases should be related to the words in the target vocabularies". In HONMeSHMapper, normalization is supplied by MeSH terminological resources (e.g. synonyms and close expressions) and by a stemmer. As a regular expression-based system HONMeSHMapper can also recognize compound MeSH terms within a window of five words. A bag-of-words approach uses the distribution of components of compound terms found in the full text. Finally, a weight is assigned to each MeSH term retrieved according to the inverse frequency of the term in the document and its position within the MeSH hierarchy.

2.2 Evaluation Corpus and Measures

The corpus used for this evaluation is composed of 82 resources randomly selected in the CISMeF catalogue. It contains about 235,000 words (1.7 Mb.). The corpus has been indexed by five professional indexers. In the literature [9], the manual indexing is considered as a gold standard to which the automatic indexing may be compared, although the inter-expert variability is high [10]. The average number of isolated keywords manually assigned to a resource in the evaluation corpus is 7.56 +/- 6.92.

The evaluation measures used are precision and recall. We also used the F-measure, which combines them with an equal weight. In the gold standard indexing used as a reference, the indexing terms consist of MeSH keyword/qualifier *pairs*. However, two of the indexing systems (NOMINDEX and HONMeSHMapper) retrieve isolated keywords. Therefore, we have focused the evaluation on the retrieval of keywords. We have considered that retrieving an isolated keyword, where the gold standard advocates the same keyword associated to a qualifier, was correct. For example, if *<hepatitis>* was retrieved where *<hepatitis/therapy>* was expected, we considered that the index term had been correctly retrieved.

3 Results

Table 1 shows the precision and recall (P-R) obtained by each system.

Table 1. Precision and recall of each system at fixed ranks

Rk	NOMINDEX	HONMeSHMapper	CISMeF- TAL -
	P – R	P – R	P – R
1	13.25 - 2.37	45.78 - 8.63	45.78 - 7.42
4	12.65 - 9.20	31.93 - 26.41	30.72 - 22.05
10	12.53 - 22.55	20.61 - 36.96	21.23 - 37.26
50	6.20 - 51.44	7.76 - 57.81	7.04 - 48.50

Figure 1 allows a comparison of the three systems through F-measure:

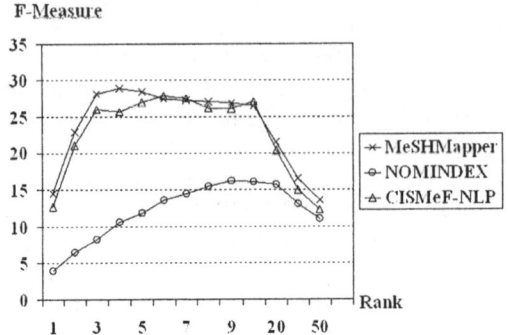

Fig. 1. Plot of F-Measure vs. fixed ranks for each indexing system

4 Discussion

Global Performances of the Systems

According to Table 1, the systems achieve at best a precision of 45% at rank 1 (HONMeSHMapper, CISMeF). HONMeSHMapper and CISMeF show a similar precision at all ranks, but the recall is higher for HONMeSHMapper. Figure 1 reflects this observation, as HONMeSHMapper achieves the best overall F-measure. MTI (Medical Text Indexer) [9] obtained a precision of 29% and a recall of 55% at rank 25 on a corpus of 273 articles. To compare the experiments, we may observe that (1) the evaluation corpus was different (scientific articles *vs.* web pages) and (2) the terminological resources or English are more comprehensive than those available in French: in 2005, about 50.000 MeSH synonyms remain to be translated into French.

Qualitative Analysis

A qualitative analysis of the terms retrieved by each system shows that the "noise" does not result from the retrieval of irrelevant terms. Most of the terms retrieved that are not selected by the human indexers are in fact either too broad (the indication on the resource content is too vague to be useful to the users) or too narrow (the concept referred is not sufficiently developed in the resource, so that users would not be satisfied with the information provided). Deciding whether the degree of specificity of each term retrieved is adequate would improve the performance of the three systems.

Perspectives

The terminological resources used by all three systems have different origins, and may be complementary. A previous evaluation of NOMINDEX [11] showed that specific updates of the lexicon could improve the system performance. Therefore, sharing resources may benefit all systems.

A recent evaluation of the American MeSH indexing system MTI [9] showed the advantage of combining different approaches (NLP & statistical methods) and filtering rules. CISMeF is currently testing the combination of the NLP system described with a statistical (k-NN) approach for keyword/qualifier pair indexing [12].

The combined approach was also evaluated on the same corpus for pair retrieval. Although the task was more difficult, the performances obtained matched those of isolated keyword retrieval. Therefore, the system resulting from the combination of NLP and statistical approaches for keyword/qualifier retrieval will be used for indexing resources to be added to the CISMeF catalogue in a semi-automatic mode. For HONMeSHMapper, the use of CISMeF manually indexed resources will allow the development of a knowledge-based approach, complementing the lexical approach already in use to suggest 5 keywords (WRAPPIN).

5 Conclusion

This paper presents a comparative evaluation of three MeSH indexing systems for French. MeSH isolated keywords were retrieved by CISMeF, HONMeSHMapper and NOMINDEX from the 82 resources of the evaluation corpus and compared to the manual gold standard. The best precision (45%) is achieved by HONMeSHMapper and CISMeF at rank 1. HONMeSHMapper shows the best overall F-measure. Sharing lexical resources used by all systems could enhance the performance. A qualitative evaluation of the indexing indicated that all systems could also be improved by judging more accurately the specificity of the terms to retrieve.

References

1. Humphrey SM., and Miller NE. Knowledge-Based Indexing of the Medical Literature: The Indexing Aid Project. J Am Soc Inf Sci, 38(3):184-96. (1987)
2. Darmoni, S.J. and Consortium VUMeF. VUMeF: Extending the French Involvement in the UMLS Metathesaurus. AMIA Annu Symp Proc. 2003;:824. (2003)
3. Néveol, A., Rogozan, A., Darmoni, S.J. : Automatic Indexing of Online Health Resources for a French Quality Controlled Gateway. In IP & M, in press. (2005).
4. Pouliquen, B., Delamarre, D., Le Beux, P., Indexation de Textes Médicaux par Extraction de Concepts et ses Utilisations, JADT'2002, St Malo, France, March 2002; (2) 617-628
5. Lenoir P., Michel JR., Frangeul C., and Chales G, Réalisation, Développement et Maintenance de la Base de Données A.D.M. Médecine informatique. 1981; 6 51--6.
6. Gaudinat A, Joubert M, Aymard S, Falco L, Boyer C, Ficschi M. WRAPIN: New Generation Health Search Engine Using UMLS Knowledge Sources for MeSH Term Extraction from Health Documentation. In Medinfo. 2004;2004:356-60.
7. Gaudinat A, Boyer C. Automatic Extraction of MeSH Terms from MEDLINEs Abstracts. Workshop on Natural Language Processing in Biomedical Applications, 2002: 53-57.
8. Cooper G, Miller R. An Experiment Comparing Lexical and Statistical Methods for Extracting MeSH Terms from Clinical Free Text. J. Am. Med. Inf. Assoc. 5, 1998: 62-75.
9. Aronson AR, Mork JG, Gay CW, Humphrey SM, Rogers WJ. The NLM Indexing Initiative's Medical Text Indexer. Medinfo. 2004;2004:268-72.
10. Funk ME., Reid CA. and Mc Googan LS. Indexing Consistency in MEDLINE. Bull. Med. Libr. Assoc. 71(2):176-183. (1983).
11. Mary V, Pouliquen B, Le Duff F, Darmoni SJ, Segui A, Le Beux P. Automatic Conceptual Indexing of French Pharmaceutical Theses. Stud Health Technol Inform. 2002;90:388-92.
12. Névéol A., Rogozan A., Darmoni SJ. Indexation Automatique de Ressources de Santé à l'Aide de Paires de Descripteurs MeSH. TALN 2005. (in press).

Populating an Allergens Ontology Using Natural Language Processing and Machine Learning Techniques

Alexandros G. Valarakos[1,2], Vangelis Karkaletsis[1], Dimitra Alexopoulou[1], Elsa Papadimitriou[1], and Constantine D. Spyropoulos[1]

[1] Software & Knowledge Engineering Lab., Inst. of Informatics and Telecomm., National Center for Scientific Research "Demokritos", 153 10 Ag. Paraskevi, Greece
{alexv, vangelis, costass}@iit.demokritos.gr

[2] Department of Information and Telecommunication Systems Engineering, School of Sciences, University of the Aegean, 83200, Karlovassi, Samos, Greece
alexv@aegean.gr

Abstract. Ontologies are becoming increasingly important in the biomedical domain since they enable the re-use and sharing of knowledge in a formal, homogeneous and unambiguous way. In the rapidly growing field of biomedicine, knowledge is usually evolving and therefore an ontology maintenance process is required to keep the ontological knowledge up-to-date. This paper presents our approach for populating a formally defined ontology for the allergen domain exploiting PubMed abstracts on allergens and using natural language processing and machine learning techniques. This approach is composed of two stages: locating initially instances of ontology concepts in the PubMed corpus, and finding at a 2nd stage instances' properties and relations between instances.

1 Introduction

The use of ontologies which describe and formalize the terminology and knowledge for a domain is an essential element for the development of information retrieval and extraction systems. For example, suppose that several different Web sites contain medical information. If these web sites share a common understanding of the structure of information through the same underlying ontologies of the terms they use, then information retrieval and extraction systems can locate and aggregate information from all these sites. Ontology construction in general involves the following steps: selection of concepts to be included in the ontology, specification of concepts' properties and relations, addition of concept instances. During the last years, several methodologies and tools for building ontologies have been presented. Concerning ontology maintenance this involves adding new instances (ontology population), as well as new concepts, properties and relations (ontology enrichment).

We have used well established tools and design principles to build an ontology in the allergens domain based on previous work and allergen related resources [20]. In this work, we present our approach for the automation of ontology population exploiting the allergens ontology built and PubMed [13] abstracts on the allergens domain and using natural language processing and machine learning techniques. We consider ontology population as an information extraction problem, where at a first stage we locate, in a domain specific corpus, ontology instances and classify them under the corresponding concepts. This is known as the named entity recognition and classification task in the language technology community, see [1]. At a second stage we find the relations between located instances and the values that fill their properties. For instance, in the allergens domain, we locate, in PubMed abstracts on allergens, instances of ontology concepts, such as the *allergen*, the *allergen source*, the *type of allergy*. At a second stage we locate the values that fill the properties of a specific allergen instance (e.g. its *molecular weight, isoelectric point*), and we find relations between them (e.g. that a specific allergen instance *occurs in* an allergen source instance and it *causes* an allergy type instance). As we noted before, this paper presents our work on ontology population focusing on the extraction of properties and relations. More specifically, section 2 provides information on existing allergen specific resources and refers to some related work on ontology population methods and relation extraction. Section 3 outlines the design principles we used for building a formally defined ontology on allergens. Section 4 presents our method for populating such an ontology extracting information from domain specific corpora employing natural language processing and machine learning techniques. Section 5 presents the experimental setting for testing our approach in the allergens domain and discusses the evaluation results. Finally, our concluding remarks and future plans are presented in section 6.

2 Related Work

Various allergen databases and lists exist and most of them are available free in the web. Their schemata are more or less similar focusing mostly to the allergen's name, the species it occurs in and the protein is associated with along with its sequence proving links to GenBank [7] and SwissProt [16]. Details on available allergen databases and data sources are given in [4]. The main problem of these schemata is related to the differences occurring in terms of their content and the meaning of database categories (semantic heterogeneity) as well as in terms of their structure (structure heterogeneity). Moreover, these schemata are highly ambiguous because they do not provide rigor definitions of the vocabulary uses, e.g. what is the meaning of source, should it be filled with allergen sources or proteins. And finally, many of them are not updated regularly, thus being out-of-date.

The above problems motivated us to build a formally defined logic-based ontology for the allergen domain [20] which could be machine exploitable. We were also concerned with the efficient maintenance of such an ontology. Various approaches based on information extraction methods have already been used for ontology population. Most of them use information extraction systems to locate the concept instances relying on manually annotated corpus [3]. We see ontology population as a bootstrapping process, where an initial manually created ontology is used to annotate the corpus which will then be used for the training of the information extraction system (the new instances found are evaluated by a human before being added in the ontology and the process starts again) [19]. Ontology population does not only concern the location of the names of new ontology instances. As we noted in the introduction, ontology population is an information extraction task, where the recognition and classification of instances represents just the 1st processing stage. All the instances properties as well as the relations between instances must be grouped together, thus resulting to a composite ontology instance.

The work presented in this paper extends our ontology population process, presented in [20], with a 2nd processing stage, that of extracting properties and relations. The problem of properties and relations extraction was examined in the 7th Message Understanding Conference [10] where it was formulated as a separate extraction task. Relation extraction is currently being studied by several researchers employing natural language processing (NLP) and/or machine learning techniques. Relation extraction in the biomedical domain has recently attracted many researchers as an application domain due to the grammatical complexities of the biomedical corpora (long sentences with coordinative and appositive structures, and clauses) and due to the large number of practical applications. In terms of the NLP techniques used in the biomedical domain these involve either full parsing [17] or shallow parsing methods [15]. Concerning machine learning techniques, these are used for pattern extraction employing lexical, syntactic and semantic features [8]. Our work is based on shallow parsing methods exploiting the semantic features extracted by the previous stage of our ontology population method (ontology instances and their synonyms). We do not employ machine learning techniques due to the limited number of examples that we could use for the training of these techniques. Machine learning based relation extraction techniques require the annotation of a large number of such relations in domain specific corpora and such corpora do not exist in the allergens domain. We must also note the complexity of the relations annotation task, in general, and mainly in the biomedical domain due to the complexity of the language used. That's why we used a corpus annotation methodology based on standard annotation practice, which involves two annotators (domain experts) and the use of detailed annotation guidelines.

3 Ontology Building

As it is presented in [20] we used well established principles and tools to design and build our ontology. We use the description logic-based ontology language, OWL [14] since logic-based languages promise more reusability, hence less cost on ontology building. In this implementation we tried to avoid the duplication (overlapping) of knowledge units[1] in the ontology. We also relied on previous

---

[1] We use the term knowledge units to refer to properties, concepts and instances of a domain ontology at the knowledge level.

work on formal biomedical relations. Two biologists and a knowledge engineer were involved in its creation and capturing knowledge from the IUIS allergen list [9] and the allergen nomenclature. The ontology was implemented using the Protégé's OWL plug-in [11].

Figure 1 illustrates the allergen domain ontology, ellipses stand for concepts whereas arrows denote ontological relations. The *"Allergens"* concept is subsumed by the *"Proteins"* concept. *"Allergens"* are linked to *"Proteins"* through the relation *"hasBiochemicalIdentityAs"*. *"Allergens"* are divided into *named* and *descriptive* ones. *"Named allergens"* are those that have a scientific name derived from the allergen nomenclature, whereas *"Descriptive Allergens"* are those that do not have a scientific name. The *"Named Allergens"* subsumes *"Isoallergens"* which subsume *"Variants"*. *"Allergen sources"* instances are connected through the *"occursIn"* relation with allergen instances. Moreover, the *"Allergen sources"* are connected with the appropriate level of the Linnaeus ontology. *"Allergens"* are linked to *"Allergies"* through the *"causes"* relation. Allergens have the *"hasVariant"* and *"hasIsoAllergen"* relations which connect

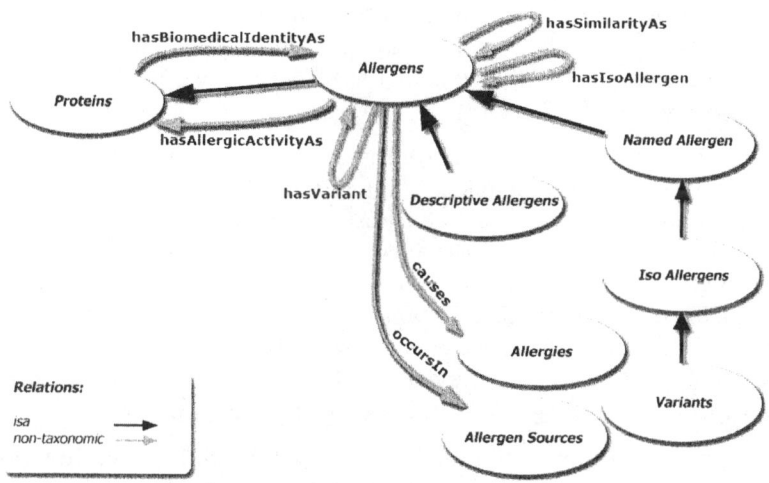

Fig. 1. Allergens' Domain Ontology (Concepts and Relations)

allergen instances with their *isoallergen* and *variant* instances. Also, allergens have the properties *"molecular weight"* and *"iso-electric point"*. Named allergens have the property *"scientific name"*, which holds the name derived from the allergen nomenclature and the *"common/former name"* which holds the name we used to have for the allergen before the allergen nomenclature system appeared. Finally, *"Proteins"* have the property *"name"* and allergen sources have the properties *"scientific"* and *"common name"*.

4 Ontology Population

Our approach [20] populates the ontology with new instances located in domain specific corpora and also enriches it with the typographic variants of its instances (different lexicalizations of the same instance) located again in the same corpora. The key idea behind this approach is that we can keep the instances of the domain ontology and their typographic variants up-to-date in a semi-automatic way, by periodically re-training an information extraction system using a domain specific corpus. The methodology is not relied on manually annotated corpus but uses the already known instances of the ontology to annotate the corpus. This work extends our ontology population approach, adding a 2nd processing stage, that of extracting the properties and the relations of located ontology instances. More specifically, our approach involves the following processing stages which were implemented using the Ellogon text engineering platform [5] and the Protégé ontology editor [12].

Ontology-Based Annotation. This stage exploits the instances in the domain ontology to automatically annotate the domain specific corpus. The annotated corpus is used by the information extraction system in the next stages for extracting new instances, their properties and relations. The ontology instances are fed to a lookup engine that finds all their occurrences in the corpus using regular expression patterns.

Recognition and Classification of Instances. A named entity recognition and classification (NERC) module is employed in this stage to locate new ontological instances. The module is trained using machine learning methods (Hidden Markov Models - HMMs) on the annotated corpus derived from the previous stage. A single HMM is trained for each property and relation as proposed in [6]. HMMs exploit tokens, intending to capture the context in which the instances of a particular concept occur. The trained NERC module is capable of recognizing new ontological instances. The extracted instances will be validated by the domain expert before being added in the updated ontology.

Knowledge Refinement. A compression-based clustering algorithm is employed in this stage for identifying typographic variants of each instance [18]. For example, the allergen source Scientific Name *'p. officinalis asparagus officinalis'* can be written as *'p. officinalis'* or the allergen scientific name *'Amb a 1'* can be written as *'Amp alpha 1'* or *'amb a I'*.

Extracting Properties and Relations. A shallow parser is used to extract the instances properties and the relations that hold between instances (and instances' properties in the case of the allergen ontology). For this purpose, it uses a set of patterns that employ lexical features (specific nouns or verbs), syntactic features (the position of the word in the sentence) and semantic features (ontology instances found in the previous stages). There are different patterns for each property and relation we try to extract. Table 1 presents the properties and relations we are interested for in the allergens case study.

Table 1. Interesting properties and relations in the allergens case study

Allergens instances' properties
Molecular Weight
Isoelectric Point
Relations between instances
hasBiochemicalIdentityAs (relates allergens and proteins)
occursIn (relates allergens with allergen sources)
causes (relates allergens with allergy types)
Relations between instances' properties
Allergen Name Scientific-Common
Allergen Source Name Scientific-Common

Validation and Insertion. At this stage the domain expert validates the extracted instances, properties and relations derived from the previous stages. He/she inserts then the validated information into the ontology. The outcome of this stage is a new version of the ontology containing knowledge extracted from the domain specific corpus. A new iteration begins with the new version of the ontology. The iterative process will stop when no more changes in the ontology are possible.

5 Experimental Setting

5.1 Corpus Annotation

This step concerns the creation of consistently annotated corpora for the training and testing of our system. The corpus annotation methodology that has been developed is comparable to standard annotation practice [2]. The annotation task is based on Annotation Guidelines that are issued for a specific domain in order to ensure a common understanding between annotators of what is to be annotated and how it should be annotated. The corpus is split and two human annotators use the guidelines in order to annotate each half. Each annotator takes then the other half, inspects the annotations produced and comments in cases of disagreements. Inter-annotator agreement is used as an indicator of the quality of the annotated corpora. Moreover consistent differences in the annotations produced can indicate which parts of the guidelines need refinement. The annotation labels come from the labels of the ontological components:

- the allergen's scientific and common/former names,
- the scientific name and common name of the allergen's source,
- the allergen's molecular weight and isoelectric point,
- the protein family to which the allergen possibly belongs or shows great homology (indicative of its biochemical function/identity) or even the protein name that happened to be an allergen and, finally,
- the type of allergy it causes.

The corpus was then annotated with information identifying the existence of the interesting properties and relations. The labels used are presented below along with some representative examples from the PubMed corpus that show the different ways used to express the same property or relation. The complexity of the language used increases the complexity of the specific information extraction task. This is also the case in other biomedical sub-domains. More specifically we use the following labels.

- those that refer to the properties of an allergen: the molecular weight (MW), and the isoelectric point (pI). Some characteristic sentences are the following: *"The N-terminal sequence of an additional **145-kDa** allergen, termed **Jun v 4**..."*, *"The molecular weights for **C13** and **C28** cloned proteins are **56,200** and **46,7000**..."*, *"...**Cav p 2** and **Cav p 1**, contained several isoforms with pI values ranging from **3.6 to 5.3**."*, *"The pI of **Pol** was in the pH region **4-6**"*.
- those that denote relations between the allergen and the allergen source, the allergen and the allergy type, the allergen and the protein name or protein family it belongs to. Such sentences are the following *"One of the clones encoded the **group 1 allergen** of **canary grass** pollen..."*, *"Cloning of the minor allergen **Api g 4** profilin from **celery (Apium graveolens)**..."*, *"...to react with serum IgE from **shrimp allergic** patients and induce immediate type skin reactions in sensitized patients."*, *"...**furfurallergic atopic dermatitis** patients (83.3%) had elevated serum levels of IgE to purified **Mal f 4**"*.
- those that denote relations between allergens properties (scientific and common names) such as *"...designated as **antigen 5 (Dol m V)**..."* and *"...the American cockroach (Periplaneta americana) **Per a 3 (Cr-PI)** allergen..."*, as well as between the allergen sources properties (scientific and common names) such as *"...the immunochemically partial identical major allergens of **Alder (Alnus glutinosa)** ..."*, *"...The complete amino acid sequences of Ag 5 from two species each of **hornets (Dolichovespula arenaria** and **maculata)**..."*, *"Sequence of the gene encoding **cat (Felis domesticus)** serum albumin."*.

5.2 Creation of the Rules

In order to assist the two domain experts during the creation of the rules, they were provided with a list of the sentences containing the characteristic phrases for each property and relation, taken from the first half of the corpus (training corpus). They made grammar rules for each sentence constructing regular expressions using lexico-syntactic and semantic information. For each property and relation, these rules were then merged and applied to the training corpus. After a few iterations, we came out with a set of rules for each property and relation. An example of such a rule that recognizes a relation between an *allergen* and an *allergy* is the following: "AllergenSource\sin\scausing\sAllergy". Another example of a rule that recognizes relation between an *allergen* and a *protein* is "[homology|homologous]\s [to|with]\s+(\w\s)*ProteinName".

5.3 Experiments

We measured the performance of our system in the task of extracting properties and relations, on a corpus annotated by the domain experts (i.e. on ideal input). The corpus was split into the training and the testing part. The training part was used for the creation and refinement of the extraction rules, whereas the testing part for evaluating the system performance. Table 2 presents the results for each property and relation As a general remark, we can say that our system presents a

Table 2. Evaluation results on the testing corpus

	Target	Correct	Incorrect	Precision	Recall
Allergen instances' properties					
Molecular Weight	38	32	9	0.78	0.84
Isoelectric Point	7	7	0	1.00	1.00
Relation between instances					
hasBiochemicalIdentityAs	80	67	7	0.91	0.84
occursIn	238	194	0	1.00	0.82
causes	18	17	0	1.00	0.94
Relations between instances' properties					
Allergen Name Scientific-Common	7	7	0	1.00	1.00
Allergen Source Name Scientific-Common	176	172	3	0.98	0.98

very good performance, in terms of both recall and precision. Precision is defined as the ratio of the information, i.e. properties and relations, extracted correctly to the number of all extracted information, whereas recall is defined as the ratio of the information extracted correctly to the number of the target information. But, at the end, what is important, is whether the system manages to fill the whole "template" correctly, that is whether it locates all the properties and relations found in the abstracts for each target allergen instance. The whole testing corpus contains 182 allergen instances. Our system managed to find correctly, either all or some of the properties and relations, in 168 out of the total 182 cases. There were 12 incorrect cases which were mainly due to the wrong sentence splitting (the general sentence splitter of Ellogon was used without any tuning to the specific corpus). In the 168 correct cases, the main problem was that the system didn't manage to locate all the information existing in the abstracts. This was mainly due to the fact that our system, in its current state, extracts properties and relations only from sentences containing instances of the allergen names or their typographic variants found in the previous processing stages. In case the information occurs in other sentences (for example, a sentence may provide input on an allergen's molecular weight without mentioning the allergen's name but just referring to it with a pronoun or other expression), this information is missed from the final "template", although it was found in the previous processing stages. A first analysis in the testing corpus showed that we missed, due to co-reference, several instances of the Molecular Weight and "isoelectric point" properties (23, 3 respectively), as well as of the Allergen Name scientific-common relation (7). The use of the co-reference module would enable us to include, also those sentences containing co-references to the instances of allergen names, increasing the performance of the information extraction system.

6 Concluding Remarks

This work proposes a 2-stage approach for automating ontology population extracting information from domain specific corpora. The 1st stage concerns the identification of new ontology instances and their typographic variants. The 2nd stage concerns the extraction of instances' properties and the relations holding between instances as well as between instances' properties. A machine learning based method is used in the 1st stage and a rule based one (shallow parsing) in the 2nd stage. Our approach was tested on a corpus of PubMed abstracts on allergens using an allergens ontology. This ontology was built using well established design principles and exploiting existing taxonomies and documents that describe the allergen nomenclature. The evaluation results were quite good, in terms of the ability of the system to extract properties and relations from sentences containing instances of allergen names and their variants. The next step is to integrate the 2nd processing stage in the iterative bootstrapping process in order to examine the whole performance of our ontology population approach. We also plan to use a co-reference analysis module in order to take into account missing information found in sentences containing co-reference to allergens names.

Concluding, we believe that our approach which combines machine learning and natural language processing techniques for ontology population is the appropriate one for this task in biomedical corpora, such as the allergen abstracts. It involves a domain expert only after the 1st processing stage, when he/she will have to create the extraction rules. The domain expert is assisted in this task since we provide him/her with the ontology-annotated abstracts and with the sentences containing the interesting properties and relations. The positive remarks we received from the two domain experts and the high performance of the created grammar support this claim. In the near future, we plan to enhance our approach with rule induction techniques in order to provide the domain expert with an initial set of rules to start experimenting with.

Acknowledgements. The authors are grateful to Prof. Brusic and his team at the Institute for Infocomm Research, Singapore, for providing the PubMed abstracts on allergens and commenting on various stages of this work.

References

1. D. Appelt. Introduction to Information Extraction. AI Communications Journal, vol. 2(3), pp. 161-172.
2. S. Boisen, M. Crystal, R. Schwartz, R. Stone, R. Weischedel. Annotating Resources for Information Extraction, In proceedings of the 2nd International Conference on Language Resources and Evaluation (LREC-2000), Athens, Greece, 2000.

3. C. Brewster, F. Ciravegna, Y. Wilks. User-centred ontology learning for knowledge management. In: 7th International Conference on Applications of Natural Language to Information Systems. Vol. 2253 of LNCS, Springer Verlag (2002).
4. V. Brusic and N. Petrovsky. Bioinformatics for Characterisation of Allergens, Allergenicity and Allergic Cross-Reactivity. Trends in Immunology 24, 225-228, 2003.
5. G. Petasis, V. Karkaletsis, G. Paliouras, I. Androutsopoulos, CD. Spyropoulos, Ellogon: A New Text Engineering Platform, In Proceedings of the 3rd International Conference on Language Resources and Evaluation (LREC-2002), Las Palmas, Spain, pp. 72-78, May, 2002.
6. D. Freitag, A. McCallum. Information extraction using hmms and shrinkage. In: Workshop on Machine Learning for Information Extraction(AAAI-99).(1999) 31-36
7. GeneBank: http://www.ncbi.nlm.nih.gov/Genbank/GenbankSearch.html
8. M.L. Huang, X.Y. Zhu, Y. Hao, D.G. Payan, K.B. Qu, and M. Li. Discovering patterns to extract protein-protein interactions from full texts. Bioinformatics,Vol. 20(18), 2004.
9. International Union of Immunological Societies: http://www.allergen.org/List.htm
10. Message Understanding Conference: http://www.itl.nist.gov/iaui/894.02/related_projects/muc/proceedings/muc_7_toc.html
11. Protégé's OWL plug-in: http://protege.stanford.edu/plugins/owl/
12. Protégé Ontology Editor: http://protege.stanford.edu/
13. PubMed: http://www.ncbi.nlm.nih.gov/entrez/query.fcgi
14. Web Ontology Language: http://www.w3.org/TR/owl-ref
15. J. Pustejovsky, J. Castano, J. Zhang. Robust Relational Parsing over Biomedical Literature: Extracting Inhibit Relations. In the Proceedings of the 7th Pacific Symposium on Biocomputing (PSB 2002). page 362-373.
16. SwissProt: http://au.expasy.org/sprot/
17. J.M. Temkin, M.R. Gilder. Extraction of protein interaction information from unstructured text using a context-free grammar.Bioinformatics 2003,vol.19.
18. A. Valarakos, G. Paliouras, V. Karkaletsis, and G. Vouros. Name-Matching Algorithm for Supporting Ontology Enrichment, In Proceedings of the Panhellenic Conference on Artificial Intelligence (SETN04), LNAI, n. 3025, pp. 381-389, Springer Verlag, 2004.
19. A. Valarakos, G. Paliouras, V. Karkaletsis, G. Vouros. Enhancing Ontological Knowledge through Ontology Population and Enrichment, In Proceedings of the 14th International Conference on Knowledge Engineering and Knowledge Management (EKAW 2004), LNAI, n. 3257, pp. 144-156, Springer Verlag, 2004.
20. A. Valarakos, V. Karkaletsis, D. Alexopoulou, E. Papadimitriou. Building an Allergens Domain Ontology and Maintaining it using Machine Learning Techniques, NCSR Technical report, 2005/7, 2005. http://www.iit.demokritos.gr/~alexv/publications/alexvTR2004-7.pdf
21. G. Zhou, J. Zhang, Z. Su, D. Shen, C. Tan. Recognizing Names in Biomedical Texts: a Machine Learning Approach, 2004.

Ontology of Time and Situoids in Medical Conceptual Modeling

Heinrich Herre and Barbara Heller[†]

Onto-Med Research Group,
Institute for Medical Informatics, Statistics,
Epidemiology (IMISE) and Institute for Informatics (IfI),
University of Leipzig, Germany,
Härtelstrasse 16-18, 04107 Leipzig
herre@informatik.uni-leipzig.de

Abstract. Time, events, changes, and processes play a major role in medical conceptual modeling. Representation of time-structures and reasoning about time-oriented medical data are important theoretical and practical research areas. We assume that a formal representation of temporal knowledge must use as a framework some top-level ontology which describes the most general categories of temporal entities. In the current paper we discuss an ontology of time and situoids which is part of the top-level ontology GFO (General Formal Ontology) being developed by the Onto-Med research group [1]. The expressive power of GFO and its usability in conceptual modeling is tested by Onto-Med by carrying out a number of case studies in several fields of medicine and biomedicine. In the present paper we report on results of reconstructing the temporal-abstraction ontology presented by Y. Shahar [2] within GFO. In carrying out this investigation it turns out that a number of aspects in [2] needs further clarification and foundation.

1 Introduction

Time, events, changes, and processes play a major role in medical conceptual modeling. Representation of time-structures and reasoning about time-oriented medical data are important theoretical and practical research areas. We assume that a formal representation of temporal knowledge must use as a framework some top-level ontology which describes the most general categories of temporal entities. There is a growing body of work of ontologies in the sense of [3], i.e. as sharable conceptual specifications and its applications in several domains [4, 5]. These developments are closely related to conceptual modeling [6, 7] and may benefit from an interdisciplinary approach [8, 9, 10]. Testing and proving the usability of top-level ontologies in conceptual modeling of real domains is an important step in establishing them as an integral part of *Ontological Engineering*.

[†] The Onto-Med research group mourns the death of its founder Barbara Heller. She died after a long illness during the work on this paper.

The current paper reports on research which is aimed at testing the top level ontology GFO in several fields of medicine and biomedicine. We discuss an ontology of time and of situoids which is part of the top-level ontology GFO (General Formal Ontology) [11]. GFO will be included in an integrated library *LibOnt* of top-level ontologies which is intended to cover all of its basic types, among them several 4D and 3D+T ontologies [12, 13]. The main purpose of *LibOnt* is to provide an integrated system of axiomatized top-level ontologies which can be used as a framework for building and representing specific ontologies pertaining to some concrete domain. The time ontology of GFO is inspired by ideas of F. Brentano [14]; situoids resemble what is sometimes called histories, and GFO-situations are ontological versions of situations in the sense of Barwise and Perry [15, 16].

The paper is structured as follows. In section 2 we present the main ideas of GFO's ontology of time, and in sections 3, 4, and 5 those categories of GFO are outlined which are relevant for the conceptual framework of the present paper. Finally, in section 6 it is shown how the temporal-abstraction ontology of Y. Shahar [2] may be reconstructed in the framework of GFO. This reconstruction is conducted by principles of ontological mappings as expounded in [17]. It turns out that a number of aspects in [2] needs further clarification and foundation.

2 Brentano Time

The time ontology expounded in this section was inspired by the ideas of Brentano [14]. We assume that time is continuous and endorse a modified and refined version of the interval-based approach of time. Following this approach, chronoids – the intervals of the classical approach – are not defined as sets of points, but as entities sui generis. Every chronoid has boundaries, which are called time-boundaries and which depend on chronoids, i.e., time-boundaries have no independent existence. Besides chronoids we introduce time-regions which are mereological sums of chronoids. We assume that time entities are related by certain formal relations, in particular the part-of relation between chronoids and time regions, denoted by *tpart*(x, y), the relations of being a (left, right) time-boundary of a chronoid, $lb(x, y)$ and $rb(x, y)$, and the relation of coincidence between two time-boundaries which is denoted by *tcoinc*(x, y).

Dealing with boundaries and the relation of coincidence is especially useful if two processes are to be modeled as "meeting" (in the sense of Allen's relation "meets"). In our opinion there are at least three conditions that a suitable model must fulfill: (a) There are two processes following one another immediately, i.e., without any gaps (b) There is a point in time where the first process ends and (c) there is a point in time where the second process starts. If, as is common practice, intervals of real numbers are used to model time intervals with reals as time points, the desired conditions cannot be satisfied. In contrast, the approach presented in GFO allows for two chronoids following immediately after one another *and* having proper starting- and ending-"points" by letting their boundaries coincide. Thus (a), (b), and (c) are preserved. An axiomatization *B(Time)* of this ontology of time – based on the relations *Chron*(x), *tpart*(x, y), *tcoinc*(x, y), $tb(x, y)$ – is presented in [18]. In [19] it is shown that the theory *B(Time)* and the theory in [20] have the same expressive power with respect to the interpretability relation, i.e. each of these theories is interpretable in the other.

3 Processes and Endurants

Material individuals are entities which are in space and time, and there is the well-known philosophical distinction between endurants and processes which is determined by their relation to time. An endurant is an object which is in time, but of which it makes no sense to say that it has temporal parts or phases; hence it is wholly present at every time-boundary of its existence and it persists through time. In our approach we make a more precise distinction between *presentials* and *processes* because it turns out that the philosophical notion of endurant combines two contradictory aspects. Based on a different distinction, there are entities which characterize others: *properties*. Furthermore, with presentials, processes and properties at hand, several "derived" categories can be discussed, among them more complex entities like *situoids* and *situations*.

Persistence is accounted for by two distinct categories: presentials and persistants. A *presential* exists wholly at a time-boundary and the relation $at(x, y)$ has the meaning "the presential x exists at time-boundary y". We assume that "at" is a functional relation, i.e. the following axiom is stipulated: $at(x, y) \wedge at(x, z) \rightarrow y = z$. This axiom raises the question of what is meant by the claim that an endurant (seemingly a philosophical analogue of our presentials) persists through time. We pursue an approach which accounts for persistence by means of a suitable universal whose instances are presentials. Such universals are called *persistants*. These do not change and they can be used to explain how presentials which have different properties at different times can nevertheless be the same.

Processes have temporal parts and develop over time, unfold in time, or perdure, and thus cannot be present at a time-boundary. Time belongs to them, because they happen in time and the time of a process is built into it. The relation between a process and a chronoid is determined by the projection function $prt(x, y)$ stating that "the process x is projected onto a chronoid y". Again we stipulate that $prt(x, y)$ is a functional relation. Yet there are two more projection relations: the relation $prt(p, c, q)$ is to be understood as follows: p is a process, c is a temporal part of the chronoid which frames p, and q is that part of p which results from the projection of p onto c. The temporal parts of a process p are exactly the projections of p onto temporal parts of the framing chronoid of p. The third relation projects processes onto time-boundaries; we denote this relation by $prb(p, t, e)$ and call the entity e, which is the result of this projection, the boundary of p at t. We postulate that the projection of a process to a time-boundary is a presential.

4 Relations, Facts, and Propositions

Relations are entities which glue together the things of the real world whereas *facts* are constituted by several related entities together with their relation. Every relation has a finite number of *relata* or *arguments* which are connected or related. Let us first consider the connection between a relation and its arguments (referring to facts on an intuitive basis). At this point, a particular fact seems to involve a relation and particular arguments. "John's being a patient of hospital A" is one fact, whereas the same "John's being a patient of hospital B" amounts to a different fact. Different particular arguments are involved in these facts, but the same relationship appears, namely "being a patient of". For this reason we assume that relations exhibit a universal character. In contrast to the extensional definition of relations in a mathematical reading, we do not consider the mere collection of the arguments with respect to a single fact as an instance of a relation. For example, the pair (John, hospital A) is not an instance of the relation "being a patient of". Instead, we assume that there are concrete entities with the power of connecting other entities (of any kind). These connecting entities are called *relators*, and they are the instances of relations. Relators themselves offer an "internal" structure which allows one to distinguish the differences in the way the arguments of a relation participate in a fact. Returning to the example, John is involved differently in the fact of being a patient of hospital A as compared to the hospital B. Exchanging John and the hospital would result in a strange sentence like "the hospital A is a patient of John". We say that John and the hospital play different roles in that relationship. Formally, this leads us to the introduction of a further type of entity: *relational roles*. A relator can be decomposed into relational roles, such that each role is a mediator between exactly one argument and the relator [21].

The simplest combinations of relators and relata are *facts*. Facts are considered as parts of the world, as entities sui generis, for example "John's being an instance of the universal Human" or "the book B's localization next to the book C" refer to facts. Furthermore, facts are frequently discussed in connection with other abstract notions like propositions (cf. [22]). However, propositions make claims which may be true or false. Therefore, truth-values are assigned to propositions and they can be logically combined. Neither is the case for facts. In analogy to atomic formulas in logic, a special type of propositions is introduced which reflects a single fact and which is called an *infon*, similar to the notion of infons in [23, 16]. We write $\langle\langle R: a_1, ..., a_n \rangle\rangle$ for the fact that a relator, i.e., an instance, of the relation R connects the entities $a_1, ..., a_n$. Preliminarily, we use $\langle R: a_1, ..., a_n \rangle$ for the corresponding infon about the same situation. Infons are the simplest type of *elementary propositions*.

To make the difference between facts and infons clear let us consider the above example. The fact of "John's being a patient of hospital A" is denoted by the symbolic structure $\langle\langle \text{Patient-of: John, A} \rangle\rangle$. In contrast, the symbolic structure $\langle \text{Patient-of: John, A} \rangle$ denotes an infon with the meaning "John is a patient of the hospital A." The difference is that the latter is a claim about the world which has an assigned truth-value and which can be logically combined with other propositions. The former simply denotes a part of the world. A deeper elaboration of the interconnections of facts, factual representations, infons, elementary propositions and propositions in general and agents in terms of an analysis of the denotation relation is to be developed in the future.

5 Situations and Situoids

Physical structures, qualities, and relators presuppose one another, and constitute complex units or wholes. The simplest units of this kind are, obviously, facts. A general configuration is an aggregate of facts. We consider a collection of presential (concrete) facts which exist at the same time-boundary. Such collections may be considered themselves as presentials, and we call them *configurations*. A *situation* is a special configuration which can be comprehended as a whole and satisfies certain conditions of unity imposed by certain universals, relations and categories associated with the situation. According to the basic assumptions of GFO, presentials have no independent existence, they depend on processes. Since configurations are presentials, too, they depend on processes. We call such processes *configuroids* [11].

Finally, there is a category of processes whose boundaries are situations and which satisfy certain principles of coherence, comprehensibility, and continuity. We call these entities *situoids;* they are the most complex integrated wholes of the world, and they have the highest degree of independence. As it turns out, each of the considered entities (including processes) is embedded into a suitable situoid. A situoid is, intuitively, a part of the world that is a coherent and comprehensible whole and does not need other entities in order to exist. Every situoid has a temporal extent and is framed by a topoid. The notion of being a coherent and comprehensible whole may be formally elucidated in terms of an *association relation* between situoids and certain categories. The notion of a *comprehensible whole* is captured in [24] by using terms of Gestalt Theorie. Furthermore, propositions are interpreted in situoids; to make this precise a basic relation |= between situoids and propositions is introduced, and "S |= p" has the meaning that the proposition p is satisfied (or true) in the situoid S. An outline of this approach is presented in [24].

6 Temporal Abstraction Ontology in the GFO-Framework

The reconstruction of ontologies in the GFO-framework is guided by the principle of ontological mappings as expounded in [17]. Ontological mappings are semantic translations which are based on top-level ontologies.

We give an overview about some aspects of the abstraction ontology in [2], which is denoted in the sequel by *AbstrOnt*, and then we sketch how these concepts/entities may be re-interpreted (reconstructed) in the framework of the time and situoid ontology of GFO. The current paper does not contain a complete analysis of all aspects of the ontology *AbstrOnt*. A full analysis of *AbstrOnt* as of other ontologies is work in progress and will be published elsewhere.

According to the GFO-approach we assume that a particular medical domain D is modeled by a class $Situ(D)$ of situoids which capture all relevant entities, relations, facts, temporal and spatial extensions of those coherent parts of the world which are related to D. We may describe $Situ(D)$ by a certain formal description $Desc(D)$ which can be understood as a GFO-category (a class in the modeling practice) whose instances contain – among others – the elements of $Situ(D)$. The pair $(Situ(D), Desc(D))$ is a kind of reference frame which is assumed to be fixed in all further considerations. Furthermore, we assume the existence of a formal language which allows to formulate the descriptions $Desc(D)$ and a set $Prop(D)$ of the relevant propositions pertaining to the class $Sit(D)$, and hence to the domain D.

6.1 Time Stamps

Time stamps, according to *AbstrOnt*, are introduced as structures which are mapped into an integer amount of an element of a set of predefined temporal granularity units.

Furthermore, a zero-point time stamp must exist, with relationship to which the time stamps are measured by using the units. This zero-point should be grounded in each domain to different absolute, real world time points. The reconstruction within GFO is carried out within a situoid S from $Situ(D)$. Let $time(S) = T$ be the chronoid onto which S is projected (which frames S). A granularity system $GS(T)$ of T is a set of chronoids being temporal parts of T, one element $c(0)$ of $GS(T)$ is fixed as a "zero point chronoid". Furthermore, we may assume a measure-function m which attaches to any chronoid c (which is a part of T) a positive real number capturing the duration of c. The set TS of time stamps can be understood as a set of symbolic structures which are interpreted by elements from $GS(T)$. All of this information can be captured in a system $TimeStamp(S) = (S, TS, f, GS(T), c(0), m)$ which is called time-stamp structure. Furthermore, we may assume a uniform way to associate to any situoid S from $Situ(D)$ a system $TimeStamp(S)$. The other conditions described in *AbstrOnt* may be defined by adding further constraints to $TimeStamp(S)$.

6.2 Time Interval

A *time interval I* in *AbstrOnt* is an ordered pair of time stamps representing the interval's endpoints. Time points are represented as zero-length intervals. In the GFO-framework there are no chronoids (intervals) of zero length but for any chronoid there exist exactly two time-boundaries. Hence time intervals are modeled by chronoids, points by time-boundaries. Since time stamps are data structures (say symbolic structures), the definition in *AbstrOnt* allows attaching time points to time stamps. In the GFO-framework it is sufficient to consider the case of associating chronoids to time stamps. Every chronoid defines two unique time-boundaries, hence, there is no need to define an interval by a pair of time stamps. In [2] it is stated that propositions are interpreted over time intervals. This seems to have no clear meaning. In our opinion propositions are interpreted in situoids (or configuroids) which themselves have a temporal extension. That means, the notion of "being interpreted over an interval" may be derived from the more fundamental notion of "being interpreted in a situoid/configuroid".

6.3 Interpretation Context

An *interpretation context*, according to *AbstrOnt*, is a proposition that, intuitively, represents a state of affairs. An example is the "drug insulin has an effect on blood glucose during this interval". And it is stated: "When interpreted over a time interval it can change the interpretation of one or more parameters within the scope of that time interval."

One problem with these definitions is that they need a sufficiently general and precise notion of "proposition" and of what it means "to be interpreted over an interval". In the GFO-framework a situoid semantics is under development which introduces so-called elementary propositions on which general propositions are built upon. In this framework the proposition "the drug has an effect on blood glucose during this interval" is an example of an elementary proposition. Propositions are interpreted, can be satisfied, in situoids S which contain as part a certain system of facts, called configuroid. Hence, the notion of context should include: a definition of the set $Prop(D)$

of (relevant) propositions pertaining to the domain D, and a precise relation of truth (satisfiability) of the propositions with respect to the systems in $Situoids(D)$. The pair $(Prop(D), Situoids(D))$ is said to be a semantic context. A step forward in carrying out such a program is presented in [24]. In *AbstrOnt* there is, furthermore, introduced the notion of a subcontext relation which is a binary relation between contexts. The subcontext relation is not clearly expounded.

6.4 Context Interval

A *context interval* is a structure $<p, I>$ consisting of an interpretation context p and a temporal interval I. Context intervals represent an interpretation context over a time interval; within the scope of that interval, it can change the interpretation of one or more parameters. P is a proposition and one has to clarify of what it means that p is interpreted over an interval I. The GFO-framework provides concepts and methods to make all these notions clear.

6.5 Event Proposition

An *event proposition* represents, according to *AbstrOnt*, the occurrence of an external volitional action or process such as "administering a drug". Events have a series of event attributes $a(i)$, and each attribute $a(i)$ must be mapped to an attribute value. There exists an is-a hierarchy of event schemas (or event types). Event schemas have a list of attributes $a(i)$ where each attribute has a domain of possible values $v(i)$. An event proposition is an event schema in which each attribute $a(i)$ is mapped to some value $v(i)$ belonging to the set $V(i)$. A part-of relation is defined over a set of event schemas. If the pair $(e(i), e(j))$ belongs to the part-of relation, then the event $e(i)$ can be a subevent of the event schema $e(j)$ (example: a clinical protocol event can have several parts, all of them are medication events). An event interval is a structure $<e, I>$ consisting of an event proposition e and a time interval I. Intuitively, e is an event proposition (with a list of attribute-value pairs), and I is as time interval over which the event proposition e is interpreted. The time interval represents the duration of the event.

In the GFO-framework we get the following interpretation. A volitional action or process *proc* is a individual which belongs to a certain situoid S. As part of reality the entity *proc* may be rather complex; surely, *proc* has a temporal extension and participants which are involved in *proc*, e.g. physicians, patients, and other entities. For the purpose of modeling we need only selected, relevant information about *proc*. This selected information is presented by a list of attributes $a(i)$ and values $v(i)$, and this list, denoted by – say – *expr(proc)*, is considered as an event proposition. In GFO *expr(proc)* is not a proposition (because it has no truth-value), but a symbolic representation of partial information about *proc*. A *event schema* can be understood, in the framework of GFO, as a category (the GFO-term for class/universal) whose instances are event expressions of the kind *expr(proc)*. Event schemas themselves are, hence, also presented by certain symbolic expressions *schemexpr*. Attributes are interpreted in GFO as property-universals whose instances have no independent existence but are associated to – are dependent on – individual entities as, e. g. objects or processes. GFO provides a framework for analyzing all possible properties of processes. In many cases so-called properties of processes are not genuine process-properties but only properties of certain presentials which are derived from processes by projecting them onto time boundaries. Since GFO provides several formal languages to represent information about real world entities, there might be information, specified in one of these languages, which cannot be represented as a list of attribute-value pairs. This implies that GFO provides means for expression of information which exceeds the possibilities of the *AbstrOnt*-framework. Furthermore, the part-of relation mentioned above is not clearly described. Part-of is defined for event-schema, i.e. in the GFO-framework, between categories (universals/classes). But what, exactly, is the meaning of that a schema expression *schemexpr*$_1$ is a part of the schema expression *schemexpr*$_2$? In GFO there is the following interpretation: every instance e_1 of *schemexpr*$_1$, which refers to a real world event *event*$_1$, is a part of an instance e_2 of *schemexpr*$_1$ referring to a real world event *event*$_2$. The final understanding of this part-of relation should be reduced to the understanding of what it means that the *event*$_1$ is a part of the *event*$_2$. The GFO-framework allows to analyze and describe several kinds of part-of relations, among them – the most natural – that *event*$_1$ is a temporal part of *event*$_2$.

6.6 Event Interval

An *event interval,* according to *AbstrOnt*, is a structure <*e, I*> consisting of an event proposition *e* and a time interval *I*. Intuitively, *e* is an event proposition (with a list of attribute-value pairs) and *I* is a time interval over which the event proposition *e* is interpreted. The time interval represents the duration of the event. In GFO this can be interpreted as follows, which shows that in the above description there is a hidden subtle ambiguity. Let *e* be the expression *expr(proc)* which refers to a real world process *proc*. If *e* is interpreted over the interval *I* then the natural meaning is that the associated process *proc* has the uniquely determined temporal extension *I* (as a chronoid). But then it is not reasonable to say that *proc* is interpreted over the duration of *I*. The other meaning is that *proc* has a temporal extension (a framing chronoid *I*) which has a certain duration *d*. But in this case the expression *e* does not refer to a unique single process *proc* but to any process satisfying the attribute-value pairs and having a temporal extension of duration *d*. In this case the expression *e* does not represent a unique process but exhibits a GFO-category (a universal/class) whose instances are individual real world processes. This consideration uncovers that we may find the same ambiguity for the notion of an event proposition as introduced above. The GFO- framework is sufficiently expressive to find the correct disambiguations of the above notions.

The remaining notions of *AbstrOnt*, like parameter schema, parameter interval, abstraction functions, abstraction, abstraction goal and others are analysed in the extended paper.

7 Conclusion

The current paper presents some results of a case study which is carried out to apply and test the GFO-framework to existing ontologies, in particular to the ontology *AbstrOnt* [2]. We hope that already our preliminary results

a) indicate that GFO is an expressive ontology which allows for the reconstruction of other ontologies like *AbstrOnt*,
b) show that several concepts and notions in *AbstrOnt* are ambiguous and are not sufficiently founded,
c) demonstrate that GFO can be used to disambiguate several definitions in *AbstrOnt* and to elaborate a better foundation for existing ontologies.

The future research of the Onto-Med group includes the reconstruction of other ontologies of the medical and biomedical domain within the framework of GFO.

Acknowledgements

We would like to thank the anonymous referees of this paper for their many useful comments that helped to improve this paper's presentation. Many thanks to the members of the Onto-Med research group for fruitful discussions. In particular we thank Frank Loebe for his effort in the editorial work of this paper.

References

1. Onto-Med Research Group: http://www.onto-med.de
2. Shahar, Y. 1994. A Knowledge-Based Method for Temporal Abstraction of Clinical Data [PhD Thesis]. Stanford University.
3. Gruber, T. R. 1993. A Translation Approach to Portable Ontology Specifications. *Knowledge Acquisition* 5(2):199-220.
4. Musen, M. 1992. Dimensions of Knowledge Sharing and Reuse. *Computer and Biomedical Research* 25(5):435-467.
5. Fensel, D., Hendler, J., Lieberman, H., Wahlster, W. (eds.) 2003. *Spinning the Semantic Web*. Cambridge: MIT Press.
6. Guarino, N. 1998. Formal Ontology and Information Systems. In: Guarino, N. (ed.) *1st International Conference (FOIS-98)*. Trento, Italy, June 6-8. p. 3-15. Amsterdam: IOS Press.
7. Guarino, N., Welty, C. 2002. Evaluating Ontological Decisions with OntoClean. *Communications of the ACM* 45(2):61-65.
8. Poli, R. 2002. Ontological Methodology. *International Journal of Human-Computer Studies* 56(6):639–664.
9. Sowa, J. F. 2000. *Knowlegde Representation - Logical, Philosophical and Computational Foundations*. Pacific Crove, California: Brooks/Cole.
10. Gracia, J. J. E. 1999. *Metaphysics and Its Tasks: The Search for the Categorial Foundation of Knowledge*. SUNY Series in Philosophy. Albany: State University of New York Press.
11. Heller, B., Herre, H. 2004. Ontological Categories in GOL. *Axiomathes* 14(1):57-76.
12. Galton, A. 2004. Fields and Objects in Space, Time, and Space-time. *Spatial Cognition and Computation* 4(1):39-68.
13. Seibt. J. 2000. The Dynamic Constitution of Things. In: Faye, J. et al. (eds.) *Facts and Events*. Poznan Studies in Philosophy of Science vol. 72, p. 241-278.
14. Brentano 1976. *Philosophische Untersuchungen zu Raum, Zeit und Kontinuum*. Hamburg: Felix-Meiner Verlag.

15. Barwise, J., Perry, J. 1983. *Situations and Attitudes*. Bradford Books. Cambridge (Massachusetts): MIT Press.
16. Devlin, K. 1991. *Logic and Information*. Cambridge (UK): Cambridge University Press.
17. Heller, B., Herre, H., Lippoldt, K. 2004. The Theory of Top-Level Ontological Mappings and Its Application to Clinical Trial Protocols. In: Günter, A. et al. (eds.) *Engineering Knowledge in the Age of the Semantic Web*, Proceedings of the 14. International Conference, EKAW 2004, Whittlebury Hall, UK, Oct 2004. LNAI vol. 3257, p. 1-14.
18. Herre, H., Heller, B. 2005. Ontology of Time in GFO, Onto-Med Report Nr. 8 Onto-Med Research Group, University of Leipzig.
19. Scheidler, A. 2004. A Proof of the Interpretability of the GOL Theory of Time in the Interval-based Theory of Allen-Hayes [BA-Thesis]. Onto-Med Report Nr. 9, 2005. Onto-Med Research Group, University of Leipzig.
20. Allen, J., Hayes, P. J. 1989. Moments and Points in an Interval-Based Temporal Logic. *Computational Intelligence* 5:225-238.
21. Loebe, F. 2003. An Analysis of Roles: Towards Ontology-Based Modelling [Master's Thesis]. Onto-Med Report No. 6. Aug 2003. Onto-Med Research Group, University of Leipzig.
22. Loux, M. 1998. *Metaphysics: A Contemporary Introduction*. New York: Routledge.
23. Barwise, J. 1989. *The Situation in Logic*. CSLI Lecture Notes, Vol. 17. Stanford (California): CSLI Publications.
24. Hoehndorf, R. 2005. Situoid Theory: An Ontological Approach to Situation Theory [Master's Thesis]. University of Leipzig.

The Use of Verbal Classification for Determining the Course of Medical Treatment by Medicinal Herbs

Leonas Ustinovichius[1], Robert Balcevich[2], Dmitry Kochin[3], and Ieva Sliesoraityte[4]

[1] Vilnius Gediminas Technical University,
LT-10223, Sauletekio al. 11, Vilnius, Lithuania,
leonasu@st.vtu.lt
[2] Public company "Natura Sanat",
LT-01114, Olandu 19-2, Vilnius, Lithuania
robert@naturasanat.com
[3] Institute for System Analysis,
117312, prosp. 60-letija Octjabrja, 9, Moscow, Russia
dco@mail.ru
[4] Vilnius University, Department of Medicine,
LT-2009, Ciurlionio 21, Vilnius, Lithuania
sliesoraityte@yahoo.com

Abstract. About 44 treatment schemes including 40 medicines prepared from Andean medicinal herbs to cure a great variety of diseases, such as cancer and other serious illnesses, have been developed. The main problem is to choose a course of medical treatment of any disease from this variety, depending on particular criteria characterizing a patient. A classification approach may be used for this purpose. Classification is a very important aspect of decision making. This means the prescription of objects to particular classes. Classified objects are described by various criteria that can be qualitatively or quantitatively evaluated. In multicriteria environment it is hardly possible to achieve this without resorting to special techniques. The paper presents a feasibility study of using verbal classification for determining a course of medical treatment, depending on a particular disease and patient's personality.

1 Introduction

There are few regions in the world where biological diversity and indigenous knowledge of the use of medicinal plants are higher than in the Peruvian Amazon [1], [2]. Although phytochemical and pharmacological information available on the region's genetic resources is limited, there is little doubt on its tremendous potential. To uncover that potential, and preserve the region´s ecosystems and societies that have lived in them for many generations will be, no doubt, one of the most important challenges for mankind in the century to come [3], [4], [5], [6].

Andean Medicine Centre is a company specialising in popularisation and propagation of knowledge about Andean phytotherapy and healing plants of South American origin. The company is located in London and has its agencies and representatives in numerous countries over the world, e.g. Germany, Poland, Italy, Lithuania, Latvia,

Czech Republic, Sweden, Peru, Bulgaria and Slovakia. Andean Medicine Centre is offering a wide range of Amazon and Andean herbal formulas and cosmetic products.

The "List of treatments" prepared by a leading Peruvian phytotherapist Professor Manuel Fernandez Ibarguen and recommended by the consultative medical team of Andean Medicine Centre is at the same time the reference book both to the AMC consultants and the patients. The major goal of the authors was to correlate ethnopharmacological data on medicinal properties of plants gathered from local inhabitants with knowledge on the ethnomedical, pharmacological, and phytochemical properties of the same plants gathered through research studies.

There is a set of 44 different treatments composed of about 40 preparations recommended for a number of diseases including such malignant diseases as cancer [7], [8], [9]. Both the duration of the treatment and the number of preparations applicable depends on a given disease, as well as on the stage of its development.

As a rule, the initial stage of all treatments is the purifying treatment, having a diuretic effect. There are some contraindications for using "Purification" like pregnancy and breastfeeding that apply to the administration of all the preparations. Some of the preparations, like Vilcacora has even more contraindications (e.g. it can not be administered during chemo- and radiotherapy as well as to patients after organ transplantation, to those treated with insulin and so on) [10], [11], [12], [13], [14].

If the abovementioned Vilcacora can not be used, it is substituted by other preparations (most often – Tahuari or Graviola).

The other most common reason for deviating from AMC course of treatment are funds the patient can spare on his/her treatment. In the case when these funds are insufficient, the consultant is obliged to suggest the use of one or two most important preparations like Vilcacora.

In choosing a particular course of treatment it is of paramount importance to base oneself on a set of criteria characterizing a patient and his/her personality. A method of classification may be used for this purpose.

Classification is a very important aspect in decision making. This means the prescription of projects to particular classes. Very often it is stated that classes in decision making are determined by the particular parameters, i.e. the efficiency of technical and technological decisions, credit value of the project, etc. Classified projects are described by assessing various efficiency criteria that could be both qualitatively and quantitatively expressed.

In fact, many different methods for solving multicriteria classification problems are widely known. ORCLASS, as an ordinary classification, was one of the first methods designed to solve these kinds of problems [15]. Then more recent methods, such as DIFCLASS [16], CLARA [17] and CYCLE, appeared [18].

The present paper describes a feasibility study of using verbal classification for determining a course of medical treatment, depending on a particular disease and patient's personality.

2 Formal Problem Statement

Given:

1. G – a feature, corresponding to the target criterion (e.g. treatment effectiveness).

2. $K = \{K_1, K_2, ..., K_N\}$ – a set of criteria, used to assess each alternative (course of treatment).

3. $S_q = \{k_1^q, ..., k_{w_q}^q\}$ – for q=1,..., N – a set of verbal estimates on the scale of criterion K_q, w_q – a number of estimates for criterion K^q; estimates in S_q are ordered based on increasing intensity of the feature G;

4. $Y = S_1 \times ... \times S_N$ – a space of the alternative features to be classified. Each alternative is described by a set of estimates obtained by using criteria $K_1, ..., K_N$ and can be presented as a vector $y \in Y$, where $y = (y_1, y_2, ..., y_N)$, y_q is an index of estimate from set S_q.

5. $C = \{C_1, ..., C_M\}$ – a set of decision classes, ordered based on the increasing intensity of feature G.

A binary relation of strict dominance is introduced:

$$P = \left\{ \begin{matrix} (x, y) \in Y \times Y \mid & \forall q = 1...N \\ x_q \geq y_q & \exists q_0 : x_{q_0} > y_{q_0} \end{matrix} \right\}. \tag{1}$$

One can see that this relation is anti-reflexive, anti-symmetric and transitive. It may be also useful to consider a reflexive, anti-symmetric, transitive binary relation of weak dominance Q:

$$Q = \{(x, y) \in Y \times Y \mid \forall q = 1... \ N, \ x_q \geq y_q\}. \tag{2}$$

Goal: on the basis of DM preferences to create imaginary $F: Y \to \{Y_i\}, i = 1, ..., M$, where Y_i – a set of vector estimations belonging to class C_i, satisfying the condition of consistency:

$$\forall x, y \in Y : x \in Y_i, y \in Y_j, (x, y) \in P \Rightarrow i \geq j. \tag{3}$$

2.1 Analytical Verbal Decision Methods for Classification of Alternatives

In this chapter some most frequently used verbal ordinal classification methods are considered. All these methods belong to Verbal Decision Analysis group and have the following common features [15]:

1. Attribute scale is based on verbal description not changed in the process of solution, when verbal evaluation is not converted into the numerical form or score.
2. An interactive classification procedure is performed in steps, where the DM is offered an object of analysis (a course of treatment). A project is presented as a small set of rankings. The DM is familiar with this type of description, therefore he/she can make the classification based on his/her expertise and intuition.
3. When the DM has decided to refer a project to a particular class, the decisions are ranked on the dominance basis. This provides the information about other classes of projects related with it by the relationship of dominance. Thus, an indirect classification of all the projects can be made based on a single decision of the DM.

4. A set of projects dominating over a considered project are referred to as domination cone. A great number of projects have been classified many times. This ensures error – free classification. If the DM makes an error, violating this principle, he/she is shown the conflicting decision on the screen and is prompted to adjust it.
5. In general, a comprehensive classification may be obtained for various numbers of the DM decisions and phases in an interactive operation. The efficiency of multicriteria classification technique is determined based on the number of questions to DM needed to make the classification. This approach is justified because it takes into consideration the cost of the DM's time and the need for minimizing classification expenses.

Let us consider several most commonly used methods in more detail.

ORCLASS [15]. This method (Ordinal CLASSification) allows us to build a consistent classification, to check the information and to obtain general decision rules. The method relies on the notion of the most informative alternative, allowing a great number of other alternatives to be implicitly assigned to various classes. ORCLASS takes into account possibilities and limitations of the human information processing system.

Method assessment: The main disadvantage of the method is low effectiveness due to the great number of questions to DM needed for building a comprehensive classification.

CLARA [17]. This method (CLAssification of Real Alternatives) is based on ORCLASS, but is designed to classify a given subset rather than a complete set of alternatives (Y space). Another common application of CLARA is classification of full set with large number of exclusions, i.e. alternatives with impossible combinations of estimations. In both cases CLARA demonstrates high effectiveness.

DIFCLASS [16]. This method was the first to use dynamic construction of chains covering Y space for selecting questions to DM. However, the area of DIFCLASS application is restricted to tasks with binary criteria scales and two decision classes.

CYCLE [18, 19]. CYCLE (Chain Interactive Classification) algorithm overcomes DIFCLASS restrictions, generalizing the idea of dynamic chain construction to the area of ordinal classification task with arbitrary criteria scales and any number of decision classes. The chain here means an ordered sequence of vectors $\langle x_1, ..., x_d \rangle$, where $(x_{i+1}, x_i) \in P$ and vectors x_{i+1} and x_i differ in one of the components.

Method assessment: As comparisons demonstrate, the idea of dynamic chain construction allows us to get an algorithm close to optimal by a minimum number of questions to DM necessary to build a complete classification. The application of ordinal classification demonstrates that problem formalization as well as introduction of classes and criteria structuring allows solution of classification problems by highly effective methods.

The method can be successfully applied to classification of investment projects when the decision classes and the criteria used are thoroughly revised.

3 Verbal Analysis of a Course of Treatment with Medicinal Herbal Products

Classification of projects is one of the multiple criteria problems within the framework of a decision making system [20], [21], [22], [23], [24], [25]. Such problems can be solved by CYCLE technique developed at the Institute of Systems Analysis of the Russian Academy of Sciences [18]. This technique allows the classification to be developed in a series of successive steps, checking the conflicting information and arriving at a general method of solution. The method described takes into account the possibilities and limitations of the human data processing system [26].

Method CYCLE
Let us consider metric $\rho(x,y)$ in discrete space Y defined as:

$$\rho(x,y) = \sum_{q=1}^{N} |x_q - y_q|. \tag{4}$$

Let us denote by $\rho(\vec{0}, y)$, i. e. the sum of vector's components, the index of vector $y \in Y$ (written as $\|y\|$). For vectors $x, y \in Y$ such that $(x, y) \in P$, let us consider a set:

$$\Lambda(x,y) = \{v \in Y | (x,v) \in Q (v,y) \in Q\}, \tag{5}$$

that is a set of vectors weakly dominating y and weakly dominated by x. Having denoted $y' = (1, \ldots, 1)$, $y'' = (w_1, \ldots, w_N)$, we can see that $\Lambda(y'', y')$ matches the entire space Y. We also introduce a set

$$L(x,y) = \left\{ v \in \Lambda(x,y) \middle| \|v\| = \frac{\|x\| + \|y\|}{2} \right\}, \tag{6}$$

that is vectors from $\Lambda(x, y)$ set equidistant from x and y (here and further division is done without remainder). We will need numerical functions $C^U(x)$ и $C^L(x)$ defined on Y, which are respectively equal to the highest and lowest class number allowable for x, that is a class for x not violating the condition of consistency (3). Let us consider vector x to be classified and belonging to class C_k, if the following condition is valid for x:

$$C^U(x) = C^L(x) = k. \tag{7}$$

Let us define the procedure $S(x)$ (spreading by dominance). It is assumed that the class of x is known: $x \in Y_k$ (that is $C^U(x) = C^L(x) = k$). Therefore, for all $y \in Y$ such as $(x, y) \in P$ and $C^U(y) > k$ function $C^U(y)$ is redefined so that $C^U(y) = k$. Similarly, for all $z \in Y$, such as $(z, x) \in P$ and $C^L(z) < k$, function $C^L(z)$ is redefined so that $C^L(z) = k$.

Basic mechanism of the CYCLE algorithm. Let us denote by $D(a, b)$ a procedure of classification on $\Lambda(a,b)$ set using the idea of dynamic construction of chains linking vectors a and b. It is assumed that $(a,b) \in P$ and classes of vectors a and b are known: $a \in Y_k, b \in Y_l$.

The algorithm is as follows:

1. For each vector $x \in L(a, b)$ the steps 2-4 are made.
2. If a class for x is unknown ($C^L(x) < C^U(x)$) then x is presented to the DM for classification. Suppose that $x \in Y_r$. The spreading by dominance $S(x)$ is being done. The condition of consistency is being checked (3).
3. If $r<k$ and $(a,x) \in P$, then perform $D(a, x)$.
4. If $r<k$ and $(x,b) \in P$, then perform $D(x, b)$.

In classifying vector x at the second step, the DM can make a mistake, and a pair of vectors $x, y \in Y$ violating the consistency condition (3) appears. Procedure R of resolving contradictions consists in the following. Let us denote the set of vectors explicitly classified by DM as E. So, while E contains a pair of vectors violating (3), such a pair is presented to DM with a proposition to change a class for one or two vectors. Then, functions C^U and C^L are redefined to their initial values and spreading by dominance $S(v)$ is done for each $v \in E$.

Generally speaking, the parameters of the algorithm including the number of questions to DM depend on the choice of vector x in the first step. The following heuristics is proposed: among all not yet classified vectors from $L(a, b)$ set the object, which explicitly dominates a maximum number of unclassified vectors is chosen. That is, one chooses the vector

$$x^* = \arg \max_{x \in L(a,b)} |\{y \in Y | (x, y) \in P \text{ or } (y,x) \in P, \rho(x, y) = 1, \quad (6)$$
$$C^L(y) < C^U(y)\}| .$$

At a very high level the CYCLE algorithm is as follows:

1. For each $v \in Y$ possible classes are set to $C^L(y) = C^U(y) = M$.
2. DM is presented vectors y' and y'', spreading by dominance $S(y')$ and $S(y'')$ is performed.
3. If classes for y' and y'' differ, then procedure $D(y'', y')$ is performed.

Algorithm features.

Statement 1. At the end of CYCLE algorithm the space Y will be fully classified, that is $\forall y \in Y \; C^L(y) = C^U(y)$.

Lemma 1. For any $x, y \in Y$, such as $(y, x) \in P$, and for any chain $\Re = \langle x,..., y \rangle$, cardinality of the set $\Re \cap L(y, x)$ equals to 1.

Statement 2. A classification made with the help of the CYCLE algorithm is consistent, implying that a condition of consistency (2) is satisfied.

4 A Classification of Chosen Medical Preparations and Description of the Main Criteria Used

A method of verbal classification may be used to analyse the treatment of 40 diseases with the suggested medicines (Fig. 1). A list of herbal medicinal products used for treating a considered disease is analysed below.

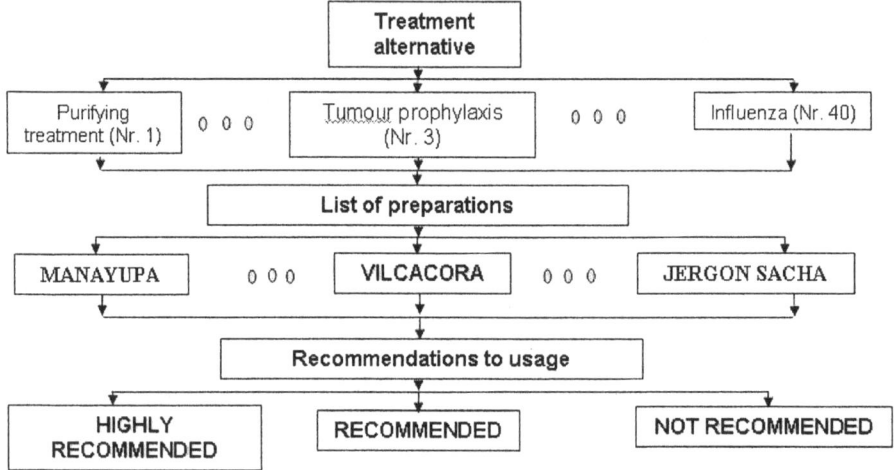

Fig. 1. General algorithm for choosing medical preparations

After a series of iterations carried out under methodological control of consultants from Public company "Natura Sanat", the following final decision classes were chosen (Fig. 2). All classes are hierarchically structured. They include a list of medicines to be used for treating a particular disease, with the following recommendations given for each medicine usage, depending on a particular patient:

1. **HIGHLY RECOMMENDED.** This medicine is highly needed for treating the patient.
2. **RECOMMENDED.** This medicine may be used for treating the patient.
3. **NOT RECOMMENDED.** This medicine should not be used for treating the patient.

Let us consider the main verbal classification principle as applied to tumour prophylaxis. The hierarchical structure of classes depends on the following criteria: patient's health condition; patient's financial condition; stage of the disease; contraindications. A more detailed description of the above groups is given below.

1. *The criterion "Patient's health condition"* includes the following definitions of patient's condition: good; satisfactory; bad. They depend on some subjective and objective patient's characteristics.
2. *The criterion "Patient's financial condition"* defines the financial state of a patient as: good; satisfactory; bad.
3. *The criterion "Stage of the disease"* defines the development of the disease.
4. *The criterion "Contraindications"* defines possible complications which may restrict the use of some medicinal products by a patient.

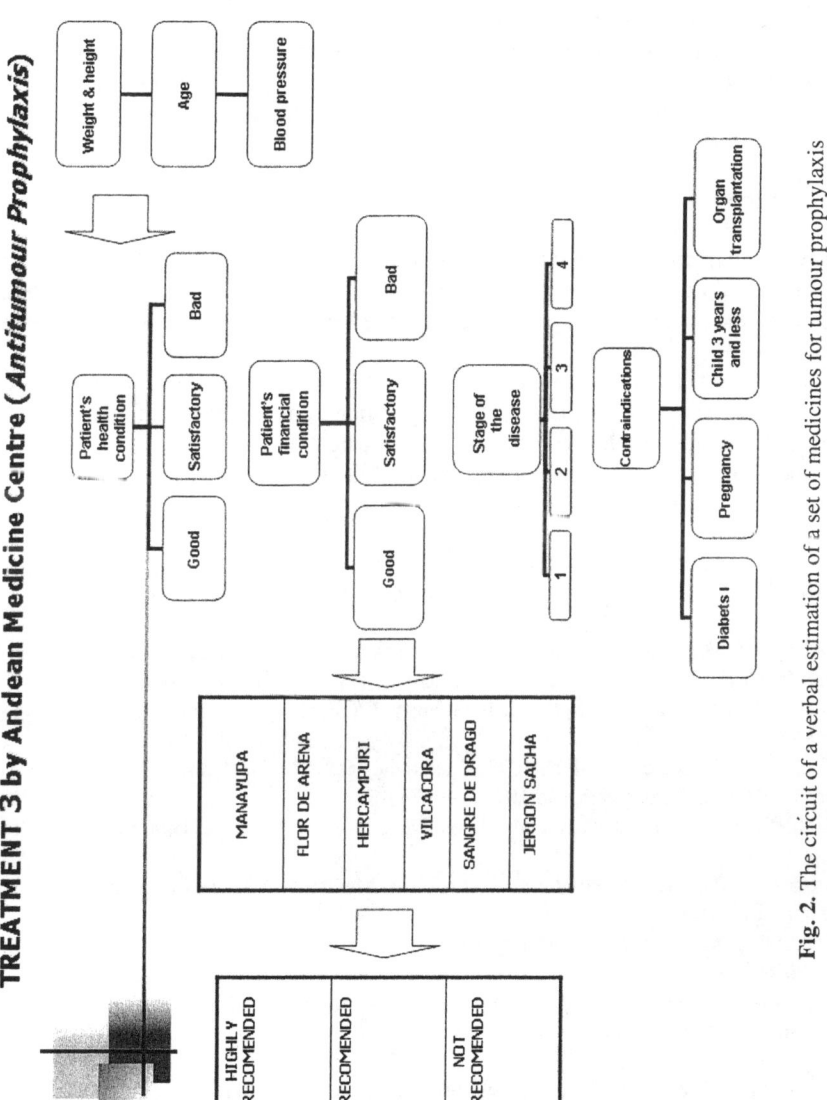

Fig. 2. The circuit of a verbal estimation of a set of medicines for tumour prophylaxis

It is now necessary to classify the medicines chosen by their multicriteria description. The results obtained should be thoroughly validated. It should be noted that for some diseases the criteria may have a two-level hierarchical structure. In this case, a classification is first built at the second level of the efficiency criteria group. The role of classes is determined by general marks made at the first level of the hierarchy. When the classification is made, these general marks are filled with concrete meaning. Then, the classification is made at the second level of the hierarchy. As a result, we get decision rules for determining various combinations of medicines for a particular patient.

The DM can determine the effectiveness of a course of treatment on the basis of the available information. It should be noted, that only the criteria of the first hierarchical level may be used. Having difficulties in assessment, the DM can use more detailed data from the second level. The possibility of using the information from the second hierarchical level exists even for some first level criteria.

5 Conclusions

A course of treatment with medicinal herbal products was defined by a verbal analysis based on the classification decision support method **CYCLE**, allowing risk evaluation according to the specified classes by the suggested criteria of determining medicine usage.

As shown by the comparative analysis, the idea of the DM dynamic chain construction allows us to get a nearly optimal algorithm by asking the minimum number of questions needed to build a comprehensive classification.

The method was validated by solving actual problems of selecting the best alternatives of the available courses of treatment for particular patients.

References

1. Richardson, M.A.: Research on Complementary/Alternative Medicine Therapies in Oncology: Promising but Challenging. J. Clin. Oncol. 17 (11 suppl.) (1999) 38–43
2. Wagner H. Phytomedicine Research in Germany.Environ. Health Perspect.1999,107:779–781
3. Matthews, H., Lucier, G., Fisher, K.: Medicinal Herbs in the United States: Research Needs. Environ. Health Perspect. 107 (1999) 733–778
4. Cassileth, B.: Complementary and Alternative Cancer Medicine. J. Clin. Oncol. 17 (11 suppl.) (1999) 44–52.
5. Artiges, A.: Pharmacopoeial Standards for Herbal Medicinal Products in Europe. Eur. Phytojournal 1 (2000) 28–29.
6. Keller, K.: EMEA Ad Hoc Working Group on Herbal Medicinal Products. Eur. Phytojournal 2000, 1: 9–16
7. Blumenthal, M (ed.): WHO Medicinal Plants Monographs, Vol. 38. HerbalGram (1997)
8. British Herbal Pharmacopoeia, 1989, Bournamouth, British Herbal Medicine Association, 255
9. Blumenthal, M (ed.): American Herbal Pharmacopoeia, Vol. 40. HerbalGram (1997)

10. Desmarchelier, C., Witting, Schaus F., Coussio, J., Cicca, G.: Effects of Sangre de Drago from *Croton lechleri* Muell.-Arg. On the Production of Active Oxygen Radicals. J. Ethnopharmacol. 58 (1997) 103-108
11. Ho, K.Y., Huang, J.S., Tsai, C.C., Lin, T.C., Hsu, Y.F., Lin, C.C.: Antioxidant Activity of Tannin Components from *Vaccinium vitis-idaea* L. J. Pharm. Pharmacol. 51 (1999) 1075-1078
12. Arnone, A., Nasini, G., Vajna de Pava, O. Merlini, L.: Constituents of Dragon's Blood. 5. Dracoflavans B1, B2, C1, C2, D1, and D2, new A-type deoxyproanthocyanidins. J. Nat. Prod. 60 (1997) 971-976
13. Quiros, C., Epperson, A., Hu, J., Holle, M.: Physiological Studies and Determination of Chromosome Number in Maca, *Lepidium meyenii*. Economic Botany 50 (1996) 216-223
14. Johns, T.: The Anu and the Maca. Journal of Ethnobiology 1 (1981) 208-211
15. Larichev, O., Mechitov, A., Moshovich, E., Furems, E.: Revealing of Expert Knowledge, Publishing House Nauka, Moscow (1989) (in Russian)
16. Larichev, O., Bolotov, A.: System DIFKLASS: Construction of Full and Consistent Bases of Expert Knowledge in Problems of Differential Classification. The Scientific and Technical Information, a series 2, Informacionie Procesi i Sist*emi* (Information Processes and Systems), 9 (1996) (in Russian).
17. Larichev, O., Kochin, D., Kortnev, A.: Decision Support System for Classification of a Finite Set of Multicriteria Alternatives. Decision Support Systems. 33 (2002) 13-21
18. Aksanov, A., Borisenkov, P., Larichev, O., Nariznij, E., Rozejnzon, G.: Method of Multicriteria Classification CYCLE and its Application for the Analysis of Credit Risk. Ekonomika i Matematiceskije Metodi(Economy and Mathematical Methods).37(2001)14-21(in Russian)
19. Larichev, O., Leonov, A.: Method CYCLE of Serial Classification of Multicriteria Alternatives. The Report of the Russian Academy of Sciences, December (2000) (in Russian)
20. Larichev, O., Moshkovich, H.: An Approach to Ordinal Classification Problems. International Transaction in Operational Research 1 (1994) 375-386
21. Larichev, O., Moshkovich, H.: Qualitative Methods of Decision Making. Nauka Fizmatlit, Moscow. (1996) (in Russian)
22. de Montgolfier, J., Bertier, P.: Approche Multicritere des Problemes de Decision. Editions Hommes et Techniques, Paris (1978) (in French)
23. Greco, S., Matarazzo, B., Slowinski, R.: Rough Sets Methodology for Sorting Problems in Presence of Multiple Attributes and Criteria. European Journal of Operational Research 138 (2002) 247-259
24. Peldschus, F., Messing, D., Zavadskas, E.K., Ustinovičius L.: LEVI 3.0 – Multiple Criteria Evaluation Program. Journal of Civil Engineering and Management, Vol 8. Technika, Vilnius (2002) 184-191
25. Ustinovičius, L., Jakučionis, S.: Multi-Criteria Analysis of the Variants of the Old Town Building Renovation in the Marketing. *Statyba* (Journal of Civil Engineering and Management), Vol. 6, Technika, Vilnius (2000) 212 – 222
26. Solso, P.: Cognitive Psychology. Trivola, Moscow (1996) (in Russian).

Case-Based Reasoning, Signal Interpretation, Visual Mining

Interactive Knowledge Validation in CBR for Decision Support in Medicine

Monica H. Ou[1], Geoff A.W. West[1], Mihai Lazarescu[1], and Chris Clay[2]

[1] Department of Computing, Curtin University of Technology,
GPO Box U1987, Perth 6845, Western Australia, Australia
{ou, geoff, lazaresc}@cs.curtin.edu.au
[2] Royal Perth Hospital, Perth, Western Australia, Australia
claycd@iinet.net.au

Abstract. In most case-based reasoning (CBR) systems there has been little research done on validating new knowledge, specifically on how previous knowledge differs from current knowledge by means of conceptual change. This paper proposes a technique that enables the domain expert who is non-expert in artificial intelligence (AI) to interactively supervise the knowledge validation process in a CBR system. The technique is based on formal concept analysis which involves a graphical representation and comparison of the concepts, and a summary description highlighting the conceptual differences. We propose a dissimilarity metric for measuring the degree of variation between the previous and current concepts when a new case is added to the knowledge base. The developed technique has been evaluated by a dermatology consultant, and has shown to be useful for discovering ambiguous cases and keeping the database consistent.

1 Introduction

Case-base reasoning (CBR) is an artificial intelligence (AI) technique that attempts to solve new problems by using the solutions applied to similar cases in the past. Reasoning by using past cases is a popular approach that has been applied to various domains, with most of the research having been focused on the classification aspect of the system. In medical applications, CBR has been used with considerable success for patient diagnosis, such as in PROTOS and CASEY [9]. However, relatively little effort has been put into investigating how new knowledge can be validated. We have developed a web-based CBR system that provides decision support to general practitioners (GPs) for diagnosing patients with dermatological problems. This paper mainly concentrates on developing a tool to automatically assist a dermatology consultant to train and validate the knowledge in the CBR system. Note that the consultants and GPs are non-computing experts.

Knowledge validation continues to be problematic in knowledge-based and case-based systems due to the modelling nature of the task. In dealing with the problem it is often desired to design a CBR system that disallows automatic updates, especially in medical applications where lives could be threatened from incorrect decisions. Normally CBR systems are allowed to learn by themselves in which the user enters the new case, compares it with those in the knowledge base and, once satisfied, adds the case to the database. In our method, the consultant needs to interactively supervise the CBR system in which the valid cases are determined by the validation tool and chosen by the consultant. The inconsistent or ambiguous cases can then be visualised and handled (modified or rejected) by the consultant. The reason for human supervision is to ensure that the decisions and learning are correct, and to prevent contradictory cases from being involved in the classification process. Adding contradictory cases into the knowledge base will negatively affect classification accuracy and data interpretation. Therefore, it is vital to constantly check and maintain the quality of the data in the database as new cases get added. The main aspects that need to be addressed are:

1. How to enable non-computing experts to easily and efficiently interact with the CBR system.
2. How to provide a simple but effective mechanism for incrementally validating the knowledge base.
3. How to provide a way of measuring the conceptual variation between the previous and new knowledge.

This paper proposes a new approach for validating the consistency of the new acquired knowledge against the past knowledge using a decision tree classifier [6], Formal Concept Analysis (FCA), and a dissimilarity metric. FCA is a mathematical theory which formulates the conceptual structure and displays relations between concepts in the form of concept lattices which comprise attributes and objects [3, 4]. A *concept* in FCA is seen as a set of objects that share a certain set of attributes. A lattice is a directed acyclic graph in which each node can have more than one parent, and the convention is that the superconcept always appears above all of its subconcepts. In addition, we derive a dissimilarity metric for quantifying the level of conceptual changes between the previous and current knowledge.

2 Related Work

FCA has been used as a method for knowledge representation and retrieval [1, 7], conceptual clustering [3], and as a support technique for CBR [2]. In [8] ripple-down rules (RDR) are combined with FCA to uncover an abstraction hierarchy of concepts and the relationship between them.

We use FCA and a dissimilarity measure approach to assist the knowledge validation process and highlight the conceptual differences between previous and current knowledge. Conceptual graph comparison has been widely studied in the area of information retrieval [5, 11, 12]. The comparison is categorised into two main parts: syntactic and semantic. Syntactic comparison uses a graphical representation, and determines their similarity by the amount of common structures shared [5, 11]. Semantic comparison measures whether the two concepts are similar to each other based on whether one concept representation can generalise the other [11, 12]. However, these techniques are not suitable for users that are non-experts in AI due to their complexity.

3 Interactive Knowledge Validation Approach in CBR

3.1 An Overview of the Knowledge Validation Process

Consider GPs using the CBR system to help in diagnosis. They generate new cases using the decision support system which are stored in the database and marked as "unchecked". This means the cases need to be checked by the consultant before deciding whether or not to add them to the knowledge base. FCA is used for checking the validity of the new cases to minimise the validation time, as the consultant is not required to manually check the rules generated by the decision tree. This is important because manual rule inspection by the human user quickly becomes unmanageable as the rule database grows in size. In most cases, if the consultant disagrees with the conclusion the correct conclusion is needed to be specified and some features in the case selected to justify the new conclusion or the instances are stored in a repository for later use.

Figure 1 presents the process of knowledge validation. It involves using J48 [10], the Weka[1] implementation of the C4.5 decision tree algorithm [6] for inducing the rules, and the Galicia[2] implementation for generating lattices. The attribute-value pairs of the rules are automatically extracted and represented as a context table which shows relations between the features and the diagnoses. The context table gets converted to a lattice for easy visualisation via the hierarchical structure of the lattices. As each new case gets added, the context table gets updated and a new lattice is generated. If adding a checked case will drastically change the lattice, the consultant is alerted and asked to confirm that the new case is truly valid given its effect on the lattice. There are three different options available to assist the consultant in performing knowledge validation:

1. A graphical representation of the lattices that enables the consultant to graphically visualise the conceptual differences.
2. A summary description highlighting the conceptual differences.
3. A measure which determines the degree of variation between lattices.

3.2 Dermatology Dataset

The dataset we use in our experiments consists of patient records for the diagnosis of dermatological problems. The dataset is provided by a consultant dermatologist. It contains patient details, symptoms and importantly, the consultant's diagnoses. Each patient is given an identification number, and episode numbers are used for multiple consultations for the same patient. Currently, the data has 17 general attributes and consists of cases describing 32 different diagnoses. Data collection is a continuous process in which new cases get added to the database.

Of interest to the consultant is how each new case will affect the knowledge base. New cases are collected in two ways: 1) The diagnosed cases provided by the GP, and 2) cases provided by the consultant. Before the consultant validates the new cases, they are marked as "unchecked" and combined with cases already in the database (previously

---

[1] www.cs.waikato.ac.nz/ml/weka [Last accessed: October 22, 2004].
[2] www.iro.umontreal.ca/galicia/index.html [Last accessed: September 10, 2004].

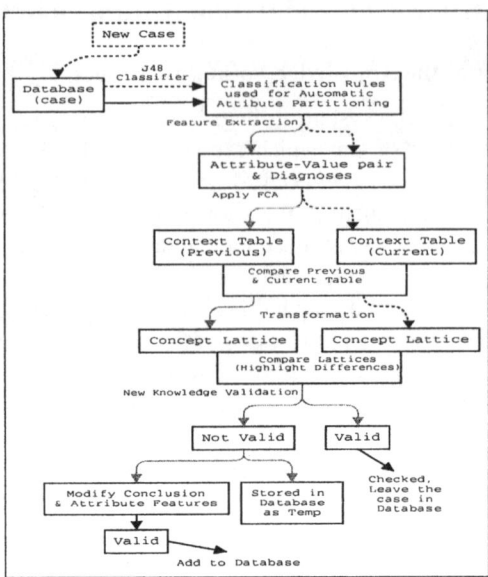

Fig. 1. Knowledge base validation

"checked") for training and generating lattices. If the lattices do not show any ambiguity this means the new cases are in fact valid and they will be updated to "checked" by the dermatologist.

3.3 Formal Context and Concept Lattices

FCA enables a lattice to be built automatically from a context table. The table consists of attribute-value pairs that are generated by the decision tree algorithm that automatically partitions the continuous attribute values into discrete values. This is because context tables need to use discrete or binary formats to represent the relations between attributes and objects. The formal context (C) is defined as follows:

Definition: A formal context $C = (D, A, I)$, where D is a set of diagnoses, A is a set of characteristics, and I is a binary relation which indicates diagnosis d has characteristic a.

Tables 1 and 2 show simple examples of formal contexts for our system using only a small number of cases for simplicity. Table 1 is derived from previously checked data which consists of 6 cases, and Table 2 is generated when a new unchecked case is added i.e. consists of 7 cases. The objects on each row represent the diagnosis D, each column represents a set of characteristics A, and the relation I is marked by "X". Note, only attributes that are relevant to a context are shown (i.e. allows discrimination), and that Table 2 shows that new attributes became relevant while others dropped. For the new unchecked case, the context table may or may not be affected to reflect the changes in characteristics used for describing the diagnoses. As can be seen from the tables, some characteristics have been introduced while some have been removed when a new

Table 1. Context table of previous data (consists of 6 cases)

Diagnoses (Concept Types)	Characteristics			
	age≤29	age>29	gender=M	gender=F
Eczema	X		X	
Psoriasis				X
PityriasisRubraPilaris		X	X	

Table 2. Context table of current data (consists of 7 cases)

Diagnoses (Concept Types)	Characteristics					
	gender=M	gender=F	lesion_status=1	lesion_status=2	lesion_status=3	lesion_status=4
Eczema	X			X	X	X
Psoriasis		X				
PityriasisRubraPilaris	X		X			

case is added due to the decision tree partitioning mechanism. In Table 1, $age \leq 29$, $age > 29$, $gender=M$, and $gender=F$ are considered to be important features for classifying *Eczema*, *Psoriasis*, and *PityriasisRubraPilaris*. However, in Table 2, $age \leq 29$ and $age > 29$ are no longer important in disambiguating the diagnoses but $lesion\_status=1$, $lesion\_status=2$, $lesion\_status=3$, and $lesion\_status=4$ are, and the characteristics $gender=M$ and $gender=F$ remain unchanged.

Conceptual changes are determined by comparing the relationships between the characteristics and the diagnoses of the current and previous context tables. However, the comparison can often be done more effectively using a lattice representation that formulates the hierarchical structure of the concept grouping. Figures 2 and 3 are built from Tables 1 and 2, respectively.

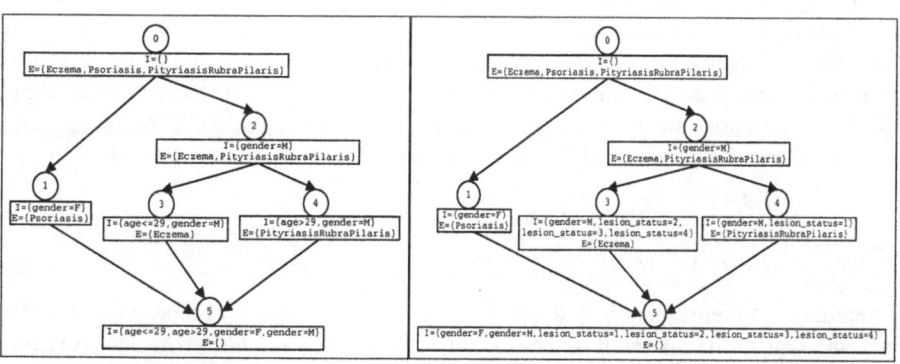

Fig. 2. Previous graph G_{t-1} (6 cases) **Fig. 3.** Current graph G_t (7 cases)

Given Table 1, the system generates a lattice shown in Figure 2. When a new case is added, a new lattice is generated. If we compare the previous and current lattices, we expect the lattices to be the same or with minor variations if changes do occur. If the concept changes significantly, the consultant needs to check if the new case is in fact valid. For each invalid case, the consultant is required to change the diagnosis or the characteristics to satisfy the new case or store it in a repository. The validation task is vitally important to prevent contradictory cases from being used in the classification process as these could lead to inaccurate diagnoses.

4 Conceptual Dissimilarity Measure

We derive a dissimilarity metric for determining the level of changes between the two lattices. Emphasis is put on illustrating the changes in the characteristics of the diagnoses. The measure is particular effective when the lattices become too large to be manually visualised by the consultant. Therefore, it is desirable to have a measure that indicates the level of changes between the current and previous lattices, and use it as a quick representation of the changes.

4.1 Highlighting Conceptual Changes Between Concept Lattices

We propose an algorithm for determining the conceptual differences between the two lattices: G_{t-1} and G_t, where $t-1$ and t represent lattices derived from previous and current cases, respectively. The algorithm determines which concepts are missing from G_{t-1} and which have been added to G_t. *Missing concepts* are determined by those present in G_{t-1} but not in G_t. Whereas, *added concepts* are those not present in G_{t-1} but present in G_t. To highlight the conceptual changes, the system displays the information such as the characteristics and diagnoses that have been ignored or added to the classification process. Based on this information the consultant does not need to manually analyse the lattice which could be time consuming and error-prone. Note in the rest of this paper the terms *lattice* and *graph* are the same.

To highlight changes, we use the concepts *extent* and *intent*. A is the extent of the concept (A, B) which comprises all the attributes (characteristics) that are valid for all the objects (diagnoses); B is the intent of the concept (A, B) which covers all the objects that are belonging to that particular concept [4]. We define the number of concepts that have the same intents in G_{t-1} and G_t as $|B(t-1)_{concept}| \cap |B(t)_{concept}|$. The number of missing concepts $n(G_{t-1})$ and added concepts $n(G_t)$ are defined as:

$$n(G_{t-1}) = |B(t-1)_{concept}| \setminus |B(t-1)_{concept}| \cap |B(t)_{concept}| \quad (1)$$

$$n(G_t) = |B(t)_{concept}| \setminus |B(t-1)_{concept}| \cap |B(t)_{concept}| \quad (2)$$

where $B(t-1)$ represents B in the previous graph G_{t-1}, and $B(t)$ represents B in the current graph G_t. However, if the results for both $n(G_{t-1})$ and $n(G_t)$ are equal to zero, this means the two graphs contain exactly the same concepts and implies that the new added cases are consistent with the previous cases in the database. In the worse case, the values of $n(G_{t-1})$ and $n(G_t)$ can be equal to the number of concepts in G_{t-1} and G_t, respectively. This implies a radical change between the two graphs and it means that the new added cases may be contradictory and need to be revised by the consultant. The values of $n(G_{t-1})$ and $n(G_t)$ provide a rough estimate of the changes in concepts between the two lattices. The locations at which the changes occur are highlighted in different colour for quick reference to the nodes in the lattice, and provide a useful indication of the number of concepts being affected. The closer the changes to the root of the lattice the more concepts get affected.

The missing and added nodes in Algorithm 1 are used as an entry point for the matching to prevent unnecessary processing of every node in the lattice. Algorithm 2 selects the lowest child node in the lattice that contains a certain extent element. The reason being the lowest child node provides the most detailed description compared to those that are higher up in the hierarchy. In a lattice, lower nodes convey more meaning than those above them.

Algorithm 1: Conceptual differences between concept lattices

```
input              : missing/added node i, G_{t-1}, and G_t.

foreach i in G_{t-1} do
    Find the parent node p of the node i
    foreach p do
        extentOfParent ← getExtent(G_{t-1}, p)
        Iterate to get each extent element e in extentOfParent
        while there are more e do
            node ← getLowestChild(p, extentOfParent)
            if node is equal to null then
                node ← node i
                Get and store the intent of node as intentG1
            else Get and store the intent of node as intentG1
            Find matched node m in G_t based on the intent of p
            if m is not equal to null then
                extentOfMatchedParent ← getExtent(G_t, m)
                node ← getLowestChild(m, extentOfMatchedParent)
                if node is equal to null then
                    node ← matched node m
                    Get and store the intent of node as intentG2
                    Highlight intent element differences between intentG1 and intentG2
                else
                    Get and store the intent of node as intentG2
                    Highlight intent element differences between intentG1 and intentG2
            else
                Get top node tn
                extentOfTopNode ← getExtent(G_t, tn)
                node ← getLowestChild(tn, extentOfTopNode)
                if node is equal to null then
                    node ← top node tn
                    Get and store the intent of node as intentG2
                    Highlight intent element differences between intentG1 and intentG2
                else
                    Get and store the intent of node as intentG2
                    Highlight intent element differences between intentG1 and intentG2
```

Algorithm 2: getLowestChild

```
input         : Node n and extent ext.
return lowest node.

Node lowest = null
Get children node of n
foreach children of node n do
    Get the children that contain extent element ext
    if lowest child with extent element ext is found then
        return lowest
```

For illustration purposes, consider the two simple examples in Figures 2 and 3. In Figure 3, suppose nodes 3 and 4 are the added nodes. If node 3 is selected for processing, then the parent node would be 2. At the parent node, the extent element *Eczema* is selected and stored. Iterate down to the lowest child node that contains *Eczema* which is node 3 with the intent elements of *gender=M, lesion_status=2, lesion_status=3 and lesion_status=4*. Then perform the matching between the two graphs. The results show that node 2 of G_{t-1} matches node 2 of G_t. Based on the stored extent element *Eczema* in G_{t-1}, iterate down to the lowest child node that contains *Eczema* which is node 3 with the intent elements of *age≤29* and *gender=M*. Compare and highlight the differences between the current and previous intent elements. In this case, the characteristics *lesion_status=2*, *lesion_status=3* and *lesion_status=4* have been introduced in G_t to give the diagnosis *Eczema* a more detailed description, but the characteristic *age≤29* has become insignificant. Repeat the same steps for node 4. The results show that in the current graph the characteristic *lesion_status=1* has become important for classifying *PityriasisRubraPilaris*, whereas the characteristic *age>29* in G_{t-1} has become insignificant. The characteristic for describing the diagnosis *Psoriasis* remains unchanged in both G_{t-1} and G_t.

4.2 Dissimilarity Metric

The measure of conceptual variation between graphs G_{t-1} and G_t when a new case is added is based on the following factors:

1. The number of diagnoses that have been affected.
2. The level in which the concept variations occur in the lattice.
3. The ratio of the characteristics of each diagnosis that have been affected.

Let $c(G_j)$ be the number of diagnoses affected after node i is removed/added to G_j, where $i = 1, 2, 3, ..., n$, and $j = t - 1, t$; n is the total number of nodes removed/added from the graphs which is calculated using Equation 1 or 2 depending on j; $C(G_j)$ is the total number of diagnoses in G_j, $a(G_{ji})$ is the number of features that exist in node i of G_{t-1} but not in G_t, and vice versa; $A(G_{ji})$ is the total number of features in node i; $md(G_j)$ is the maximum depth of G_j; and $d(G_{ji})$ is the depth of node i from top of the graph to the current position of the node. The variation measure $v(G_j)$ for each graph is:

$$v(G_j) = \begin{cases} v_1(G_j) & : md(G_j) = 1 \text{ and } d(G_{ji}) = 0 \\ v_2(G_j) & : md(G_j) = 1 \text{ and } d(G_{ji}) \neq 0 \\ v_3(G_j) & : md(G_j) > 1 \end{cases} \quad (3)$$

where $v(G_j) = \{v_1(G_j)|v_2(G_j)|v_3(G_j)\}$, and $v_1(G_j)$, $v_2(G_j)$ and $v_3(G_j)$ are defined as:

$$v_1(G_j) = \sum_{i=0}^{n} \frac{c(G_j)}{C(G_j)} \cdot \frac{a(G_{ji})}{A(G_{ji})} \cdot \frac{md(G_j) - d(G_{ji})}{md(G_j) * (n+1)}$$

$$v_2(G_j) = \sum_{i=0}^{n} \frac{c(G_j)}{C(G_j)} \cdot \frac{a(G_{ji})}{A(G_{ji})} \cdot \frac{1}{n+1}$$

$$v_3(G_j) = \sum_{i=0}^{n} \frac{c(G_j)}{C(G_j)} \cdot \frac{a(G_{ji})}{A(G_{ji})} \cdot \frac{md(G_j) - d(G_{ji})}{md(G_j) * n}$$

The total dissimilarity measure $d(G)$ between G_{t-1} and G_t is then defined as:

$$d(G) = v(G_{t-1}) + v(G_t) \quad (4)$$

The dissimilarity measure between the two graphs falls into the range of $[0, 1]$. The lower the value of $d(G)$ the higher the consistency since there is less variation between the two graphs. If $d(G) = 0$, the new cases are consistent with the previous cases. In the worse case, the value of $d(G)$ is close to or equal to 1, implying the new added cases contradict the previous cases. This might be because there are not enough cases to disambiguate some diagnoses, or the diagnoses are classified using different sets of characteristics.

We use the examples in Figures 2 and 3 to illustrate how the dissimilarity measure is calculated. Based on G_{t-1}, $v(G_{t-1}) = 0.111$ with $c(G_{t-1}) = 2$; $C(G_{t-1}) = 3$; $a(G_{t-1(1)})/A(G_{t-1(1)}) = 0.5$ and $a(G_{t-1(2)})/A(G_{t-1(2)}) = 0.5$; $md(G_{t-1}) = 3$; and $d(G_{t-1(1)}) = 2$ and $d(G_{t-1(2)}) = 2$. Graph G_t has $v(G_t) = 0.139$ with $c(G_t) = 2$; $C(G_t) = 3$; $a(G_{t(1)})/A(G_{t(1)}) = 0.75$ and $a(G_{t(2)})/A(G_{t(2)}) = 0.5$; $md(G_t) = 3$; and $d(G_{t(1)}) = 2$ and $d(G_{t(2)}) = 2$. Thus, applying Equation 4 we get $d(G) = 0.25$ which implies *significant change* according to the classifications that are defined in Table 3.

Table 3. Dissimilarity values categorization

Rank	Category	Dissimilarity Values
1	No change	0.00 - 0.10
2	Slight change	0.10 - 0.15
3	Significant change	0.15 - 0.50
4	Major change	0.50 - 0.90
5	Radical change	0.90 - 1.00

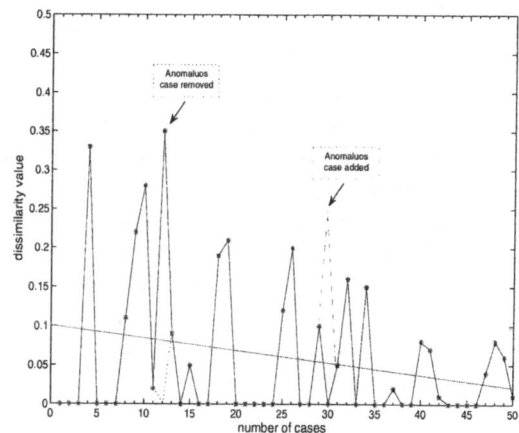

Fig. 4. Dissimilarity values vs. number of new cases

4.3 Results

Discussion with the consultant revealed the effectiveness of the proposed techniques. First, the consultant recommended the grouping of the dissimilarity values into 5 different categories shown in Table 3. The categories provide a qualitative measure of the changes ranked from "No change" to "Radical change". The value of less than 0.10 is considered as "No change", since the variations between the two graphs are not significant enough to have a major effect on the results.

The evaluation process involved analysing how the quality of the existing cases in the database is affected by the update process. It is important to note that the decision tree classifier built from the cases gives 100% correct classification and hence the lattices reflect perfect classification. First, we considered the case where no consultant interaction occurred and allowed the CBR to incrementally add new cases. Figure 4 shows the dissimilarity values as each new case is added. As can be seen, there are significant and minor variations between the previous and current concepts as we incrementally update the database (indicated by the variations in the dissimilarity values). This is expected since the decision tree classifier repartitions the attributes to get the best classification, causing the context tables to change and hence change the lattices.

In general, the dissimilarity values decrease as the number of cases used for training increase. The decreasing trend shows the CBR system increases the consistency, and this means the classifier is becoming more stable and generalising better. This is shown by the linear regression line that indicates a steady decrease as new cases are added. To check for consistency of the results, the cases are randomly added to the lattice one by one. After a number of trials, the results are similar to those shown in Figure 4 with decreasing regression lines.

Rerunning the updating process with the consultant present reveals that the high values in dissimilarity in Figure 4 closely match the consultant's perceptions of the new cases as they are added. For the two large peaks at case 4 and case 12 in Figure 4, the consultant examined the inconsistency, and observed some anomalies in case 12 and modified the features accordingly leading to lower ambiguity (represented by the dotted line). The reason for many of the anomalies is because of the GPs' and consultants' interpretation of the symptoms. This can be quite subjective and the checking of the cases reduces these anomalies[3]. Case 4, however, is considered to be valid and no modification has been made. The increase in the dissimilarity value at case 4 is due to the repartitioning of existing attributes plus some new ones selected for describing the reoccurring diagnosis *Psoriasis* (i.e. already existed in the database).

To further illustrate this, we randomly chose case number 30 having the dissimilarity value of zero, and modified its characteristics to determine whether the value does increase to show the fact that the modified case is no longer valid. The result shows a significant increase in the dissimilarity value (represented by the dashed line) which suggests that the case is no longer valid or consistent with other cases in the database, and this leads to a slight decrease in the accuracy of the decision tree classifier.

5 Conclusions

This paper presents a technique that enables the domain expert to interactively supervise and validate the new knowledge. The technique involves using concept lattices to graphically present the conceptual differences, a summary description highlighting the conceptual variations, and a dissimilarity metric to quantify the level of variations between the current and previous cases in the database. The trials involved having the consultant interactively revise the anomalous cases by modifying the characteristics and the diagnoses that are likely to cause the ambiguity. The results show that dissimilarities match a number of actual processes. First, when the lattices change significantly but the decision tree classifier is giving 100% classification as each new diagnosis is added. Second, when there is a problem in the data for a new case requiring consultant interaction.

---

[3] Note this can also deal with other factors such as errors in data entry.

Acknowledgements

The research reported in this paper has been funded in full by a grant from the AHMAC/SCRIF initiative administered by the NHMRC in Australia.

References

1. P. Cole, R. Eklund and F. Amardeilh. Browsing Semi-structured Texts on the Web using Formal Concept Analysis. *Web Intelligence*, 2003.
2. B. Díaz-Agudo and P. A. Gonzalez-Calero. Formal Concept Analysis as a Support Technique for CBR. *Knowledge-Based System*, 7(1):39–59, March 2001.
3. B. Ganter. Computing with Conceptual Structures. In *Proc. of the 8th International Conference on Conceptual Structure*, Darmstadt, 2000. Springer.
4. B. Ganter and R. Wille. *Formal Concept Analysis: Mathematical Foundations*. Springer, Heidelberg, 1999.
5. M. Montes-y Gómez, A. Gelbukh, A. López-López, and R. Baeza-Yates. Flexible Comparison of Conceptual Graphs. In *Proceedings of the 12th International Conference and Workshop on Database and Expert Systems Applications*, pages 102–111, Munich, Germany, 2001.
6. J. Ross. Quinlan. *C4.5 Programs for Machine Learning*. Morgan Kaufmann Publishers, USA, 1993.
7. D. Richards. Visualizing Knowledge Based Systems. In *Proceedings of the 3rd Workshop on Software Visualization*, pages 1–8, Sydney, Australia, 1999.
8. D. Richards. The Visualisation of Multiple Views to Support Knowledge Reuse. In *Proceedings of the Intelligent Information Processing (IIP'2000) In Conjunction with the 16th IFIP World Computer Congress WCC2000*, Beijing, China, 2000.
9. I. Watson. *Applying Case-Based Reasoning: Techniques for Enterprise Systems*. Morgan Kaufmann Publishers, USA, 1997.
10. I. Witten and E. Frank. *Data Mining: Practical Machine Learning Tools and Techniques with Java Implementations*. Morgan Kaufmann Publishers, USA, 2000.
11. P. Z. Yeh, B. Porter, and K. Barker. Using Transformations to Improve Semantic Matching. In *Proceedings of the International Conference on Knowledge Capture*, pages 180–189, Sanibel Island, FL, USA, 2003.
12. J. Zhong, H. Zhu, J. Li, and Y. Yu. Conceptual Graph Matching for Semantic Search. In *Proceedings of the 10th International Conference on Conceptual Structures: Integration and Interfaces*, pages 92–106, Borovets, Bulgaria, 2002.

Adaptation and Medical Case-Based Reasoning Focusing on Endocrine Therapy Support

Rainer Schmidt[1] and Olga Vorobieva[1,2]

[1] Institute for Medical Informatics and Biometry, University of Rostock,
D-18055 Rostock, Germany
rainer.schmidt@medizin.uni-rostock.de
[2] Setchenow Institute of Evolutionary Physiology and Biochemistry,
St.Petersburg, Russia

Abstract. So far, Case-Based Reasoning has not become as successful in medicine as in some other application domains. One, probably the main reason is the adaptation problem. In Case-Based Reasoning the adaptation task still is domain dependent und usually requires specific adaptation rules. Furthermore, in medicine adaptation is often more difficult than in other domains, because usually more and complex features have to be considered. We have developed some programs for endocrine therapy support, especially for hypothyroidism. In this paper, we do not present them in detail, but focus on adaptation. We do not only summarise experiences with adaptation in medicine, but we want to elaborate typical medical adaptation problems and hope to indicate possibilities how to solve them.

1 Introduction

Case-Based Reasoning (CBR) has become a successful technique for knowledge-based systems in many domains, while in medicine some more problems arise to use this method. A CBR system has to solve two main tasks [1]: The first one is the retrieval, which is the search for or the calculation of similar cases. For this task much research has been undertaken. The basic retrieval algorithms for indexing [2], Nearest Neighbor match [3], pre-classification [4] etc. have already been developed some years ago and have been improved in the recent years. So, actually it has become correspondingly easy to find sophisticated CBR retrieval algorithms adequate for nearly every sort of application problem.

The second task, the adaptation means modifying a solution of a former similar case to fit for a current problem. If there are no important differences between a current and a similar case, a solution transfer is sufficient. Sometimes just few substitutions are required, but usually adaptation is a complicated process. While in the early 90th the focus of the CBR community lay on retrieval, in the late 90th CBR researchers investigated various aspects of adaptation. Though theories and models for adaptation [e.g. 5, 6] have been developed, adaptation is still domain dependent. Usually, for each application specific adaptation rules have to be generated.

Since adaptation is even more difficult in medicine, we want to elaborate typical medical adaptation problems and we hope to show possibilities how to solve them.

2 Medical Case-Based Reasoning Systems

Though CBR was not as successful in medicine as in some other domains so far, several medical systems have already been developed which at least apply parts of the Case-Based Reasoning method. Here we do not want to give a review of all these systems (for that see [7, 8, 9]), but we intend to show the main developments concerning adaptation in this area.

2.1 Avoiding the Adaptation Problem

Some systems avoid the adaptation problem, because they do not apply the complete CBR method, but only a part of it, namely the retrieval. These systems can be divided into two groups, retrieval-only systems and multi modal reasoning systems.

Retrieval-only systems are mainly used for image interpretation, which is mainly a classification task [10]. However, retrieval-only systems are not only used for image interpretation, but for other visualisation tasks too, e.g. for the development of kidney function courses [11] and for hepatitic surgery [12].

Multi modal reasoning systems apply parts of different reasoning methods. From CBR they usually incorporate the retrieval step, often to calculate or support evidences [13], e.g. in CARE-PARTNER [14] CBR retrieval is used to search for similar cases to support evidences for a rule-based program.

2.2 Solving the Adaptation Problem

So far, only a few medical systems have been developed that apply the complete CBR method. In these systems three main techniques are used for adaptation: adaptation operators or rules, constraints, and compositional adaptation. Furthermore, abstracting from specific single cases to more general prototypical cases sometimes supports the adaptation.

Adaptation rules and operators. One of the earliest medical expert systems that use CBR techniques is CASEY [16]. It deals with heart failure diagnosis. The most interesting aspect of CASEY is the ambitious attempt to solve the adaptation task. Since the creation of a complete rule base for adaptation was too time consuming, a few general operators are used to solve the adaptation task. Since many features have to be considered in the heart failure domain and since consequently many differences between cases can occur, not all differences between former similar cases and a query case can be handled by the developed general adaptation operators. So, if no similar case can be found or if adaptation fails, CASEY uses a rule-based domain theory.

However, the development of complete adaptation rule bases never became a successful technique to solve the adaptation problem in medical CBR systems, because the bottleneck for rule-based medical expert systems, the knowledge acquisition, occurs again.

Constraints. A more successful technique is the application of constraints. In ICONS, an antibiotics therapy adviser [17], adaptation is rather easy, it is just a reduction of a list of solutions (recommended therapies for a similar, retrieved case) by constraints (contraindications of the query patient).

Another example for applying constraints is a diagnostic program concerning dysmorphic syndromes [18]. The retrieval provides a list of prototypes sorted according to their similarity in respect to the current patient. Each prototype defines a diagnosis (dysmorphic syndrome) and represents the typical features for this diagnosis. The provided list of prototypes is checked by a set of explicit constraints. These constraints state that some features of the patient either contradict or support specific prototypes (diagnoses).

A typical task for applying constraints is menu planing [19], where different requirements have to be served: special diets and individual factors, not only personal preferences, but also contraindications and demands based on various complications.

Compositional adaptation. A further successful adaptation technique is compositional adaptation [20]. In TA3-IVF [21], a system to modify in vitro fertilisation treatment plans, relevant similar cases are retrieved and compositional adaptation is used to compute weighted averages for the solution attributes.

In TeCoMed [22], an early warning system concerning threatening influenza waves, compositional adaptation is applied on the most similar former courses to decide whether a warning against an influenza wave is appropriate.

Abstraction. As one reason for the adaptation problem is the extreme specificity of single cases, the generalisation from single cases into abstracted prototypes [18] or classes [23] may support the adaptation. The idea of generating more abstract cases is typical for the medical domain, because (proto-) typical cases directly correspond to (proto-) typical diagnoses or therapies. While in GS.52 all prototypes are organised on the same level, in MNAOMIA [23], a hierarchy of classes, cases, and concepts with few layers is used. MEDIC [24], a diagnostic reasoner on the domain of pulmonology, consists of a multi-layered hierarchy of schemata, of scenes, and of memory organisation packets of individual cases.

3 Adaptation Problems in Endocrinology Diseases Therapy Support

We have developed an endocrine therapy support system for a children's hospital. The architecture is shown in figure 1, for technical details see [25]. Here, we focus on adaptation problems within it to illustrate general adaptation problems in medicine.

All body functions are regulated by the endocrine system. The endocrine gland produces hormones and secrets them in blood. Hypothyroidism means that a patient's thyroid gland does not produce enough thyroid hormone naturally. If hypothyroidism is undertreated, it may lead to obesity, brachicardia and other heart diseases, memory loss and many other diseases [26]. Furthermore in children it causes mental and physical retardation. If hypothyroidism is of autoimune nature, it sometimes occurs in combination with further autoimune diseases such as diabetes. The diagnosis hypothyroidism can be established by blood tests. The therapy is inevitable: thyroid hormone replacement by levothyroxine. The problem is to determine the therapeutic dose, because the thyroxin demand of a patient follows only very roughly general schema and so the therapy must be individualised [27]. If the dose is too low, hypothyroidism is undertreated. If the dose it too high, the thyroid hormone concentration is also too high, which leads to hyperactive thyroid effects [26, 27].

There are two different tasks of determining an appropriate dose. The first one aims to determine the initial dose, while later on the dose has to be updated continuously during a patient's lifetime. Precise determination of the initial dose is most important for newborn babies with congenital hypothyroidism, because for them every week of proper therapy counts.

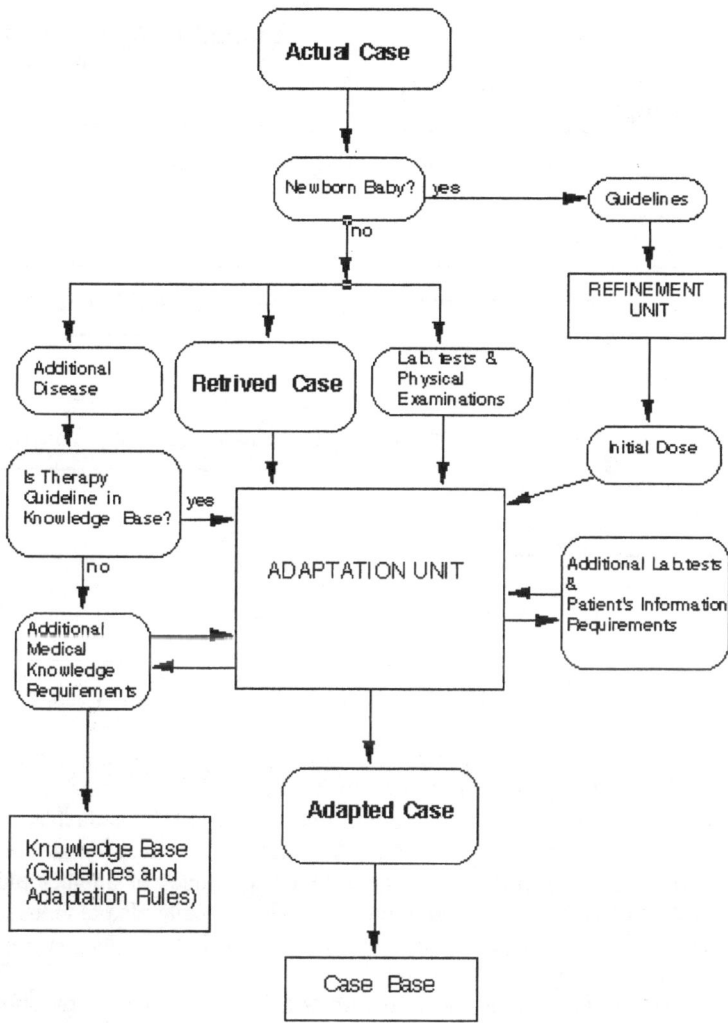

Fig. 1. Architecture of our endocrine therapy support system

3.1 Computing an Initial Dose

For the determination of an initial dose (fig. 2), a couple of prototypes, called guidelines, exist, which have been defined by commissions of experts. The assignment of a patient to a fitting guideline is obvious because of the way the

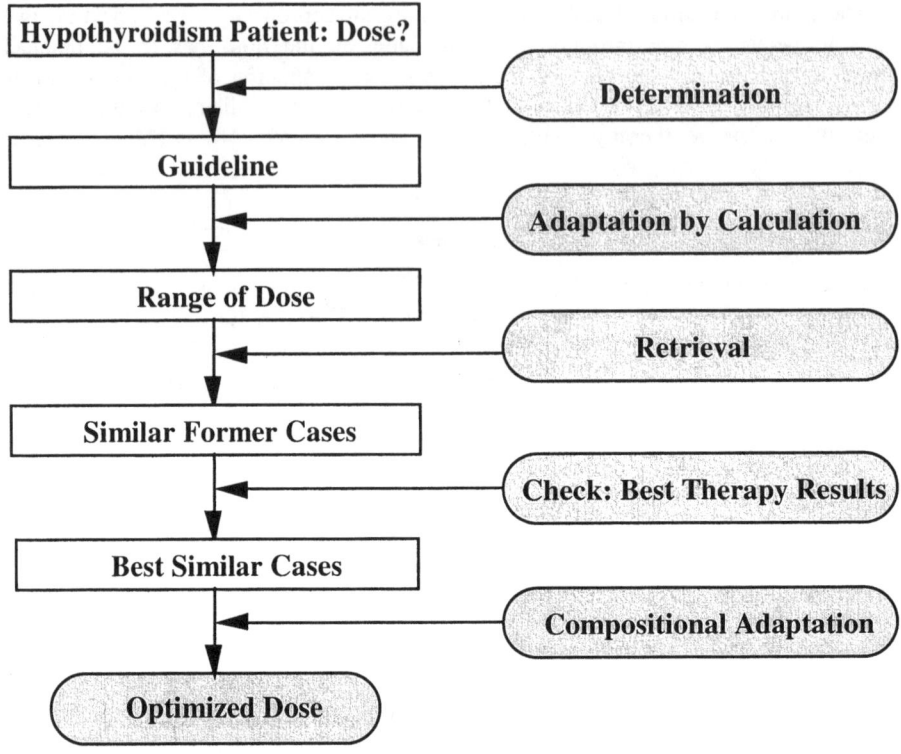

Fig. 2. Determination of an initial dose

guidelines have been defined. With the help of these guidelines a range for good doses can be calculated.

To compute an optimal dose, we retrieve similar cases with initial doses within the calculated ranges. Since there are only few attributes and since our case base is rather small, we use Tversky's sequential measure of dissimilarity [28]. On the basis of those of the retrieved cases that had best therapy results an average initial therapy is calculated. Best therapy results can be determined by values of another blood test after two weeks of treatment with the initial dose. The opposite idea to consider cases with bad therapy results does not work here, because bad results may be caused by various reasons.

So, to compute an optimal dose recommendation, we apply two forms of adaptation. First, a calculation of ranges according to guidelines and patients attribute values. Secondly, we use Compositional Adaptation. That means, we take only similar cases with best therapy results into account and calculate the average dose for these cases, which has to be adapted to the query patient by another calculation.

Example for computing an initial dose. The query patient is a newborn baby that is 20 days old, has a weight of 4 kg and is diagnosed for hypothyroidism. The guideline for babies about 3 weeks age and normal weight recommend a levothyroxine therapy with a daily dose between 12 and 15 µg/kg. So, because the baby weighs 4 kg, a range of 48-60 µg is calculated. The retrieval provides similar cases that must have doses within the calculated range. These cases are restricted to those where after two weeks treatment less than 10 µU/ml thyroid stimulating hormone could be observed. Since these remaining similar cases are all treated alike, an average dose per kg is computed which subsequently is multiplied with the query patient's weight to deliver the optimal daily dose.

3.2 Updating the Dose in a Patient's Lifetime

For monitoring the patient, three laboratory blood tests have to be made. Usually the results of these tests correspond to each other. Otherwise, it indicates a more complicated thyroid condition and additional tests are necessary. If the tests show that the patient's thyroid hormone level is normal, it means that the current levothyroxine dose is OK. If the tests indicate that the thyroid hormone level is too low or too high, the current dose has to be increased resp. decreased by 25 or 50 µg [26, 27]. So, for monitoring adaptation is just a simple calculation according to well-known standards.

Example. Figure 3 shows an example of a case study. We compared the decisions of an experienced doctor with the recommendations of our system. The decisions are based on the basic laboratory tests and on lists of observed symptoms. Intervals between two visits are approximately six months.

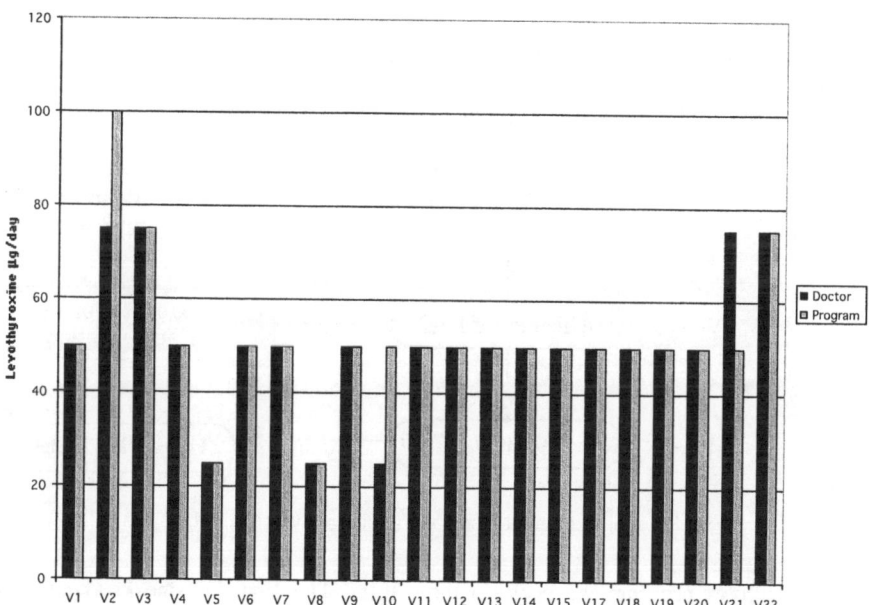

Fig. 3. Dose updates recommended by our program compared with doctor's decision. V1 means the first visit, V2 the second visit etc

In this example there are three deviations, usually there are less. At the second visit (v2), according to laboratory results the levothyroxine should be increased. Our program recommended a too high increase. The applied adaptation rule was not precise enough. So, we modified it. At visit 10 (v10) the doctor decided to try to decrease the dose. The doctor's reasons were not included in our knowledge base and since his attempt was not successful, we did not alter any adaptation rule. At visit 21 (v21) the doctor increased the dose because of some minor symptoms of hypothyroidism, which were not included in our program's list of hypothyroidism symptoms. Since the doctors decision was probably right (visit 22), we added these symptoms to the list of hypothyroidism symptoms of our program.

3.3 Additional Diseases or Complications

It often occurs that patients do not only have hypothyroidism, but they additionally suffer from further chronic diseases or complications. So, the levothyroxine therapy has to be checked for contraindications, adverse effects and interactions with additionally existing therapies. Since no alternative is available to replace levothyroxine, if necessary additionally existing therapies have to be modified, substituted, or compensated (fig. 4) [26, 27].

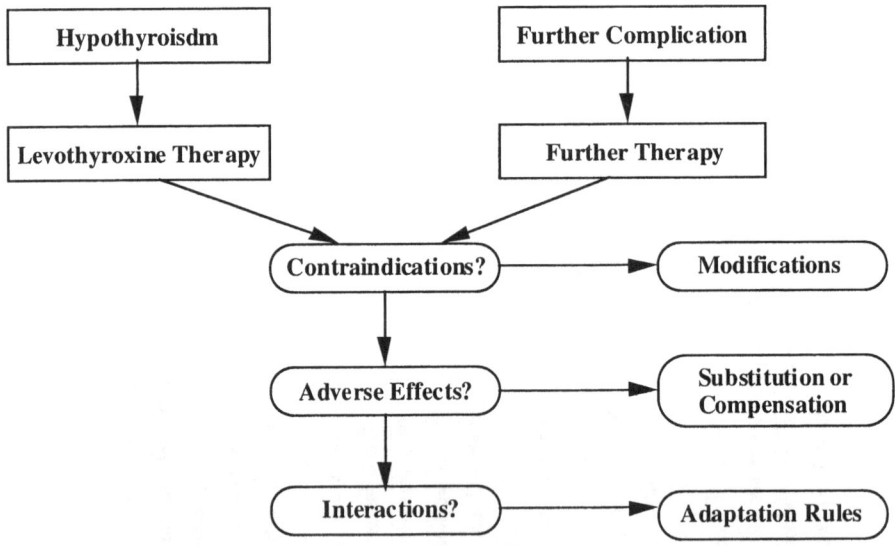

Fig. 4. Levothyroxine therapy and additionally existing therapies

In our support program we perform three tests. The first one checks if another existing therapy is contraindicated to hypothyroidism. This holds only for very few therapies, namely for specific diets like soybean infant formula, but they are typical for newborn babies. Such diets have to be modified. Since no exact knowledge is available how to do it, our program just issues a warning saying that a modification is necessary.

The second test considers adverse effects. There are two ways to deal with them. A further existing therapy has either to be substituted or it has to be compensated by another drug. Since such knowledge is available, we have implemented corresponding rules for substitutional resp. compensational adaptation.

The third test checks for interactions between both therapies. Here we have implemented some adaptation rules, which mainly attempt to avoid the interactions. For example, if a patient has heartburn problems that are treated with an antacid, a rule for this situation exists that states that levothyroxine should be administered at least 4 hours after or before an antacid. However, if no adaptation rule can solve such an interaction problem, the same substitution rules as for adverse effects are applied.

4 Conclusion: Adaptation Techniques for Medical Therapy Problems

Our intention is to undertake first steps in the direction of developing a methodology for the adaptation problem for medical CBR systems. However, we have to admit that we are just at the beginning. Furthermore, our experience concerning the adaptation problem is mainly based on therapeutic tasks. Indeed, in contrast to ideas of many computer scientists, doctors are much more interested in therapeutic than in diagnostic support programs.

So, in this paper, we firstly reviewed how adaptation is handled in medical CBR systems and secondly enriched the experiences by additional examples from the endocrinology domain, where we have recently developed support programs.

For medical therapy systems, that intend to apply the whole CBR cycle, at present we can summarise useful adaptation techniques (fig. 5). However, most of them are promising only for specific tasks.

Abstraction. from single cases to more general prototypes seems to be a promising implicit support. However, if the prototypes correspond to guidelines they may even explicitly solve some adaptation steps (see section 3.1).

Compositional Adaptation. at first glance does not seem to appropriate in medicine, because it was originally developed for configuration [20]. However, it has been successfully applied for calculation therapy doses (e.g. in TA3-IVF [21] and see section 3.1.).

Constraints. are a promising adaptation technique too, but only for a specific situation (see section 2.2), namely for a set of solutions that can be reduced by checking e.g. contraindications (in ICONS) or contradictions (in GS.52).

Adaptation rules. The only technique that seems to be general enough to solve many medical adaptation problems is the application of adaptation rules or operators. The technique is general, but unfortunately the content of such rules has to be domain specific. Especially for complex medical tasks the generation of adaptation rules often is too time consuming and sometimes even impossible.

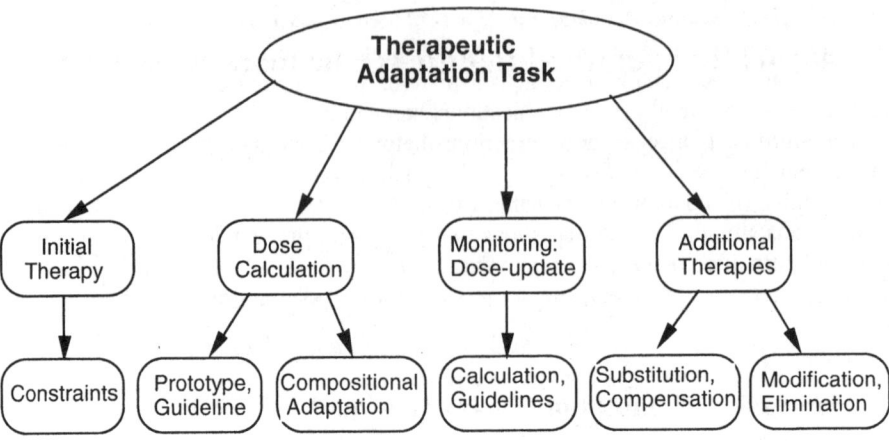

Fig. 5. A task oriented adaptation model

However, for therapeutic tasks some typical forms of adaptation rules can be made out, namely for substitutional and compensational adaptation (e.g. section 3.3.), and for calculating doses (e.g. section 3.2.). So, a next step might be an attempt to generate general adaptation operators for these typical forms of adaptation rules.

References

1. Aamodt, A., Plaza, E.: Case-based reasoning: Foundational issues, methodological variations, and system approaches. AI Communications 7 (1) (1994) 39-59
2. Stottler, R. et al.: Rapid retrieval algorithms for case-based reasoning. In: Proc of 11th Int Joint Conference on Artificial Intelligence, Morgan Kaufmann Publishers, San Mateo (1989) 233-237
3. Broder, A.: Strategies for efficient incremental nearest neighbor search. Pattern Recognition 23 (1990) 171-178
4. Quinlan, J.: C4.5, Programs for Machine Learning. Morgan Kaufmann Publishers, San Mateo (1993)
5. Bergmann, R., Wilke, W.: Towards a new formal model of transformational adaptation in case-based reasoning. In: Gierl L, Lenz, M. (eds.): Proceedings of th German Workshop on CBR. University of Rostock (1998) 43-52
6. Fuchs,B.,Mille, A.: A knowledge-level task model of adaptation in case-based reasoning. In: Althoff, K.-D. et al. (eds.): Case-Based Reasoning Research and Development, Proc. of 3rd Int Conference. Springer, Berlin (1999) 118-131
7. Gierl, L., Bull, M., Schmidt, R.: CBR in Medicine. In: Lenz, M. et al., Case-Based Reasoning Technology, From Foundations to Applications. Springer, Berlin (1998) 273-297
8. Schmidt, R., Montani, S., Bellazzi,E., Portinale, L., Gierl, L.: Case-Based Reasoning for Medical Knowledge-based Systems. Int J Med Inform 64 (2-3) (2001) 355-367
9. Nilsson M, Sollenborn M: Advancements and trends in medical case-based Reasoning: An overview of systems and system developments. In: Proc of FLAIRS, AAAI Press (2004) 178-183

10. Perner, P.: Why Case-Based Reasoning is Attractive for Image Interpretation. In: Aha, D., Watson, I. (eds.): Case-Based Reasoning Research and Development, Proc 4th Int Conference. Springer, Berlin (2001) 27-43
11. Schmidt, R. et al.: Medical multiparametric time course prognoses applied to kidney function assessments. Int J Med Inform 53 (2-3) (1999) 253-264
12. Dugas M.: Clinical applications of Intranet-Technology. In: Dudeck, J. et al. (eds.): New Technologies in Hospital Information Systems. IOS Press, Amsterdam (1997) 115-118
13. Montani, S. et al.: Diabetic patient's management expoiting Case-based Reasoning techniques. Computer Methods and Programs in Biomedicine 62 (2000) 205-218
14. Bichindaritz, I. et al.: Case-based reasoning in CARE-PARTNER: Gathering evidence for evidence-based medical practice. In: Smyth, B., Cunningham, P. (eds.): Advances in Case-Based Reasoning, Proc of 4th European Workshop. Springer, Berlin (1998) 334-345
15. Koton, P.: Reasoning about evidence in causal explanations. In: Kolodner, J. (ed.): First Workshop on CBR. Morgan Kaufmann Publishers, San Mateo (1988) 260-270
16. Schmidt, R., Gierl, L.: Case-based Reasoning for Antibiotics Therapy Advice: An Investigation of Retrieval Algorithms and Prototypes. Artificial Intelligence in Medicine 23 (2) (2001) 171-186
17. Gierl, L., Stengel-Rutkowski, S.: Integrating consultation and semi-automatic knowledge acquisition in a prototype-based architecture: Experiences with Dysmorphic Syndromes. Artificial Intelligence in Medicine 6 (1994) 29-49
18. Petot, G.J., Marling, C., Sterling, L.: An artificial intelligence system for computer-assisted menu planing. Journal of American Diet Assoc 98 (9) (1998) 1009-10014
19. Wilke, W., Smyth, B., Cunningham, P.: Using Configuration Techniques for Adaptation. In: Lenz, M., Bartsch-Spörl, B., Burkhard, H.-D., Wess, S. (eds.): Case-Based Reasoning Technology, From Foundations to Applications. Springer, Berlin (1998) 139-168
20. Jurisica, I. et al: Case-based reasoning in IVF: prediction and knowledge mining. Artificial Intelligence in Medicine 12 (1998) 1-24
21. Schmidt, R., Gierl, L.: Prognostic Model for Early Warning of Threatening Influenza Waves. In: Minor, M., Staab, S. (eds.): Proc 1st German Workshop on Experience Management. Köllen, Bonn (2002) 39-46
22. Bichindaritz, I.: From cases to classes: Focusing on abstraction in case-based reasoning. In: Burkhard, H.-D., Lenz, M. (eds.): Proc 4th German Workshop on CBR. Humboldt University Berlin (1996) 62-69
23. Turner, R.: Organizing and using schematic knowledge for medical diagnosis. In: Kolodner, J. (ed.): First Workshop on CBR. Morgan Kaufmann Publishers, San Mateo (1988) 435-446
24. Schmidt, R., Vorobieva, O., Gierl L.: Adaptation problems in therapeutic case-based reasoning systems. In: Palade, L., Howlett, R.J., Jain, L.(eds.): Knowledge-Based Intelligent Information and Engineering Systems, Springer, Berlin (2003) 992-999
25. Hampel, R.: Diagnostik und Therapie von Schilddrüsenfunktionsstörungen. UNI-MED Verlag, Bremen (2000)
26. DeGroot, L.J.: Thyroid Physiology and Hypothyroidsm. In: Besser, G.M., Turner, M. (eds.): Clinical endocrinilogy. Wolfe, London (1994) (Chapter 15)
27. Tversky, A.: Features of similarity. Psychological review 84 (1977) 327-352

Transcranial Magnetic Stimulation (TMS) to Evaluate and Classify Mental Diseases Using Neural Networks

Alberto Faro[1], Daniela Giordano[1], Manuela Pennisi[2], Giacomo Scarciofalo[1], Concetto Spampinato[1], and Francesco Tramontana[1]

[1] Dipartimento di Ingegneria Informatica e Telecomunicazioni, Università di Catania,
viale A., Doria 6, 95125 Catania, Italy
{afaro, dgiordan, gscarcio, cspampin, ftramont}@diit.unict.it
[2] Dipartimento di Neuroscienze, Università di Catania, Policlinico Città Universitaria,
via S.Sofia 78, 95123 Catania, Italy
mpennisi@mail.it

Abstract. The paper proposes a methodology based on a neural network to process the signals related to the hands movements in response to the Transcranial Magnetic Stimulation (TMS) in order to diagnose the pathology and evaluate the treatment of the patients affected by demency diseases. First a time-frequency analysis of such signals is carried out to identify the main signal variables that characterize the demency diseases. Then these variables are processed by a neural network in order to classify the responses into four classes: healthy subjects, people affected by Subcortical Ischemic Vascular Dementia (SIVD) and/or Alzheimer. A comparison between the proposed method and a fuzzy approach previously developed by the authors is presented.

1 Introduction

Early diagnosis and effective therapy are decisive for a successful treatment of patients affected by highly critical diseases. However, current medical practices lack quantitative methods able to diagnose with a given confidence type and degree the mental diseases such as Alzheimer and Subcortical Ischemic Vascular Dementia (SIVD). The paper aims at overcoming this limit by a two step methodology. First the relevant variables that may reveal the type and the degree of the mental diseases are identified. The second step is to find a non-linear model based on the mentioned variables that allows us to identify by a neural network the type of disease and to express a quantitative evaluation of the patient status in terms of fuzzy quantifiers (e.g., SIVD at an initial stage, very advanced Alzheimer disease, and so on).

Several variables and experiments may be used for discovering the type and the degree of the mental disease, e.g., the average values of EEG signals or appropriate tests related to cognitive and physical abilities. In the paper the Transcranial Magnetic Stimulation (TMS) is taken into account since it may be used for both diagnosis and therapy [1]. Sect.2 briefly recalls the main features of the TMS and how it is currently administered for the treatment of patients affected by mental diseases [2]. In sect.3 a time-frequency analysis is carried out in order to identify what variables related to the responses of the patients to TMS are useful to characterize the mental diseases. In sect.4 all these variables are given as input to a supervised neural network in order to classify people in four classes, i.e., healthy people, people affected by Alzheimer and/or SIVD. In this section a comparison is carried out between this method and a fuzzy approach previously developed by the authors [3] to point out the advantages of integrating the two approaches into a two steps methodology: the first step deals with the disease identification by a neural network, the second step aims at evaluating the degree and the effect of the TMS based therapy by fuzzy logic.

2 Transcranial Magnetic Stimulation (TMS)

TMS produces a modification of the neuronal activity related to a defined brain area stimulated by the variable magnetic field generated by a coil [4]. Such magnetic field induces an electrical flow in the brain that goes towards the limbs and determines some involuntary movements of the legs and of the hands [5]. The movements of the limbs in response to TMS are measured by an ElectroMyoGraph (EMG).

TMS is painless and its positive effect consists of an increase in the physical and cognitive performances of the brain activity of the people affected by dementia. Since after a certain period of time such neural activity returns to the initial conditions, it is useful to have a method to identify when TMS should be administered anew to reactivate the neural activity. To gain some insight about the patient conditions from the muscles response to TMS, the tests are conducted according to a protocol consisting of three phases: "Bi-Stim-Before", "R-Stim" and "Bi-Stim-After".

In phase "Bi-Stim-Before", two stimulations are given to the subject; the first acts as a conditioning stimulus, the second acts as the testing stimulus. The muscular responses to be compared with the ones obtained after the repetitive stimulation are taken and stored by the EMG. In phase "R-Stim", a repetitive stimulation is administered to the subject for a certain period of time (e.g., one repetitive stimulation session per day for 15 days). The patient is stimulated for about 30 minutes by a magnetic field at a stimulation frequency between 1 Hz and 30 Hz depending on the pathology. In phase "Bi-Stim-After", the patient is stimulated as in phase "Bi-Stim-Before".

By comparing the signals obtained from the hand movements before and after a repetitive stimulation, it is possible to evaluate the subject's status. In healthy subjects the signals before and after R-stim are more or less the same, whereas in the people affected by dementia such signals differ. Data on the muscular responses are collected during the mentioned Bi-Stim phase varying the delay between the first and the second stimulus. Such delay is called Inter-Stimulus time Interval (ISI). Six ISIs have been tested (i.e., 0,1,2,5,7,10 ms). For each ISI nine tracks have been stored, for a total of 54 stimulations per subject.

After the R-Stim phase, a second bi-stimulation phase (i.e., Bi-Stim-After phase) is carried out to evaluate if the subject is healthy and if the R-Stim phase has produced the envisaged positive effect for patients affected by dementia. To give a quantitative basis to such a comparison, it is necessary to identify the values of the muscular response that may be useful to characterize the subject status. To this aim an analysis of the signals related to the mentioned muscular movements in the time-frequency domain and using the Wavelet transform is carried out in the next section.

3 Variables Characterizing the Mental Diseases

The variables related to the signals detected by EMG in the mentioned TMS tests are assumed to concur to characterize the mental diseases if they show different values before and after the repetitive stimulation for the patients affected by dementia, since they remain unchanged for the healthy people. To diagnose the type and the degree of the dementia it is useful to have more than one relevant variables since in absence of an explicit model, the only way to obtain a characterization of the dementia is to put into correspondence dementia type and degree with a particular combination of the mentioned variables and related values. In the following we discuss what variables may be used for this aim.

To find the variables relevant to characterize the dementia diseases we have taken into account several variables defined on the EMG tracks, as for example, the following ones: latency L, amplitude A, Max and Min module of the Fast Fourier Transform (FFT), Max and Min module of the Hilbert transform. The relevance check for each of these variable was performed by first finding the average track for a given value of ISI and then by verifying, ISI by ISI, if the variable values after R-Stim differ from the ones assumed by the same variable before R-Stim. This check has been performed for each variable by a simple inspection of a graphic consisting of two curves: one formed by the values of the variable in the 9 stimulations before R-stim and the other formed by the values of the variable in the 9 stimulations after R-stim.

Interestingly, this allowed us not only to identify the variables relevant for this study on the mental diseases, but also to find that the stimulations for ISI > 5 are not useful for treating the patients. The following table points out that this effect is valid for all the variables taken into account, thus we limit our study to EMG tracks with ISI ≤ 5. In such table the symbols ↑, ↓ and ≈ respectively indicate that the variables after R-stim increase, decrease, or do not change.

Table 1. Changes in the variables after the repetitive stimulation at different ISIs

	A	L	FFT Mod.Max	FFT Mod.Min	HT Mod.Max	HT Mod.min
ISI 1	↑	↓	↑	↓	↓	↑
ISI 2	↑	↓	↑	↓	↓	↑
ISI 5	↑	↓	↑	↓	↓	↑
ISI 7	≈	≈	↑	≈	≈	↓
ISI 10	↑	≈	≈	↓	≈	≈

For a better characterization of the EMG tracks it has been decided to take into account also the Continuous Wavelet Transform (CWT) of the signals detected before and after R-stim. What makes CWT interesting is that it is able to point out details of the signals that are difficult to evaluate by using the classical time-frequency analysis, such as rapid variability or slow evolution. A comparison between the CWT of the signals detected before and after R-stim is then able to point out regularities or difference that cannot be detected by using other methods. In this way it is possible to diagnose difficult dementia cases that cannot be detected by Fourier or Hamilton transform. To this aim, after having computed the CWT for the signals related to the various ISI, a cross-correlation has been carried out between the set of values related to the phase before and the one related to the phase after R-Stim. We have found that the maximum of such cross-correlation for a patient affected by dementia is at the highest ISI being very low (near to zero) the cross-correlation at the lowest ISI. Healthy people have shown a high cross-correlation for any ISI. This confirms that stimulations at highest ISI are not useful for the patient's treatment and that CRW is an effective variable to be take into account to diagnose mental diseases.

4 Classifying Mental Diseases: Neural Networks Versus Fuzzy Logic

The choice of the variables to be given as inputs to a neural network is particularly important since considering variables that are not relevant for the study may cause high imprecision in classifying the cases. Thus the preprocessing phase discussed in the previous section is necessary for a successful classification of the patients. The variables that have a low cross-correlation between the values taken before and after the repetitive stimulation for the patients affected by dementia while they show high cross-correlation for the healthy people are the following: Latency, Amplitude, FFT Max Module, FFT Min module, Min module of the Hilbert transform, Max cross-correlation of the Wavelet transform. The difference between the values of these variables with respect to the same ISI before and after the repetitive stimulation are given as inputs to the multilayer neural network consisting of six inputs and two outputs neurons. A hidden layer consisting of 20 neurons proved sufficient to make the neural network generalize from the learned examples. The output neurons classify the cases into four classes as follows: None, Alzheimer, SIVD and Mixed Dementia. Table 2 shows the success rate obtained in diagnosing the pathology by using the neural networks in comparison with the findings the authors obtained in another study using fuzzy logic, where the same input variables, except the one dealing with the Wavelet transform, were taken into account.

Table 2. Success rate in the diagnosis of the pathology

Pathology	Using neural networks	Using fuzzy logic
None	90 %	90%
Alzheimer	92,7%	92.5%
SIVD	95%	92.5%
Mixed dementia	87%	90%

The comparison shows that the neural network approach is more appropriate to classify crisp cases, i.e., healthy people and people affected by Alzheimer or SIVD, whereas the fuzzy logic based approach is more appropriate in discovering mixed dementia. These results refer to twenty cases. Validation of the success rate will be done with the larger number of cases that currently are being collected. Two other important user requisites have to be taken into account, i.e., the simplicity in obtaining the right information and the possibility of gaining useful quantitative evaluation for both the diagnosis and the therapy. The first requisite can be easily satisfied by a neural network with a crisp codification of the classes to recognize, whereas the fuzzy approach can be suitably used to express quantitative/qualitative rules that are enough to support medical decisions as for example "the patient is affected by an early demency that may treated by frequent sessions of TMS". For this reason it may be convenient to integrate neural network and fuzzy logic in a unique methodology as follows: first the patient's condition is evaluated with the help of a neural network, then the fuzzy approach is applied to have hints about the diagnosis and therapy.

5 Concluding Remarks

The paper has shown that the responses to the transcranial magnetic stimulations (TMS) can be used effectively to classify mental diseases by using both neural networks and fuzzy classifiers. The neural networks classification shows better performance to classify crisp cases (i.e. no mental disease, SIVD, Alzheimer), whereas the fuzzy logic is more suitable when one is interested in having some measurements about the mental disease, e.g., to identify the disease's stages or if the disease is due to both SIVD and Alzheimer. An integration of the two classification methods could be very effective. A way to increase the success rate is to increase the number of the inputs by taking into account variables related to other practices, e.g., EEG signals, genetic information and so on. Adding to the fuzzy classifier information related to the wavelet transform could increase its success rate. This is for further study.

References

1. Handbook of TMS. Edited by Pascual-Leone, A. et alii Arnold, London (2001)
2. Iramina, K., Maeno, T., Kowatari, Y., Ueno, S.: Effects of Transcranial Magnetic Stimulation on EEG Activity, IEEE Transactions on Magnetics, Vol. 38, N. 5 (2002)
3. Faro, A., Giordano, D., Pennisi, M., Scarciofalo, G., Spampinato, C., Tramontana F.: A Fuzzy System to Analyze SIVD Diseases using TMS, Int. J. Signal Processing N.2 (2005)
4. Pepin JL., Bogacz D., de Pasqua V., Delwaide PJ.: Motor Cortex Inhibition is not Impaired in Patients with Alzheimer's Disease: Evidence from Paired Transcranial Magnetic Stimulation, J. Neurological Sciences.Vol.170 N.2 (1999)
5. Ruohonen, J., Ollikainen, M., Nikouline, V., Virtanen, J., Ilmoniemi, R.J.: Coil Design for Real and Sham Transcranial Magnetic Stimulation, IEEE Transactions on Biomedical Engineering , Vol.47 N.2 (2000)

Towards Information Visualization and Clustering Techniques for MRI Data Sets

Umberto Castellani[1], Carlo Combi[1], Pasquina Marzola[2], Vittorio Murino[1], Andrea Sbarbati[2], and Marco Zampieri[1]

[1] Dipartimento di Informatica - Università di Verona
[2] Dipartimento di Scienze Morfologiche Biomediche - Università di Verona

Abstract. The paper deals with the integrated use of Information Visualization techniques and clustering algorithms to analyze Magnetic Resonance Imaging (MRI) data sets. The paper also describes the criteria we followed in designing and implementing the prototype, according to the above approach. Finally, some preliminary results are given for the considered medical application.

1 Introduction

The research interest on visualization and analysis of multidimensional data has grown rapidly during the last decade [2]. Focusing on medical applications, several activities require the visual investigation and analysis of images, video, and graphs [1]. In this paper we aim at integrating the use of Information Visualization (IV) techniques and data mining algorithms for the analysis of Magnetic Resonance Imaging (MRI) data sets. Preclinical and clinical evaluation of the efficacy of antiangiogenic compounds poses new problems to researchers because the traditional criterion for assessing the response of a tumor to a treatment, based on the measurement of tumor size reduction, is no longer valid [3]. Dynamic Contrast Enhanced MRI (DCE-MRI) techniques play a relevant role in this field [3]. DCE-MRI with macromolecular contrast agents has been used to measure characteristics of tumor microvessels such as transendothelial permeability (kPS) and fractional plasma volume (fPV) that are accepted surrogate markers of tumor angiogenesis [3]. In order to improve the analysis of such kind of data, an efficient and effective visual application has been developed with respect to the main IV criteria and methodologies. Moreover, a *cluster analysis* on kPS and fPV parameters space has been introduced by adopting a bayesian approach based on the combined application of *K-Means* algorithm and *Bayesian Information Criterion* (BIC)[4]. The main contribution consists of merging the cluster analysis and *linked brushing* visualization method by switching between the MRI volumetric space and the parameter space.

2 Information Visualization

Graphical tools for visualizing data or knowledge are very useful for human perception [2]. In order to design and develop an effective IV application, the *visualization process* needs to be carefully defined: (i) raw data are transformed into intermediated representations (*Data transformation*); (ii) transformed data need to be represented by effective visual structures (this phase is called *visual mapping*). Visual structures are characterized by the *spatial substrate*, the *graphical objects or marks*, and the *connection and enclosure* [2]. Finally, (iii) the last step of the visualization process consists of *View transformations*: the visual structures are interactively modified in order to improve the perception of the analyzed data. An effective example of view transformation is *linked brushing*, i.e., the cursor passing over one location creates visual effects to other markers.

3 The DCE-MRI Data Set

Aim of DCE-MRI experiments is to determine non invasively the fractional plasma volume (fPV) of tumor tissue and the endothelial permeability (kPS) of tumor vasculature, accepted surrogate markers of angiogenesis. HT-20 human colon carcinoma fragments were implanted subcutaneously in the flank of 10 nude mice [3]. The dynamic evolution of the Signal Intensity in MR images is analyzed using a two compartments tissue model in which the contrast agent can freely diffuse between plasma and interstitial space. kPS and fPV values are obtained pixel by pixel by fitting the theoretical expression to experimental data. In this work the experiments were performed in order to assess the antiangiogenic effect of a specific drug. Data analysis was adapted from [3] for the special case of a macromolecular contrast agent.

4 Cluster Analysis

In order to reduce manual interventions in identifying different parts of the considered parametric maps, the classic K-Means [4] algorithm has been combined with the Bayesian Information Criterion, aiming at automatically estimating the number of classes K and the derived clusters. The main idea consists of computing different clusterizations by running K-Means by changing the value of K, and use the BIC criteria to evaluate each of them. The implemented procedure is a simplified version of the X-Means algorithm proposed by Pelleg and Moore in [4]: assume we are given the data set D and a family of alternative clusterizations M_j or *models*. Different models correspond to solutions with different K values of K-Means. For example M_2 means the clusterization obtained from the 2-Means (i.e., K-Means with $K = 2$). Furthermore, K-Means can be modelled by spherical Gaussians [4].

A posteriori probability $P_r(M_j|D)$ is used to score the models. In order to approximate the posteriors, up to normalization, the Kass and Wasserman [4] formula is defined as:

$$BIC(M_j) = \hat{l}_j(D) - \frac{p_j}{2} \log R \qquad (1)$$

where $\hat{l}_j(D)$ is the *log-likelihood* of data according to the j-th model and taken at the maximum likelihood point, p_j is the number of independent parameters in M_j and $R = |D|$. The maximum likelihood estimate (MLE) is applied for the variance, under the identical spherical Gaussian assumption [4].

In order to estimate automatically the K value, the K-Means algorithm is performed several times by incrementing the value K. At each computation, the BIC evaluation of the obtained clusterization is calculated. As usual, a gaussian behavior is assumed for the BIC evaluation, so that the maximum is obtained when the BIC value ceases to increase.

5 The Proposed Application: *Visual MRI*

The proposed application, named *Visual MRI*, allows the visualization of different representations of the MRI data set with respect to the selected spatial substrate. Four spatial substrates have been defined: the physical space, the kPS and fPV spaces, and the *joined* parameter space.

- **physical space**: The physical space is a volumetric space. As usual for MRI data set, data are visualized through a 2D image (the *MRI* image) that is obtained by selecting a slice of the whole volume.
- **kPS and fPV spaces**: The considered parameters kPS and fPV, previously described, are derived from the MRI slices applying the pharmacokinetics model introduced in [3]. Two parameter maps are derived that represent the kPS and fPV spaces, respectively.
- *joined* **parameter space**: In order to obtain a joined representation of the kPS and fPV maps, a further parameter space is defined. Two quantitative axes have been introduced (kPS for horizontal and fPV for vertical axis). Then, the physical image has been scanned and for each pixel x_i the two values kPS_i and fPV_i are observed. Thus, after the projection of all the 2D points $p_i(kPS_i, fPV_i)$ the *joined* parameter space is obtained.

According to the proposed IV approach the visual interface of the *Visual MRI* application has been thoroughly designed. The main available options are:

- **parameter map extraction**. The kPS and fPV parameter maps can be extracted by a suitable button.
- *joined* **parameter space projection and clustering**. The joined parameter space can be displayed and clusters are automatically detected.
- **brushing**. The user can switch between the physical and the parameter space. A sort of *bidirectional* linked brushing has been proposed. Indeed, by selecting a region into the physical space, the parameter distribution on the parameter space is highlighted (*straight* linked brushing). On the other hand, by clustering the parameter space, the corresponding regions on the physical space appear (*reverse* linked brushing).

Figure 1 shows an example of the use of the *Visual MRI* application. The tumoral area is manually selected. Figure 1 (left) shows the selected area. Then, the pharmacokinetics model is applied and the parameter maps are extracted (with respect to selected area). Figure 1 (right) shows the two parameter maps.

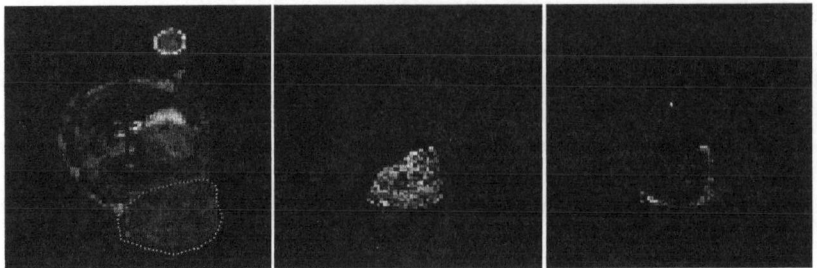

Fig. 1. Selected region by ROI operator (left) and kPS (middle), fPV (right) maps

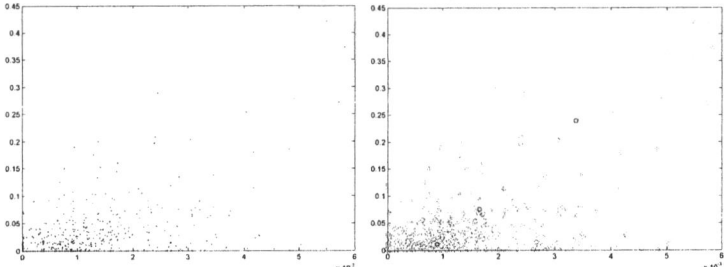

Fig. 2. Parameter space before and after cluster detection

Fig. 3. Tumoral regions detected by the reverse linked brushing

Therefore, the selected region is mapped into the *joined* parameter space and the more significative clusters are collected by carrying out the automatic cluster detector operator. Figure 2 shows the parameter space before and after cluster detection, respectively. This phase realizes a *straight* linked brushing (from physical space to *joined* parameter space). Therefore, selected clusters are reprojected into the physical space by evidencing some slice regions of the cancer area. This phase realizes a *reverse* linked brushing (from *joined* parameters space to physical space). Figure 3 highlights the tumoral regions inferred by the proposed approach: in the present experimental model, cluster analysis provides a subdivision of the tumor tissue in three clusters. The first cluster (left part of Figure 3) contains in general a limited number of pixels characterized by the highest values of fPV. The second cluster (middle part of Figure 3) contains an intermediate number of pixels located in the external part of the tumor. The third cluster (right part of Figure 3) contains most pixels of the image and covers the whole interior of the tumor; pixels belonging to the last cluster are characterized by low values of fPV. It is worth noting that from the medical point of view this is an interesting result since the regions detected by reverse linked brushing correspond to typical subdivision of the tumoral area observed in this kind of tumors by histology [3].

6 Conclusions

In this paper a new application for MRI data analysis is proposed aiming at improving the support of medical researchers in the context of cancer therapy: preliminary results have shown the effectiveness of the *Visual MRI* application for the comprehension of dependencies between the analyzed parameters and the known tumoral regions. The information visualization criteria have been carefully considered and implemented. Furthermore, data mining techniques have been introduced by defining a simplified version of the X-Mean algorithm for cluster analysis.

References

1. J. Bemmel and M. A. Musen. *Handbook of medical informatic*. Springer, 2002.
2. S.K. Card, J.D. Mackinglay, and B. Shneiderman. *Readings in Information Visualization - Using Vision to Think*. Morgan Kaufmann, San Francisco, 1999.
3. Marzola P., Degrassi A., Calderan L., Farace P., Crescimanno C., Nicolato E., Giusti A., Pesenti E., Terron A., Sbarbati A., Abrams T., Murray L., and Osculati F. In vivo assessment of antiangiogenic activity of su6668 in an experimental colon carcinoma model. *Clin. Cancer Res.*, 2(10):739–50., 2004.
4. Dan Pelleg and Andrew Moore. X-means: Extending K-means with efficient estimation of the number of clusters. In *Proc. 17th International Conf. on Machine Learning*, pages 727–734. Morgan Kaufmann, San Francisco, CA, 2000.

Computer Vision and Imaging

Electrocardiographic Imaging: Towards Automated Interpretation of Activation Maps

Liliana Ironi and Stefania Tentoni

IMATI - CNR, via Ferrata 1, 27100 Pavia, Italy

Abstract. In present clinical practice, information about the heart electrical activity is routinely gathered through ECG's, which record electrical potential from just nine sites on the body surface. However, thanks to the latest technological advances, body surface potential maps are becoming available, as well as epicardial maps obtained noninvasively from body surface data through mathematical model-based reconstruction methods. Such maps can capture a number of electrical conduction pathologies that can be missed by ECG's analysis. But, their interpretation requires skills that are possessed by very few experts. The Spatial Aggregation (SA) approach can play a crucial role in the identification of patterns and salient features in the map, and in the long-term goal of delivering an automated map interpretation tool to be used in a clinical context. In this paper, the focus is on epicardial activation isochrone maps. The salient features that characterize the heart electrical activity, and visually correspond to specific geometric patterns, are defined, extracted from the epicardial electrical data, and finally made available in an interpretable form within a SA-based framework.

Keywords: imaging, qualitative reasoning, spatial reasoning, electrocardiology.

1 Introduction

During the last decade, noninvasive functional imaging techniques, such as computerized tomography and magnetic resonance, have increasingly replaced pure anatomical imaging for medical diagnosis as they are capable to provide both very detailed anatomical images and spatio-temporal measures of physiological parameters that characterize the activity of different organ areas. In Electrocardiology, unfortunately, similar directly applicable techniques are not yet available. Nevertheless, the heart electrical function may be noninvasively evaluated by reconstructing spatio-temporal information of the epicardial activity from body surface mapping.

The research effort currently devoted to the development of novel methods for electrocardiographic imaging [1] is strongly motivated by the intrinsic diagnostic limitations of traditional electrocardiograms (ECG's), for which, however, an interpretative rationale is well-established. Infact, ECG's provide only a low resolution projection on the chest surface of the heart electrical activity: on the one hand, due to the distance of the electrodes from the cardiac bioelectric sources, the informative content of the electrical signals recorded on the chest is necessarily weak. On the other hand, when probing is limited to a small number of sites on the chest, as in clinical ECG's protocols, a few electrical conduction pathologies (arrythmias, infarcts, Wolf-Parkinson-White syndrome just to cite some) may remain undetected.

A higher resolution projection of the cardiac electrical activity is obtained by body surface mapping (BSM): electrical potential is simultaneously recorded from a few hundreds of sites on the entire chest surface over a complete heart beat [2]. But, the most of information useful to localize anomalous conduction sites is got when mappings of the significant physical variable values are given, and visualized, as close as possible to the heart where such phenomena originate, and where any necessary surgical intervention has to be extremely focussed.

Thanks to the latest advances in scientific computing, given as inputs (i) body surface potentials and (ii) the geometric relationship between the chest and the heart, epicardial electrical data may be noninvasively reconstructed by using mathematical models and numerical inverse procedures [3, 4]. Moreover, mathematical models are crucial to highlight, through numerical simulation, the links between the observable patterns (effects) and the underlying bioelectric phenomena (causes). Although still progressively being improved, the interpretative rationale for electrocardiac maps defined by expert electrocardiophysiologists with the helpful support of applied mathematicians is significant enough to be actually used. However, its introduction into the clinical practice is not yet at hand because the ability to both extract salient visual features from electrocardiographic maps and relate them to the underlying complex physiological phenomena still belongs to very few experts [2]. Thus, the need to bridge the gap between the established research outcomes and clinical practice.

This paper describes a piece of work that fits into a long-term research project aimed at delivering an automated electrocardiac map interpretation tool to be used in a clinical context. To this end, Qualitative Reasoning (QR) methodologies, and the Spatial Aggregation (SA) approach can play a crucial role in the identification of spatio-temporal patterns and salient features in the map. Let us remind that the application of QR methods is not new in Electrocardiology as demonstrated by a number of automated interpretation tools of traditional ECG's [5, 6, 7, 8].

SA is a computational framework specifically designed for reasoning about spatially distributed data [9, 10, 11], and provides a suitable ground to capture spatio-temporal adjacencies at multiple scales. Its hierarchical strategy in aggregating spatial objects to abstract a field at different levels emulates the way experts usually perform imagistic reasoning and reason about fields, that is (1) searching for regularities, and (2) abstracting structural information about the underlying physical processes. In outline, SA transforms a numeric input field into a multi-layered symbolic description of the structure and behavior of the physical variables associated with it. This results from successive transformations of lower-level objects into more and more abstract ones by exploiting distinctive qualitative equivalence properties shared by neighbor objects. This paper is focussed on activation time maps at epicardial level, as they are a synthetic representation of the spatio-temporal aspects of the propagation of the electrical excitation. It describes how the most significant features that characterize such phenomena and reveal either their normality or abnormality, such as wavefront breakthrough and extinction regions, minimum and maximum propagation velocity, are defined within the SA conceptual framework, abstracted from the epicardial electrical data, and made readily available for reasoning tasks.

2 Describing Ventricular Excitation Through Features Abstracted from the Activation Map

Experimental and model-based studies recently carried out show that the spread of the excitation within the heart is not uniform: both anisotropic conductivity properties and the fiber structure of the tissue affect the wavefront propagation. To investigate this spatio-temporal process electrocardiologists use a well-established parameter that is also important for the diagnosis of cardiac rhythm, namely the activation time.

Definition 1. Let $\mathbf{x}$ be a point of the myocardium $\Omega \subset R^3$. The *activation time* $\tau(\mathbf{x})$ is the instant at which the excitation front reaches $\mathbf{x}$, causing it to depolarize.

Definition 2. An *activation map* is a contour map of the activation time built on a reference surface, where each contour line aggregates all and none but the points that depolarize at the same instant.

Since wavefront propagation is a 3D process, which is quite difficult to be visualized within the volume Ω, activation maps are built on reference surfaces, usually the external/internal boundaries of Ω (epicardial/endocardial surfaces, respectively), but also transverse and longitudinal intramural sections. The activation time can be either experimentally measured by advanced optical techniques, or computed from the epicardial potential data when these are available over a whole beat. Activation maps contain a lot of information about the wavefront structure and propagation: subsequent isochrones represent the wavefront kinematics as a sequence of snapshots. The isochrone distributions are complex, with several distinct areas showing different propagation patterns that the expert analysis may reveal: the locations on the considered surface where wavefront breaks through and vanishes, the local fiber direction, the wavefront propagation pathways, and the regions with high, low or null conductivity. Thus, such kinds of maps have a clear and strong diagnostic value: by comparison with a nominal activation map, anomalous conduction patterns and regions with altered conductivity can be easily detected and classified.

Herein, we consider simulated data obtained by one of the sophisticated mathematical models of the ventricular excitation that take into account both fiber architecture

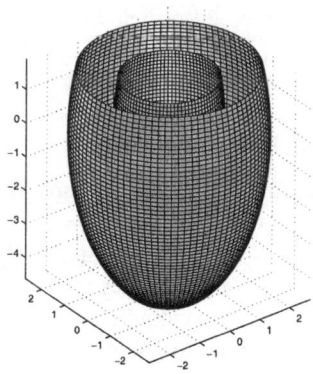

Fig. 1. Model ventricle 3D geometry: the mesh is shown on the most external and internal ventricle layers

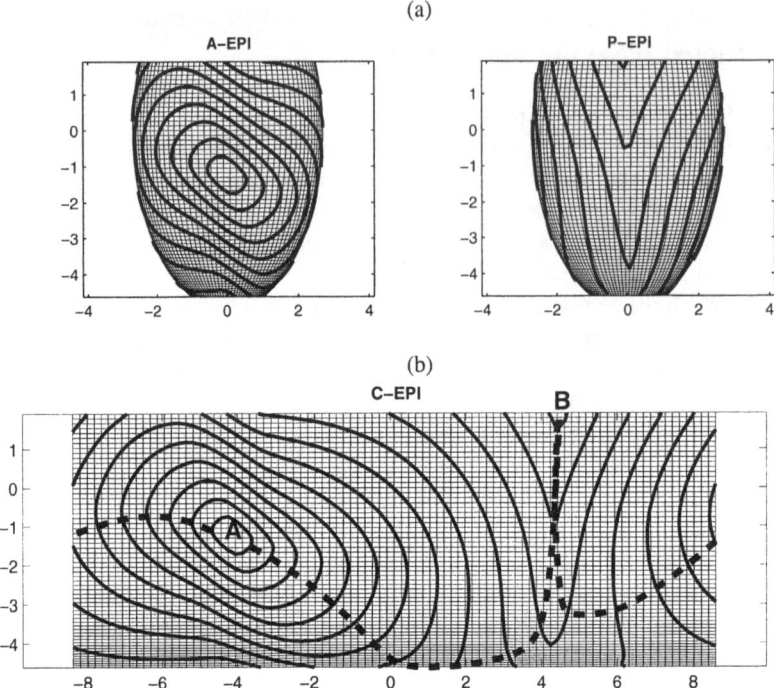

Fig. 2. (a) Anterior and posterior orthogonal projections of the activation map (solid thick lines) drawn on the external boundary of the 3D mesh (thin lines). (b) Cylindrical projection of the same isomap; maximum velocity propagation pathways (thick dashed lines) from wavefront breakthrough (A) to extinction (B) locations are sketched

and conduction anisotropy available in the literature [12, 13, 14, 15]. Figure 1 illustrates a 3D simplified ventricular geometry. Its discretization was carried out by 90 horizontal sections, 61 angular sectors on each section, and 6 radial subdivisions of each sector. A numerical simulation, based on an anisotropic bidomain model of the ventricle tissue, was carried out on this mesh [15], and for each node $\mathbf{x}_i$ the activation time τ_i was computed to provide us with input data.

2.1 The Feature Extraction Problem

Contour lines are the first result from processing the input activation time data. Figure 2 highlights what are the pieces of information that we want to extract from contour maps. Figure 2(a) shows the anterior and posterior orthogonal projections of the activation map on the external ventricle boundary. In order to have a unique global view with minimal spatial distortion, we consider a cylindrical projection of this map (Fig.2 (b)). Reasoning on panel (b), the expert would: i) identify point A where the excitation starts from, ii) identify regions where contours are more scattered/dense as regions where propagation is faster/slower, iii) sketch the maximum velocity propagation pathway towards the site B where excitation vanishes. Therefore, the *feature extraction problem* is equivalent to the following one: given the activation time field, build an activation map, and search for those geometric patterns or spatial objects that characterize salient aspects of the wavefront propagation process. More precisely,

- given in INPUT:
  - the discretized geometry data, i.e. the set of the surface mesh nodes $\Omega_h = \{\mathbf{x}_i\}_{i=1..N}$,
  - the activation data $\{\tau_i\}_{i=1..N}$, where $\tau_i = \tau(\mathbf{x}_i)$,
  - a time step $\Delta\tau$ to uniformly scan the time range $[0, T]$;
- provide as OUTPUT:
  - the sequence of wavefront snapshots: $\mathcal{I}_k = \{\mathbf{x} \mid \tau(\mathbf{x}) = k\Delta\tau\}_k$, $k = 1, .., n_\tau$
  - the wavefront breakthrough region: $\mathcal{R}_b = \{\mathbf{x} \mid \tau(\mathbf{x}) = \min \tau\}$
  - the wavefront extinction region: $\mathcal{R}_e = \{\mathbf{x} \mid \tau(\mathbf{x}) = \max \tau\}$
  - the propagation velocity patterns.

2.2 The Spatial Aggregation Framework

The problem above, i.e. the extraction of both wavefront structure and propagation from raw epicardial data, is solved through a sequence of intermediate representations that gradually identify the geometric patterns, the spatial relations between them, and the global dynamical behavior. The adopted ontological framework is that one underlying the Spatial Aggregation approach: geometric patterns, or *spatial objects*, are built up from a given input field by applying an iterative procedure that transforms lower-level abstract objects, called *spatial aggregates*, into ones at a higher abstraction level. Neighborhood relations play a crucial role in extracting the necessary structural and behavioral information for performing a specific task: on the one hand, intra-relations bind a set of contiguous spatial aggregates into a single object; on the other hand, inter-relations highlight the connectivity and interactions between the spatial objects aggregated at the previous level. The former kind of relation is called *strong adjacency*, and the latter one *weak adjacency*. In outline, the overall process iterates three main steps: *aggregate*, *classify*, and *redescribe*. The aggregate procedure makes the spatial contiguity between field primitive objects explicit by encoding it in a *neighborhood graph* (n-graph). Then, the application of a strong adjacency relation on contiguous elements represented by the n-graph defines equivalence classes characterized by a distinctive property. The equivalence classes are finally transformed into new higher-level spatial objects through the *redescribe* operator. The three steps are repeated until the desired structural and behavioral information is obtained.

The hierarchical structure of the whole set of built spatial objects allows us to state a bi-directional mapping between higher and lower-level aggregates, and, then, it facilitates the identification of the piece of information relevant for a specific task.

3 Extracting Wavefront Structure from Epicardial Data

The isochrone shapes and distributions built on ventricular external and internal surfaces, and on intramural sections, define the wavefront structure. Then, its reconstruction turns into 2D contouring problems.

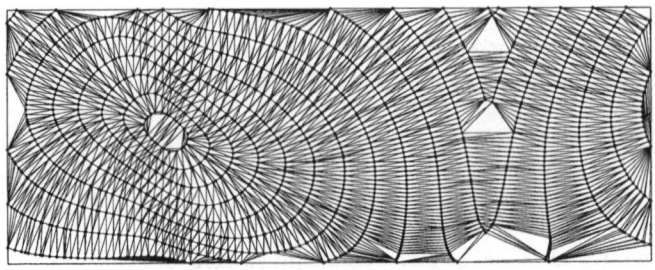

Fig. 3. Isopoints (dots) and their ngraph (thin solid lines)

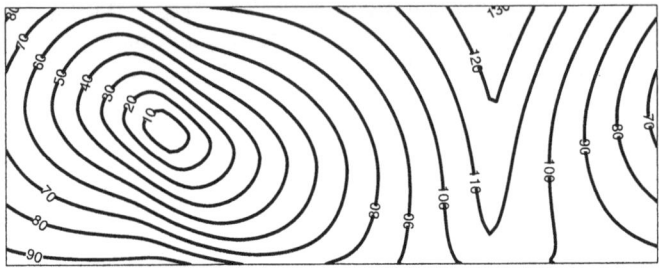

Fig. 4. Isochrones abstracted as strong adjacencies between isopoints

3.1 From Epicardial Data to Activation Isochrone Maps

Proper definitions and algorithms to soundly tackle the contouring task for generic geometrical domains within the SA framework have been given and discussed in [16]. In outline, SA contouring is performed in four main steps:

1. Pre-processing of the activation data to generate the set of isopoints $\mathcal{P}$ for the required levels. The set $\mathcal{P}$ is built by comparison of the values at the mesh nodes with the required levels, and by linear interpolation of mesh nodal values.
2. Definition of the spatial contiguities between isopoints, i.e. construction of the n-graph $\mathcal{N}_\mathcal{P}$ (Fig. 3). The resulting n-graph must ensure that the spatial contiguity of points in $\mathcal{N}_\mathcal{P}$ also respects their nearness in terms of the associated functional values: a Delaunay triangulation is accordingly adjusted to guarantee a proper representation.
3. Classification of the contiguous isopoints represented in $\mathcal{N}_\mathcal{P}$. $\mathcal{P}$ is partitioned into equivalence classes that are built by applying a strong adjacency relation based on topological adjacency properties rather than on a metric distance.
4. Construction of the isocurves (Fig. 4). The equivalent classes defined at the previous step are redescribed as polylines, whose vertices are isopoints and whose edges are instances of the strong adjacency relation holding between them. Let us observe that a single wavefront snapshot $\mathcal{I}_k$ may consist of more connected components $\mathcal{I}_k^{i_k}$ (see, for example, the isocurve labelled 80 in Fig. 4). Thus, $\mathcal{I}_k = \cup_{i_k=1,..,n_k} \mathcal{I}_k^{i_k}$, where n_k is the number of connected components.

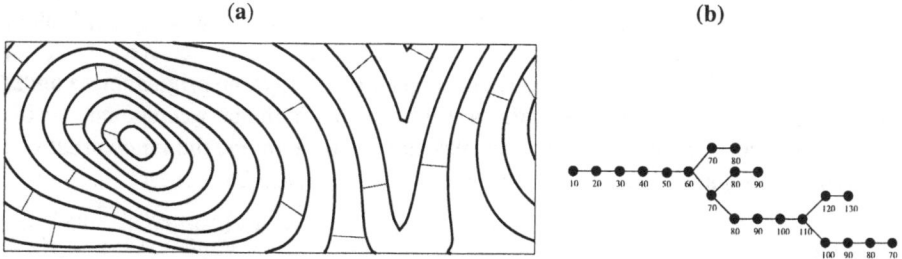

Fig. 5. (a) Spatial, and (b) symbolic representation of $\mathcal{N}_\mathcal{I}$

3.2 Spatial Adjacency Relations Between Isochrones

To identify the salient features that characterize wavefront propagation, steps analogous to 2-4 given above are iterated until the relevant pieces of information are made available at the desired high-level as aggregate objects. Then, after isochrones $\mathcal{I}_k$ have been abstracted by exploiting both contiguity and strong adjacency between isopoints, the next step deals with the construction of a neighborhood graph, $\mathcal{N}_\mathcal{I}$, that encodes curves contiguity. To this end, a straightforward strategy consists in exploiting weak adjacency relations between isochrone constituent isopoints.

Definition 3. Given the set of isopoints $\mathcal{P}$ and their n-graph $\mathcal{N}_\mathcal{P}$, we say that $x, y \in \mathcal{P}$ are *weakly adjacent* if they are contiguous within $\mathcal{N}_\mathcal{P}$ but not strongly adjacent.

Definition 4 (*n-graph of isochrones*). Two isochrones $\mathcal{I}'$ and $\mathcal{I}''$, with respective time labels τ', τ'', are contiguous if:

1) $|\tau' - \tau''| = \Delta\tau$, and
2) there exists at least one couple of isopoints x, y weakly adjacent, where $x \in \mathcal{I}'$ and $y \in \mathcal{I}''$.

Spatial contiguity between isocurves is then represented by $\mathcal{N}_\mathcal{I}$ that encodes any one of these weak connections. Figure 5 depicts a spatial (panel A) and a symbolic (panel B) representation of $\mathcal{N}_\mathcal{I}$. In the latter representation, graph nodes represent isochrone connected components, and edges state neighborhood relations between them.

Let us emphasize that the graph $\mathcal{N}_\mathcal{I}$ encodes both a spatial contiguity relation and a temporal order between isochrones.

4 Extracting Wavefront Propagation from Isochrone Maps

The ordered time sequence of the wavefront snapshots, their velocity properties, as well as the breakthrough and extinction regions are the features that define the wavefront propagation as it is observed on the surface considered.

4.1 Breakthough and Extinction Regions

The *breakthrough* and *extinction* regions where excitation arises and, respectively, vanishes are easily characterized as the subsets $\mathcal{R}_b$ and $\mathcal{R}_e$ of Ω_h which are earliest and last activated.

Let us define a *quantity space* of the time variable: $\mathcal{Q}_\tau = \{\tau_{min}\ \tau_{med}\ \tau_{max}\}$, and a mapping $q : [0, T] \rightarrow \mathcal{Q}_\tau$.

Let us consider the lowest-level spatial objects defined by the original mesh nodes $\Omega_h = \{\mathbf{x}_i\}$. Then, the mesh itself defines the spatial contiguity between points, i.e. the related n-graph, and new spatial objects are abstracted by applying the following strong adjacency relation:

Definition 5. $\mathbf{x}_i$, $\mathbf{x}_j \in \Omega_h$ are *similarly-activated* if they are contiguous within the mesh AND $q\tau(\mathbf{x}_i) = q\tau(\mathbf{x}_j)$.

As a consequence, $\mathcal{R}_b$, $\mathcal{R}_e$ are the redescribed objects that correspond to the earliest-activated (τ_{min}) and last-activated (τ_{max}) classes. In Figure 6 such regions are labelled A and B, respectively. In this case, B is one single point, located on the top edge of the surface boundary beyond the last contour, while A consists of a whole mesh element whose vertices coincide with the sites where the electrical stimulus was applied.

4.2 Propagation Velocity Bands: A Qualitative Approach

As the spatio-temporal progression of the isochrones, encoded by $\mathcal{N}_\mathcal{I}$, is available, we can identify another important feature of the excitation process, that is the wavefront velocity patterns. This is achieved in two main steps (1) by identifying isochrone segments characterized by the same qualitative velocity value, and (2) by classifying them in accordance with their propagation direction. Let us remind that the wavefront motion is a 3D process, therefore the velocity here considered is the wavefront apparent surface velocity along the outward normal to the front. If $\mathbf{x} \in \mathcal{I}_k$, its velocity $\mathbf{v}(\mathbf{x})$ is directed as the outward normal to $\mathcal{I}_k$, and has a magnitude $v(\mathbf{x}) = 1/|\nabla\tau(\mathbf{x})|$, where $\nabla\tau(\mathbf{x})$ is the gradient of $\tau(\mathbf{x})$ and is numerically approximated.

Algorithm 1. *The wavefront fragment extraction algorithm.*

Let us define a *quantity space* $\mathcal{Q}_v = \{v_{min}\ v_{med}\ v_{max}\}$ of qualitative values that velocity magnitude may assume.
For each given isochrone I:

1. Denote by $v(I)$ the velocity magnitude range.
2. Define a mapping $\mu^I : v(I) \rightarrow \mathcal{Q}_v$.

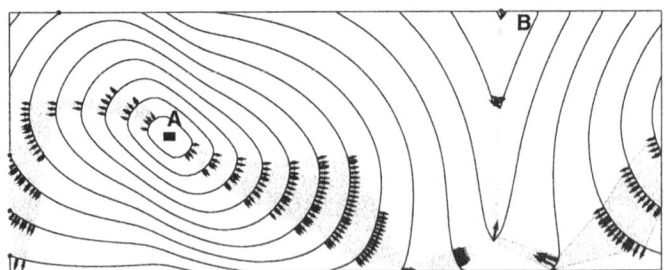

Fig. 6. A, B respectively denote breakthrough and extinction regions. Wavefront fragments qualitatively characterized by v_{max} are represented by the set of velocity vectors plotted in their constituent isopoints. Maximum propagation velocity bands are filled in gray

3. Consider the isochrone constituent points, whose spatial contiguity is encoded by their strong-adjacency graph $\mathcal{N}_\mathcal{P}|_I$, and define the following relation between them:
   Definition. $\forall \mathbf{x}, \mathbf{y} \in I$ contiguous within $\mathcal{N}_\mathcal{P}|_I$, we say that they have the same velocity if $\mu^I v(\mathbf{x}) = \mu^I v(\mathbf{y})$.
4. Apply the above relation, build velocity equivalence classes, and call each new object a *front fragment*.
5. Repeat points 1-4 for all isochrones.
6. Denote by $\mathcal{W}$ the set of all the generated front fragments.

A front fragment is spatially represented by the set of velocity vectors associated with its constituent points. Spatial contiguity of front fragments is inherited from $\mathcal{N}_\mathcal{I}$ and encoded in $\mathcal{N}_\mathcal{W}$ by making each fragment contiguous to all the fragments of contiguous isochrones. Since the constituent points of a front fragment w have the same qualitative velocity value, we can refer to such value as the front fragment velocity magnitude $\nu_w \in \mathcal{Q}_v$.

Algorithm 2. *The propagation velocity pattern extraction algorithm.*

1. Define the *propagation direction* of a front fragment $w \in \mathcal{W}$ as the direction of the vector $\mathbf{u}(w) := \sum_{\mathbf{x} \in w} \mathbf{v}(\mathbf{x})$.
2. Define a *similarly advancing* relation in $\mathcal{W} \times \mathcal{W}$ to highlight velocity homogeneities:
   Definition. $\forall w, w' \in \mathcal{W}$ contiguous within $\mathcal{N}_\mathcal{W}$, we say that they are related if they are advancing in a similar direction and with same qualitative velocity magnitude:
$$\mathbf{u}(w) \cdot \mathbf{u}(w') > 0 \text{ AND } \nu_w = \nu'_w.$$
3. Build equivalence classes and abstract them as new objects, called *velocity bands*.

Figure 6 shows the front fragments qualitatively characterized by ν_{max}, and the resulting ν_{max}-bands as gray-filled regions.

5 Conclusions

This paper focuses on the extraction, from activation time data given in surface mesh nodes, of spatial objects at different abstraction level that correspond to salient features of wavefront structure and propagation, namely activation map, front fragments, and propagation velocity bands. The work is done within the SA conceptual framework, and exploits both numerical and qualitative information to define a neat hierarchical network of spatial relations and functional similarities between objects. Such a network provides a robust and efficient way to qualitatively characterize spatio-temporal phenomena. In our specific case, it allows us to identify the locations where the wavefront breaks through or vanishes, its propagation patterns, regions with electrical conductivity properties qualitatively different. Such pieces of information are essential in a clinical context to diagnose ventricular arrhythmias as they can localize possible ectopic sites and highlight abnormal propagation of the excitation wavefront, such as slow conduction, conduction block, and reentry. With the aim of building a diagnostic tool, more work needs also to be done to identify such phenomena, and to extract additional temporal information from sequences of isopotential maps built from epicardial potential data. Further work will design and implement methods to automatically interpret activation maps, and to compare the features extracted from different raw epicardial data sets, either simulated or measured.

References

1. Ramanathan, C., Ghanem, R., Jia, P., Ryu, K., Rudy, Y.: Noninvasive electrocardiographic imaging for cardiac electrophysiology and arrythmia. Nature Medicine (2004) 1–7
2. Taccardi, B., Punske, B., Lux, R., MacLeod, R., Ershler, P., Dustman, T., Vyhmeister, Y.: Useful lessons from body surface mapping. Journal of Cardiovascular Electrophysiology **9** (1998) 773–786
3. Colli Franzone, P., Guerri, L., Tentoni, S., Viganotti, C., Baruffi, S., Spaggiari, S., Taccardi, B.: A mathematical procedure for solving the inverse potential problem of electrocardiography. Analysis of the time-space accuracy from in vitro experimental data. Math.Biosci. **77** (1985) 353–396
4. Oster, H., Taccardi, B., Lux, R., Ershler, P., Rudy, Y.: Noninvasive electrocardiographic imaging: reconstruction of epicardial potentials, electrograms, and isochrones and localization of single and multiple electrocardiac events. Circulation **96** (1997) 1012–1024
5. Bratko, I., Mozetic, I., Lavrac, N.: Kardio: A Study in Deep and Qualitative Knowledge for Expert Systems. MIT Press, Cambridge, MA (1989)
6. Weng, F., Quiniou, R., Carrault, G., Cordier, M.O.: Learning structural knowledge from the ECG. In: ISMDA-2001. Volume 2199., Berlin, Springer (2001) 288–294
7. Kundu, M., Nasipuri, M., Basu, D.: A knowledge based approach to ECG interpretation using fuzzy logic. IEEE Trans. Systems, Man, and Cybernetics **28** (1998) 237–243
8. Watrous, R.: A patient-adaptive neural network ECG patient monitoring algorithm. Computers in Cardiology (1995) 229–232
9. Yip, K., Zhao, F.: Spatial aggregation: Theory and applications. Journal of Artificial Intelligence Research **5** (1996) 1–26
10. Bailey-Kellogg, C., Zhao, F., Yip, K.: Spatial aggregation: Language and applications. In: Proc. AAAI-96, Los Altos, Morgan Kaufmann (1996) 517–522
11. Huang, X., Zhao, F.: Relation-based aggregation: finding objects in large spatial datasets. Intelligent Data Analysis **4** (2000) 129–147
12. Henriquez, C.: Simulating the electrical behavior of cardiac tissue using the bidomain model. Crit. Rev. Biomed. Engr. **21** (1993) 1–77
13. Henriquez, C., Muzikant, A., Smoak, C.: Anisotropy, fiber curvature, and bath loading effects on activation in thin and thick cardiac tissue preparations: Simulations in a three-dimensional bidomain model. J. Cardiovasc. Electrophysiol. **7** (1996) 424–444
14. Roth, B.: How the anisotropy of the intracellular abd extracellular conductivities influences stimulation of cardiac muscle. J. Mathematical Biology **30** (1992) 633–646
15. Colli Franzone, P., Guerri, L., Pennacchio, M.: Spreading of excitation in 3-D models of the anisotropic cardiac tissue. II. Effect of geometry and fiber architecture of the ventricular wall. Mathematical Biosciences **147** (1998) 131–171
16. Ironi, L., Tentoni, S.: On the problem of adjacency relations in the spatial aggregation approach. In Salles, P., Bredeweg, B., eds.: Seventheen International Workshop on Qualitative Reasoning (QR2003). (2003) 111–118

Automatic Landmarking of Cephalograms by Cellular Neural Networks

Daniela Giordano[1], Rosalia Leonardi[2], Francesco Maiorana[1],
Gabriele Cristaldi[1], and Maria Luisa Distefano[2]

[1] Dipartimento di Ingegneria Informatica e Telecomunicazioni, Università di Catania,
Viale A. Doria 6, 95125 Catania, Italy
{dgiordan, fmaioran, gcristal}@diit.unict.it
[2] Istituto di II Clinica Odontoiatrica, Policlinico Città Universitaria, Via S. Sofia 78,
95123 Catania, Italy
{rleonard, mdistefa}@unict.it

Abstract. Cephalometric analysis is a time consuming measurement process by which experienced orthodontist identify on lateral craniofacial X-rays landmarks that are needed for diagnosis and treatment planning and evaluation. High speed and accuracy in detection of craniofacial landmarks are widely demanded. A prototyped system, which is based on CNNs (Cellular Neural Networks) is proposed as an efficient technique for landmarks detection. The first stage of system evaluation assessed the image output of the CNN, to verify that it included and properly highlighted the sought landmark. The second stage evaluated performance of the developed algorithms for 8 landmarks. Compared with the other methods proposed in the literature, the findings are particularly remarkable with respect to the accuracy obtained. Another advantage of a CNN based system is that the method can either be implemented via software, or directly embedded in the hardware, for real-time performance.

1 Introduction

Cephalograms are lateral skull (craniofacial) X-radiographs. Cephalometric radiography was introduced in research and clinical orthodontics because with skull radiographs taken under standardized conditions, the spatial orientation of different anatomical structures inside the skull can be studied more thoroughly by means of linear and angular measurements [1]. Information derived from the morphology of dental, skeletal and soft tissue of the cranium can be used by specialists for the orthodontic planning and treatment. The standard practice is to locate certain characteristic anatomical points, called landmarks, on a lateral cephalogram. Orthodontic treatment effects can be evaluated from the changes between the pre- and post-treatment measurement values. With serial cephalometric radiographs, growth and development of craniofacial skeleton can also be predicted and studied. The major sources of error in cephalometric analysis include radiographic film magnification, variation in tracing, measuring, recording and landmarks identification [2], [3]. The inconsistency of landmarks identification depends on the experience and training of the clinician.

Automated approaches to landmarks identification are widely demanded, both to speed-up this time consuming manual process that can take up to thirty minutes and also to improve on the measurements accuracy, since both inter-rater and intra-rater variability of error measurements can be quite high, especially for those landmarks more difficult to locate. Since the first approaches to automated landmarking, the major issues that have been pointed out are: 1) the landmarks detection rate, given the great variability in morphology and anatomical structures of the skull, and in the quality of the X-rays, and 2) the accuracy level that the proposed methods are able to achieve. Accuracy is a crucial issue since measurements are considered precise when errors are within 1 mm (the mean estimating error of expert landmarking identification has been reported to be 1.26 mm [4]); measurements with errors within 2 mm are considered acceptable, and are used as a reference to evaluate the recognition success rate, although the former level of precision is deemed desirable [5]. As a consequence of these requirements, the methods proposed so far have been criticized as not applicable for standard clinical practice (e.g., [6], [7]). The novelty of the approach proposed in this paper is the application of CNNs (Cellular Neural Networks) [8], which is a new paradigm for image processing, together with landmark specific algorithms that incorporate the knowledge for point identification. The method is suitable for hardware coding for fast, real time performance. The remainder of the paper is organized as follows. Section 2 reviews previous approaches to automated landmarks identification. Section 3 outlines the fundamentals of CNNs. Section 4 illustrates the developed prototype and the CNN templates that have been used. Section 5 reports the experimental evaluation of the method and discusses the results, by comparing the achieved accuracy with the other methods. In the conclusions, factors that can lead to further performance improvements are discussed.

2 Automated Cephalometric Landmarks Identification

This section briefly reviews the approaches used for landmarks detection. Because not all the mentioned studies report assessment of their method, a detailed comparison with respect to the accuracy and number of landmarks detected, where possible, is delayed to section 4, after our approach has been illustrated.

The first attempts to develop an automatic landmark detection system were based on the use of filters to minimize noise and enhance the image, on the Mero-Vassay operator for edge detection, and on line-following algorithms guided by prior knowledge, introduced in the system by means of simple ad hoc criteria, and on the resolution pyramid technique to reduce processing time [9], [10], [11]. A knowledge-based system, based on a blackboard architecture was proposed in [12]; as in the previously mentioned works, due to the rigidity of the knowledge-based rules used, the results were highly dependent on the quality of the input images. A different approach to landmark detection is based on the use of pattern-matching techniques. Mathematical morphology was used in [13] to locate directly the landmarks on the original images. To make detection more robust and accurate, the system searched for several structures, assured to maintain an almost exact geometrical relation to the landmark. However, these structures can only be determined for a small number of landmarks. Spatial spectroscopy was used in [14]. The main disadvantage of the system is that it applies only a pattern detection step thus false detections can arise far from the expected landmark location, dramatically reducing the system accuracy. Recently, to solve this problem, neural networks together with genetic algorithms have been used to search for sub-images containing the landmarks [15]. A model of the grey-levels around each point was generated and matched to a new image to locate the points of interest. Accuracy of this method was assessed in [6]. Fuzzy neural networks have been used in [16] and in [17] (in conjunction with template matching), whereas [18] have used Pulse Coupled Neural Networks. Active shape models (ASMs) were used in [7]. ASMs model the spatial relationships between the important structures, and match a deformable template to the structure in an image. Accuracy is not sufficient for completely automated landmarking, but ASMs could be used as a time-saving tool to provide a first landmarks location estimate. Similarly, in [19] small deformable models are applied to areas statistically identified to predict landmark position. The method proposed in this paper is based on CNNs (Cellular Neural Networks), which are described in the next section.

3 Cellular Neural Networks

Cellular Neural Networks (CNNs) afford a novel paradigm for image processing [8]. A CNN array is an analog dynamic processor in which the processing elements interact with a finite local neighborhood, and there are feedback, but not recurrent connections. The basic unit of a CNN is called cell (or neuron), and contains linear and non linear circuitry. Whereas neighboring cells can directly interact, the other ones are indirectly influenced by the propagation effect of the temporal-continuous dynamics typical of CNNs. Every neuron implements the same processing functions and this property makes CNNs suitable for many image processing algorithms, by working on a local window around each pixel.

A cell in a matrix of M × N is indicated by C (i,j). The neighborhood radius of the interacting cells is defined as follows:

$$N_r(i,j) = \{C(k,h): \max(|k-i|, |h-j|) \leq r, 1 \leq k \leq M; 1 \leq h \leq N\} \quad (1)$$

CNN dynamics is determined by the following equations, where x is the state, y the output, $u_{k,l}$ is the input and I the threshold (bias):

$$\dot{x}_{i,j} = -x_{i,j} + \sum_{C(k,h) \in N_r(i,j)} A(i,j,k,h) y_{kh}(t) + \sum_{C(k,h) \in N_r(i,j)} B(i,j,k,h) u_{kh}(t) + I \quad (2)$$

$$y_{i,j} = \frac{1}{2}(|x_{i,j} + 1| - |x_{i,j} - 1|) \quad (3)$$

A is known as feedback template and B is known as control template. The parameters of the templates A and B correspond to the synaptic weights of a neural network structure. In equation (2) we must specify the initial condition $x_{i,j}(0)$ for all cells and the boundary condition for those cells that interact with other cells outside the CNN array. Initial state influences only transient solution, while the boundary conditions influence the steady state solution. With CNNs several processing tasks can be accomplished and they can be programmed via templates; libraries of known templates for typical image processing operations are available [20].

A key advantage is that the inherently parallel architecture of the CNN can be implemented on chips, known as CNN-UM (CNN Universal Machine) chips, that allow computation times three orders of magnitude faster than classical DSP and where CNN based medical imaging can be directly implemented [21],[22].

Various CNN models have been proposed for medical image processing. In [21] the 128×128 CNN-UM chip has been applied to process Xrays, CT images and MRI of the brain, in the telemedicine scenario. Aizenberg et al. [22] discuss two classes of CNNs, in particular binary CNNs and Multivalued CNNs, and their use as filtering and image enhancement. Whereas classical solution for edge detection by means of operators such as Laplace, Prewitt, Sobel have the disadvantage of being imprecise in case of a small difference between brightness of the neighbor objects, binary CNNs can obtain precise edge detection, whereas multivalued linear filtering can be used for global frequency correction [22].

4 Cephalometric Landmarks Identification by CNNs

The tool developed for automated landmarking is based on a software simulator of a CNN of 512 × 480 cells, which is thus able to map an image of 512 × 480 pixels, with 256 grey levels, scaled in the interval −1 1, where −1 corresponds to white and 1 to black. Using a fixed resolution allows to make positional considerations useful during the detection process. Compliant input images were obtained from digital or scanned X-rays by selecting an area proportional to the required dimension (e.g.. 1946x1824) and by using a reduction algorithm with a good colour balance (e.g., smart resize), and converting the image to grey scale. The system uses different types of CNNs on the scanned cephalogram: first to pre-process the image and eliminate the noise, then it proceeds with a sequence of steps in which identification of the landmarks coordinates is done, for each point, by appropriate CNN templates followed by the application of landmark-specific algorithms. The tool has been designed to detect 12 landmarks, which are essential to conduct a basic cephalometric analysis: Menton, B point, Pogonion, M point, Upper incisal, Lower incisal, Nasion, A Point, ANS, Orbitale, Gonion, Sella. The tool interface is shown in Fig. 1.

The CNNs are simulated under the following conditions: 1) Initial state: every cell has a state variable equal to zero ($x_{ij}=0$); Contour condition: $x_{ij}=0$ (Dirichlet contour). All feedback templates (A) used in this work are symmetrical, which ensures that operations reach a steady state, although in our approach we exploit the transient solutions provided by the CNNs. For these reasons number of cycles and integration steps become important information for point identification. The tool may run in two modalities: one is entirely automated, in the other one each point can be identified by modifying the input parameters of the CNN (templates, number of cycles, bias and integration step). This latter modality is appropriate for tuning the system, because, for example, X-rays with high luminosity could need less cycles or a less sharpening template. If not mentioned otherwise, we consider bias=0; integration step=0.1; cycle 60. In the following we exemplify the methodology.

Automatic Landmarking of Cephalograms by Cellular Neural Networks 337

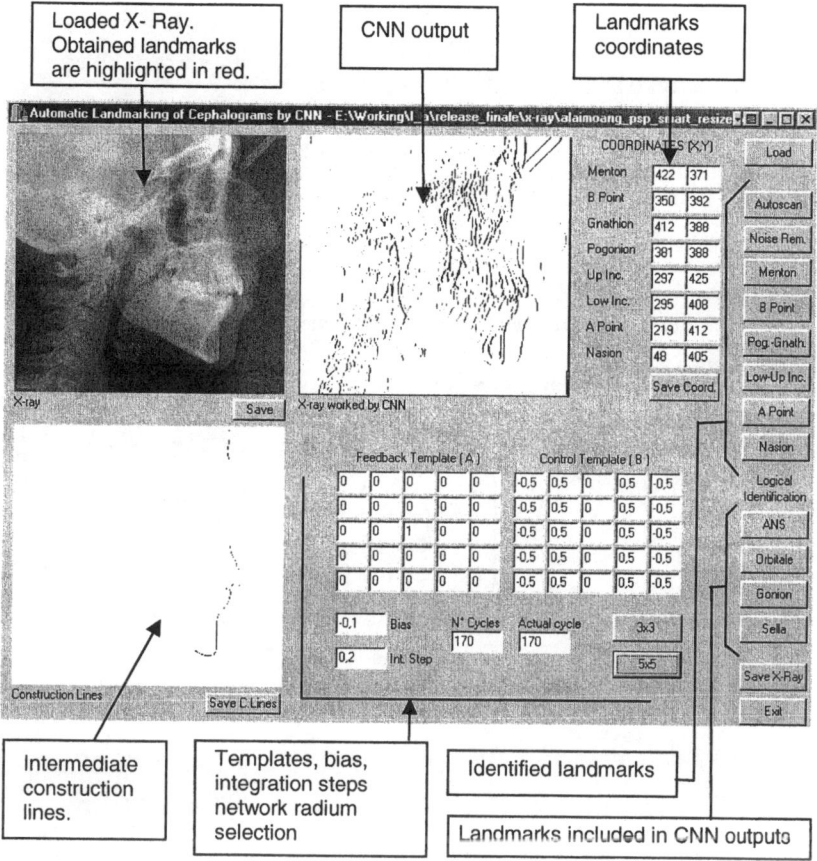

Fig. 1. Tool interface

In order to find the landmarks we used two methods: the first method tries to find the front bone profile and in this line picks up the point of interest: Menton, B Point, Pogonion and M point. With this method, each landmark extraction depends on the previous one. For this reason accuracy becomes worse after each extraction: the best accuracy is obtained for Menton, the worse for Point M. The effect of template application is exemplified in figures 2 and 3, where the used templates and the CNN outputs are reported. For the next four landmarks (Upper and Lower Incisal, A Point and Nasion) the method is different since we try to find each one almost independently from the others. Since the incisors configuration variability is high, in this prototype we have worked with the configuration where the up incisor is protruding with respect to the inferior one. After noise removal two processes are possible: the first one uses the left control template, the second one uses the right control template reported in Fig. 3. In both cases we used bias = -0.1; integration step = 0.2 and 60 cycles. With these templates we try to light up both incisors. The

$$A = \begin{pmatrix} 0 & 0 & 0 & 0 & 0 \\ 0 & 0 & 0 & 0 & 0 \\ 0 & 0 & 1 & 0 & 0 \\ 0 & 0 & 0 & 0 & 0 \\ 0 & 0 & 0 & 0 & 0 \end{pmatrix}; \quad B = \begin{pmatrix} 1 & 1 & 1 & 1 & 1 \\ 0 & 0 & 0 & 0 & 0 \\ 0 & 0 & 0 & 0 & 0 \\ 0 & 0 & 0 & 0 & 0 \\ -1 & -1 & -1 & -1 & -1 \end{pmatrix};$$

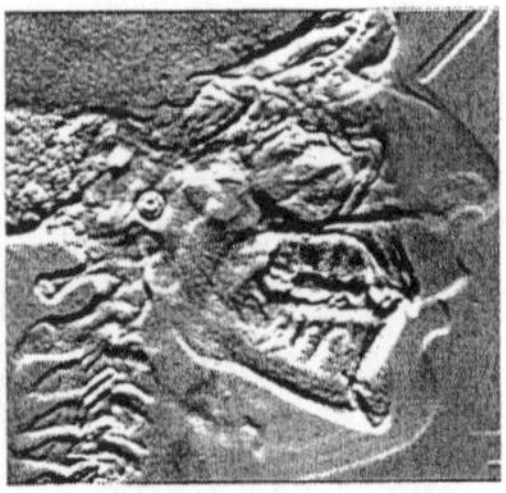

Fig. 2. Templates and CNN output for menton (n.cycles=30)

$$A = \begin{pmatrix} 0 & 0 & 0 \\ 0 & 1 & 0 \\ 0 & 0 & 0 \end{pmatrix}; \quad B = \begin{pmatrix} 1 & 1 & 0 \\ 1 & 0 & -1 \\ 0 & -1 & -1 \end{pmatrix};$$

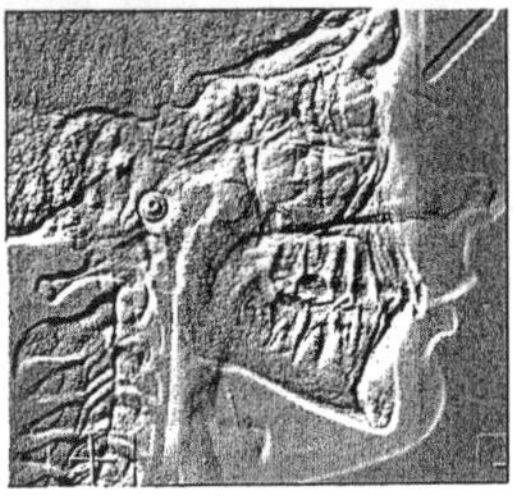

Fig. 3. Templates and CNN output for chin curvature (n.cycles=80)

$$B = \begin{pmatrix} 0 & 0 & 0 & 0 & 0 \\ 0 & 0 & 0 & 0 & 0 \\ 1 & 0 & 0 & 0 & -1 \\ 1 & 0 & 0 & 0 & -1 \\ 0 & 0 & 0 & 0 & 0 \end{pmatrix} \quad B = \begin{pmatrix} 0 & 0 & 0 & 0 & 0 \\ 0 & 0 & 0 & 0 & 0 \\ 2 & 0 & 0 & 0 & -2 \\ 2 & 0 & 0 & 0 & -2 \\ 0 & 0 & 0 & 0 & 0 \end{pmatrix}$$

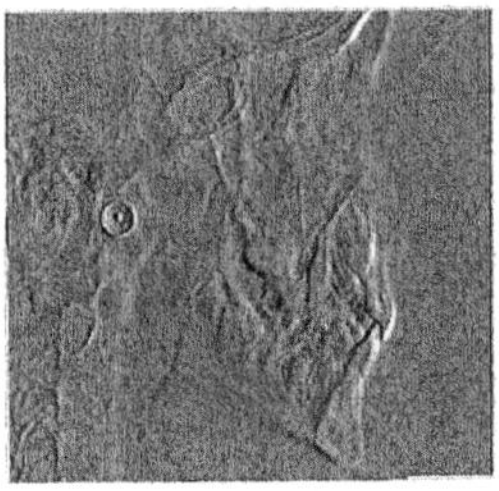

Fig. 4. Control Templates and CNN output for incisors (n.cycles=60)

extraction algorithm used is more robust and more efficient if the up incisor edge is higher than the lower incisor. In order to find Nasion we used four templates (Fig.4). The first two are used for X-ray with a good contrast: the first one when the nasion is in white and the second one when the nasion is in black. The second pair of templates was used for contour sharpening. In all cases we used bias = -0.1; integration step = 0.2 and 60 cycles. To extract A point we started from knowledge of upper incisal, which is a landmark extracted quite accurately. In this case, template selection is guided by a local evaluation of the X-ray brightness. After simulation with the chosen template we used two algorithms to find our point: the decision about which point to choose in this case is left to the user and his or her knowledge of the morphology.

$$B = \begin{pmatrix} 1 & 0 & 0 & 0 & -1 \\ 0 & 1 & 0 & -1 & 0 \\ 1 & 0 & 0 & 0 & -1 \\ 0 & 0 & 0 & 0 & 0 \\ 0 & 0 & 0 & 0 & 0 \end{pmatrix}$$

White template

$$B = \begin{pmatrix} -2{,}5 & 0 & 0 & 0 & 2{,}5 \\ 0 & -2{,}5 & 0 & 2{,}5 & 0 \\ -2{,}5 & 0 & 0 & 0 & 2{,}5 \\ 0 & 0 & 0 & 0 & 0 \\ 0 & 0 & 0 & 0 & 0 \end{pmatrix}$$

Black template

$$B = \begin{pmatrix} 2 & 0 & 0 & 0 & -2 \\ 0 & 2 & 0 & -2 & 0 \\ 2 & 0 & 0 & 0 & -2 \\ 0 & 0 & 0 & 0 & 0 \\ 0 & 0 & 0 & 0 & 0 \end{pmatrix}$$

Sharp White template

$$B = \begin{pmatrix} -3 & 0 & 0 & 0 & 3 \\ 0 & -3 & 0 & 3 & 0 \\ -3 & 0 & 0 & 0 & 3 \\ 0 & 0 & 0 & 0 & 0 \\ 0 & 0 & 0 & 0 & 0 \end{pmatrix}$$

Sharp Black template

Fig. 5. Control Templates and CNN output for Nasion

5 Experimental Evaluation

Twelve landmarks were chosen for preliminary assessment of the prototype, and a set of 97 digital X-rays was landmarked by an expert orthodontist, who consulted with another independent expert on dubious cases. Assessment was carried out in two stages. The first stage assessed the image output of the CNN to verify that it included the sought landmark. This was done by visual inspection from the same expert who landmarked the X-rays. Over 97 cases, 29 cases (30%) led to CNN outputs in which some edges were overly eroded. This implies that the number of processing cycles in these cases needs to be reduced.

The second stage evaluated performance of the developed algorithms for 8 landmarks, on a sample of 26 cases (50%) randomly selected from a new set obtained from the previous one after eliminating the cases that had not been taken into consideration by the algorithms, (e.g., very young patients with deciduous teeth, cases with inverse bite or overbite).

The coordinates of each point found by the program were compared to expert landmarking, and the Euclidean distance of the found landmark from the reference one was computed. Following the standard, points with a distance less than 2mm were considered successfully located. Table 1 reports the findings, specifying for each point the percentage of cases located within 1mm precision, and those falling in the range 1 to 2 mm. To facilitate comparison with other experimental findings the distribution of the points in the surroundings of the valid interval, i.e. from 2 to 3mm, and over, is also reported. To compute the mean error for some points the outliers were eliminated. The error distribution is not normal but highly skewed towards the lower side of the range, however outliers that were within the range typically found in the literature, were left; this leads to a conservative estimation. Thus the overall success rate of our method is estimated in two cases, i.e., a) the reduced sample, and b) the overall sample size. The first one is suitable if some way of automatically detecting outliers is devised, so that the program does not offer a solution instead of offering an imprecise one. Table 1 reports the results.

The overall mean success rate is 85%. Best detection performances were on menton and on upper incisor, and lowest performances were A point and B point. Remarkably, 73% of the found landmarks were within 1 mm precision.

Table 1. Experimental results for 8 landmarks

Landmark	N.	Mean error (mm)	MD	SD	≤1 (mm)	>1;≤2 (mm)	Imprecise cases ≤3 (mm)	>3 (mm)	Success Rate	Success Rate (overall sample)
Upper incisor	25	.48	.25	.60	88%	8%	4%	-	96%	92%
Lower incisor	23	.92	.67	.94	66%	26%	4%	4%	92%	81%
Nasion	24	1.12	.76	1.11	70%	17%	-	13%	87%	81%
A Point	24	1.34	1.06	.82	58%	21%	17%	4%	79%	73%
Menton	26	.62	.33	.82	85%	7%	4%	4%	92%	92%
B Point	24	2.00	.42	3.3	71%	8%	-	21%	79%	73%
Pogonion	26	.87	4.0E-02	1.34	73%	8%	8%	11%	81%	81%
M Point	26	1.25	.33	1.68	69%	8%	8%	15%	77%	77%

6 Discussion

There are some methodological issues that must be taken into account in carrying out a comparison with the findings reported in the literature. There are differences in the sample, in the set of points chosen, and also in the way of reporting. However, some considerations can be done. With respect to the studies that report the error distribution, a major finding of this study is that we have improved detection performance. For example, the study of Liu et al.[6] found that the errors of their automatic landmarking system were statistically different from those made by the expert for identifying A point, B point, pogonion, menton, upper and lower incisal edge. In particular they report the following mean error: A point 4.29±1.56; B point 3.69±1.55; Pogonion 2.53±1.12; Menton 1.90±0.57; Upper incisal 2.36±2.01; Lower incisal 2.86±1.24. With exception of the B point, ours finding are comparable to the distribution of the human mean error reported in the same study; moreover, there is a remarkable difference in the percentage of cases with mean error less than 1mm, which in our case is 73% and in [6] is 8%. Our mean errors are smaller also compared to Rudolph et al. [14], who reports the following mean error: A point 2.33±2.63; B point 1.85±2.09; Pogonion 1.85±2.26; Menton 3.09±3.46; Upper incisal 2.02±1.99; Lower incisal 2.46±2.49. Table 2 summarizes the comparisons.

Table 2. Comparison of the accuracy of approaches to automated landmarking

Work and Ref.	Sample size	N. Landmarks and accuracy	Techniques
Parthasarathy et al. (1989) [10]	5	9 landmarks, 58% < 2mm, (18%<1mm) mean error: 2.06 mm	Resolution piramid Knowledge based line extractor
Tong et al. (1990) [11]	5	17 landmarks, 76%< 2mm mean error: 1.33 mm	Resolution pyramid Edge enhancement Knowledge-based extraction
Cardillo et al. (1994) [13]	40	20 landmarks, 75% < 2mm mean error: not reported	Pattern matching
Rudolph et al. (1998) [14]	14	15 landmarks, 13% <2mm mean error: 3,07 mm	Spatial spectroscopy Statistical pattern recognition
Liu et al. (1999) [6]	38	13 landmarks, 23% < 2mm (8% <1mm), mean error: 2,86 mm	Multilayer Perceptron Genetic Algorithms
Hutton et al. (2000) [7]	63	16 landmarks, 35% < 2mm (13% < 1mm) mean error: 4,08	Active Shape Models
El-Feghi et al. (2003) [16]	200	20 landmarks, 90% <2mm mean error: not reported	Fuzzy neural network
Innes et al. (2002) [18]	109	3 landmarks, 72% <2mm, mean error: not reported	PCNN : pulse coupled neural networks
Our Work	26	8 landmarks, 85%<2mm (73% < 1mm) mean error: 1.07	Cellular Neural Networks Knowledge based landmark extraction

7 Conclusions

There are basically two classes of methods to tackle cephalometric landmark detection: edge-based and region-based. Appraisal of previous works does not demonstrate a superiority of one on the other, rather they have relative advantages over certain landmarks, and indeed integration has been suggested [6]; however, in both cases, precision is not suitable for their application to clinical practice. This paper has shown that a method based on CNNs and landmark-specific search algorithms affords a better, suitable precision. Furthermore, CNNs are versatile enough to be used also for the detection of landmarks that are not located on edges, but on regions, e.g., the Sella, thus the approach is unifying, and lends itself to implementation on a CNN-UM. Future research will be devoted to find suitable templates and algorithms for detection of other landmarks that are used in more sophisticated cephalometric analyses, and to make the overall approach more robust by prior classification of the X-rays based on the morphologies of key anatomical structures, i.e., nasion, maxilla and symphysis, and bite typologies and on classification of the X-rays with respect to brightness. This information is useful both for a targeted selection and/or tuning of the CNN template(s) to apply before launching the landmark extraction algorithm, and for optimization of these extraction algorithms.

References

1. Broadbent, B.H.: A New X-Ray Technique and its Application to Orthodontia. Angle Orthod. 51 (1981), 93-114
2. Kenneth, H.S., Tsang, S., Cooke, M.S.: Comparison of Cephalometric Analysis Using a Non-Radiographic Sonic Digitizer. European Journal of Orthodontics 21 (1999) 1-13
3. YiJ.Chen, S.K.Chen ,H.F.Chang, Chen, K.C.: Comparison of Landmark Identification in Traditional vs Computer-Aided Digital Cephalometry. Angle orthod. 70 (2000) 387-392
4. Baumrind, S., Frantz, R.C.: The Reliability of Head Film Measurements Landmark Identification. American Journal Orthod. 60, 2 (1971) 111-127
5. Rakosi, T.: An Atlas and Manual of Cephalometric Radiography. Wolfe Medical Publications, London, 1982
6. Liu, J., Chen, Y., Cheng, K.: Accuracy of Computerized Automatic Identification of Cephalometric Landmarks. American Journal of Orthodontics and Dentofacial Orthopedics 118 (2000) 535-540
7. Hutton, T.J., Cunningham. S., Hammond, P.: An Evaluation of Active Shape Models for the Automatic Identification of Cephalometric Landmarks. European Journal of Orthodontics, 22 (2000), 499-508
8. Chua, L.O., Roska, T.: The CNN Paradigm. IEEE TCAS, I, 40 (1993), 147-156
9. Levy-Mandel, A.D., Venetsamopolus, A.N., Tsosos, J.K.: Knowledge Based Landmarking of Cephalograms. Computers and Biomedical Research 19, (1986) 282-309
10. Parthasaraty, S., Nugent, S.T., Gregson, P.G., Fay, D.F.: Automatic Landmarking of Cephalograms. Computers and Biomedical research, 22 (1989), 248-269
11. Tong, W., Nugent, S.T., Jensen, G.M., Fay, D.F.: An Algorithm for Locating Landmarks on Dental X-Rays. 11th IEEE Int. Conf. on Engineering in Medicine & Biology (1990)
12. Davis, D.N., Taylor, C.J.: A Blackboard Architecture for Automating Cephalometric Analysis. Journal of Medical Informatics, 16 (1991) 137-149
13. Cardillo, J., Sid-Ahmed, M.A.: An Image Processing System for Locating Craniofacial Landmarks. IEEE Trans. On Medical Imaging 13 (1994) 275-289
14. Rudolph, D.J., Sinclair, P.M., Coggins, J.M.: Automatic Computerized Radiographic Identification of Cephalometric Landmarks. American Journal of Orthodontics and Dentofacial Orthopedics 113 (1998) 173-179
15. Chen, Y., Cheng, K., Liu, J.: Improving Cephalogram Analysis through Feature Subimage Extraction. IEEE Engineering in Medicine and Biology (1999) 25-31
16. El-Feghi, I.; Sid-Ahmed, M.A.; Ahmadi, M.: Automatic Localization of Craniofacial Landmarks for Assisted Cephalometry. Circuits and Systems, 2003. ISCAS '03. Proc. International Symposium on, 3 (2003), 630-633
17. Sanei, S., Sanaei, P., Zahabsaniesi, M.: Cephalograms Analysis Applying Template Matching and Fuzzy Logic. Image and Vision Computing 18 (1999) 39-48
18. Innes, A., Ciesilski, V., Mamutil, J., Sabu, J. : Landmark Detection for Cephalometric Radiology Images Using Pulse Coupled Neural Networks. In H. Arabnia and Y.Mun (eds.) Proc. Int. Conf. on Artificial Intelligence, 2 (2002) CSREA Press
19. Romaniuk, M., Desvignes, M., Revenu, M., Deshayes, M.J. : Linear and Non-Linear Models for Statistical Localization of Landmarks. Proceedings IEEE 16th International Conference on Pattern Recognition 4 (2002) 393-396
20. Roska, T. et alii: CSL CNN Software Library. 1999 Budapest, Hungary
21. Szabo, T., Barsi, P., Szolgay, P. Application of Analogic CNN Algorithms in Telemedical Neuroradiology. Proc. 7th IEEE International Workshop on Cellular Neural Networks and their Applications, 2002. (CNNA 2002). 579 – 586
22. Aizemberg, I, Aizenberg, N., Hiltner, J., Moraga, C., Meyer zu Bexten, E.: Cellular Neural Networks and Computational Intelligence in Medical Image Processing. Image and Vision Computing 19 (2001) 177-183

Anatomical Sketch Understanding: Recognizing Explicit and Implicit Structure

Peter Haddawy[1], Matthew Dailey[2], Ploen Kaewruen[1], and Natapope Sarakhette[1]

[1] Asian Institite of Technology
[2] Sirindhorn International Institute of Technology, Thammasat University

Abstract. Sketching is ubiquitous in medicine. Physicians commonly use sketches as part of their note taking in patient records and to help convey diagnoses and treatments to patients. Medical students frequently use sketches to help them think through clinical problems in individual and group problem solving. Applications ranging from automated patient records to medical education software could benefit greatly from the richer and more natural interfaces that would be enabled by the ability to understand sketches. In this paper we take the first steps toward developing a system that can understand anatomical sketches. Understanding an anatomical sketch requires the ability to recognize what anatomical structure has been sketched and from what view (e.g. parietal view of the brain), as well as to identify the anatomical parts and their locations in the sketch (e.g. parts of the brain), even if they have not been explicitly drawn. We present novel algorithms for sketch recognition and for part identification. We evaluate the accuracy of the recognition algorithm on sketches obtained from medical students. We evaluate the part identification algorithm by comparing its results to the judgment of an experienced physician.

1 Introduction

Sketching is ubiquitous in medicine. Physicians commonly use sketches as part of their note taking in patient records and to help convey diagnoses and treatments to patients. Medical students frequently use sketches to help them think through clinical problems and to facilitate communication with other students when participating in group problem solving. Applications ranging from automated patient records to medical education software could benefit greatly from the richer and more natural interfaces that would be enabled by the ability to understand sketches. Our particular interest in sketch understanding stems from our work on the COMET collaborative intelligent tutoring system for medical problem-based learning (PBL) [12]. COMET provides a collaborative environment in which students from disparate locations can work together to solve clinical reasoning problems. It generates tutorial hints by using models of individual and group problem solving. The system provides a multi-modal interface that integrates text and graphics so as to provide a rich communication channel between the students and the system, as well as among students in the group. While COMET has already proven itself useful [13], it still does not support the full range of interaction that occurs in human-tutored PBL sessions. In particular, it does not support interaction through sketches. From observation of PBL sessions at Thammasat University Medical School we have found that students typically sketch anatomical structures on the white board while solving a problem. The sketches are used to help think through the problem and as an artifact to support communication among the students. Consider the following scenario:

> A group of students in a PBL session is given a problem concerning unconsciousness due to a car accident. One student sketches the brain. Thinking about direct impact to the head, another student annotates the sketch to indicate a contusion in the area where the frontal lobe should be, although the frontal lobe was not explicitly drawn. The tutor understands this annotation and encourages the students to also consider damage to the brain stem by pointing to that part of the sketch and saying "think about what is going on here as well".

Supporting this kind of interaction requires several capabilities. First is the ability to recognize what anatomical structure or structures have been sketched and from what perspective (e.g. parietal view of the brain). Next is the ability to identify anatomical parts of the sketched structure (e.g. frontal lobe of the brain), even if they have not been explicitly drawn. Finally is the ability to understand annotations on the sketch and to be able to effectively use the sketch as a medium of communication in a dialogue. In this paper we address the first two issues. We present a novel approach to sketch recognition that combines the use of shape context matching [3] belongie:shape together with continuous Naive Bayes classification. The approach is robust and is insensitive to scaling. Next we present an algorithm that uses shape context matching in yet another way to identify the parts of the anatomical structure. The algorithm works even if the proportions in the sketch are not anatomically correct and whether or not the anatomical parts have been explicitly drawn. We evaluate the sketch recognition algorithm on a collection of sketches by medical students of various views of the brain, heart, and lungs. Our algorithm achieves a recognition accuracy of 73.6%, far above the baseline random classification accuracy of 12.5%. We evaluate the part identification algorithm by comparing its results to those of an experienced physician. Location, orientation, size, and shape of the parts identified by the physician and the algorithm are in close agreement.

2 Related Work

The last few years has seen a tremendous increase in interest in sketch-based interfaces. Applications include computer-aided design, knowledge acquisition, and image retrieval. Researchers in this area emphasize that the informalness of sketches is important because it communicates that fact that the ideas being represented are still rough and thus invites collaboration and modification.

Clean, precise-looking diagrams created by most graphics programs can produce an impression of more precision than was intended and can lead to a feeling of commitment to a sketch as originally drawn [9, 7]. We now discuss a few systems that are representative of the state-of-the-art.

The Electronic Cocktail Napkin [7] is a general-purpose sketching program that provides trainable symbol recognition, parses configurations of symbols and spatial relations, and can match similar figures. It recognizes a symbol by comparing its features — pen path, number of strokes and corners, and aspect ratio — with a library of stored feature templates. Applications developed using the system include a visual bookmark system, an interface to simulation programs, and an HTML layout design tool.

SILK [10] is a sketching tool for developing user interfaces. SILK recognizes seven basic widgets, as well as combinations of widgets. To recognize a widget, SILK first identifies primitive components using a statistical classifier learned from examples. SILK recognizes four single-stroke primitive components: rectangle, squiggly line, straight line, and ellipse. Once components are identified, they are passed to an algorithm that detects spatial relationships among primitive and widget components. These include containment, closeness, and sequence. SILK finally uses a set of rules to identify widgets from primitive components. In an evaluation with twelve users, SILK achieved a widget recognition accuracy of 69%. SILK supports use of five single-stroke gestures for editing sketches: cross, circle, squiggly line, spiral, and angle (for insertion). Designers can create storyboards by drawing arrows from any screen's graphical objects, widgets, or background to another screen. SILK has a run mode in which it can simulate the functioning of the widgets and the transitions between screens.

ASSIST [2] supports sketching and simulation of simple 2-dimensional mechanical systems. ASSIST recognizes the user's sketch by identifying patterns that represent mechanical parts, leveraging off the fact that mechanical engineering has a fairly concrete visual vocabulary for representing components. ASSIST uses a three-stage procedure to choose the most likely interpretation for each stroke. First it matches the stroke to a set of templates to produce the set of possible interpretations, e.g. circle or rectangle. Next it ranks the interpretation using heuristics about drawing style and mechanical engineering. Finally, the system chooses the best consistent overall set of interpretations and displays this to the user. ASSIST supports editing of the sketch through the use of gestures. At any time during the design process, the user can run a simulation of the design being sketched.

In an effort to attain immediate practical functionality as well as broad domain independence, Forbus and Usher [5] take a very different approach to sketching. Their sKEA system does not address the recognition issue, focusing rather on qualitative reasoning about the spatial relations among objects and on analogical comparison of sketches containing multiple objects. They avoid the recognition problem by requiring the user to indicate when he begins and finishes drawing a new object as well as the interpretation of the object. The interpretation is selected from a pull-down menu.

The work reported in this paper is the first application of sketch-based interfaces to intelligent tutoring that we know of, and also the first in a medical domain other than image retrieval [1]. The motivation behind the use of sketching in medical tutoring is similar to that previously mentioned, namely that sketching supports collaboration and encourages modification. But in addition, sketching in medical PBL is valuable because it gives students practice in recalling anatomical structure. A menu-based drawing interface would not provide such practice. The issues involved in recognizing anatomical sketches are significantly different from those of recognizing design diagrams. Most of the previous work in sketching starts by recognizing primitive components such as lines, circles, and corners. This works fine for domains such as mechanical engineering and user interface design, but anatomical sketches are rather amorphous complex structures which may be sketched with more or less detail. This complexity and lack of a well-defined set of primitive components demands a very different approach to object recognition. Fortunately, the anatomical recognition problem is eased by the fact that by convention 2-dimensional depictions of anatomical structures are only shown from eight standard views. We have five external views corresponding to the sides of a cube: anterior, posterior, superior, inferior, lateral (2 sides); and three internal views corresponding to the three cutting planes: sagittal, coronal, axial. This fact is exploited by our recognition algorithm, described next.

3 Recognizing Structure and Parts

We call our prototype system UNAS[1] for UNderstanding Anatomical Sketches. We divide the task of understanding a sketch into two subtasks: identifying *what* the sketch portrays, then identifying the relevant *parts* of the sketch.

Without constraints, this problem would be extremely difficult, if not impossible. Fortunately, the fact that 2-dimensional anatomical sketches are always drawn from one of eight standard views allows us to cast the problem of identifying what a sketch portrays as a *classification* problem: given an image of a sketch $\mathcal{I}$, find the class $y = f(\mathcal{I}) \in \{1, \ldots, K\}$ to which the image belongs. The set of possible classes corresponds to the set of standard views of anatomical structures, e.g., "parietal view of the brain" and "internal view of the lungs." With enough labeled examples $\{(\mathcal{I}_1, y_1), \ldots, (\mathcal{I}_m, y_m)\}$, it is possible to construct a classifier $\hat{y} = h(\mathcal{I})$ that predicts the unknown true class $y = f(\mathcal{I})$ given a previously unseen $\mathcal{I}$.

Once we assume the class y that sketch $\mathcal{I}$ belongs to, we must then *segment* the sketch into regions corresponding to anatomical parts. Since every instance of a standard anatomical view contains the same parts, the task is well-defined: attach a label $z \in \{1, \ldots, L_y\}$ to every pixel in $\mathcal{I}$. Here the set of possible

---

[1] Unas was the last king of the 5th dynasty of ancient Egypt. The interpretation of the bas-relief scenes on the inside of his tomb remains a challenge to this day.

labels corresponds to the set of anatomical parts normally visible in view y, e.g., "temporal lobe" and "parietal lobe."

In the preliminary experiments reported upon in this paper, we have made the following simplifying assumptions:

- Each image $\mathcal{I}$ contains exactly one anatomical structure, e.g. brain, lungs, heart.
- Sketches may not contain annotations or extraneous parts.
- Each sketch is complete (there are no major parts left out).

In future work, we plan to relax all of these assumptions.

For the classification problem, we take the Bayesian maximum a posteriori (MAP) approach: measure a finite set of features $x_1, \ldots, x_n$ from $\mathcal{I}$ then select the class

$$\hat{y} = \arg\max_y P(y \mid \mathbf{x})$$

where

$$P(y \mid \mathbf{x}) \propto P(\mathbf{x} \mid y) P(y).$$

$P(\mathbf{x} \mid y)$ is the likelihood of feature vector $\mathbf{x}$ given class y, and $P(y)$ is the prior probability of class y. We estimate the parameters of statistical model $P(\mathbf{x} \mid y)$ from training data, and in the experiments reported in this paper, we assume uniform priors $P(y)$. In some contexts, such as a PBL session, however, the priors could be chosen to reflect our prior knowledge that, for example, in a head injury case study, sketches of the brain are more likely than sketches of the lungs.

The MAP classifier just described requires a set of features and a model for the data likelihood. In our scheme, feature x_i for sketch $\mathcal{I}$ is the dissimilarity between $\mathcal{I}$ and template image $\mathcal{T}_i$ according to Belongie et al.'s Shape Context measure [3]. Ideally, the set of templates $\mathcal{T}_i$ contains several examples of each class. Our model for the data likelihood is the well-known Naive Bayes model

$$P(\mathbf{x} \mid y) = \prod_i P(x_i \mid y).$$

The model is "naive" in that it assumes the feature values x_i are statistically conditionally independent given y, even though they generally are not.

Once our Naive Bayes classifier picks the best class $\hat{y}$ for a given input sketch $\mathcal{I}$, the next step is to segment the sketch into regions. Our system first warps the input sketch into correspondence with a pre-labeled *canonical* template $\mathcal{T}_{\hat{y}}^*$ for class $\hat{y}$, assigns labels to sketch points using the labels in $\mathcal{T}_{\hat{y}}^*$, finds the boundary of each region, then labels each pixel in the sketch according to which region it falls into.

We compute point correspondences between $\mathcal{I}$ and $\mathcal{T}_{\hat{y}}^*$ using (once again) Belongie et al.'s Shape Context algorithm [3]. We then use the point correspondences to estimate a mapping between arbitrary points in the sketch and template using the Thin Plate Spline (TPS) model [4]. To identify the boundary of each region, we transfer the labeled points from $\mathcal{T}_{\hat{y}}^*$ to $\mathcal{I}$ then connect those points using a simple traveling salesperson algorithm [8].

In the rest of this section, we describe the sketch classification and segmentation algorithms in more detail.

3.1 Sketch Classification

As previously described, the basic features in our Naive Bayes classifier are dissimilarities between the input sketch image $\mathcal{I}$ and each of a set of template images $\mathcal{T}_i$. The particular dissimilarity measure we use is Belongie et al.'s Shape Context (SC) measure [3]. SC represents a shape as a set of points sampled from the shape's contours. Each sample point is represented by a coarse histogram of the other points surrounding it. To determine the dissimilarity of two shapes, SC first finds a correspondence between the sampled points in the two shapes. Then the total dissimilarity between the shapes is simply the sum of the dissimilarities of the sample points.

For each template image, we convert the raw grayscale or color image to a line drawing then In either case, we randomly sample N_s points from the resulting "edge" image. For each point p_i, we obtain the SC histogram by counting the number of pixels falling into N_b log-polar bins around p_i then normalizing the bin counts (so the sum of the bin counts is 1). The width of the bin template is adjusted to be proportional to the mean squared distance between points, to make the resulting histograms invariant to the scale of the image.

For a new sketch, we perform the same sampling and SC histogram computation steps, then find the optimal correspondence between the sketch sample points and the template's sample points. The dissimilarity between two normalized SC descriptors is the simply the χ^2 test statistic. Given the (square) dissimilarity matrix for the sketch and template SC histograms, the optimal correspondence is the permutation of the sketch points minimizing the summed dissimilarity of the matched points. This corresponds to a weighted bipartite graph matching problem and is solved in $O(N_s^3)$ time using the Hungarian method [11]. Once we obtain the optimal assignment, the final dissimilarity x_i between sketch $\mathcal{I}$ and template $\mathcal{T}_i$ is the sum of the N_s individual point-matching costs.

After computing the dissimilarities x_i between sketch $\mathcal{I}$ and templates $\mathcal{T}_i$, UNAS forms the feature vector $\mathbf{x} = [x_1, \ldots, x_n]^T$, which is then input to the sketch classifier.

UNAS assumes each of the probability densities $P(x_i \mid y)$ used in the Naive Bayes classifier is a Gaussian with mean $\mu_{y,i}$ and standard deviation $\sigma_{y,i}$. The classifier's $2nK$ parameters $\mu_{y,i}, \sigma_{y,i}$ are estimated directly from a training set containing an equal number of example sketches from each class.

Once UNAS obtains the MAP estimate $\hat{y}$ for the class of $\mathcal{I}$, the next step is to segment the sketch into regions corresponding to anatomical parts. We describe the details of the segmentation procedure next.

3.2 Sketch Segmentation

As previously described, the first step in segmentation is to align sketch $\mathcal{I}$ with the canonical labeled template $\mathcal{T}_{\hat{y}}^*$ for class $\hat{y}$. To align the sketch with the template, UNAS first uses Shape Context as described above to find a set of N_s point correspondences $(x_i, y_i) \leftrightarrow (x_i', y_i')$ between the sketch and the template. These correspondences are then used to fit a thin plate spline (TPS) model [4] mapping $\mathcal{T}_{\hat{y}}^*$ to $\mathcal{I}$. TPS fits a smooth function $f_x(x,y)$ mapping the template points (x_i, y_i) to the x coordinates x'_i of the sketch points, and another smooth function $f_y(x,y)$ mapping the template points to the y coordinates y'_i of the sketch points. The fitted functions f_x and f_y model the deformation of thin steel plates constrained to interpolate the observed values x'_i and y'_i, respectively. However, since sampling introduces noise, and the Hungarian assignment method does not attempt to impose any spatial regularity constraints, strict interpolation is not desirable. Belongie et al. [3] introduce a regularization factor into the minimization that penalizes excessively warped transformations. The quality of the final transform can be iteratively improved by repeating the correspondence estimation and transform estimation steps, using the results of the previous step as a starting point. In our experiments, we iterate the process 6 times. The result is a smooth mapping from every point in $\mathcal{T}^*_{\hat{y}}$ to a point in $\mathcal{I}$.

The canonical templates $\mathcal{T}^*_y$ are derived from drawings in medical atlases, for which the ground truth segmentation is known. When we sample and compute the SC histograms for each canonical template, we also associate (by hand) a set of labels with each sampled point. The labels indicate which regions (anatomical parts) each point belongs to. Since the sampled points correspond to edges in the original image, they often delineate boundaries between two regions; in these cases, the points are assigned the labels of both regions.

We initiate the segmentation process by simply copying the labels of the template points (x_i, y_i) to the corresponding points $(f_x(x_i, y_i), f_y(x_i, y_i))$ in $\mathcal{I}$. Now the task is to use these points to compute a closed boundary for each region of $\mathcal{I}$. Under certain conditions described by Giesen [6], solutions to the *traveling salesperson tour problem* (TST) accomplish exactly this task.

We use Giesen's insight for curve reconstruction in UNAS. For each anatomical part label $z_i \in \{1, \ldots, L_{\hat{y}}\}$ for view $\hat{y}$, UNAS collects the set of projected boundary points for region z_i and runs a traveling salesperson algorithm [8] to "connect the dots." The result is a simple polygon approximating the boundary of region z_i in $\mathcal{I}$.

The final step, after the region boundaries have been determined, is to use those boundaries to assign a unique label z to each pixel of $\mathcal{I}$. UNAS tests each pixel for membership in each polygonal region using the technique of segment intersections: if an arbitrary ray from pixel p intersects an odd number of the polygon's sides, it is inside the polygon; otherwise, it is outside the polygon.

This concludes our description of the classification and segmentation algorithms employed by UNAS. In the next section, we describe an empirical evaluation of the approach.

4 Evaluation

We evaluated the sketch classification algorithm by building a Naive Bayes classifier for the brain, heart, and lungs and evaluating its accuracy in classifying sketches. We chose the following eight views:

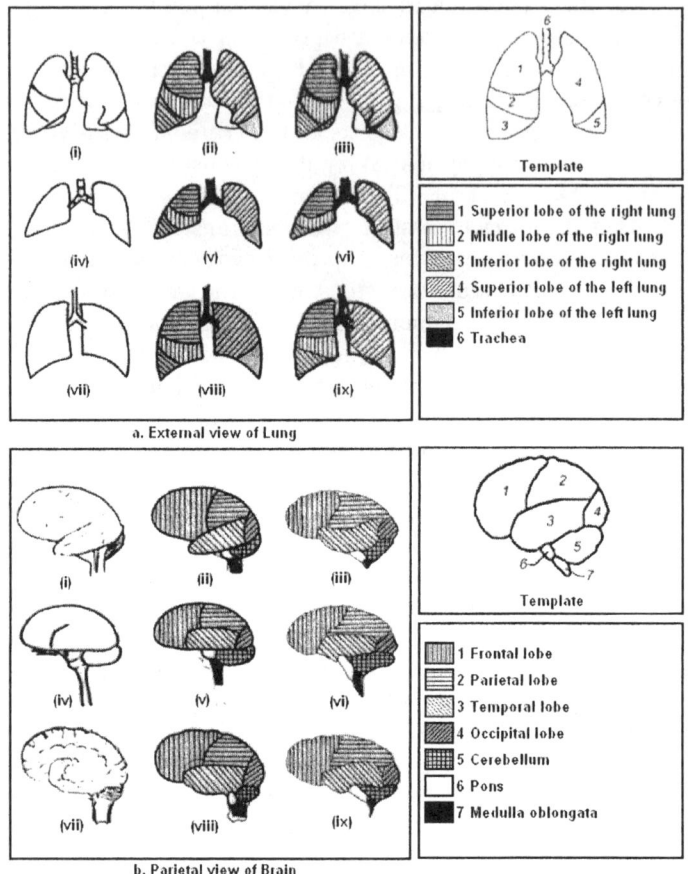

Fig. 1. Medical student sketches (first column) with corresponding segmentations produced by a physician (second column) and by UNAS (third column). The templates used by the segmentation algorithm are shown in the upper right corners

- Brain: parietal (lateral), sagittal, basal (inferior)
- Heart: anterior, posterior, interior (coronal)
- Lung: anterior, interior (coronal)

These views were chosen because they are the standard views from which these organs are typically drawn. We collected 300 sketches from 48 medical students in their second to sixth years of study. The sketches were vetted for quality by a physician and we eliminated those that the physician could not identify. This was done because we do not expect our recognition algorithm to perform better than an experienced physician and because low quality sketches are unlikely to be useful as templates. This left us with 272 sketches. We then chose an equal number of sketches for each view, resulting in 30 sketches for each view or a total of 240 sketches. For each view we randomly separated the sketches into 70% (21 sketches) for training and 30% (9 sketches) for testing. All the 168 sketches in the training set were potential templates in the Naive Bayes classifier. To this set we added six medical atlas illustrations for each view, resulting in a total of 216 candidate templates. The 168 sketches in the training set were used to compute the means $\mu_{y,i}$ and variances $\sigma_{y,i}$ of eight conditional Gaussian distributions $P(x_i \mid y)$ for each candidate template T_i. Using all the templates would result in a classifier with unacceptably slow running time and also may not yield the highest classification accuracy. So we conducted feature selection by performing a best-first search through the space of all subsets of templates. Each subset resulted in a different Naive Bayes classifier, that was evaluated on a validation set, using 7-fold cross validation (to evenly divide the training set of 21 sketches per view). The best performing classifier contained 24 templates. This classifier had a total classification accuracy of 73.6% on the test set, far above the baseline random classification accuracy of 12.5%. The accuracy for each class ranged from the lowest value of 55.6% for the brain parietal and heart posterior views to the highest of 88.9% for the heart anterior and lung external views.

We evaluated the sketch segmentation algorithm by comparing its segmentation to that of an experienced physician on three sketches each of the external view of the lungs and the parietal view of the brain. We chose three qualitatively different sketches for each organ. Each sketch used was correctly recognized by UNAS. The segmentation results are shown in Figure 1. The first column shows the sketches, the second column is the physician's segmentation, and the last column is UNAS's segmentation. The segmentations produced by UNAS and by the physician agree quite closely on all sketches. For example, in the first sketch of the lung (i) the student drew a protrusion below the superior lobe of the left lung that is not normally drawn in the external view. Both the physician and UNAS correctly did not include this as part of the superior lobe. The segmentations produced by UNAS differ from of those of the physician in two primary respects. When internal parts are drawn slightly incorrectly, the physician still segments following the lines in the sketch. In contrast, UNAS attempts to correct the sketch. This can be seen by comparing the superior lobe of the left lung in viii and ix, and the cerebellum in viii and ix. The other difference is that because the thin-plate spline transformation is applied globally, sometimes parts get warped too much, for example the pons in segmentation vi.

5 Conclusions and Future Research

The results from our initial prototype system are encouraging but much work remains to be done in order to realize the functionality described in our motivating example. We are currently gathering sample sketches of more anatomical structures to expand the scope of UNAS. We also plan to compare the recognition accuracy and segmentation results of UNAS to those of physicians with varying levels of experience. On the algorithm side, several improvements and extensions can be made. The accuracy of the recognition algorithm can be improved. A first step is to use a more sophisticated search for feature selection since the feature space seems to contain many local maxima. A next step is to relax the Gaussian assumption in the Naive Bayes model, but this will require more examples. Other machine learning techniques that direclty use similarity information, such as support vector machines with similarity kernels, are promising and should be tried. We have assumed that a sketch includes only one anatomical structure but sketches often contain multiple structures as well as incompletely drawn structures. Generalizing our approach to handle this will possibly require adding spatial reasoning abilities. In addition to understanding the sketch, UNAS should be able to understand annotations commonly used in medicine, such as arrows, circles, crosses, darkened regions, and clusters of dots. For this we are exploring the use of hidden Markov models, which tend to work well for such relatively simple symbols. The final step will be to integrate UNAS into the COMET intelligent tutoring system.

References

1. Dean, D., Buckley, P., Bookstein, F., Kamath, J., Kwon, D., Friedman, L., Lys, C.: Three dimensional MR-based morphometric comparison of schizophrenic and normal cerebral ventricles. Vis. In Biom. Computing, Lecture Notes in Comp. Sc., pp. 363-372, 1996.
2. Styner, M., Gerig, G., Pizer, S., and Joshi, S.: Automatic and robust computation of 3D medial models incorporating object variability. International Journal of Computer Vision 55(2/3), pp. 107-122, 2003.
3. Brechbuhler, C., Gerig, G. and Kubler, O.: Parameterization of closed surfaces for 3D shape description. Computer Vision, Graphics, Image Processing: Image Understanding, Vol. 61, pp. 154-170, 1995.
4. Kelemen, A., Szekely, G., Gerig, G.: Elastic Model based Segmentation of 3D Neuroradiological Data Sets. IEEE Transaction on Med. Im., Vol. 18, No. 10, pp. 823-839, 1999.
5. Geric, G.: http://www.cs.unc.edu/~gerig/pub.html.
6. Gibson, SFF., Mirtich, B.: A survey of deformable modeling in computer graphics. MERL-A Mitsubishi Electric Research Laboratory, TR-97-19, 1997.
7. McInerney, T., Terzopoulos, D.: Deformable models in medical images analysis: a survey. Medical Image Analysis, Vol. 1, No. 2, pp. 91-108, 1996.
8. Fisher, R. A.: The use of multiple measurements in taxonomic problems. Annals of Eugenics, Vol. 7, pp. 179-188, 1936.
9. Vapnik, V. N.: The Nature of Statistical Learning Theory, Springer, 1995.
10. Karabassi, E. A., Papaioannou, G. and Theoharis, T.: A Fast Depth-Buffer-Based Voxelization Algorithm. Journal of Graphics Tools, ACM, Vol. 4, No. 4, pp. 5-10, 1999.
11. Choi, S.M., Kim, M.H.: Shape Reconstruction from Partially Missing Data in Modal Space. Computers & Graphics, Vol. 26, No. 5, pp. 701-708, 2002.
12. Bathe, K.: Finite Element Procedures in Engineering Analysis. Prentice-Hall: Englewood Cliffs, NJ.
13. Zhang, Z.: Iterative point matching for registration of freeform curves and surfaces. International Journal of Computer Vision, Vol. 13, No.2, pp. 119-152, 1994.

Morphometry of the Hippocampus Based on a Deformable Model and Support Vector Machines

Jeong-Sik Kim[1], Yong-Guk Kim[1], Soo-Mi Choi[1], and Myoung-Hee Kim[2]

[1] School of Computer Engineering, Sejong University, Seoul, Korea
smchoi@sejong.ac.kr
[2] Dept. of Computer Science and Engineering,
Ewha Womans University, Seoul, Korea
mhkim@ewha.ac.kr

Abstract. This paper presents an effective representation scheme for the statistical shape analysis of the hippocampal structure and its shape classification: Morphometry of the hippocampus. The deformable model based on FEM (Finite Element Method) and ICP (Iterative Closest Point) algorithm allows us to represent parametric surfaces and to normalize multi-resolution shapes. Such deformable surfaces and 3D skeletons extracted from the voxel representations are stored in the Octree data structure. And, it will be used for the hierarchical shape analysis. We have trained SVM (Support Vector Machine) for classifying between the control and patient groups. Results suggest that the presented representation scheme provides various level of shape representation and SVM can be a useful classifier in analyzing the statistical shape of the hippocampus.

1 Introduction

Anatomical structure of the hippocampus in the human brain provides important information for the medical diagnosis. For instance, it is known that an abnormal shape of the hippocampus involves with neurological diseases such as epilepsy, schizophrenia, and Alzheimer's diseases [1]. In order to estimate shape deformation of the hippocampus by computer, it is essential to select an efficient shape representation scheme. Then, a powerful classifier is used to discriminate a patient group from the normal one.

In general, there are two approaches for the 3D shape analysis of the hippocampus: the global and local methods. The former approach focuses on the volume changes of the whole area of the 3D shape, and then investigates the correlation between the shape changes and its neurological disease. The latter approach is often adopted in planning a surgery and diagnosing a certain disease that may be related to the hippocampus 3D shape abnormality.

Often, 3D shape of the human organ is analyzed according to the skeleton-based description such as Medial Representation (M-rep) [2] or the surface-based representation such as Spherical Harmonic basis function (SPHARM) [3], which represents spherical topology of the shape and acquires a hierarchical description of the parametric surfaces. However, this representation scheme can be applied to only the object with a spherical structure. Gerig et al., have done numerous studies (see [5] for the list), identifying statistical shape abnormalities of different neuroanatomical structures using SPHARM and M-rep.

It seems that the parameterized model is useful for the statistical analysis of the shape since it is able to represent the global as well as the local shapes. Such model is constructed by using a deformable modeling. Several attempt to reconstruct the shape of objects and to track their motion [6,7] are based on physics-based deformable models. The merit of such approaches stems not only from their ability to exploit knowledge about physics to disambiguate input data, but also from their capacity to interpolate and smoothen raw data based on prior assumptions on material properties, noise and so on.

Once, the 3D shape of any organ is represented according to the above methods, we need to discriminate its shape normality using the machine learning method, by which one can train a classifier that able to discriminate between the control and abnormal groups. Such classifiers can be categorized into 1) parametric vs. non-parametric and 2) linear vs. non-linear. The most commonly used algorithm is the PCA (Principle Components Analysis) algorithm, which is a linear classifier. Similarly, FLD (Fisher Linear Discriminant) [8] is a linear and parametric classifier. Artificial Neural network based on back-propagation algorithm can be adopted as an effective non-linear classifier. Recently, SVM (Support Vector Machine) [9] turn out to be a powerful classifier since it guarantees to converge to an optimal solution even for small set of training sample.

In this paper, we use a deformable model for accurate similarity estimation for the global shape changes of the hippocampus, and the skeleton extracted from the hippocampal volume is used for the local shape analysis. Then, SVM will be adopted for an accurate classification method between normal controls and neurological patients.

The rest of this paper is organized as follows. Section 2 describes the surface and skeletal representation for 3D shape analysis of hippocampal structures and Section 3 shows the hierarchical shape similarity. Section 4 illustrates the implementation of the SVM-based classifier. Experimental results and discussion are given in Section 5 and some conclusions and future works are given in Section 6.

2 The Surface and Skeleton Representation for Shape Analysis

In this section, we describe how to represent the shape of the hippocampal structure based on a deformable model and skeletal representation. Initially, we segment the hippocampal structure from the MRI of the brain. Then, we reconstruct the deformable model by fitting to the surface points extracted from the images. The 3D skeletal representation is generated by using depth-buffer based voxelization [10], which makes easier to extract a skeleton as well as relate to the original medical images. Both representations are used for the measurement of shape similarity explained in Section 3.

2.1 The Deformable Surface Representation

The procedure for creating the deformable model for the hippocampal structure is illustrated in Fig. 1.

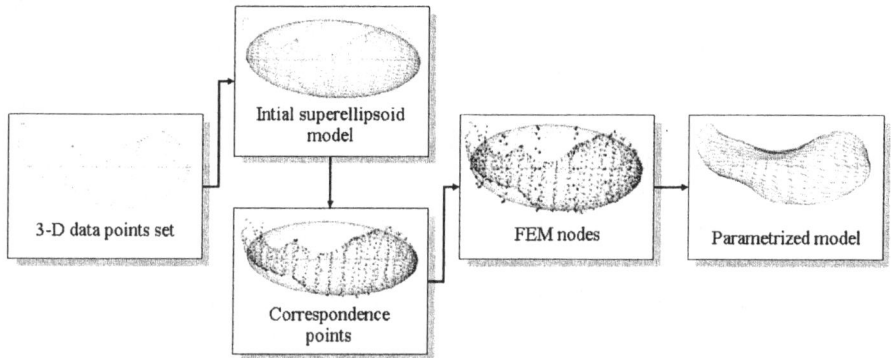

Fig. 1. Overall procedure for creating the deformable model

First, we find the center of mass of the hippocampal structure and its principal axes of the surface points. Then we create an initial superellipsoid and triangulate it. Here, we use a single 3D blob element proposed as suggested in [11]. This element has the same size and orientation as the initial reference shape. The triangulation is carried out with the desired resolution and then we adopt the vertices of meshes to the FEM nodes. Using Galerkin's surface interpolation approach [12], we can find the relationship between the blob element's displacements at any point and the nodal point displacements. It alleviates problems caused by irregular sampling of feature points. We use a 3D Gaussian function as a shape function. The function allows us to generate the efficient deformed shape with an iterative way. Eq. (1) is the 3D Gaussian basis interpolation functions:

$$h_i(x,y,z) = \sum_{k=1}^{n} q_{ik} g_k(x,y,z), g_i(x,y,z) = e^{-[(x-x_i)^2/2\sigma_x^2 + (y-y_i)^2/2\sigma_y^2 + (z-z_i)^2/2\sigma_z^2]} \tag{1}$$

where n is the number of FEM nodes and q_{ik} is the coefficient satisfying the property of interpolation function [12].

In order to achieve the physics-based shape deformation, we compute the mode shape vectors which are derived from the equilibrium equation for simulating the dynamic behavior of an object, and here they are the generalized eigenvectors of the dynamic equilibrium equation without damping:

$$MU'' + KU = 0, \ U = \phi \sin w(t - t_0) \tag{2}$$

where U is a $3n \times 1$ vector of the $(\Delta x, \Delta y, \Delta z)$ displacements of the n nodal points relative to the object's center of mass. ϕ, t, t_0 is the vector of order n, the time variable, and the time constant, respectively. w is a constant identified to represent the frequency vibration of the vector ϕ. M and K are $3n \times 3n$ matrices describing the mass and material stiffness, respectively. Eq. (2) may be interpreted as assigning a certain mass to each nodal point and a certain material stiffness between nodal points without damping. 3D mass matrix M can be computed directly from the interpolation matrix H and ρ is the mass density. The 3D stiffness matrix K is calculated by Eq. (3) where B is the strain displacement matrix and C is the material matrix. The strain displacement matrix B is obtained by appropriately differentiating and combining rows of the element interpolation matrix H. The material matrix C expresses the material's particular stress-strain law.

$$M = \int_V \rho H^T H \, dV \quad and \quad K = \int_V B^T C B \, dV \qquad (3)$$

Eq. (2) can be transformed into a form that is not only less costly but also allows a closed-form solution by mode superposition. To diagonalize the equation, the modal matrix Φ is used. U is transformed into modal displacements $\widetilde{U}$ by $U = \Phi \, \widetilde{U}$. Because M and K are normally symmetric positive definite, they can be diagonalized by Φ.

The mode shape vectors form an orthogonal object-centered coordinate system for describing feature locations. We transform the mode shape vectors into nodal displacement vectors and iteratively compute the new position of the points on the deformable model using 3D Gaussian interpolation functions. We can get the final deformed positions if the energy value is below the threshold or the iteration count is over the threshold.

2.2 The 3D Skeletal Representation

3D skeletonization is a process for replacing the complex 3D model with the discrete structure including the low level representation. Since the multiresolution skeletons are extracted from intermediate binary voxels using depth-buffers [10], it is relatively easy to extract a skeleton as well as to compare to the original medical image.

Our method consists of four steps. First, we divide a voxel space into 2D slices along the y-axis. At this time, we compute the centroid of the object boundary for each slice, and then we interpolate the initial centroids in order to generate skeleton points which each point has uniform distance. Finally, we fit the skeleton and the mesh model using the skeleton normalization method. Fig. 2 shows the algorithm for the skeletonization process. In Fig. 3, (a) is the depth buffer images (or depth-maps). A depth buffer image is generated for each face of the bounding box of a 3D model by parallel-projecting the object onto it. The left two columns are six depth-maps of the left hippocampus of a normal control and the right two columns are six depth-maps of an epileptic patient. Fig 3 (b) shows the binary voxel images of the left hippocampus of a normal

Step 1. Divide 3D voxel space into n slices along y-axis (y is the longest axis).
Step 2. For each slice S_i,
1) Compute a center point C_i from the object boundary of each slice.
2) Consider C_i as an element of the skeleton, and then store it.
Step 3. For each pair of skeletal points (C_i, C_j) // $j=i+1$ ($0 \leq i \leq n-1$)
1) Compute Euclidean_Dist(C_i, C_j).
2) If(Euclidean_Dist$(C_i, C_j) >$ *threshold*) Interpolate (C_i, C_j) using *threshold*

Fig. 2. The algorithm for the skeletonization process

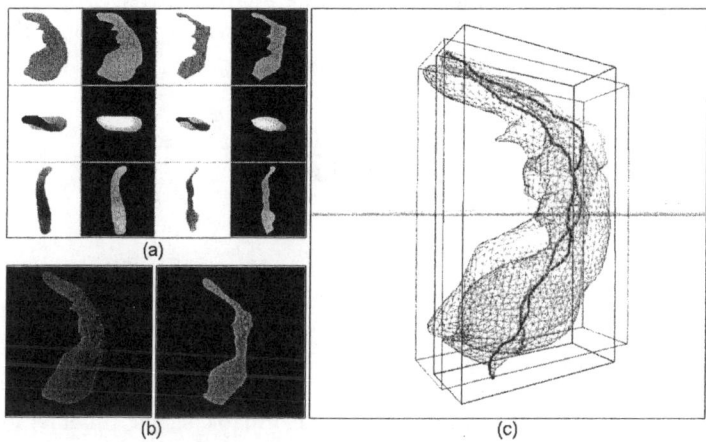

Fig. 3. The result of the skeletonization of the hippocampus: (a) depth-maps; (b) binary voxels; (c) superimposition of the surface models and the skeletons

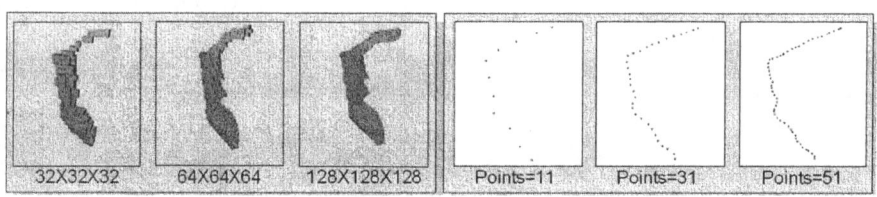

(a) multiresolutional voxels   (b) multiresolutional skeletons

Fig. 4. The result of multiresolutional voxels and skeletons

control (left) and an epileptic patient (right), respectively. Fig 3 (c) shows the result of comparing two surface models of the hippocampus with its skeletons.

In order to reduce the computation time for constructing the shape representation as well as for estimating the shape similarity, the multi-resolution approach to the voxels and skeletons representation is useful. As we specify the resolution of the skeleton or voxels, we can get multi-resolution representations. That result is shown in Fig. 4.

3 The Hierarchical Shape Similarity

To reduce the computation time for the similarity estimation and to capture the local shape difference with a hierarchical fashion, the deformable surface and skeletal represenations are integrated by the Octree structure. The Octree is a data structure to represent objects in 3D space, automatically grouping them hierarchically and avoiding the representation of empty portion of the space. Given the reconstructed parametric representation, it has to be placed into a canonical coordinate system, where the position, orientation are normalized.

To normalize the position and rotation, we adapt the Iterative Closest Point (ICP) algorithm proposed by Zhang et al. [13] in which they apply a free-form curve representation to the registration process.

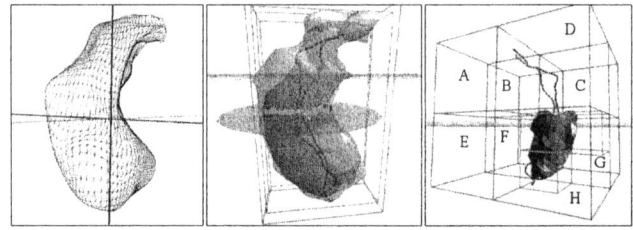

Fig. 5. Shape similarity estimation: (left) the deformable shape; (middle) local shape similarity using skeleton point picking; (right) Octree-based hierarchical similarity

After normalizing the shape, we estimate the shape difference by computing the distance for the sample meshes extracted from the deformable meshes using the L_2 norm metric. The L_2 norm is a metric to compute the distance between two 3D points by Eq. (4), where x and y represents the centers of corresponding sample meshes.

$$L_2(x,y) = \left(\sum_{i=0}^{k} |x_i - y_i|^2 \right)^{\frac{1}{2}} \quad (4)$$

Fig. 5 shows the results of shape similarity computation between the hippocampal structures of a normal control and an epilepsy patient. Fig. 5 (left) shows the parametric representation of the hippocampus. Fig. 5 (middle) and (right) show how to compare two hippocampal shapes based on the proposed Octree and skeletal scheme. It is possible to reduce the computation time in comparing two 3D shapes by picking a certain skeletal point (Fig. 5(middle)) or by localizing an Octree node (Fig. 5(right)) from the remaining parts. It is also possible to analyze the more detail region by expanding the resolution of the Octree, since it has a hierarchical structure. The result of shape comparison is displayed on the surface of the target object using color-coding.

4 An SVM-Based Classifier

Once the feature vectors are extracted from the deformable model, they can be used to analyze the shape differences between populations, for example, normal controls and epilepsy patients. In this section, we briefly describe our approach based on discriminative modeling method using SVM [9]. First, we train a classifier for labeling new examples into one of the two groups. Each training data set is composed of coordinates for the deformable meshes. We then extract an explicit description for the differences between two groups captured by the classifier. This method is to detect statistical differences between two populations. In order to acquire the optimal solution, it is important to select a good classifier function. SVM is known to be robust and free from the over-fitting problem.

Given a training data set $\{(x_k, y_k), 1 \leq k \leq n\}$, where x_k are observations and y_k are corresponding groups, and a kernel function $K : \mathbb{R}^n \times \mathbb{R}^n \mapsto \mathbb{R}$, the SVM classification function :

$$y_k(x) = \sum_{k=1}^{n} a_k y_k K(x, x_k) + b \qquad (5)$$

where the coefficients a_k and b are determined by solving a quadratic optimization problem that is constructed by maximizing the margin between the two classes. For the non linear classification, we employ the commonly used Polynomial Function $K(x, x_k) = (x \cdot x_k + 1)^d$ (where the kernel K of two objects x and x_k is the inner product of their vectors in the feature space, parameter d is the degree of polynomial). In order to estimate the accuracy of the resulting classifier and decide the optimal parameters in the non-linear case, we use cross-validation. To obtain error, recall, and precision, we evaluate the performances for three types of SVM kernels (i.e. polynomial, RBF, sigmoid) and the linear case. Results are described in Section 5.

5 Experimental Results

In order to analyze whether the 3D hippocampus shape extracted from MR brain images is included in normal controls or epilepsy patients. First, we have experimented with the reconstruction method on points clouds obtained from the meshes. A surface representation is acquired through the marching cube algorithm. The deformable modeling algorithm is applied for the 3D meshes models. We implemented the SVM-based classifier and estimated its performance. For these experiments, we collected two template 3D models (normal control and epileptic patient) from the real MRI. And we also generate 80 deformed models using a modeling tool.

To estimate the capacity of our deformable modeling method, we constructed 80 deformed models. Fig. 6 shows hippocampus shapes reconstructed with the different number of vibration modes. Our method is robust to model non-distributed model. Fig. 7 shows the result of the deformable models generated by different iteration stage.

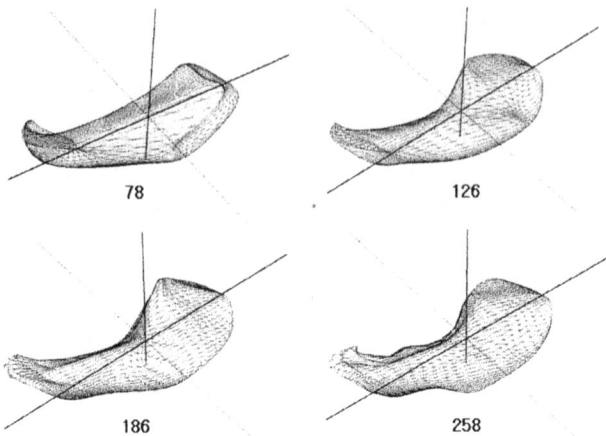

Fig. 6. The deformable model reconstruction of the hippocampus depending on the vibration modes

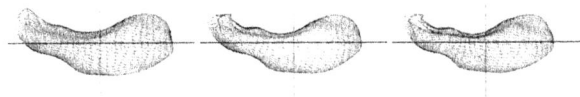

Fig. 7. The result of the deformable models generated by different iteration stage: (left) iteration=1; (middle) iteration=2; (right) iteration=3

We measured 80 Euclidean distances between skeleton points and sampled surface points as a feature vector set for discriminating between normal hippocampus group and epilepsy hippocampus group. In our experiment, 80 training sets are composed of 40 normal cases and 40 abnormal cases. In order to implement the SVM classifiers, four kernels were tested; linear, RBF, polynomial, sigmoid functions. The cross-validation technique is used in order to overcome the problem of small training sets. So we were able to execute 10 learning and 10 test processes from 80 training sets (learning: 72 cases, testing: 8 cases). Fig. 8 illustrates the result of the training test for four different kernels. Results suggest that the polynomial kernel outperformed the others.

Table 1 summarizes the result of local shape differences by comparing the 3D shapes between the reference models (P_L and N_R) and deformed targets (T1~T4), respectively. P_L is an abnormal left hippocampus in epilepsy and N_R is a normal right hippocampus. As shown in Fig. 5, we are able to evaluate the qualitative result of the shape difference at specific region and to control the hierarchical analysis using the Octree structure (i.e. upper-front-right, bottom-front-left, upper-back-left, and the bottom region, respectively). In Fig. 5(right), we can confirm that the node H of the Octree can be divided into detailed regions and be analyzed in hierarchical fashion. In Table 1, the values in bold type represent the significantly deformed area of the hippocampus model and so

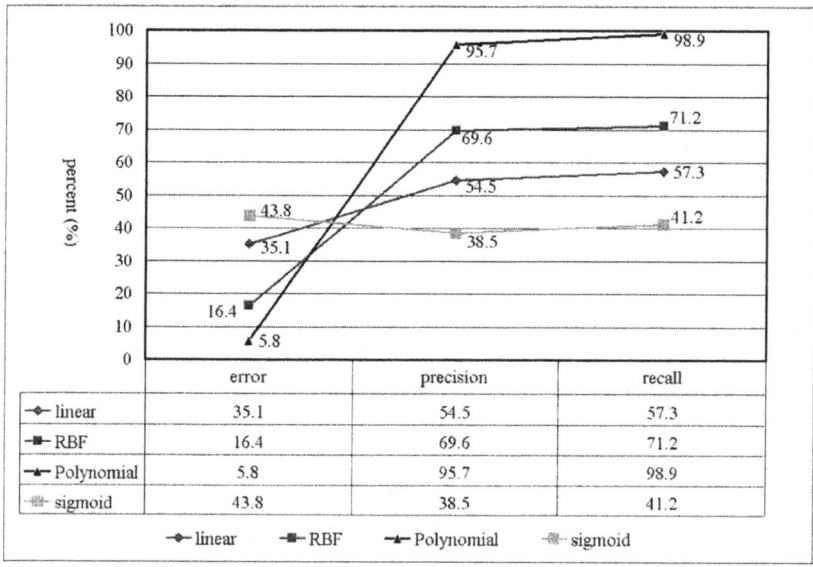

Fig. 8. The result of the training test using SVM for four types of kernels

Table 1. The result of local shape analysis based on the Octree structure: each column (A~H) represents the sub-space of the Octree and each row shows the shape difference between each pair of models

	A	B	C	D	E	F	G	H
P_L:T1	0.15	0.77	0.84	**3.15**	0.00	0.00	0.00	0.15
P_L:T2	1.20	0.00	0.00	0.00	**3.12**	2.00	1.00	1.44
N_R:T3	0.06	**1.02**	0.06	0.00	0.00	0.12	0.00	0.00
N_R:T4	0.00	0.00	0.00	0.00	**1.54**	**1.31**	**1.31**	**1.54**

we observe that the similarity error at deformed region is higher than at other regions. As shown in Table 1, our method is able to discriminate the global shape difference and is also able to distinguish a certain shape difference at a specific local region in a hierarchical fashion.

6 Conclusions

This paper presents a new method for 3D shape analysis based on a deformable model and a SVM classifier. The present method is invariant under translation, rotation of models and is robust to non-uniformly distributed and incomplete data sets. A modal model based on the FEM physics is constructed from points cloud data using vibration modes and can be utilized to the statistical shape modeling. As we integrate the parametric representation and the multi-resolution skeletons into the Octree structure, we can estimate the global and local shape similarity of the hippocampus. In addition, the ICP based normalization provides fast registration by a coarse-to-fine strategy and helps to overcome the alignment problem derived from the parametric shape representation. We have adopted a SVM-based classifier for the discrimination task. Results suggest that polynomial kernel outperforms the others. To ensure a more reliable result, we need to collect more experimental data for the subject controls and the epilepsy patients.

Acknowledgements

We would like to thank Prof. Seung-Bong Hong and Woo-Suk Tae in Samsung Medical Center for giving useful comments. This work was supported by grant No. (R04-2003-000-10017-0) from the Korea Research Foundation.

References

1. Dean, D., Buckley, P., Bookstein, F., Kamath, J., Kwon, D., Friedman, L., Lys, C.: Three dimensional MR-based morphometric comparison of schizophrenic and normal cerebral ventricles. Vis. In Biom. Computing, Lecture Notes in Comp. Sc., pp. 363-372, 1996.
2. Styner, M., Gerig, G., Pizer, S., and Joshi, S.: Automatic and robust computation of 3D medial models incorporating object variability. International Journal of Computer Vision 55(2/3), pp. 107-122, 2003.
3. Brechbuhler, C., Gerig, G. and Kubler, O.: Parameterization of closed surfaces for 3D shape description. Computer Vision, Graphics, Image Processing: Image Understanding, Vol. 61, pp. 154-170, 1995.
4. Kelemen, A., Szekely, G., Gerig, G.: Elastic Model based Segmentation of 3D Neuroradiological Data Sets. IEEE Transaction on Med. Im., Vol. 18, No. 10, pp. 823-839, 1999.
5. Geric, G.: http://www.cs.unc.edu/~gerig/pub.html.
6. Gibson, SFF., Mirtich, B.: A survey of deformable modeling in computer graphics. MERL-A Mitsubishi Electric Research Laboratory, TR-97-19, 1997.
7. McInerney, T., Terzopoulos, D.: Deformable models in medical images analysis: a survey. Medical Image Analysis, Vol. 1, No. 2, pp. 91-108, 1996.
8. Fisher, R. A.: The use of multiple measurements in taxonomic problems. Annals of Eugenics, Vol. 7, pp. 179-188, 1936.
9. Vapnik, V. N.: The Nature of Statistical Learning Theory, Springer, 1995.
10. Karabassi, E. A., Papaioannou, G. and Theoharis, T.: A Fast Depth-Buffer-Based Voxelization Algorithm. Journal of Graphics Tools, ACM, Vol. 4, No. 4, pp. 5-10, 1999.
11. Choi, S.M., Kim, M.H.: Shape Reconstruction from Partially Missing Data in Modal Space. Computers & Graphics, Vol. 26, No. 5, pp. 701-708, 2002.
12. Bathe, K.: Finite Element Procedures in Engineering Analysis. Prentice-Hall: Englewood Cliffs, NJ.
13. Zhang, Z.: Iterative point matching for registration of freeform curves and surfaces. International Journal of Computer Vision, Vol. 13, No.2, pp. 119-152, 1994.

Automatic Segmentation of Whole-Body Bone Scintigrams as a Preprocessing Step for Computer Assisted Diagnostics

Luka Šajn[1], Matjaž Kukar[1], Igor Kononenko[1], and Metka Milčinski[2]

[1] University of Ljubljana, Faculty of Computer and Information Science,
Tržaška 25, SI-1001 Ljubljana, Slovenia
{luka.sajn, matjaz.kukar, igor.kononenko}@fri.uni-lj.si
[2] University Medical Centre in Ljubljana, Department for Nuclear Medicine,
Zaloška 7, SI-1525 Ljubljana, Slovenia
metka.milcinski@kclj.si

Abstract. Bone scintigraphy or whole-body bone scan is one of the most common diagnostic procedures in nuclear medicine used in the last 25 years. Pathological conditions, technically poor quality images and artifacts necessitate that algorithms use sufficient background knowledge of anatomy and spatial relations of bones in order to work satisfactorily. We present a robust knowledge based methodology for detecting reference points of the main skeletal regions that simultaneously processes anterior and posterior whole-body bone scintigrams. Expert knowledge is represented as a set of parameterized rules which are used to support standard image processing algorithms. Our study includes 467 consecutive, non-selected scintigrams, which is to our knowledge the largest number of images ever used in such studies. Automatic analysis of whole-body bone scans using our knowledge based segmentation algorithm gives more accurate and reliable results than previous studies. Obtained reference points are used for automatic segmentation of the skeleton, which is used for automatic (machine learning) or manual (expert physicians) diagnostics. Preliminary experiments show that an expert system based on machine learning closely mimics the results of expert physicians.

1 Introduction

Whole-body scan or bone scintigraphy is a well known clinical routine investigation and one of the most frequent diagnostic procedures in nuclear medicine. Indications for bone scintigraphy include benign and malignant diseases, infections, degenerative changes ... [2]). Bone scintigraphy has high sensitivity and the changes of the bone metabolism are seen earlier than changes in bone structure detected on radiograms [15].

The investigator's role is to evaluate the image, which is of poor resolution due to the physical limitations of gamma camera. There are approximately 158 bones visible on both anterior and posterior whole-body scans [10]. Poor quality and the number of bones to inspect makes it difficult and often tedious work. Some research on automating the process of counting bone lesions has been done, but only few studies attempted to automatically segment individual bones prior to the computerized evaluation of bone scans [6; 7; 1].

1.1 Related Work

First attempts to automate scintigraphy in diagnostics for thyroid structure and function were made in 1973 [11]. Most of the research on automatic localization of bones has been done at the former Institute of medical information science at the University of Hildesheim in Germany from 1994 to 1996. The main contribution was made by the authors Berning [7] and Bernauer [6] who developed semantic representation of the skeleton and evaluation of the images. Benneke [1] realized their ideas in 1996.

Yin and Chiu [13] tried to find lesions using a fuzzy system. Their preprocessing of scintigrams includes rough segmentation of six parts with fixed ratios of the whole skeleton. Those parts are rigid and not specific enough to localize a specific bone. Their approach for locating abnormalities in bone scintigraphy is limited to point-like lesions with high uptake.

When dealing with lesion detection other authors like Noguchi [10] have been using merely intensity thresholding and manual lesion counting or manual bone ROI (region of interest) labeling. Those procedures are only sufficient for more obvious pathologies whereas new emerging pathological regions are overlooked.

2 Aim and Our Approach

The aim of our study was to develop a robust method for segmenting whole-body bone scans to allow further development of automatic algorithms for bone scan diagnostics of individual bones.

We have developed the algorithm for detecting extreme edges of images (peaks). Here, respective skeletal regions are processed in the following order: shoulders, head, pelvis, thorax and extremities. The experience with automatic processing is presented. Several image processing algorithms are used such as binarization, skeletonization, Hough's transform, Gaussian filtering [4], least square method and ellipse fitting in combination with background knowledge of anatomy and scintigraphy specialities.

In everyday practice, when a bone is identified, it is diagnosed by the expert physician according to several possible pathologies (lesions, malignom, metastasis, degenerative changes, inflammation, other pathologies, no pathologies). This process can be supported by using some machine learning classifier [9] which produces independent diagnoses. As an input it is given a suitably parameterized bone image, obtained from detected reference points. As an output it assigns the bone to one of the above pathologies. It can therefore be used as a tool to give physician an additional insight in the problem.

3 Materials and Methods

3.1 Patients and Images

Retrospective review of 467 consecutive, non-selected scintigraphic images from 461 different patients who visited University Medical Centre in Ljubljana from October 2003 to June 2004 was performed. Images were not preselected, so the study included standard distribution of patients coming to examination in 9 months. 19% of the images were diagnosed as normal, which means no pathology was detected on the image. 57% of the images were diagnosed with slight pathology, 20% with strong pathology and 2% were classified as super-scans.

Images also contained some artifacts and non-osseous uptake such as urine contamination and medical accessories (i.e. urinary catheters) [5]. In addition, segmentation was complicated by the radiopharmaceutical site of injection. Partial scans (missing a part of the head or upper/lower extremities in the picture) were the case in 18% of the images. There were also adolescents with growth zones (5% of the images), manifested as increased osteoblastic activity in well delineated areas with very high tracer uptake.

3.2 Bone Scintigraphy

All patients were scanned with gamma camera model Siemens MultiSPECT with two heads with LEHR (Low Energy High resolution) collimators. Scan speed was 8cm per minute with no pixel zooming. 99m-Tc-DPD (Techneos^R) was used. Bone scintigraphy was obtained about 3h after intravenous injection of 750 MBq of radiopharmaceutical agent. The whole body field was used to record anterior and posterior views digitally with resolution of 1024 x 256 pixels. Images represent the counts of detected gamma rays in each spatial unit with 16-bit grayscale depth.

3.3 Detection of Reference Points

Bone scans are very different (Figure 3) one from another even though the structure and position of bones is more or less the same. In practice many scans are only partial because only a determined part of the body is observed or due to the scanning time limitations. In our study we have observed that only on two images out of 467 the shoulders were not visible. Many other characteristic parts could have been missing in images more often (i.e. head, arms, one or both legs). We have chosen shoulders as the main reference points to start with, which means they are supposed to be visible in the images. Second and the last assumption is the upward orientation of the image. This assumption is not limiting since all scintigraphies are made with same orientation.

In order to make the detection of reference points faster and more reliable we have tried to automatically detect intuitive peaks which would represent edges and would cover roughly also the reference points. With normal Canny edge filter too many peaks were obtained. Our approach is based on orthogonal two-way Gaussian filtering [16].

Low image intensities (count level) acquired in typical studies are due to the limited level of radioactive dosage required to ensure patient's safety. They make bone scans look distorted. Bone edges are more expressive after we filter images with some averaging algorithm (i.e. wavelet based, median filter, Gaussian filter) [4]. We have used Gaussian filter so that the detection of peaks was more reliable.

Both images, anterior and posterior, are simultaneously processed in the same detection order and in each step the detected reference points visible on both images are compared and corrected adequately.

Detected points from the anterior image are mirrored to the posterior and vice versa. Some bones are better visible on anterior and some on posterior images due to the varying distances from both collimators. This improves the calculation of circles, lines and ellipses with least square method (LSM).

The order in which the reference points were detected was determined by using knowledge of human anatomy as well as physicians' recommendations. They are represented as a list of parameterized rules. Rule parameters (e.g. thresholds, spatial and intensity ratios, ...) were initially set by physicians and further refined on a separate tuning set. (e.g. iliumStart(*spineLocation*, *iliumROI*) :- shift *iliumROI* (width: shoulder width * 0.8, height: 10 pixels) starting at 60% of the estimated spine length downwards and stop when there are more than 3 peaks inside the *iliumROI* or the *iliumROI*'s average itensity changes more than 80% regarding the previous *iliumROI*. iliumBone(*iliumCircleParam*) :- spine(*spineLocation*), iliumStart(*spineLocation*, *iliumROI*), extend *iliumROI*'s height to its width, narrow *iliumROI* with dynamic binarization, apply LSM on peaks inside *iliumROI*, run LSM iterations until all peaks are covered with the *iliumCircleParam* ring (in each run remove peaks lying outside the ring).) More details can be found in [16].

Shoulders. They are the only part of the body that is assumed to be present in every image in the upper part on both sides. The algorithm just searches for the highest detected peak on both sides of the image. The next step is to locally shift the candidate points with local maximum intensity tracing to the outermost location. Only in 5 images out of 467 shoulders were not found correctly due to the tilted head position.

Pelvic Region (Ilium Bone, Pubis Bone, Great Trochanter of Femur). The most identifiable bone in pelvic region is ilium bone which has higher uptake values than it's neighboring soft tissue. Ilium bone has circular shape in the upper part and it is therefore convenient for circle detection with LSM method. This bone is well described with already detected peaks as shown in Figure 1(b). Ilium position is roughly estimated with regions of interest (ROIs) which are found on the basis of skeleton's anticipated ratios and reference points found up to this step of detection.

The pelvis is located at the end of the spine and has approximately the same width as shoulders. In order to find the pelvis, the calculation of the spine position is required. This is done with a beam search (Figure 1(a)). The anticipated spine length is determined from the distance between shoulders. Beam starting point is the middle point of the shoulders and it's orientation is perpendicular to the shoulder line. The angle at which the beam covers most peaks, is a rough

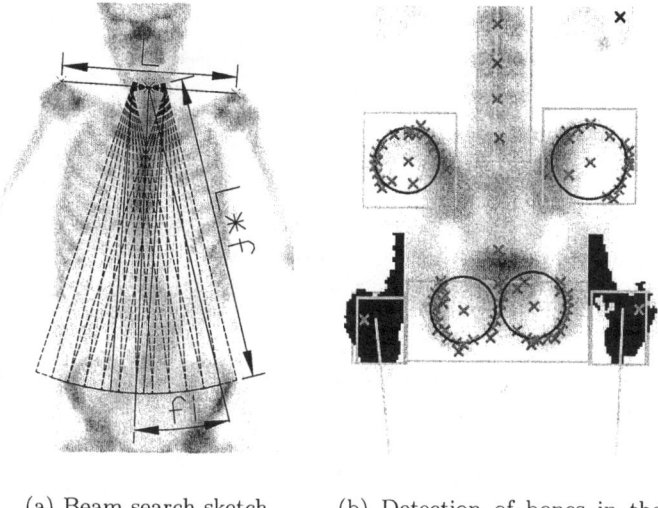

(a) Beam search sketch (b) Detection of bones in the pelvic region

Fig. 1. Beam search and detection in pelvic region

estimation of spine direction since there is most of the uptake in the vertebrae and hence peaks are dense in that region.

Pubis bone is detected by estimating the pubis ROI using detected ilium location, distance between detected ilium circles and their inclination. The experimentally determined ROI's size is narrowed and additional vertical peaks are added and circles detected as shown in Figure 1(b).

Head and Neck. When at least image orientation and the location of the shoulders are known, some part of the neck or even head is visible since they are between the shoulders. Finding the head is not difficult but its orientation is, especially in cases where a part of the head in scan is not visible. The most reliable method for determining head orientation and position is ellipse fitting of the head contour determined by thresholding. Neck is found by local vertical shifting of a stripe determined by the ellipse's semiminor axis (position and orientation).

Thoracic Part (Vertebrae, Ribs). Vertebrae have more or less constant spatial relations, the only problem is that on a bone scintigraphy only a planar projection of the spine is visible. Since the spine is longitudinally curved, the spatial relations vary due to different longitudinal orientation of the patients. Average vertebrae relations have been experimentally determined from normal skeletons.

Ribs are the most difficult skeleton region to detect since they are quite unexpressive on bone scans, their formation can vary considerably and their contours [14] can be disconnected in the case of stronger pathology (Figure 2).

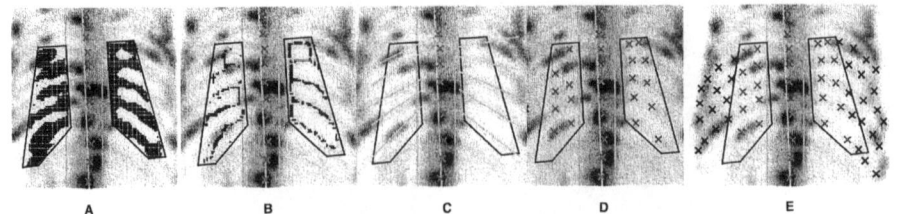

Fig. 2. Rib detection steps example on a skeleton with strong pathology. Rib ROI is binarized (A), binarized image is skeletonized (B), Hough transform of linear equation is calculated on skeleton points (C), reference points are estimated using results of the Hough transform (D), rib contours are individually followed by the contour following algorithm (E)

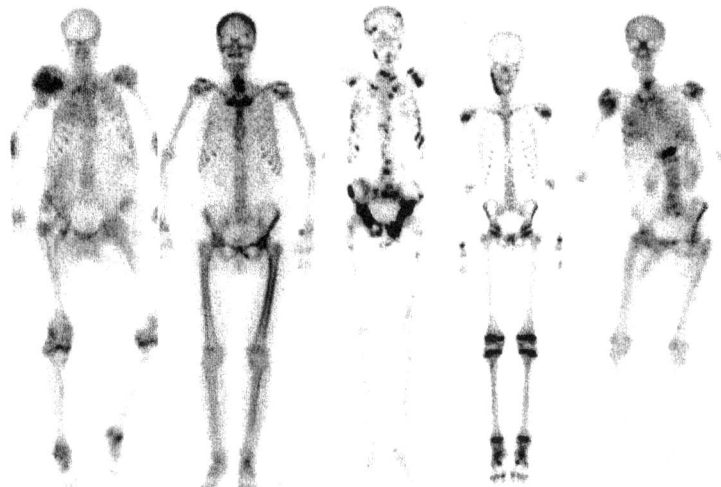

Fig. 3. Examples of body scan variety

Lower and Upper Extremities (Femur, Knee, Tibia, Fibula, Humerus, Elbow, Radius, Ulna). They are often partly absent from whole-body scan because of limited gamma camera detector width. In our patients, a maximum of 61cm width is usually not enough for the entire skeleton. The regions of humerus, ulna and radius as well as femur, tibia and fibula bone are located with the use of controlled beam search. The beam lengths can be estimated from skeletal relationships (i.e. femur length is estimated as 78% of the distance between the neck and ilium bone center). The detection is designed so that a part or all of the extremities and/or the head may not be visible.

3.4 Diagnosing Pathologies with Machine Learning

When all reference points are obtained, every bone is assigned a portion of original scintigraphic image, according to relevant reference points. Obtained image is parameterized by using the ArTeX algorithm [8]. It uses association rules to describe images in rotation-invariant manner. Rotation invariance is very important in our case since it accounts for different patients' positions inside the camera.

Bones were described with several hundreds of automatically generated attributes. They were used for training the SVM [12] learning algorithm. In our preliminary experiments pathologies were not discriminated, i.e. bones were labelled with only two possible diagnoses (no pathology, pathology). In 19% of patients no pathology or other artifacts were detected by expert physicians. In the remaining 81% of the patients at least one pathology or artifact was observed.

4 Results

4.1 Segmentation

Approximately half of the available images were used for tuning rule parameters to optimize the recognition of the reference points and another half to test it. All 246 patients examined from October 2003 to March 2004 were used as the tuning set and 221 patients examined from April 2004 to June 2004 were used as the test set. In the tuning set there were various non-osseous uptakes in 38.9% of the images, 47.5% images with the visible injection point and 6.8% images of adolescents with the visible growth zones. Similar distribution was found in the test set (34.5% non-osseous uptakes, 41.0% visible injection points and 2.85% adolescents). Most of the artifacts were minor radioactivity points from urine contamination in genital region or other parts (81.4% of all artifacts) whereas only few other types were observed (urinary catheters 13%, artificial hips 4% and lead accessories 1.6%). We have observed that there were no ill-detected reference points in adolescents with the visible growth zones since all the bones are homogenous, have good visibility and are clearly divided with growth zones. Results of detecting reference points on the test set are shown in the Table 1.

4.2 Machine Learning Results

From our complete set of 467 patients, pathologies were thoroughly evaluated by physicians only for 268 patients. These 268 patients were used for evaluation of

Table 1. False reference point detection on test set. Both frequencies and percentages are given

Bone	no pathology		slight pathology		strong pathology		super-scan		all	
	46		133		39		3		221	
ilium	0		2	0.9%	6	2.7%	1	0.5%	9	4.1%
pubis	2	0.9%	3	1.4%	2	0.9%	0		7	3.2%
trochanter	0		1	0.5%	0		0		1	0.5%
shoulder	0		0		1	0.5%	0		1	0.5%
extremities	5	2.3%	11	5.0%	0		0		16	7.2%
spine	0		2	0.9%	1	0.5%	0		3	1.4%
ribs	11	5.0%	17	7.7%	3	1.4%	0		31	14.0%
neck	2	0.9%	4	1.8%	0		0		6	2.7%

Table 2. Experimental results with machine learning on two-class problem

Bone group	Classification accuracy	spec.%	sensit.%
Cervical spine	75,9	80,0	77,8
Feet	83,8	84,1	68,0
Skull posterior	94,7	88,2	100,0
Ilium bone	87,3	87,6	82,8
Lumbal spine	71,4	75,7	65,4
Femur and tibia	88,9	84,6	73,3
Pelvic region	92,2	90,7	85,0
Ribs	98,1	92,5	91,7
Scapula	91,4	90,9	90,9
Thoracic spine	82,0	79,2	61,5
AVG	**86,6**	**85,4**	**79,6**

machine learning approach by using ten-fold cross validation. Results are shown in Table 2. The bones were grouped in ten relevant bone regions defined by the reference points. Classification accuracy was obtained for a two-class problem.

5 Discussion

The testing showed encouraging results since the detection of proposed reference points gave excellent results for all bone regions but the extremities, which was expected.

We have paid special attention to the images with partial skeletons since it is often the case in clinical routine (in our study 18% of the images were partial and no particular problem appeared in detecting) and a robust segmentation algorithm should not fail on such images. The detection of ribs showed to be the most difficult, yet that was expected. Results show that in 14% to 20% of images there were difficulties in detecting the ribs. This usually means one rib is missed or not followed to the very end which we intend to improve in the future. In the present system such reference points can be manually repositioned by the expert physicians.

Automatically detected reference points can be used for mapping a standard skeletal reference mask, which is to our belief the best way to find individual bones on scintigrams since bone regions are often not expressive enough to follow their contour. An example of such mask mapping is shown in Figure 4.

While our experimental results with machine learning are quite good one must bear in mind that they were obtained for a simplified (two class) problem. Simply extending a problem to a multi-class paradigm is not acceptable in our case, as the bone may be assigned several different pathologies at the same time. A proper approach, the one we are currently working on, is to rephrase a problem to the multi-label learning problem, where each bone will be labelled with a nonempty subset of all possible labels [17; 3].

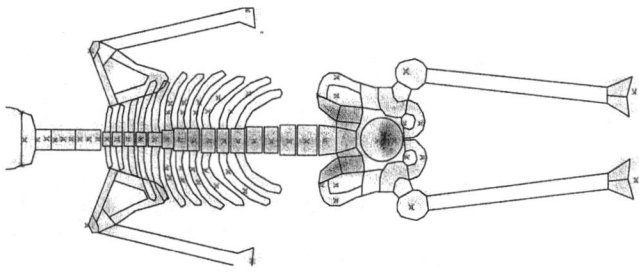

Fig. 4. Example of mapped standard skeletal mask with the detected reference points

6 Conclusion

The presented computer-aided system for bone scintigraphy is a step forward in automating routine medical procedures. Some standard image processing algorithms were tailored and used in combination to achieve the best reference point detection accuracy on scintigraphic images which have very low resolution. Poor quality, artifacts and pathologies necessitate that algorithms use as much background knowledge on anatomy and spatial relations of bones as possible in order to work satisfactorily. This combination gives quite good results and we expect that further studies on automatic scintigraphy diagnosing using reference points for image segmentation will give more accurate and reliable results than previous studies, negligent to the segmentation. This approach opens a new view on automatic scintigraphy evaluation, since in addition to detection of point-like high-uptake lesions there are also:

- more accurate and reliable evaluation of bone symmetry when looking for skeletal abnormalities. Many abnormalities can be spotted only when the symmetry is observed (differences in length, girth, curvature etc.),
- detection of lesions with low-uptake or lower activity due to metallic implants,
- possibility of comparing uptake ratios among different bones,
- more complex pathology detection with combining pathologies of more bones (i.e. arthritis in joints)
- possibility of automatic reporting of bone pathologies in written language.

Machine learning approach in this problem is in a very early stage, so its usefulness in practice cannot yet be objectively evaluated. However, preliminary results are encouraging and switching to the multilabel learning framework may make them even better.

Acknowledgement

This work was supported by the Slovenian Ministry of Higher Education, Science and Technology through the research programme P2-0209. Special thanks to nuclear medicine specialist Jure Fettich at the University Medical Centre in Ljubljana for his help and support.

References

[1] Benneke A. Konzeption und Realisierung Eines Semi-Automatischen Befundungssystems in Java und Anbindung an ein Formalisiertes Begriffssystem am Beispiel der Skelett-Szintigraphie. Diplom arbeit, Institut für Medizinische Informatik, Universität Hildesheim, mentor Prof. Dr. D.P. Pretschner, 1997.

[2] Hendler A. and Hershkop M. When to Use Bone Scintigraphy. It Can Reveal Things Other Studies Cannot. *Postgraduate Medicine*, 104(5):54–66, 11 1998.

[3] McCallum A. Multi-Label Text Classification with a Mixture Model Trained by EM. In *Proc. AAAI'99 Workshop on Text Learning*, 1999.

[4] Jammal G. and Bijaoui A. DeQuant: a Flexible Multiresolution Restoration Framework. *Signal Processing*, 84(7):1049–1069, 7 2004.

[5] Weiner M. G., Jenicke L., Mller V., and Bohuslavizki H. K. Artifacts and Non-Osseous Uptake in Bone Scintigraphy. Imaging Reports of 20 Cases. *Radiol Oncol*, 35(3):185–91, 2001.

[6] Bernauer J. Zur Semantischen Rekonstruktion Medizinischer Begriffssysteme. Habilitationsschrift, Institut für Medizinische Informatik, Univ. Hildesheim, 1995.

[7] Berning K.-C. *Zur Automatischen Befundung und Interpretation von Ganzkörper-Skelettszintigrammen.* PhD thesis, Institut für Medizinische Informatik, Universität Hildesheim, 1996.

[8] Bevk M. and Kononenko I. Towards Symbolic Mining of Images with Association Rules: Preliminary Results on Textures. In Brito P. and Noirhomme-Fraiture M., editors, *ECML/PKDD 2004: proc. of the workshop W2 on symbolic and spatial data analysis: mining complex data structures*, pages 43–53, 2004.

[9] Kukar M., Kononenko I., Grošelj C., Kralj K., and Fettich J. Analysing and Improving the Diagnosis of Ischaemic Heart Disease with Machine Learning. *Artificial Intelligence in Medicine*, 16:25–50, 1999.

[10] Noguchi M., Kikuchi H., Ishibashi M., and Noda S. Percentage of the Positive Area of Bone Metastasis is an Independent Predictor of Disease Death in Advanced Prostate Cancer. *British Journal of Cancer*, (88):195–201, 2003.

[11] Maisey M.N., Natarajan T.K., Hurley P.J., and Wagner H.N. Jr. Validation of a Rapid Computerized Method of Measuring 99mTc Pertechnetate Uptake for Routine Assessment of Thyroid Structure and Function. *J Clin Endocrinol Metab*, 36:317–322, 1973.

[12] Cristianini N. and Shawe-Taylor J. *An Introduction to Support Vector Machines and Other Kernel-Based Learning Methods.* Cambridge University Press, 2000.

[13] Yin T.K. and Chiu N.T. A Computer-Aided Diagnosis for Locating Abnormalities in Bone Scintigraphy by a Fuzzy System With a Three-Step Minimization Approach. *IEEE Transactions on Medical Imaging*, 23(5):639–654, 5 2004.

[14] Kindratenko V. *Development and Application of Image Analysis Techniques for Identification and Classification of Microscopic Particles.* PhD thesis, Universitaire Instelling Antwerpen, Departement Scheikunde, 1997.

[15] Müller V., Steinhagen J., de Wit M., and Bohuslavizki H. K. Bone Scintigraphy in Clinical Routine. *Radiol Oncol*, 35(1):21–30, 2001.

[16] Šajn L., Kononenko I., Fettich J., and Milčinski M. Automatic Segmentation of Whole-Body Bone Scintigrams. Technical report, Faculty of Computer and Information Science, University of Ljubljana, Nov. 2004. URL http://lkm.fri.uni-lj.si/papers/Skelet.pdf.

[17] Shen X., Boutell M., Luo J., and Brown C. Multi-Label Machine Learning and its Application to Semantic Scene Classification. In *Proceedings of the 2004 International Symposium on Electronic Imaging (EI 2004)*, San Jose, California, 2004.

Knowledge Management

Multi-agent Patient Representation in Primary Care

Chris Reed[1,2], Brian Boswell[2], and Ron Neville[2,3]

[1] Division of Applied Computing University of Dundee, Dundee DD1 4HN, UK
[2] Calico Jack Ltd, Argyll House, Dundee DD1 1QP, UK
[3] Westgate Health Centre, Charleston Dr., Dundee DD2 4AD
{chris, brian, ron}@calicojack.co.uk

Abstract. Though multi-agent systems have been explored in a wide variety of medical settings, their role at the primary care level has been relatively little investigated. In this paper, we present a system that is currently being piloted for future rollout in Scotland that employs an industrial strength multi-agent platform to tackle both technical and sociological challenges within primary care. In particular, the work is motivated by several specific issues: (i) the need to widen mechanisms for access to primary care; (ii) the need to harness technical solutions to reduce load not only for general practitioners, but also for practice nurses and administrators; (iii) the need to design and deploy technical solutions in such a way that they fit in to existing professional activity, rather than demanding changes in current practice. With direct representation of individuals in health care relationships implemented in a multi-agent system (with one multi-functional agents representing each patient, doctor, nurse, pharmacist, etc.) it becomes straightforward first to model and then to integrate with existing practice. It is for this reason that the system described here successfully widens access for patients (by opening up novel communication channels of email and SMS texting) and reduces load on the practice (by streamlining communications and semi-automating appointment arrangement). It does this by ensuring that the solution is not imposed on, but rather, integrated with what currently goes on in primary care. Furthermore, with agents responsible for maintaining audit trails for the patients they represent, it becomes possible to see elements of the electronic patient record (EPR) emerging under agent control. This EPR can be extended through structured interaction with the practice system (here, we examine the GPASS system, the market leader in Scotland), to allow rich agent-agent and agent-human interactions. By using multi-agent design and implementation techniques, we have been able to build a solution that integrates both with individuals and extant software to successfully tackle real problems in primary care.

1 Introduction

Increasingly, research in multi-agent systems is exploring the advantages offered by the emerging multi-agent software engineering paradigm (see, for example [13]). By focusing on the relationship between an entity in the real world (an individual, a relationship, an organisation, a datum) and its corresponding entity in the "electronic world" (an agent, a relationship between agents, a set of agents, a datum), design can become easier and quicker [4]. The process of teasing out complex and intricate stakeholder relationships in real world domains is not made harder by the restrictions and assumptions of the implementation paradigm. As a result, interesting multi-agent based models of complex social structures have started to emerge [22].

The health care system is a perfect example. It offers extremely rich interdependent sets of relationships, stakeholders, rights, requirements and agendas that, though interesting for the modeller, have proved an enormous challenge for the deployment and uptake of practical IT systems [15]. It is an environment subject to constant change of workforce, 'clients', and infrastructure, often with a zero tolerance of error. The challenge for multi-agent systems presented by the complexities of health care has been well documented (see e.g. [10, 12, 16]) and has provided a rich field for research, but primary care - and its own unique set of issues - is often omitted from these investigations. The work described here harnesses agentive representation and techniques from agent oriented programming in tackling some of these features of primary care.

2 Background

Patients, politicians and health care professionals all agree that Patient Centred Care is a good thing, but translation of concept to reality has yet to be achieved [23]. The fields of health and computing share the common jargon of 'user friendly', accessible, and flexibility and so it is unsurprising that agents have been touted for patient-centered health care.

One of the earliest examples of work examining the role of multi-agent systems in health care is offered by the AADCare architecture [10]. The focus of the work presented there, and of the broader context in which it was conducted (*viz.*, the DILEMMA project), is upon appropriate theorem proving in decision support systems that have to deal with complex, incomplete, inconsistent and potentially conflicting data. The agent component is designed to support the distribution of clinical 'tasks' amongst players in the system, in a manner similar to the much earlier Contract Net protocol for automated task distribution [24]. A prototype of the AADCare system as a whole was implemented for the management of cancer patients in the UK NHS system, though the extent of deployment and its subsequent success is unreported. Crucially, access for the patient to their medical record, and the unification of record components across different health services for an individual patient was not a focus for AADCare in either implementation or theory, and therefore mostly side-steps issues of patient-centered health care.

The Guardian Angel project [8] represents a "manifesto" developed since 1994 that tackles the patient-centered approach head on. Some elements of the manifesto have lead to implementation, of which the earliest was the Personal Internetworked Notary and Guardian project, PING [21]. Although that work mentions "agents" in passing, its focus is upon implementing basic security mechanisms for (conceptually) centralised data stored using XML. It makes no use of the agent oriented, peer-to-peer approach in either design or implementation. The motivating concepts, described in [14] however, are precisely those addressed in the current work: the need to balance patient access and security; the need to reduce fragmentation in medical records; the need for IT infrastructure to be interoperable; etc.

In the context of UK health care, Pouloudi and Reed [20] offer a relatively early example of using multi-agent systems to represent and model interactions in the NHS in an attempt to build a realistic foundation for integrative systems. The work combines intra-agent representational concepts with inter-agent communication and relationship structures in modelling the interactions between stakeholder relationships in patient data. The model there was theoretical and unimplemented.

More recently, the Advanced Computational Lab at Cancer Research UK has built multi-agent models of the same sorts of complex relationships specifically in the context of cancer, from initial patient contact with their GP through various stages of care and maintenance [2; 7]. They employ the mature COGENT and PRO*forma* tools and the tried-and-tested Domino model of agent architecture, but still the focus is squarely upon the interacting agencies of the health system, for which the patient is simply a customer.

Moreno *et al.* [16] describes a system that moves closer to the ideal of patient centered involvement and access. In their HeCaSe system, patients have an interface that supports appointment booking and various static configuration parameters. It is, however, focused only on the interaction between patients and initial, primary care consultations, and is run from PC clients. Crucially from a deployment point of view, it requires doctors to switch to a new system.

Finally, it is worth noting that perhaps the largest impact of multi-agent systems in health care to date has been in specifically targeted applications that focus on particular functions of the health system. So, for example, there are prototypes and demonstrators of multi-agent system applications in areas such as organ transplant [6; 17], antibiotic prescription [9], pharmacy in general [3], protocol monitoring [1], proactive information provision in anaesthesia [11], data flow in Leukemia management [12] and others (such as those in the special issue, volume 27 issue 3, of *AI in Medicine*). These examples are clinician centred attempts to streamline existing processes. Thus multi-agent systems as a tool is having an impact in many areas. But this is peripheral to the argument that we hope to make here, namely, that multi-agent systems as a paradigm fits the goal of patient-centered health care perfectly not only at a conceptual level, but also in implementation and deployment.

3 Multi-agent Systems for Patient-Centered Health Care

The concept of **agentiverepresentation** is implicit in very many agent-based models of real world structures, and even entire agent based methodologies such as Gaia [25]. The idea is simply that one component in the real world is represented by a single corresponding agent in the system. This idea is now also starting to gain traction in the commercial world [4]. In the medical domain, agentive representation means agents representing general practitioners, consultants, pharmacists, and, of course, patients.

To build systems that are to be deployed in real health care situations, it is important that the infrastructure meets and exceeds a range of basic expectations of the users with respect to various aspects such as security, scaling and reliability. In the work described here, we have selected the JUDE platform [5] for reasons of flexibility and robustness. The architecture of agents in JUDE is simple in that each agent is equipped with a set of generic functionality (such as basic reasoning and communication) that can then be augmented with additional modular functionality as needed.

The system implements the patient-centered approach by equipping agents representing patients with all the functionality they require to represent their corresponding patient in the electronic health care world. So for example, the patient agent can access data on that patient held in different locations and by different parties. The patient agent can communicate with the local surgery to organise appointments. The patient agent can access information on pharmacy location and availability. And, of course, the patient agent can communicate with, and be contacted by, the patient themselves. This communication can make use of whatever channels may happen to be available at a given moment – from web to SMS. But every time, and in every case, the patient is simply communicating with their own, persistent, agent.

Detailing the implementation in full is beyond the scope of this paper, but it is useful to offer depth in a subset of the functionality and go on to show how this functionality is deployed and fitted in to existing primary care processes.

3.1 An Example: Reducing DNA Rates

In this currently live trial, patient agents are equipped with the ability to interact with agents representing individuals in a GP surgery, including the receptionist and GP. One agent-mediated interaction is the process of booking and confirming appointments. The appointments process is a current area of interest in practice management, since a substantial proportion of valuable GP time is wasted as a result of people who book appointments but then subsequently do not attend (DNA). Reducing the DNA rate offers practical and substantial advantages to GPs and practices in the UK.

The current model is to allow patients to ring the practice receptionist and negotiate verbally to arrange an appointment time convenient for both GP and patient. In some cases, as described above, some or all of this process may be conducted by email instead of over the telephone.

An agent-based solution offers a technical improvement whilst integrating with existing practice to minimise barriers to use. A patient's agent is responsible for intervening in some or all of the communication between the patient and the practice, and is responsible for reminding the patient of upcoming appointments. A patient is allocated an agent in the system following consent agreement. At that point, the patient can send a text message or an email to their agent, which, in either case, then communicates with the agent representing the practice receptionist. The receptionist's agent then communicates with the receptionist through the most appropriate means – at the moment, that is email. The negotiation is conducted in this way between patient and receptionist until agreement on appointment time is met. (It is unreasonable to expect patients to be using an electronic diary, and thus it is not possible to automate the patient end of the negotiation process. Similarly, it is important to keep the receptionist in the loop, and so automating that end is also counterproductive.) When agreement is reached, the receptionist confirms the appointment through a web interface provided by the receptionist's agent. That agent then informs the patient's agent of the confirmed appointment time. At 24 hours before the appointment, the patient's agent sends a reminder (currently by SMS). At two hours before the appointment is due, the patient's agent sends a second reminder. If the patient does not reply to that second reminder, thereby failing to confirm that they still intend to keep the appointment, the patient's

Multi-agent Patient Representation in Primary Care   379

agent will inform the receptionist's agent of a problem. In this case, the receptionist's agent will take some default action, which is currently to email the receptionist suggesting that the appointment be cancelled and the time freed up.

Figure 1, above, summarises an example interaction, demonstrating the various communication mechanisms (text, email and web, indicated by the icons on the

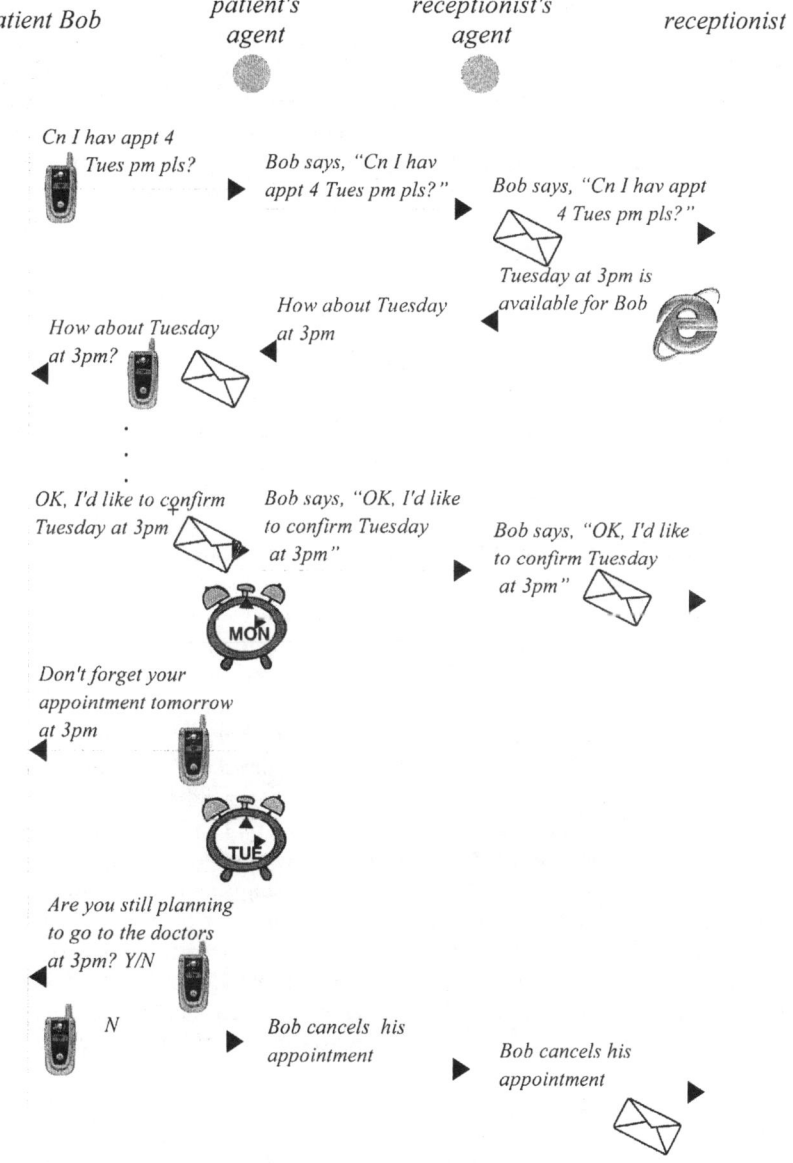

Fig. 1. Sample Interaction

interaction arrows), the simple proactive work of the patient's agent, and the involvement of the receptionist and patient in the system.

There are many practical advantages offered by introducing agents into the loop, both in the current system and for its future development. First, robustness is improved by having state information maintained explicitly in the agents – so, for example, if an SMS message fails to be delivered, an agent can retry, use a different communication medium (such as email) or at least alert appropriately (such as warning the receptionist). Second, message routing in general becomes transparent – the receptionist need not be concerned with a patient's decision to have communications delivered through one medium (SMS) rather than another (email). Third, as explored in the next section, agents represent a natural and simple means of offering audit and tracing facilities. Fourth, agents in the framework are extensible on the fly; as discussed below, developing and deploying new functionality is straightforward. Fifth, for some services, patient anonymity is vital; agents provide a natural decoupling that can preserve such anonymity. Finally, looking further to the future, MAS provides a natural mechanism for representing real world relationships that can be exploited in routing messages.

4 Realities of Using a Multi-agent System in Primary Care

The published work on MAS applications in health care understandably concentrates on the computing methodology and on the need to design software around complex health care problems. It will become increasingly important to involve the people using the system – clinicians and patients - in future developments. Research into any new technology, including MAS, must look at subtle patient centred issues. Innovations need to be based around what people actually want to use. Multi-agent systems have the potential to support an ongoing dialogue between doctor and patient. Research must therefore include an ongoing dialogue to plan and implement findings. The "Do Not Attend" component of the system described in the previous section is adopted as an exemplar by which to follow through this process. By drawing on previous experience of integrating new technology into the patient-facing side of primary care [18; 19], the design of pilot trials and ethical approval for those trials has been achievable. The current deployment is based around 'as needed' creation of agents for up to 100 patients who volunteer to take part in the trial. Text messaging based appointment booking is offered as an extra service.

For the receptionist, all interaction with the system, and with patients using the system is through a simple web interface and email, both of which are familiar and non-threatening. The interface between the system and patients is text messaging, with which all who sign up are very familiar. Finally, the interface between the system and additional components (such as GPs) is built around email, again fitting in with existing practices. As a result, introduction of the service has been straightforward and has hit no major problems.

Clearly, the system, its deployment and its uptake are in very early days, but the current status marks an important milestone. The key step that has been taken is to provide each individual patient with an agent that interacts, on the patient's behalf, with agents representing health care professionals. With this scenario engineered and deployed, and with the dynamic upgrade facilities in JUDE (whereby new functionality can be deployed to existing agents without needing to "reboot" either the systems or those agents that are upgraded), it is relatively easy to map out a programme of rolling development and deployment of patient-centered services.

With appointment booking and reminders in place, the next step is to integrate another burdensome practice task: repeat prescription ordering. Ordering repeat prescriptions is, in the UK and other health systems, a task initiated by a patient who has a long-term need for prescription drugs. It requires a GP to sign off, which takes both GP time, and a physical appointment, involving both travel and time for the patient, as well as practice overhead in the form of receptionist time for booking. With agents representing all the parties, it becomes relatively simple for the request to be routed from the patient to the GP, confirmed (or otherwise) by the GP, and then forwarded to the appropriate pharmacist, from where the patient can collect their prescription. Of course this is far from the first time that a proposal has been tabled for streamlining this process, nor is it the only IT-based solution. The novelty lies in that it is exactly the same system as is currently used for appointment booking, made available for repeat prescription ordering by virtue of the direct representation of the people involved and the relationships between them. One of the additional benefits that arises "for free" with the approach is an audit trail at the individual patient level, so that health care professionals and patients can track where a request is in the system so cutting out unnecessary phone calls to the practice or pharmacist. Also, with the advent of electronic prescribing, our agent system represents a solution anchored to existing practice systems.

5 An EPR Under Agent Control?

In Scotland, well over 80% of primary care practices have adopted the GPASS system to manage patient data and other practice functions[1]. With a wide variety of proposals for electronic patient record (EPR) management currently under discussion and development, integration with primary care systems is a key concern. GPASS, like many of its competitors, does provide programmatic access to the data it stores, via mediated SQL queries. Such a clean interface makes it a good starting point for investigating the alignment of the notion of an EPR with that of one agent for every patient.

The EPR can be analysed to yield a key subset of patient medical information which has general utility for both patients and health-care professionals. This subset contains information regarding a patient's significant clinical events, current prescribed medication (both acute, and repeat), key indicators such as tobacco and alcohol history, and their age, height, weight and body mass index. Together with primary personal information – name, address, date-of-birth, and CHI (unique health service number) – this constitutes what we call the Core Clinical Summary (CCS).

The information which makes up the CCS is stored in the MS SQL database which acts as the data store for the GPASS clinical system. In order to access the information required to construct the CCS, a JUDE module was developed for use by the appropriate agents to log into and make the relevant queries to GPASS, from

---

[1] See http://www.gpass.co.uk

which those agents might then construct the CCS accordingly. Figure 2 summarises the mechanisms by which this information is extracted in response to a patient initiated request.

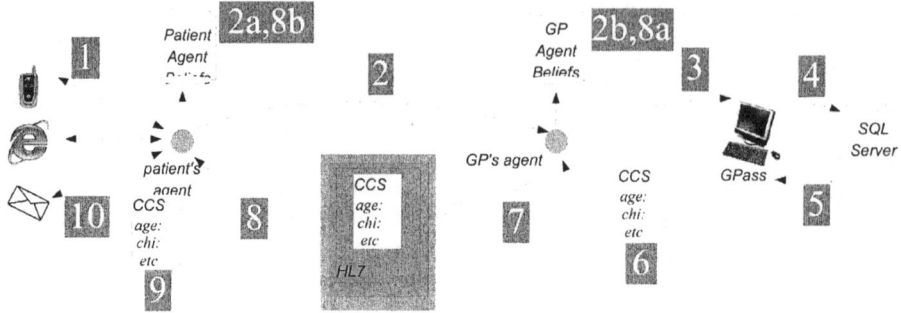

Fig. 2. Sample Patient-Agent-GP-GPASS interaction

In this example, at (1), the patient requests some part of CCS data via the web, email or their mobile. Then, at (2), the patient's agent requests CCS from the GP's agent, and by the implemented semantics of the inter-agent communication language, the patient's agent (2a) and GP's agent (2b) update their respective belief sets to reflect that the request was made. This update is defined by the semantics of the J-ACL communication language implemented in JUDE [5]. At (3) the GP's agent logs in to GPASS clinical system and then makes set of requests to GPASS for patient information. In turn, GPASS calls into the SQL database (4) which returns the appropriate patient data (5). At (6) the GP's agent then uses that data to construct the CCS which it then embeds in the appropriate nested wrappers of a well formed HL7 message for subsequent transmission (7). At (8), the GP's agent informs the patient's agent with the CCS, again leading to updates in the belief sets of the GP's agent (8a) and patient's agent (8b). Finally, at (9) the patient's agent extracts CCS from HL7 wrappers and at (10) transmits CCS data to the appropriate device (where what is appropriate is determined through rich contextual reasoning). This same architecture also fits snugly into a more radical, long-term and ambitious picture in which patient agents have ultimate responsibility for maintaining an up-to-date picture of EPRs.

The ability of a patient to have to hand their own medical information via entirely ordinary devices, promotes the position of patient as genuine stakeholder in their own health care. The information available to patients via the CCS allows them to accurately inform their lifestyle using straightforward mechanisms, and on their terms. So, for example, a patient can easily match their recollection of past clinical events with the corresponding sections of their CCS. Further, in situations where clinical systems are not available (e.g., an accident in a remote location) the patient themselves has the means to provide key information (such as allergies, or current medications) to assist the health care professional.

Putting the patient in a position where they can easily interact proactively with their representation in the health care system also supports more interactive relationships between health care providers and patients. For GP's (and other health care professionals), the MAS based primary care solution provides all parties from all aspects of health care with a single point of contact to the patient, *viz.*, the patients agent. Whilst providing GPs with mobile access to CCS records may be convenient (immediately prior to house calls, for example), in positions where urgent access to medical information is vital, such as an emergency situation with an incapacitated patient outwith the health care infrastructure, the ability for the patient's agent to be accessed for information in the CCS (such as current medication regimes or illnesses) offers the potential for significant advantages.

6 Conclusions and Directions

The focus of this work is on the design, implementation, deployment and evaluation of initially very simple solutions to very real problems that despite their simplicity nevertheless use a full, mature, industrial-strength multi-agent system that can not only tackle the simple problems as they scale numerically, but also incrementally take on an ever more significant role, tackling ever more complex problems that demand ever more of the underlying technology.

Multi-agent systems have great potential to transform the process, and possibly even the outcome, of medical care. It is important that innovation goes hand in hand with evaluation. Our own next steps are to evaluate the outcomes of the pilot trial in designing larger scale trials which are based upon enriched functionality within individual agents. It is a logical extension to offer a MAS-based text message/email/web service including appointment booking, repeat prescription ordering and provision of clinical advice. Qualitative work will explore the views, aspirations and experiences of people who chose to use this service, with the first component of this work – health care staff interviewing – already almost complete. Quantitative work will measure when and how often people use the service, and the impact that the service has on the functioning of the practice. It will be important to look at the language and exchange of information in any patient – doctor text dialogue. Preliminary technical work and evaluation will then allow a larger cluster randomised trial to proceed in several practices involving hundreds of patients.

Multi-agent systems are likely to transform health care within the next decade. At a basic level the very nature of a consultation between a patient and a health care professional will need to be re-defined. At a more sophisticated level, patients will have the opportunity to integrate health-related activity and decision making into everyday behaviour. Professionals will be able to support and advise patients in a completely new and different way. The effect of these changes on health outcome needs to be addressed. The reactions of people using and working within the health service need to be explored. The major barrier to the implementation of multi-agent systems in health care may not be technical, but attitudinal, and it is this aspect that needs to be brought in to every stage of the development and deployment lifecycle.

References

1. Alsinet, T., Ansotegui, C., Bejar, R., Fernandez, C., Manya, F.: Automated monitoring of medical protocols, Art. Int. in Med. 27(3) (2003) 367-392
2. Black, E.: Using Agent Technology to Model Complex Organisations AgentLink 12 (2003)

3. Calabretto, J.P., Couper, D., Mulley, B., Nissen, M., Siow, S., Tuck, J., Warren, J.: Agent Support for Patients and Community Pharmacists, Proc. of the 35th HICSS, IEEE (2002)
4. Calico Jack: Multi-Agent Systems in Mobile Telecommunications Networks, Calico Jack White Paper #2004/01 (2004)
5. Calico Jack: "An Introduction to the Jackdaw University Development Environment", Calico Jack Developer Documentation (2004)
6. Calisti, M., Funk, P., Biellman, P., Bugnon, T.: Multi-Agent System for Organ Transplant Management, in (Moreno & Nealon, 2003) 199-212
7. Fox, J., Beveridge, M., Glasspool, D.: Understanding intelligent agents: analysis and synthesis, AI Communications 16 (3) (2003) 139-152
8. GA, http://www.ga.org Guardian Angel website, last updated 15 March 2002.
9. Godo, L., Puyol-Gruart, J., Sabater, J., Torra, V., Barrufet, P., Fabregas, X.: A multi-agent systems approach for monitoring the prescription of restricted use antibiotics, Art. Int. in Med. 27(3) (2003) 259-282.
10. Huang, J., Jennings, N.R., Fox, J.: An Agent-based Approach to Health Care Management. Applied Artificial Intelligence 9 (4) (1995) 401-420
11. Knublauch, H., Rose, T., Sedlmayr, M.: Towards a Multi-Agent System for Pro-Active Information Management in Anaesthesia. In Proc. of the Workshop on Autonomous Agents in Health Care at Agents 2000, Barcelona, Spain 2000.
12. Lanzola, G. Gatti, L. Falasconi, S., Stefanelli, M.: A Framework for Building Co-operative Software Agents in Medical Applications. Art. Int. in Med., 16(3) (1999) 223-249
13. Luck, M., Ashri, R. & D'Inverno, M.: *Agent-Based Software Development*, Artech 2004.
14. Mandl, K.D., Szolovits, P., Kohane, I.S.: Public Standards and Patients' Control: How to Keep Electronic Medical Records Accessible But Private. BMJ 322 (2001) 283-287.
15. Mark, A., Pencheon, D., Elliott, R.: Demanding Healthcare. Intl. J. of Health Planning & Mgmt. 15 (2000) 237-253
16. Moreno, A., Isern, D., Sanchez, D.: Provision of Agent-Based Healthcare Services, AI Comms. 16 (3) (2003) 167-178
17. Moreno, A., Valls, A., Bocio, J.: Management of Hospital Teams for Organ Transplant Coordination, Proc. of AIME 2001 (2001)
18. Neville R.G., Greene A.C., McLeod J., Tracy A., Surie J.: Mobile phone text messaging can help young people manage asthma. BMJ 2002 325 600
19. Neville R.G., McCowan C., Pagliari H.C., Mullen H., Fannin A.: E-mail Consultations in General Practice (in press)
20. Pouloudi A., Reed, C.A.: Towards a Multi-agent representation of stakeholder interests in NHSnet, Proc. PAAM98 (1998) 393-407
21. Riva, A., Mandl, K.D., Oh, D.H., Nigrin, D.J., Butte, A., Szolovits, P., Kohane, I.S.: The Personal Internetworked Notary and Guardian. Intl. J. of Med. Informatics 62 (2001) 27-40
22. Sabater, J., Sierra, C.: Reputation and Social Network Analysis in Multi-Agent Systems, Proc. AAMAS 2002, ACM Press.
23. White Paper – Patients as Partners in Care: A Plan for Action a Plan for Change HMSO (2003) The Scottish Executive
24. Smith, R.G.: The Contract Net Protocol: High Level Communication and Control in a Distributed Problem Solver. IEEE Trans. Computers 29 (12) (1980) 1104-1113
25. Wooldridge, M., Jennings, N.R., Kinny, D.: The Gaia Methodology for Agent-Oriented Analysis and Design. J. of Auton. Agents and Multi-Agent Systems 3 (3) (2000) 285-312

Clinical Reasoning Learning with Simulated Patients

Froduald Kabanza[1] and Guy Bisson[2]

[1] Department of Computer Science, University of Sherbrooke,
Sherbrooke, Québec J1K2R1, Canada
kabanza@usherbrooke.ca
[2] Faculty of Medicine, University of Sherbrooke,
Sherbrooke, Québec J1K2R1, Canada
Guy.Bisson@Usherbrooke.ca

Abstract. In this paper we introduce *clinical reasoning automata* to model states and transitions about different cognitive processes that occur during a clinical reasoning activity. A state of the automaton represents a particular process in a complex patient diagnosis using influence diagrams encoding clinical knowledge about the case. Transitions model switch between diagnosis cognitive processes, such as collecting evidences, formulating hypothesis or explicitly asking for assistance at a given point during the reasoning process. That way, we can efficiently model tutoring feedback hints for clinical reasoning learning that are based not only on the clinical knowledge, but also on the sequencing of the tutoring processes.

1 Introduction

Medical diagnostic problems that are the focus of clinical reasoning are examples of complex decision making problems for which solutions depend not only upon clinical knowledge and medical experience, but also on well drilled strategies for collecting evidences about pathologies, analyzing them, formulating hypotheses and evaluating them based on collected evidences. Clinical reasoning learning (CRL) in medicine deals with teaching medical students to acquire the basics of such cognitive strategies and to apply them [6].

In many medical schools, CRL is taught using a problem-based learning approach (PBL). Students, in small groups (typically six to eight students) are presented a patient case and asked to diagnose it and propose a treatment or a management plan. Under the supervision of an instructor, students will usually formulate initial hypotheses just after getting a brief presentation of the case, under the form of a textual problem statement, a live encounter with a patient simulated by a student playing a patient scenario prepared by the instructor, or a live encounter with a real patient recruited from a clinic or hospital. Then they will begin to collect evidences by asking questions to the patient (e.g., the motive of the consultation, in which parts of the body he is experiencing problems, how long and frequently the symptoms occur, his life style, and so on), then they will proceed with a directed physical exam (e.g., sensing reflexes) and after that order laboratory/imaging tests (e.g., urine tests, blood tests,

X-rays or MRI). The evidences are analyzed and then the hypotheses are reevaluated to discard those not fitting with the analysis, to keep those still uncertain, and to collect again new evidences in order to discard or confirm remaining hypotheses or generate new ones. This process of evidence collection, evidence analysis, hypothesis evaluation and hypothesis reformulation is iterated until the students are able to narrow their list of probable hypotheses to the one or two most probable diagnosis.

Students conduct their investigation based upon their declarative knowledge they have learned in PBL sessions and also on similar cases they have already seen in clinical settings or in previous CRL sessions. The clinical knowledge linking symptoms to diseases is at least in part a probabilistic exercise whereas the actions used to collect evidences (i.e., questions, physical exams and lab tests) involve tradeoffs about costs, harm to the patient, and the value of the information obtained from the tests with regard to the current hypotheses. The instructor uses his own experience and knowledge to provide hints to the students during their investigation and sometimes to comment on variant of similar cases.

Because of the cognitive complexity of CRL, it is crucial that students have a varied, very well organized and structured knowledge base, and be exposed to as many cases as possible in their curriculum, since this is mostly an experience-based learning process. To foster the acquisition of their clinical reasoning skills, it is mandatory that the CRL involves small group sizes. However, this requires that a lot of instructors be available, yet for the most part these instructors are also physicians and/or researchers, hence with very limited availability, particularly given today severe shortage of physicians in most countries.

Many medical schools are therefore turning towards the use of software simulations to support at least in part the CRL activities. One possible strategy is to keep an affordable number of CRL courses directly supervised by instructors and to have students practice on computer-based cases that are variants of those learned in classes, in groups or individually, with the assumption that computer-based cases will require little supervision by instructors or no supervision at all if the computer has enough intelligence capabilities to automatically provide the required feedback to students.

Providing feedback to students in computer-based CRL requires a system that not only is able to assess the student's strengths and weaknesses of his clinical reasoning process to solve a patient case, but is also able to apply metacognitive strategies to identify and correct flaws in his reasoning strategies, for instance, with regard to how he interleaves evidence collection and the hypothesis formulation processes. However, computer-based CRL systems proposed to date focus mostly on providing feedback with regard to the application of declarative clinical knowledge, with very little emphasis on feedback related to cognitive strategies about the sequencing of clinical reasoning sub-processes [3,4,9,10].

DxR is one of the most used commercial CRL software with a database of about a hundred clinical cases, covering both patient diagnosis and management [3]. However, DxR has no built-in student's model other than a simple decision tree checking whether the student has reached the correct diagnosis within a given deadline and has considered all relevant hypotheses. The decision tree is explicitly specified by the instructor who authors the case. Consequently, students using DxR autonomously learn mostly by reinforcement as the decision tree indicates whether they have the right hypotheses or not, but with little ongoing feedback about their reasoning processes. Other commercial CRL systems such as VIPS have the same limitations [10].

The Adele [4] and COMET [9] systems provide more advanced automated tutoring feedback by using an influence diagram (i.e., a Bayesian network with actions and action utilities) to model the clinical knowledge about the patient. In fact the influence diagram represents expert knowledge about how symptoms probabilistically relate to diseases and how evidence-collect actions or clinical-knowledge-apply actions relate to evidences. It is essentially the same kind of Bayesian networks used in medical decision support systems to recommend diagnosis, to collect new evidences, or treatment to clinicians in real-life cases [7,8]. The generation of tutoring feedbacks is done by comparing the recommendations obtained from the network, to actions, evidences or hypotheses found by the students, and by providing hints accordingly.

More specifically, at any step of the interaction between the student and the CRL interface that simulates a patient, we can recognize the evidence collected by the student and we can also determine the hypothesis he is currently working on, either by asking them to the student directly, or by inferring them. Thus, given the current evidences as collected by the student we can use Bayesian inference algorithms to determine the most likely hypotheses from the expert point of view and compare them with the hypotheses currently inferred by the student. Based on the comparison, we can for example give hints to the student about whether he is on the right track or not, or give hints that will put him on the right track. Conversely, given the current hypotheses collected by the student, we could use again Bayesian inference algorithms to determine the most valuable evidences to collect next, and exploit this information to give hints about which evidences to collect next and how.

However, this approach does not model CRL strategies about how to interleave and refine the different phases of evidence collection, evidence analysis, hypothesis evaluation and hypothesis reformulation. An instructor supervising CRL will provide hints not just aimed at instructing the student how to apply clinical knowledge, but also hints aimed at sharing with him his "rules of thumb" about how to interleave the different phases of evidence collection, evidence analysis, hypothesis evaluation and hypothesis reformulation. For instance, he may remind the student of the appropriate time to stop the current phase of evidence collection in order to re-evaluate his hypotheses. He may also explain why at a given step it's better to collect evidences that rule out one current hypothesis rather than evidences that confirm a current active hypothesis, for instance as a measure to minimize the cost of evidence collection and not jeopardize the patient health. He may also intervene at certain points to provide structured knowledge about variant cases related to the one under study. For instance after a student has correctly interpreted evidences gathered from a lab test based on the current patient's data, the instructor may discuss patient cases for which the same test results would have yield a different interpretation. Such strategic interventions are not easily conveyed by Bayesian networks; in fact none of the above systems addresses them.

We introduce *clinical reasoning automata* (CRA) in our model on top of influence diagrams to fill this gap. These are hybrid finite state automata representing allowed sequences and refinements of the different phases of evidence collection, evidence analysis, hypothesis evaluation and hypothesis reformulation. The automaton has a finite number of states, but each state represents a clinical reasoning sub-process, that is, the system continues to evolve within a state, hence the qualification "hybrid". A process modeled by a state has access to a global influence diagram encoding clinical knowledge as in Adele [4] and COMET [9], and local state-based production rules to provide feedback. This provides a means for modeling sequenced feedback rules, and also leads to a modular specification of tutoring feedbacks.

In the next section we present the system that we are currently developing to simulate patients and foster clinical reasoning cognitive strategies. Then we discuss the modeling of tutoring feedbacks using CRA. After a conclusion, we discuss future developments.

2 Patient Simulation System

Our patient simulator, TeachMed, has a graphic user interface (GUI) that provides functionalities similar to DxR [3] and VIPS [10]. The student GUI allows the student to select a patient case, access the patient's medical record, interview the patient, proceed with a physical exam on a 3D model of the patient (Fig. 1), interact with a laboratory module to order tests (Fig. 2), and finally treat and manage the patient. Instructors use another GUI to author patient cases.

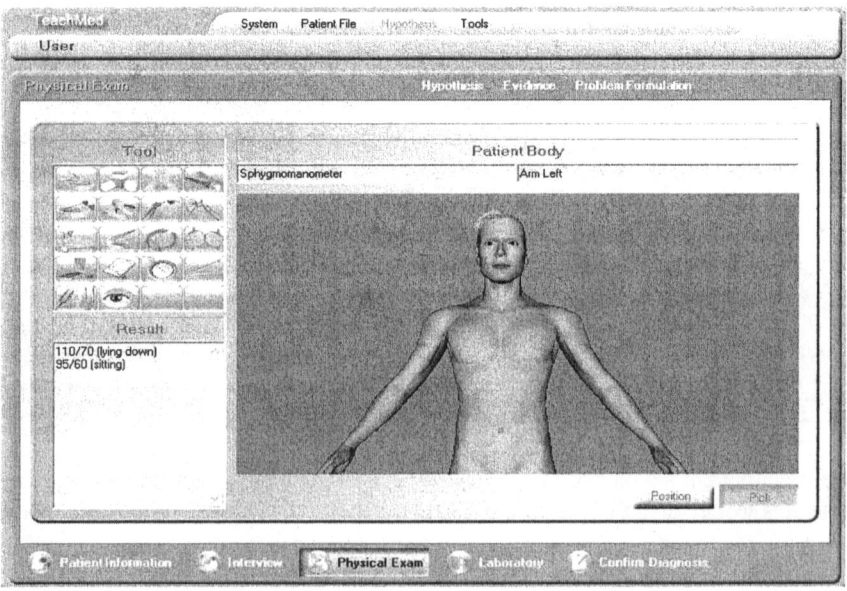

Fig. 1. The student decides to take the patient's blood pressure

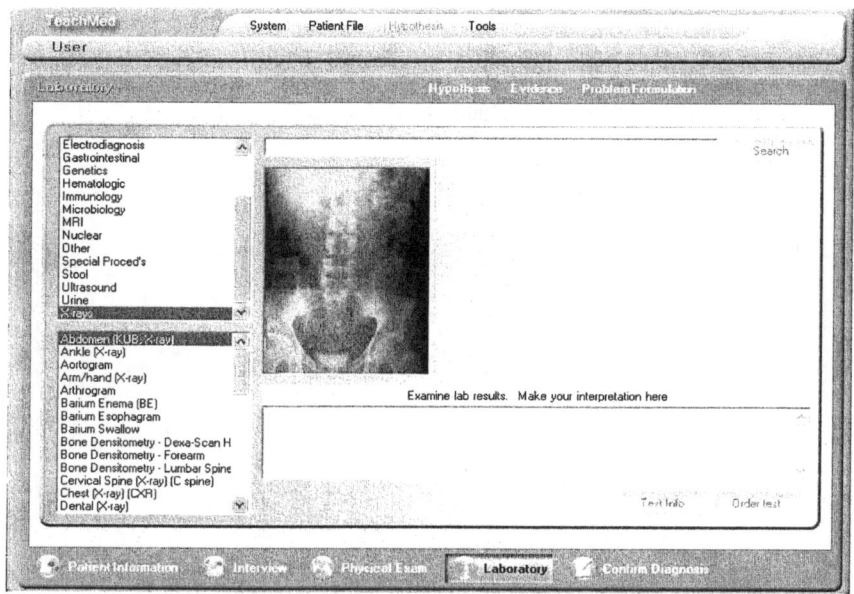

Fig. 2. Abdominal plain x-ray ordered by the student

3 Automated Tutor

A key component of TeachMed is an automated tutor that monitors the student's actions to provide rapid feedback. Tutoring feedback is implemented based on a *clinical influence diagram*, the *current system state*, *feedback rules* triggered by the current system state, and a *clinical reasoning automaton* that sequences clinical reasoning sub-processes and corresponding feedback rules.

3.1 Clinical Influence Diagram and Bayesian Inference Processes

A clinical influence diagram is a Bayesian network encoding the clinical diagnostic knowledge from an expert point of view. It specifies causal links between evidences, symptoms and pathologies (with corresponding probability distributions), as well as actions that investigate these symptoms (with corresponding utilities). Fig. 3 shows a fragment of an influence diagram we use for a case of acute diarrhea. Probabilities and utility specifications are omitted for clarity. The fragment illustrates only some nodes with few evidence-collection actions (questions to the patient and lab tests). The entire model for the diarrhea case contains 70 nodes, including physical exam actions and curriculum-knowledge application actions to collect evidences.

The influence diagram is implemented using Smile Bayesian network library [2]. Evidences gathered by the student are recorded into a *student evidence table*. Given this table, we use Smile library to compute the posterior probability for a set of hypotheses from the expert point of view and rank them according to their likelihood, that is, the *expert hypothesis table*. Intuitively, assuming the influence diagram correctly models the expert clinical knowledge, the expert would infer these hypotheses from the given evidences. On the other hand, based on his evidence table, the student will infer his own hypothesis table (i.e., the *student hypothesis table*) which may or may not match the expert hypothesis table.

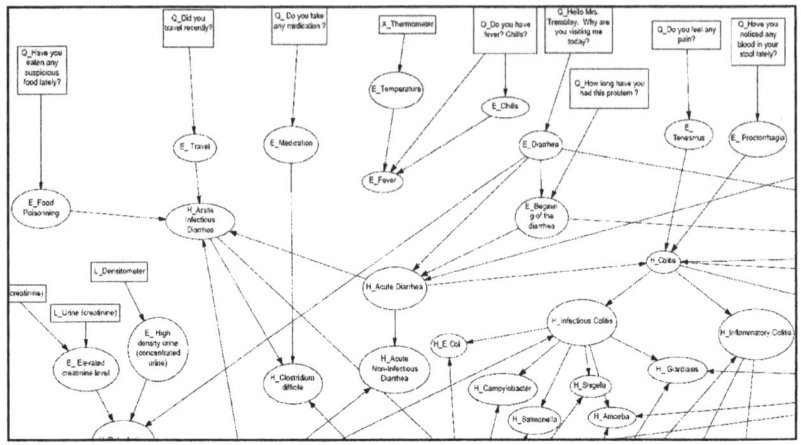

Fig. 3. Fragment of the Bayesian network for the acute diarrhea case

In principle, the next best evidence-gathering process should be one yielding a value of information that exceeds the cost of gathering information. However, in general it is very difficult to express the utilities of evidence-gathering actions with a level of accuracy that takes into account all possible evidence observations [7,8]. Therefore, we do not rely entirely on the utilities specified for evidence-gathering actions to provide feedback about the next evidence-gathering process. Rather we use these utilities as heuristic input to feedback rules that provide the actual hints about the next evidence-gathering steps. More specifically, based on the current student's evidence and hypothesis tables, we use Smile library to compute evidence-collection actions and store them into a *next student evidence-action table*, on top of which we can express facts that are preconditions of feedback rules. For instance, we can specify a feedback rule stating that "if not acute-infection-diarrhea and urine test's value of information is less than blood test no more by x threshold, then perform urine test".

In order to provide feedback TeachMed needs to determine the current hypothesis the student is trying to confirm or reject (i.e., the *student's hypothesis goal*) or the current evidence he is trying to collect (i.e., the *student's evidence goal*). We could obtain this information by simply asking it to the student, but this would result in too much intervention, disturbing the tutoring strategy, particularly for advanced students who just need occasional help. Instead, based on the observed student's actions (i.e., questions he asks, physical exams he makes, or lab tests he orders), we use Smile library to infer the evidence he is trying to collect, similarly for the student's hypothesis goal. If the output of this goal recognition is below a validity threshold, we prompt a question to the student to get directly from him the goal he is working on. If the recognition output is a list of at most three elements with valid probability above the threshold, the question looks like "are you trying to establish x, y or z?" Otherwise, the question is a direct one such as "what hypothesis are you trying to establish?"

3.2 Student Model and Model Tracer

TeachMed maintains a *student model*, reflecting the student's progress information inferred from the influence diagram as explained above (i.e., student evidence table, expert evidence table, student's hypothesis table, the student's hypothesis goal, and the student's evidence goal), and student's input for feedback request (e.g., the student can ask TeachMed to help him decide between two interpretations of a lab test). A process, called the *student's model tracer*, monitors the student's actions and periodically invokes the update processes described above to maintain the student's model.

3.3 Feedback Rules and Feedback Generator

The *feedback generator* is a process that periodically checks the current student's model to trigger tutoring feedback to the student, using production rules that are preconditioned on data in the student's model and having consequents that are tutoring hints. These are "teaching" expert rules and can be as efficient as the available teaching expertise allows.

To illustrate, a feedback rule of the form "if student-asks-help (interpret, test, results) then hint-test-interpretation (test, results)" will trigger a hint helping the student about the interpretation of a lab test. Following Andes' approach [5], hints are implemented using template-based heuristic dialogues, with slots replaced by data in the student's model. With the previous example, TeachMed will engage a tree-structured dialog with the student by asking him his impressions about the interpretation and issuing hints until the dialog concludes in the correct interpretation. Feedback rules can also be triggered by TeachMed initiative by having rules with antecedents based upon the evaluation of the student's progress as reflected by the student's model.

3.4 Clinical Reasoning Automaton

A *clinical reasoning automaton* (CRA) is a state transition system that abstracts the evolution of the student's model under the student's actions. The feedback generator starts in a given state of the automaton. In the current state, it is synchronized with the model tracer monitoring the student's actions, focusing on one sub-goal, and using a set of feedback rules to help the student. A transition to a new state switches the sub-goal and the feedback rules to those of the new state. From another perspective, a state of the CRA represents a sub-process of the clinical reasoning (e.g., the student is collecting evidence for "Acute Diarrhea"). Therefore, a CRA state is a dynamic state in that, the student's model continues to evolve; for example, the evidence and hypothesis table continue to change under the student's actions. A transition signals the occurrence of an event that is sufficiently interesting (from the point of view of a given tutoring strategy) to switch a context (e.g., the student's has finished collecting evidences for the current student's evidence goal). More formally, a CRA is a hybrid automaton [1], consisting of:

- A finite set of variables (composing the student's model), a *time* variable (counting the time elapsed in a state), and possibly additional variables defined by the patient-case author (e.g., a student performance variable).
- A finite set of states, consisting of the variables (*time* and student's model variables remain implicit), feedback rules and functions about each variable evolution in the state.
- A start state.
- A finite set of transition between states.

A transition is a triplet of the form "*(u, test, v)*", where *test* is a Boolean expression over variables in state *u* (implicit and/or explicit), possibly involving author-defined Boolean functions over these variables. The transition means that if the *test* holds (i.e., the transition is enabled), then the feedback generator moves into state *v*. If many transitions are simultaneously enabled, then it moves in a nondeterministic fashion into one of the successor states.

The author must define functions determining the evolution of the variables he specifies. For the built-in variables, the functions are defined as follows. The time variable is initialized to zero upon entering the state and is automatically incremented as time passes. The variables in the student's model are updated by the *model tracer*.

There is no explicit notion of accepting a run for a task automaton. Goodness or badness of runs is conveyed to the learner via the feedback given in states. However, it's possible to implement rules with a side effect of updating a performance score for the student. One can also specify transitions to states in which the feedback indicates complete success for the task or complete failure.

Assuming that we are in a state monitoring the student collecting evidence for some symptom, we can have an outgoing transition labeled "hypothesis-goal-changed" (i.e., the model tracer has established that the student has switched to another hypothesis) to a state in which we watch whether the student remembers to reformulate his hypotheses. In this new state, if a student attempts any action not related to the evaluation and re-formulation of his hypotheses he will get feedback hints aimed at making him remember why at this stage he should reformulate his hypotheses. It could be possible to express this feedback without using a CRA transition to a new state, but then this will result in complex, unstructured feedback rules that not only become difficult to maintain, but also are executed less efficiently since at every stage the system has a large number of rules to consider. In contrast, CRA feedback rules only depend on states and in the current state there are only few of them to consider, that is, those active in that state. It is possible to encode feedback rules that depend on a trace (i.e., a sequence of states), by defining a variable that records relevant part of the trace into a state and specifying feedback rules that have facts in their antecedents that depend on the current value of the variable.

4 Experiments

TeachMed is still under development and so far has been tested on simple scenarios. To illustrate the use of CRA, at given point the student may be asking a series of questions to the patient focusing on one particular hypothesis among his current list, to confirm or reject it. We say that this is the working hypothesis. Usually it's not a good idea to switch the focus of the working hypothesis back and forth without exhausting all relevant questions on the current working hypothesis, until more evidences are introduced in to make re-activation of the hypothesis relevant. Therefore, whenever the student asks a question that is irrelevant to the working hypothesis, we determine whether he has changed his working hypothesis without explicitly stating it (hence the question may actually be relevant to the new working hypothesis). In this case, we check whether he has exhausted all questions related to the working hypothesis at this point. We have two possibilities: (a) if he has indeed exhausted all relevant questions, a feedback message is displayed asking him to formulate his new working hypothesis, with a transition to a new state of the CRA, activating feedback rules for hypothesis formulation; (b) otherwise, Teachmed initiates a dialogue with him aimed at making him realize that there are still evidences to collect using questions, for the current working hypothesis.

The following dialogue illustrates (a). Some answers of the simulated patient to questions by the student are omitted to make it short. There is no natural language processing contrary to what the dialogue may suggest. Student's questions are used for a keyword search into a database of questions and matched ones are displayed for the student to pick one of them corresponding to the question he actually wants to ask.

Collected Evidence:	Acute lower abdominal pain
Working Hypothesis:	Urinary infection
Student (Question):	"Any fever?"
Student (Question):	"Could you describe your pain?"
Student (Question):	"Is it worse on one side?"
Student (Question):	"How many times did you urinate since the beginning of your pain?"
Student (Question)	"Do you have a burning sensation on urination?"
Student (Question):	"Do you have a sexual partner?"
Tutor:	Is this question relevant to the hypothesis you are working with? (Yes / No - I'm examining another hypothesis.)
Student:	No - I'm examining another hypothesis.
Tutor:	Formulate your hypothesis.

5 Conclusion

In our medical school, CRL are currently conducted live in small groups of eight students under the supervision of a professor who is a domain expert. One student is picked to play the role of a patient and another plays the role of the physician. The remaining students are observers but also actively participate in the discussion. The patient student behaves according to instructions prepared by the professor on paper based on pedagogical objectives that are fixed by the curriculum committee. The school is planning to start using TeachMed to complement these simulations in the winter of 2006. The students will use TeachMed in an autonomous mode.

Besides this forthcoming deployment of TeachMed in our medical curriculum, future work includes the implementation of an interface between TeachMed and a real-world health record containing information about patients and how they were treated. As noted by Gertner et al. in their physics tutoring system [5], a Bayesian network implicitly models solutions, but not the solution process itself. Yet, being able to model the solution process can improve the quality of feedback given to the student. A similar observation holds in CRL, with the difference that the solving process is harder to formalize other than giving general strategies about the interleaving of the different clinical reasoning sub-processes. Nevertheless, we feel that the possibility of having one expert-solution, albeit not encompassing all experts' solutions, can be exploited to provide enriched feedback. In the more trivial case, we could illustrate the solution to the student as one example of expert's approach. Given that an electronic heath-record does not contain clinical reasoning traces, but contains just the solutions (i.e., the diagnosis and the patient treatment), the challenge will be to find techniques for inferring expert solving processes from expert solutions.

References

1. Alur, R., Courcoubetis, C., Henzinger, T., and Po. H.: Hybrid automata: an algorithmic approach to the specification and verification of hybrid systems. In: Proceedings of Hybrid Systems. Lecture Notes in Computer Science, Vol. 736, Springer Verlag, (1993):209-229.
2. Druzdzel, M.: SMILE: Structural Modeling, Inference, and Learning Engine and GeNIE: A Development Environment for Graphical Decision-Theoretic Models. In Proceedings of the Eleventh Conference on Innovative Applications of Artificial Intelligence, (1999) 902-903. (See http://www.sis.pitt.edu/~genie/ for system download).
3. DxR Clinician: http://www.dxrgroup.com/
4. Ganeshan, R., Johnson, L., Shaw, E. and Wood, B.: Tutoring Diagnostic Problem Solving. In: Proceedings of Conference on Intelligent Tutoring Systens, Lecture Notes in Computer Science, Vol. 1839, (2000) 33-42
5. Gertner, A., Conati, C. and VanLehn, K.: Procedural help in Andes: Generating Hints Using a Bayesian Network Student Model. In: Proceedings of National Conference on Artificial Intelligence, AAAI Press, (1998)106-111.
6. Gruppen, L. and Frohna, A.: Clinical Reasoning. International Handbook of Research in Medical education. Kluwer Academic (2000) 205-230
7. Heckerman, D., Horvitz, E. and Nathwani, B.: Towards Normative Expert Systems: Part I. The Pathfinder Project. In: Methods of Information in Medecine (1992): 90-105.
8. Onisko, A., Lucas, P. and Druzdzel M.: Comparison of Rule-Based and Bayesian Network Approaches in Medical Diagnostic Systems. In: Proceedings of the Eighth {Annual Conference on Artificial Intelligence in Medicine, Lecture Notes in Computer Sciences, vol. 2101, Springer Verlag, (2001): 281-292.
9. Suebnukarn, S. and Haddawy, P. Collaborative Intelligent Tutoring System for Medical Problem-Based Learning. In: Proceedings of the Ninth Conference on Intelligent User Interfaces, (2004)14-21.
10. VIPS: Virtual Internet Patient Simulator: https://www.swissvips.ch/fr/index.htm

Implicit Learning System for Teaching the Art of Acute Cardiac Infarction Diagnosis*

Dmitry Kochin[1], Leonas Ustinovichius[2], and Victoria Sliesoraitiene [2,3]

[1] Institute for System Analysis,
117312, prosp. 60-letija Octjabrja, 9, Moscow, Russia
dco@mail.ru
[2] Vilnius Gediminas Technical University,
LT-10223, Sauletekio al. 11, Vilnius, Lithuania
leonasu@st.vtu.lt
[3] Vilnius University Children hospital Rehabilitation and education centre,
LT-08406, Santariskių 7, Vilnius, Lithuania
viktorijaslie@one.lt

Abstract. There are two types of knowledge – declarative (theoretical) and procedural (practical skills). While the former knowledge may be acquired by reading books, the latter requires long intensive practice. The majority of computer-aided learning systems teach declarative knowledge only. This paper presents basic ideas of building intellectual computer systems for teaching procedural expert knowledge, such as medical diagnostic skills. Two sub-problems are under consideration – the elicitation of experienced physician's decision rules and the construction of the computer system for teaching these rules. Such systems utilize the principle of implicit learning. The authors present the methodology of practical realization of these ideas in application of teaching the art of acute cardiac infarction diagnosis.

1 Introduction

There are two types of knowledge – declarative and procedural. Declarative knowledge includes theories, facts and data. It can be described in books. The most illustrative example of declarative knowledge is a textbook.

Procedural knowledge is the ability to apply declarative knowledge in practice. A person who acquired mastery in any professional field is called *expert*. To become an expert one requires at least 10 years of intensive practice as well as guidance by an experienced tutor [1, 8].

One of the approaches to shortening this time is computerized learning systems. They allow intensifying the learning process, increasing the motivation of novices and

---

* This work is supported by the Scientific Programs "Mathematical Modeling and Intelligent Systems", "Fundamentals of Information Technology and Systems" of the Russian Academy of Sciences; the projects 04-01-00290, 05-01-00666 of the Russian Foundation for Basic Research; the grant 1964.2003.1 of the President of the Russian Federation for the support of the prominent scientific schools.

facilitating the job of a tutor. However, the majority of modern learning systems teach only declarative knowledge, that is appear to be just an interactive textbook. Of course, in many cases, such learning systems allow students to learn better due to more "alive" presentation of the material, but still, on the completion of learning the student doesn't have enough practical skills and requires additional practice.

In order to build a learning system we have to solve two problems [5]:

1. To build a knowledge base imitating the knowledge of the given expert.
2. To transfer this knowledge base to a novice, thus teaching him/her to solve practical problems like experts.

In this paper we consider a particular approach to the construction of the learning systems for teaching *procedural knowledge*, allowing a novice to gain the experience of solving practical tasks in learning. We present the methodology of learning system application to teaching the art of Acute Cardiac Infarction (ACI) diagnosis.

2 Building the Knowledge Base

To solve the first problem, we can use *expert classification* approach [6, 2], allowing us to build a comprehensive and consistent knowledge base in an individual knowledge field for a relatively short time. This approach was first developed by Oleg Larichev [6] and is designed for the problems where an expert assigns different objects to different classes. The medical diagnosis perfectly suits this model. A doctor assigns a patient (object) described by a set of distinct attributes (symptoms) to a particular class (diagnosis). Contrary to machine learning methods, this approach results in precise knowledge base, because all decisions affecting the base are manually made by an interviewed expert. Let us formally state the problem of expert classification.

1. G – a property, corresponding to the target criterion of the problem (for example, presence of the specific disease and degree of its development).
2. $K = \{K_1, K_2, ..., K_N\}$ – a set of attributes (such as groups of symptoms), by which each object (patient) is evaluated.
3. $S_q = \{k_1^q, k_2^q, ..., k_{\omega_q}^q\}$ for $q = 1, ..., N$ – a set of verbal attribute values on the scale of attribute K_q; ω_q – number of values for K_q; values in S_q are *in descending order* by typicality for the property G. That is, for each S_q there is defined linear reflexive antisymmetric transitive relation Q_q: $\left(k_i^q, k_j^q\right) \in Q_q \Leftrightarrow i \leq j$. For example, in application to ACI diagnosis, we have an attribute "Age" with values ("Older than 30 years", "Younger than 30 years"). Age more than 30 is more typical of ACI.
4. $Y = S_1 \times S_2 \times ... \times S_N$ – a Cartesian product of attribute scales defining a space of object states to be classified. Each object is described by a set of values for attributes $K_1, ..., K_N$ and can be represented by a vector $y \in Y$, where $y = (y_1, y_2, ..., y_N)$, y_q equals the index of the corresponding value in S_q.
5. $L = |Y| = \prod_{q=1}^{N} \omega_q$ – Cardinality of Y.

6. $C = \{C_1, C_2, ..., C_M\}$ – a set of decision classes in descending order by intensity of the property G. On the C set there is defined linear reflexive antisymmetric transitive relation Q_C: $(C_i, C_j) \in Q_C \Leftrightarrow i \leq j$. With respect to ACI, there are three classes: "ACI", "Possible ACI, but additional study is required" and "No ACI (may be another disease)". The classes are ordered by the degree of intensity of ACI in the class formulation.

Let us introduce binary relation of the dominance:

$$P = \left\{ (\mathbf{x}, \mathbf{y}) \in Y \times Y \,\middle|\, \forall q = 1...N \ \ x_q \geq y_q \ \ \grave{e} \ \ \exists q_0 : x_{q_0} > y_{q_0} \right\} \quad (1)$$

Required: to build with the help of the expert a reflection $F: Y \rightarrow \{Y_i\}, i = 1...M$, such that $Y = \bigcup_{l=1}^{M} Y_l$; $Y_l \cap Y_k = \emptyset, \ k \neq l$ (where Y_i – a set of vectors, belonging to class C_i), satisfying the consistency condition:

$$\forall x, y \in Y : x \in Y_i, y \in Y_j, (x, y) \in P \Rightarrow i \geq j \quad (2)$$

The knowledge base is comprehensive in the sense that *any* possible combination of values of diagnostic attributes is contained within the base along with its class (diagnosis). And it is logically consistent as long as condition (2) is satisfied.

The method solving this problem uses the expert as the only information source. To assign an object to a class the method requires questioning the expert. In general, to assign each object to a class, the expert would need to consider all objects. However, utilizing relations (1) and (2) it is possible to build a far more efficient procedure [0], when the majority of objects are classified indirectly. For example, provided that the expert assigned an object with moderate dyspnea to class ACI, then we can judge that the object with the same symptoms, but asthmatic fit, should also be assigned to class ACI, because the asthmatic fit is more typical to ACI than moderate dyspnea.

To build a comprehensive knowledge base of ACI diagnosis using method CLARA (SAC) [0] (about 2500 real-life combinations of symptoms), the expert was directly presented with only 250 clinical situations. Analyzing the knowledge base it is possible to reveal decision rules defining the whole classification [4, 6].

3 Implicit Learning

The goal of learning is the creation of subconscious rules in the long-term memory of a young specialist, which would allow him/her to make decisions identically to an expert. One of the first learning system used rule-based learning. A student was presented with diagnostic rules for memorizing, and then the system asked him/her to diagnose hypothetic patients. If the student made a mistake, the system showed the correct decision rule.

This scheme being perfect for solving standard mathematical problems was ineffective in teaching the art of medical diagnosis. It was discovered that learning by explicitly specified decision rules did not develop any clinical thinking based on the analysis of patient descriptions, but led to routine logic and arithmetic manipulations. Forgetting only a small fragment of a rule produced catastrophic results in the knowledge verification tests.

The way out of the deadlock became the idea that one should not try to "transmit" the decision rules of the expert to the novice, but should rather help the novice to "grow" them on his/her own by using human abilities for implicit learning. Research in this interesting direction of cognitive psychology was aimed at solving abstract test problems like the artificial grammar [3]. In such problems the subject was presented with different sets of symbols generated by some rule, and the task was to recognize whether this unknown rule is applied in control sets of the verification test. The unique feature of knowledge acquired in this way was the fact that subjects kept the acquired skills for several years without being able to verbalize the rule itself.

We redesigned the computer system for the new paradigm. The system does not show the rules anymore, but only presents a series of hypothetic patients (randomly selected from the knowledge base), asking a student for a diagnosis (Fig. 1). Experimenting with the new system brought very interesting results. During the whole course of learning (two days, four hours a day), every student (the students of the Russian Academy of the Post-diploma Education and young physicians of the Botkin hospital of Moscow) solved about 500 tasks of different complexity. During the verification test the subjects gave 90-100% answers identical to the expert's

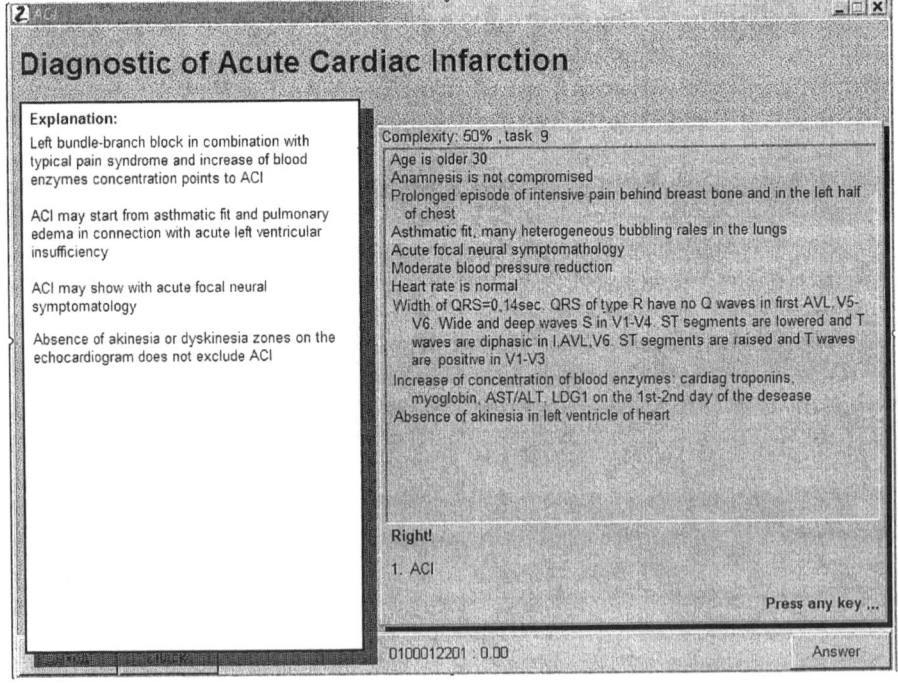

Fig. 1. The learning system with the comment on a diagnostic task solution

answers, but failed, as well as the expert, to verbalize the decision rules describing their decisions [7].

It should be noted that this method of teaching, based on students' creative analysis of their own decisions and comparing them to expert decisions, helps them not just start solving diagnostic problems at a higher quality level, but significantly improve their clinical thinking.

The teaching methodology developed includes gradual increasing of tasks complexity depending on the progress of a student, theoretical course in ACI, comments to the mistakes of a student.

4 Conclusion

This paper presents basic ideas of building the intellectual computer systems for teaching procedural expert knowledge. The system contains the knowledge base built with the help of a prominent expert. This base is used to pick sample tasks during the learning process. The system utilizes the principle of implicit learning to transfer knowledge to a student. Implicit learning results in better and longer memorizing than rule-based approaches.

Such systems can be used for training young specialists as well as for retraining specialists experienced in other knowledge fields who could acquire expert skills in lesser time and with fewer fatal mistakes.

New computer systems create the conditions for developing a new type of university education aimed at preparing young specialists possessing not only theoretical knowledge, but also practical skills.

References

1. *Ericsson K.A., Lehnmann A.C.* Expert and Exceptional Performance: Evidence of Maximal Adaptation to Task Constraints. Annual Review of Psychology. 1996. V. 47. pp. 273-305.
2. *Kochin D.Yu., Larichev O.I., Kortnev A.V.* Decision Support System for Classification of a Finite Set of Multicriteria Alternatives, Journal of Decision Support Systems 33 (2002), pp. 13-21
3. *Reber A.S.* Implicit Learning of Artificial Grammars. Journal of Verbal Learning and Verbal Behaviour. 1967. V. 77. pp. 317-327
4. *Asanov A.A., Kochin D.Yu.* The Elicitation of Subconscious Expert Decision Rules in the Multicriteria Classification Problems. CAI-2002. Conference proceedings. Vol. 1, pp. 534-544. M.: Fizmatlit, 2002. (in Russian)
5. *Larichev O.I., Brook E.I.,* The Computer Learning as the Part of University Education. Universitetskaya Kniga, №5, 2000, pp. 13-15 (in Russian)
6. *Larichev O.I., Mechitov A.I., Moshkovich E.M., Furems E.M.* Expert Knowledge Elicitation. M.: Nauka, 1989 (in Russian)
7. *Larichev O.I., Naryzhniy E.V.* The Computer Learning of the Procedural Knowledge. Psyhologicheskiy Zhurnal, 1999, V. 20, № 6, pp. 53-61 (in Russian)
8. *Peldschus, F., Messing, D., Zavadskas, E.K., Ustinovičius L.*: LEVI 3.0 – Multiple Criteria Evaluation Program. Journal of Civil Engineering and Management, Vol 8. Technika, Vilnius (2002) 184-191

Which Kind of Knowledge Is Suitable for Redesigning Hospital Logistic Processes?

Laura Măruşter and René J. Jorna

Faculty of Management and Organization, University of Groningen,
PO Box 800, 9700 AV Groningen, The Netherlands

Abstract. A knowledge management perspective is rarely used to model a process. Using the cognitive perspective on knowledge management in which we start our analysis with events and knowledge (bottom-up) instead of with processes and units (top-down), we propose a new approach for redesigning hospital logistic processes. To increase the care efficiency of multi-disciplinary patients, tailored knowledge in content and type that supports the reorganization of care should be provided. We discuss the advantages of several techniques in providing robust knowledge about the logistic hospital process by employing electronic patient records (EPR's) and diagnosis treatment combinations (DTC's).

1 Introduction

Due to the application of information technology and the promotion of changing the structure in certain organizations, business processes need to be redesigned, an approach coined as Business Process Reengineering [1]. As changes occur in the business environment, the existing process is at risk of becoming misaligned and consequently less effective. To increase the capabilities of enterprises to learn faster through their processes, strategies have been proposed that construct knowledge management systems around processes to: (i) increase their knowledge creating capacity, (ii) enhance their capacity to create value, and (iii) make them more able to learn [2]; in other words "... knowledge management (KM) can be thought of as a strategy of business process redesign" [2]. Modelling and redesigning a business process involves more than restructuring the workflow; therefore business professionals need to learn how to describe, analyze, and redesign business processes using robust methods.

Using the KM perspective, we make distinctions between content and form of knowledge. Concerning the *content* of knowledge, we are providing support for people to analyze, model and reorganize the hospital logistic processes with the new knowledge that can be distilled from electronic patient records (EPR's) and from diagnosis treatment combinations (DTC). With respect to the *forms* (types) of knowledge, a classification consisting of sensory, coded and theoretical knowledge has been used, based on the ideas of Boisot [3] and using the insights of cognitive science [4]. *Sensory knowledge* is based on sensory experience; it is very difficult to code. *Coded knowledge* is a representation based on a conventional relation between the representation and that which is being referred to. Coded knowledge contains all types of signs or symbols, expressed either as texts, drawings, or mathematical formulas. A person who is able to explain why certain pieces of knowledge belong together possesses *theoretical knowledge* concerning this specific knowledge domain. Theoretical knowledge is often used to identify causal relations (i.e. if-then-relations).

Employing the knowledge categorization defined by van Heusden&Jorna [5] (i.e. sensory, coded and theoretical knowledge), we propose a KM perspective for redesigning a business process which consists of:

1. Knowledge creation. Raw data are first converted into coded knowledge, then this knowledge is used to provide theoretical knowledge about the logistic hospital process.
2. Knowledge use and transfer. New theoretical knowledge can be used for analyzing, diagnosing and reorganizing the logistic hospital process. Because of its codification, it can be easily transferred to other people, or from one part of the organization to another one.

The paper is organized as follows: in Section 2 we describe two forms of knowledge conversion and the creation of new knowledge about the treatment process in a hospital. In Section 3 we illustrate how newly created knowledge can be used to reorganize the hospital logistic process. We conclude our paper with directions for further research in Section 4.

2 Knowledge Conversion. New Knowledge About Patients

The number of patients who require the involvement of different specialisms is increasing because of the increasing specialization of doctors and an aging population. Special arrangements have emerged for these patients; however, the specialisms comprising these centers are based on the specialists' perceptions. In other words, specialists have a certain sensory knowledge about what specialisms should form a center, which eventually could be supported by some quantitative information (e.g. frequencies of visits), but knowledge expressed in models or rules is missing. Given some criteria for selecting patients, we use the records of 3603 patients from Elisabeth Hospital, Tilburg, The Netherlands. The collected data refer to personal characteristics (e.g. age, gender), policlinic visits, clinical admissions, visits to radiology and functional investigations.

Medical specialists need knowledge expressed in explicit models (i.e. theoretical knowledge) as a base for creating multi-disciplinary units, where different specialisms coordinate the treatment of specific groups of patients. However, the information existing in electronic patient records (EPR's) needs to be distilled in a meaningful way. We obtain the needed knowledge by converting (i) **raw data** into **coded knowledge** (RD$\Rightarrow$CK) and (ii) **coded knowledge** into **theoretical knowledge** (CK$\Rightarrow$TK).

2.1 The Development of Logistic Patient Groups

For the first type of conversion RD⇒CK, we use the idea of operationalizing the logistic complexity by distinguishing six aggregated logistic variables, developed in [6]. Theoretical knowledge provides knowledge expressed as causal and structural relations. This knowledge is necessary when taking decisions for re-organizing hospitals. For the second type of conversion CK⇒TK, we refer again to [6]. First, two valid clusters are identified: one cluster for "moderately complex" patients, and another cluster for "complex" ones. Second, a rule-based model is induced to characterize these clusters. As general characteristic, patients from the "moderately complex" cluster have visited up to three different specialists, while patients from the cluster "complex" have visited more than three different specialists [6].

2.2 Discovering the Process Models for Patient Logistic Groups

Theoretical knowledge expressed in clear-cut patient logistic groups and their rule-based characterizations do not provide enough understanding and arguments for (re-)organizing multi-disciplinary units. To better understand the treatment process, we need insight into the logistic process model. Modelling an existing process is often providing a prescriptive model, that contains what "should" be done, rather than describing the actual process. A modelling method closer to reality is using the data collected at runtime, recorded in a process log, to derive a model explaining the events recorded. This activity is called *process discovery* (or *process mining*) (see [7]).

Employing the process discovery method using Petri net formalism, described in [8], we construct process models for patients from the "moderately complex" and "complex" cluster. Thus, we convert coded knowledge (the process executions recorded in the process logs) into theoretical knowledge. In Figure 1 (a) the discovered Petri net model using only medical cases from the cluster "moderately complex" is shown. On every possible path, at most three different specialisms are visited, e.g. "CHR, INT" or "CRD, NEUR, NRL" (the visits for functional investigations/radiology are not counted as specialisms)[1].

Using the process discovery method, we obtain insights into "aggregated" process models for the patients belonging to "moderately complex" and "complex" clusters. We want to be more patient-oriented, that is to obtain insights at the individual patient level. We obtain theoretical knowledge expressed as *instance graphs*, which is a graph where each node represents one log entry of a specific instance [9]. The advantage of this technique is that it can look at individual or at grouped patient instances. In Figure 1 (b) we construct the instance graph for a selection of 5 "moderately complex" patients (the instance graph has been produced with ProM software, version 1.7 [10]). Moreover, we can see the

---

[1] The node labels mean: CHR - surgery, CRD - cardiology, INT - internal medicine, NRL - neurology, NEUR - neurosurgery, FNKT (FNKC) - functional investigations. RONT (ROEH, RMRI, RKDP, ROZA) - radiology.

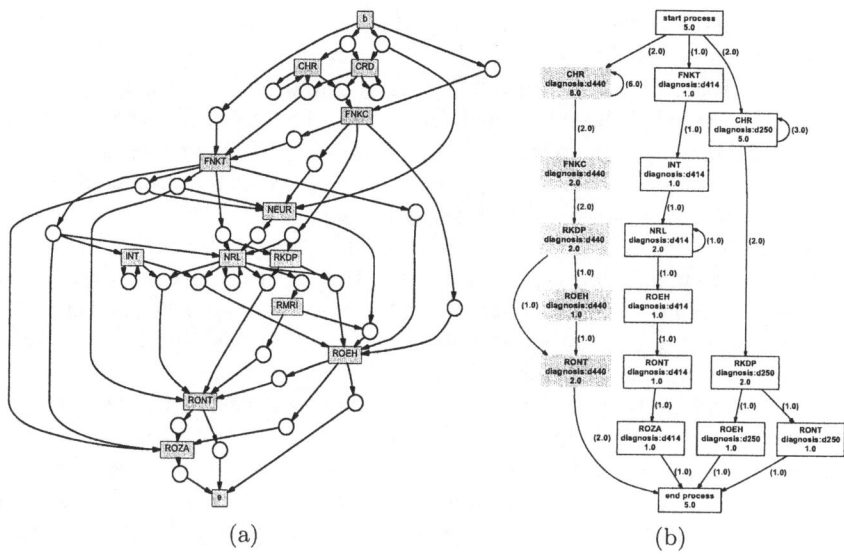

Fig. 1. The discovered process models. The Petri net model for cluster "moderately complex" (a) patients. The instance graph for 5 patients in the "moderately complex" cluster (b)

hospital trajectory of patients with specific diagnoses. For example, in Figure 1 (b), we can inspect the path of patients with diagnosis "d440" - atherosclerosis.

3 Knowledge Use and Transfer

For a better coordination of patients within hospitals, new multi-disciplinary units have to be created, where different specialisms coordinate the treatment of specific groups of patients. According to our results, two units can be created: for "moderately complex" cases, a unit consisting of CHR, CRD, INT, NRL and NEUR would suffice. "Complex" cases need additional specialisms like OGH, LNG and ADI. The discovered process models show that both processes contain parallel tasks. When treating multi-disciplinary patients, many possible combinations of specialisms appear in the log, due to a complex diagnosis process. Without patient clustering, it would be difficult to distinguish between patients, which leads to unnecessary resource spending (e.g. for "moderately complex" cluster).

Concerning the content of knowledge, it is possible to analyze, model and reorganize the hospital logistic processes in combination with the knowledge that can be distilled from Electronic Patient Records (EPR) (concerning illnesses, treatments, pharmaceutics, medical histories) and from Diagnosis Treatment Combinations (DTC). DTC's are integrated in such a way that hospitals can predict within ranges how long a patient with a certain illness will remain in the hospital.

The first issue concerning knowledge types is that much sensory knowledge - or behavioral activities of doctors and nurses - of the medical domain has to be converted into coded knowledge. EPR's and DTC's are designed from theoretical knowledge about the medical domain. The integration of sensory and theoretical knowledge via codes continues, however with increasing resistance of the medical profession. The second issue concerns the distillation of sensory, coded and theoretical knowledge from EPR's and DTC's, which are about the medical domain, into sensory and theoretical knowledge of the logistic processes.

The already mentioned clustering within the logistic processes and the methodology we explained can be of help, but the transfer of sensory and theoretical knowledge from the one content domain to another completely different content domain is very difficult. On one hand, the knowledge that triggers important decisions should be transparent, understandable and easy to be checked by all involved parties; reorganizing an institution implies difficult decisions and high costs. Therefore, our approach provides robust theoretical knowledge of a highly abstract kind of the logistic hospital process. On the other hand, the newly developed coded and theoretical knowledge transferred to people, may even lead to a new development in behavior.

4 Conclusions and Further Research

In this paper we proposed a KM approach for redesigning a business process, by employing the knowledge categorization defined by van Heusden&Jorna [5]. Our strategy focuses on (i) knowledge creation and (ii) knowledge use and transfer. We illustrated our approach by considering the treatment process of multi-disciplinary patients, that require the involvement of different specialisms for their treatment. The problem is to provide knowledge for reorganizing the care for these patients, by creating new multidisciplinary units. First, we identified patients groups in need of multi-disciplinary care. The clustering of the complexity measures obtained by converting raw data into coded knowledge, resulted into new pieces of knowledge: two patient's clusters, "complex" and "moderately complex". Second, we found the relevant specialisms that will constitute the ingredients of the multi-disciplinary units. We converted coded knowledge into theoretical knowledge, by building instance graphs for a selection of "moderately complex" patients, and Petri net process models for the treatment of "complex" and "moderately complex" patients. This theoretical knowledge provides insights into the logistic process and supports the reorganization of the care process. Our approach is meant to be more patient-oriented, in the sense of reducing redundant and overlapping diagnostic activities, which will consequently decrease the time spent in the hospital and shorten the waiting lists.

As future research, we will concentrate on EPR and DTC. These kinds of data structures will give more possibilities to improve the logistic processes and can be used to inform the patient better about the medical issues and treatment sequences.

References

1. Davenport, T., Short, J.: The New Industrial Engineering: Information Technology and Business Process Redesign. Sloan Management Review **31** (1990) 11–27
2. Sawy, O., Robert A. Josefek, J.: Business Process as Nexus of Knowldge. In: Handbook of Knowledge Management. International Handbooks on Information Systems. Springer (2003) 425–438
3. Boisot, M.: Information Space: A Framework for Learning in Organizations, Institutions and Culture. Routledge (1995)
4. Jorna, R.: Knowledge Representations and Symbols in the Mind. Tübingen: Stauffenburg Verlag (1990)
5. van Heusden, B., Jorna, R.: Toward a Semiotic Theory of Cognitive Dynamics in Organizations. In Liu, K., Clarke, R.J., Andersen, P.B., Stamper, R.K., eds.: Information, Organisation and Technology. Studies in Organizational Semiotics. Kluwer, Amsterdam (2001)
6. Măruşter, L., Weijters, A., de Vries, G., Bosch, A.v., Daelemans, W.: Logistic-based Patient Grouping for Multi-disciplinary Treatment. Artificial Intelligence in Medicine **26** (2002) 87–107
7. Aalst, W., van Dongen, B., Herbst, J., Maruster, L., Schimm, G., Weijters, A.: Workflow Mining: A Survey of Issues and Approaches. Data and Knowledge Engineering **47** (2003) 237–267
8. Măruşter, L.: A Machine Learning Approach to Understand Business Processes. PhD thesis, Eindhoven University of Techology, The Netherlands (2003)
9. van Dongen, B., van der Aalst, W.: Multi-phase Process Mining: Building Instance Graphs. In Atzeni, P., Chu, W., Lu, H., Zhou, S., Ling, T., eds.: Conceptual Modeling - ER 2004. LNCS 3288, Springer-Verlag (2004) 362–376
10. : Process Mining. http://tmitwww.tm.tue.nl/research/processmining/ (2004)

Machine Learning, Knowledge Discovery and Data Mining

Web Mining Techniques for Automatic Discovery of Medical Knowledge

David Sánchez and Antonio Moreno

Department of Computer Science and Mathematics,
University Rovirai Virgili (URV),
Avda. Països Catalans, 26. 43007 Tarragona (Spain)
{david.sanchez, antonio.moreno}@urv.net

Abstract. In this paper, we propose an automatic and autonomous methodology to discover taxonomies of terms from the Web and represent retrieved web documents into a meaningful organization. Moreover, a new method for lexicalizations and synonyms discovery is also introduced. The obtained results can be very useful for easing the access to web resources of any medical domain or creating ontological representations of knowledge.

1 Introduction

The World Wide Web is an invaluable tool for researchers, information engineers, health care companies and practitioners for retrieving knowledge. However, the extraction of information from web resources is a difficult task due to their *unstructured definition*, their *untrusted sources* and their *dynamically changing nature*.

To tackle these problems, we base our proposal is the *redundancy of information* that characterizes the Web, allowing us to detect important concepts and relationships for a domain through statistical analysis. Moreover, the exhaustive use of web search engines is a great help for selecting "representative" resources and getting global statistics of concepts; they can be considered as our particular "experts".

So, in this paper we present a *methodology to extract knowledge from the Web to build automatically structured representations in the form of taxonomies of concepts and web resources for a domain*. Moreover, if named entities for a discovered concept are found, they are considered as *instances*. During the building process, the most representative web sites for each subclass or instance are retrieved and categorized according to the topic covered. With the final hierarchy, an *algorithm for discovering different lexicalizations and synonyms of the domain keywords* is also performed, which can be used to widen the search. A prototype has been implemented and tested in several knowledge areas (results for the *Disease* domain are included).

The rest of the paper is organised as follows: section 2 describes the methodology developed to build the taxonomy and classify web sites. Section 3 describes a new approach for discovering lexicalizations and synonyms of terms. Section 4 explains the way of representing the results and discusses the evaluation with respect to other systems. The final section contains the conclusions and proposes lines of future work.

2 Taxonomy Building Methodology

The algorithm is based on analysing a significant number of web sites in order to find important concepts by studying the *neighbourhood* of an initial *keyword*. Concretely, in the English language, the immediate anterior word for a keyword is frequently *classifying* it (expressing a semantic specialization of the meaning), whereas the immediate posterior one represents the *domain* where it is applied [5].

More concretely, it queries a web search engine with an initial keyword (e.g. *disease*) and analyses the obtained web sites to retrieve the previous (e.g. *heart disease*) and posterior words (e.g. *disease treatment*). Previous words are analysed to distinguish if they will be considered as future subclasses or concrete instances into the taxonomy. In order to perform this differentiation, we take into consideration the way in which named entities are presented: English language distinguishes named entities through capitalisation [5]. More in detail, the method analyses the first web sites returned by the search engine when querying the instance candidates and counts the number of times that they are presented with upper and lower letters. Those which are presented in capital letters in most cases will be selected as instances (see some examples in Table 1).

Table 1. Examples of named entities (instances) found for several classes of the obtained taxonomy for the *Disease* domain (100 web documents evaluated for each candidate)

Class	Instance	Full name	Conf.
Chronic	Wisconsin	*Wisconsin Chronic Disease Program*	92.59
Lyme	American	*American Lyme Disease Foundation*	81.69
Lyme	California	*California Lyme Disease Association*	83.33
Lyme	Connecticut	*Connecticut Lyme Disease Coalition*	100.0
Lyme	Yale	*Yale University Lyme Disease Clinic*	87.23
Mitochondrial	European	*European Mitochondrial Disease Network*	100.0
Parkinson	American	*American Parkinson Disease Association*	87.5

Regarding to subclass candidates, a statistical analysis is performed, taking into consideration their relevance in the whole Web for the specific domain. Concretely, the web search engine is queried with the new concepts and relationships found (e.g. *"heart disease"*) and the estimated amount of hits returned is evaluated in relation to the initial keyword's measure (hits of *"disease"*). This web scale statistic combined with other local values obtained from the particular analysis of individual web resources are considered to obtain a relevance measure for each candidate and reject extreme cases (very common words or misspelled ones). Only the most relevant candidates are finally selected (see Fig. 1). The selection threshold is automatically computed in function on the domain's generality itself. For each new subclass, the process is repeated recursively to create deeper-level subclasses (e.g. *coronary heart disease*). So, at each iteration, a *new* and *more specific* set of relevant documents for the subdomain is retrieved. Each final component of the taxonomy (classes and instances) stores the set of URLs from where they have been selected.

Regarding to the posterior words of the keyword they are used to categorize the set of URLs associated to each class (see Fig. 2). For example, if we find that for a URL associated to the class *heart disease*, this keyword is followed by the word *prevention*, the URL will be categorized with this *domain of application*.

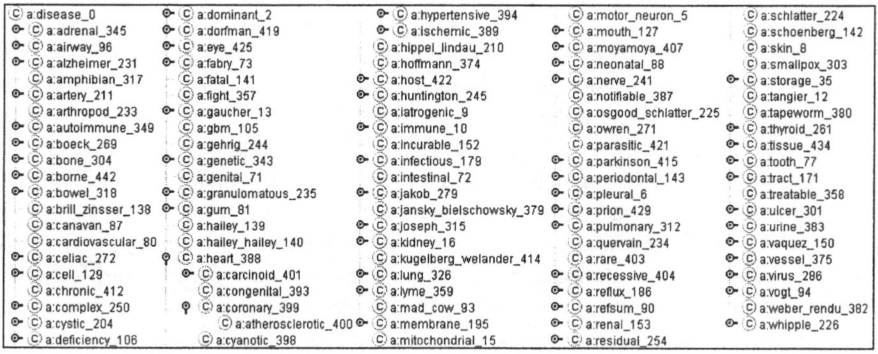

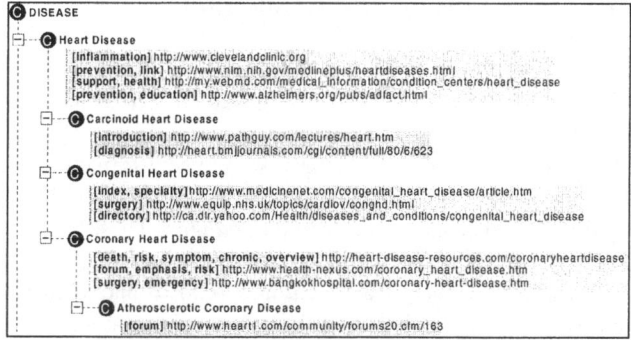

Fig. 1. *Disease* taxonomy visualized on Protégé: numbers are class identifiers

Fig. 2. Examples of categorized URLs for the *Heart* subclasses of *Disease*

When dealing with polysemic domains (e.g. *virus*), a semantic disambiguation algorithm is performed in order to group the obtained subclasses according to the specific word sense. The methodology performs a clusterization process of those classes depending on the amount of coincidences between their associated URLs sets.

Finally, a refinement is performed to obtain a more compact taxonomy: classes and subclasses that share a high amount of their URLs are merged because we consider them as closely related. For example, the hierarchy *"jansky->bielschowsky"* results in *"jansky_bielschowsky"*, discovering automatically a *multiword* term.

3 Lexicalizations and Synonyms Discovery

A very common problem of keyword-based web indexing is the use of different names to refer to the same entity (*lexicalizations* and *synonyms*). The goal of a web search engine is to retrieve relevant pages for a given topic determined by a keyword, but if a text doesn't contain this specific word with the same spelling as specified it will be ignored. So, in some cases, a considerable amount of relevant resources are omitted. In this sense, not only the different morphological forms of a given keyword are important, but also synonyms and aliases.

We have developed a novel methodology for discovering lexicalizations and synonyms using the taxonomy obtained and, again, a web search engine. Our approach is based on considering the longest branches (e.g. *atherosclerotic coronary heart disease*) of our hierarchy as a contextualization constraint and using them as the search query ommiting the initial keyword (e.g. *"atherosclerotic coronary heart"*) for obtaining new webs. In some cases, those documents will contain equivalent words for the main keyword just behind the searched query that can be candidates for lexicalizations or synonyms (e.g. *atherosclerotic coronary heart disorder*). From the list of candidates, those obtained from a significant amount of multiword terms are selected as this implies that they are comonly used in the particular domain. For example, for the *Disease* domain, some alternative forms discovered are: *diseases, disorder(s), syndrome* and *infection(s)*.

4 Ontology Representation and Evaluation

The final hierarchy is stored in a standard representation language: OWL. The *Web Ontology Language* is a semantic markup language for publishing and sharing ontologies on the World Wide Web [2].

Regarding to the evaluation of taxonomies, we have performed evaluations of the first level of the taxonomies for different sizes of the search computing, in each case, the *precision* and the number of *correct results obtained*. These measures have been compared to the ones obtained by a human-made directory (Yahoo), and automatic classifications performed by web search engines (Clusty and AlltheWeb). For the *Disease* domain (see Fig. 3), comparing to Yahoo, we see that although its *precision* is the highest, as it has been made by humans, the number of results are quite limited. The automatic search tools have offered good results in relation to *precision*, but with a very limited amount of correct concepts obtained.

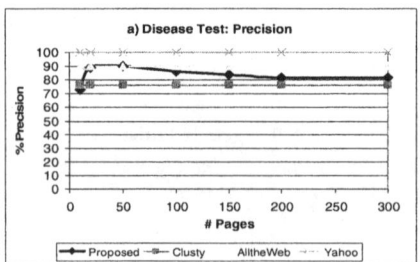 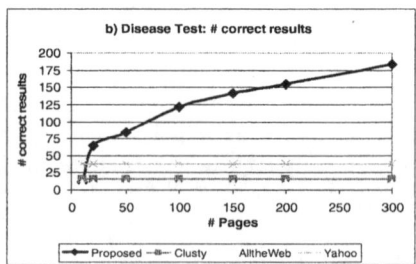

Fig. 3. Evaluation of results for the *Disease* domain for different sizes of web corpus

For the named-entities discovered, we have compared our results to the ones returned by a *named-entity detection package trained for the English language* that is able to detect with high accuracy some word patterns like *organisations, persons*, and *locations*. For illustrative purposes, for the *Disease* domain, we have obtained a precision of a 91%.

5 Related Work, Conclusions and Future Work

Several authors have been working in the discovery of taxonomical relationships from texts and more concretely from the Web. In [1, 6] authors propose approaches that rely in previously obtained knowledge and semantic repositories. More closely related, in [4] authors try to enrich previously obtained semantic structures using web-scale statistics. Other authors using this approach are [3], that learn taxonomic relationships, and [7], for synonyms discovery.

In contrast, our proposal does not start from any kind of predefined knowledge and, in consequence, it can be applied over domains that are not typically considered in semantic repositories. Moreover, the automatic and autonomous operation eases the updating of the results in highly evolutionary domains.

In addition to the advantage of the hierarchical representation of web sites for easing the accessing to web resources, the taxonomy is a valuable element for building machine processable representations like *ontologies*. This last point is especially important due to the necessity of ontologies for achieving interoperability in many knowledge intensive environments like the Semantic Web [1].

As future work, we plan to study the discovery of non-taxonomical relationships through the analysis of relevant sentences extracted from web resources (*text nuggets*), design forms of automatic evaluation of the results and study the evolution of a domain through several executions of the system in different periods of time to extract high level valuable information from the changes detected in the results.

Acknowledgements

This work has been supported by the "*Departament d'Universitats, Recerca i Societat de la Informació*" of Catalonia.

References

1. Agirre, E., Ansa, O., Hovy, E., and Martinez, D.: Enriching very large ontologies using the WWW. Workshop on Ontology Construction (ECAI-00). 2000.
2. Berners-lee T., Hendler, J., Lassila O.: The semantic web. Available at: http://www.sciam.com72001/050lissue/0501berners-lee.html
3. Cimiano, P. and Staab, S.: Learning by Googling. SIGKDD, 6(2), pp. 24-33. 2004.
4. Etzioni, O., Cafarella, M., Downey, D., Kok, S., Popescu, A., Shaked, T., Soderland, S. and Weld, D.: Web Scale Information Extraction in KnowItAll. WWW2004, USA. 2004.
5. Grefenstette G.: SQLET: Short Query Linguistic Expansion Techniques. In: Information Extraction: A Multidisciplinary Approach to an Emerging Information Technology, volume 1299 of LNAI, chapter 6, 97-114. Springer. SCIE-97. Italy, 1997.
6. Navigli, R. and Velardi, P.: Learning Domain Ontologies from Document Warehouses and Dedicated Web Sites. In Computational Linguistics, Volume 30, Issue 2. June 2004.
7. Turney, P.D.: Mining the Web for synonyms: PMI-IR versus LSA on TOEFL. In Proceedings of the Twelfth European Conference on Machine Learning. 2001.

Resource Modeling and Analysis of Regional Public Health Care Data by Means of Knowledge Technologies

Nada Lavrač[1,2], Marko Bohanec[1,3], Aleksander Pur[4], Bojan Cestnik[5,1],
Mitja Jermol[1], Tanja Urbančič[2,1], Marko Debeljak[1],
Branko Kavšek[1], and Tadeja Kopač[6]

[1] Jožef Stefan Institute, Jamova 39, SI-1000 Ljubljana, Slovenia
[2] Nova Gorica Polytechnic, Nova Gorica, Slovenia
[3] University of Ljubljana, Faculty of Administration, Ljubljana, Slovenia
[4] Ministry of the Interior, Štefanova 2, Ljubljana, Slovenia
[5] Temida, d.o.o. Ljubljana, Slovenia
[6] Public Health Institute, Celje, Slovenia

Abstract. This paper proposes a selection of knowledge technologies for health care planning and decision support in regional-level management of Slovenian public health care. Data mining and statistical techniques were used to analyze databases collected by a regional Public Heath Institute. Specifically, we addressed the problem of directing patients from primary health care centers to specialists. Decision support tools were used for resource modeling in terms of availability and accessibility of public health services for the population. Specifically, we analyzed organisational aspects of public health resources in one Sovenian region (Celje) with the goal to identify the areas that are atypical in terms of availability and accessibility of public health services.

1 Introduction

Regional Public Health Institutes (PHIs) are an important part of the system of public health care in Slovenia. They are coordinated by the national Institute of Public Health (IPH) and implement actions aimed at maintaining and improving public health in accordance with the national policy whose goal is an efficient health care system with a balanced distribution of resources in different regions of Slovenia.

The network of regional PHIs, coordinated by the national IPH, collect large amounts of data and knowledge that need to be efficiently stored, updated, shared, and transferred to help better decision making. These problems can efficiently be solved by appropriate *knowledge management* [6], which is recognized as the main paradigm for successful management of networked organizations [2, 3]. Knowledge management can be supported by the use of knowledge technologies, in particular by *data mining* and *decision support* [4].

This paper describes applications of data mining and decision support in public health care, carried out for the Celje region PHI within a project called MediMap. The main objective was to set up appropriate models and tools to support decisions concerning regional health care, which could later serve as a reference model for other regional PHIs. We approached this goal in two phases: first, we analyzed the available data with data mining techniques, and second, we used the results of data mining for a more elaborate study using decision support techniques. In the first phase we focused on the problem of directing the patients from primary health care centers to specialists. In the second phase we studied organisational aspects of public health resources in the Celje region with the goal to identify the areas that are atypical in terms of availability and accessibility of public health services. Some of the achieved results are outlined in Sections 2 and 3, respectively. Section 4 provides the summary and conclusions.

2 Selected Results of Statistical and Data Mining Techniques

In order to model the Celje regional health care system we first wanted to better understand the health resources and their connections in the region. For that purpose, data mining techniques were applied to the data of eleven community health centers. The dataset was formed of three databases:

- the health care providers database,
- the out-patient health care statistics database (patients' visits to general practitioners and specialists, diseases, human resources and availability), and
- the medical status database.

To model the processes of a particular community health center (the patient flow), data describing the directing of patients to other community health centers or specialists were used. Similarities between community health centers were analyzed according to four different categories: (a) patients' age, (b) patients' social status, (c) the organization of community health centers, (d) their employment structure.

For each category, similarity groups were automatically constructed using four different clustering methods. Averages over four clustering methods per category were used to detect the similarities between the community health centers of the Celje region. The similarities of community health centers were presented and evaluated by

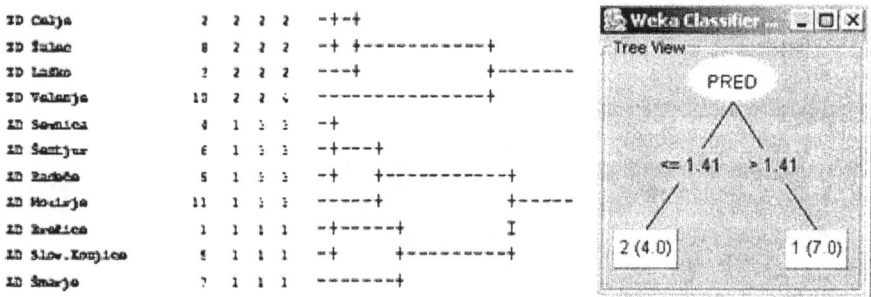

Fig. 1. Left: Results of hierarchical clustering of community health centers. Right: A decision tree representation of the top two clusters, offering an explanation for the grouping

PHI Celje domain experts, as described in more detail in [5]. An illustration of clusters, generated by agglomerative hierarchical clustering using the Ward's similarity measure, based on four categories (a)-(d), is given in Figure 1.

In order to get the descriptions of particular groups, a decision tree learning technique was used. The decision tree in Figure 1 shows that the most informative attribute, distinguishing between the groups of health centers, is category (a) - the age of patients. Community health centers in which pre-school children (PRED) constitute more than 1.41 % of all visits to the center form Cluster 1 (consisting of seven health centers). The experts' explanation is that these centers lack specialized pediatrician services, hence pre-school children are frequently treated by general practitioners.

3 Selected Results of Decision Support Techniques

The key issues of the second phase of the project were the detection of outliers and the analysis of causes for different availability and accessibility of services. Out of several analyses carried out, two of them are described in this section: (1) analysis of pharmacy capacities, and (2) analysis of availability of public health care resources.

Analysis of Pharmacy Capacities. explored the regional distribution of pharmacies and the detection of atypical cases. Capacity deviations were observed by comparing the demand (population) with the capacity of pharmacies, where the capacity computation is the result of a weighted average of several parameters: infrastructure (evaluated by the number of pharmacies) and human resources (evaluated by the number of pharmacists of low and high education level and the number of other staff).

Hierarchical multi-attribute decision support system DEXi [1] was used for the evaluation of composed criteria from the values of low-level criteria. Hierarchical structuring of decision criteria by DEXi is shown in Figure 2. Qualitative aggregation of the values of criteria is based on rules, induced from human-provided cases of individual pharmacy evaluations.

Figure 3 shows the capacity deviations of pharmacies in the Celje region, where the X axis denotes the actual number of people (city inhabitants), and the Y axis is the capacity of pharmacies. Atypical pharmacies are those deviating from the diagonal (Žalec and Velenje), while other five regional pharmacies (Celje, Šmarje and three others in the lower-left corner of Figure 3) are balanced in terms of the requirement-capacity tradeoff.

Attribute	Scale
Appropriateness of pharmacies	over-developed; appropriate; *under-developed*
├─Expected requirements	low; decreased; medium; increased; *high*
│ └─Number of inhabitants	15000-25000; 25000-35000; 35000-45000; 45000-55000; *55000-65000*
└─Capacity of pharmacies	inadequate; adequate; good; v_good; *excellent*
├─Infrastructure	basic; good; *excellent*
│ └─Number of pharmacies	to_4; 4-8; *9_more*
└─Human resources	inadequate; adequate; good; *excellent*
├─Pharmacists, Low education	1; *2*
├─Pharmacists, High education	to_20; 20-60; 61-100; *101_more*
└─Other staff	to_2; 2-10; *11_more*

Fig. 2. The structure and value scales of criteria for the evaluation of the appropriateness of pharmacies in terms of requirements and capacity

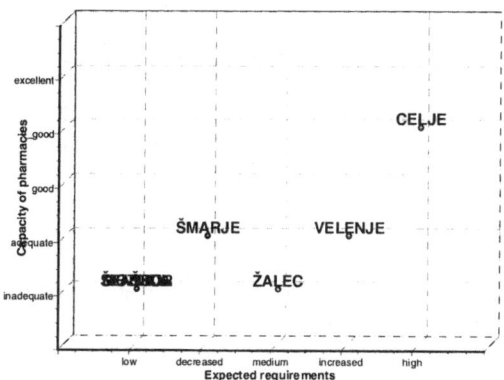

Fig. 3. Analysis of pharmacy capacity deviations in the Celje region

Analysis of the Availability of Public Health Care Resources. was carried out to detect local communities that are underserved concerning general practice health care.

We evaluated 34 local communities in the Celje region according to criterion $AHSP_m$ – the Availability of Health Services (measured in hours) for Patients from a given community (c), considering the Migration of patients into neighbouring communities – computed as follows:

$$AHSP_m = \frac{1}{p_c} \sum_i a_i p_{ci} \qquad (1)$$

In $AHSP_m$ computation, a_i is the available time of health care services (i) per person, defined as the ratio of total working time of health care services and total number of visits, p_c is the total number of accesses of patient from community (c), and p_{ci} is the number of accesses of patient from community (c) to health service (i).

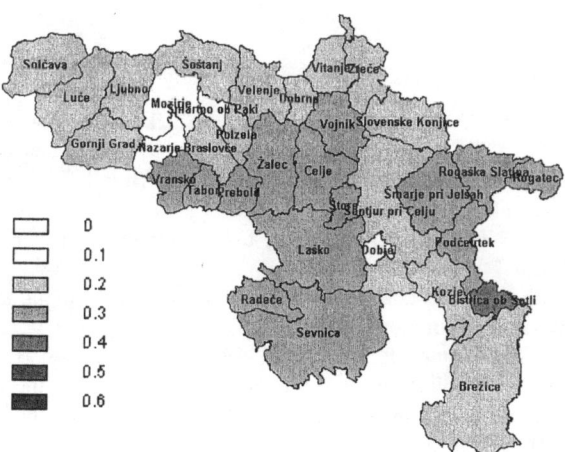

Fig. 4. Availability of health services for patients from the communities in the Celje region, considering the migration of patients to neighboring communities ($AHSP_m$) for year 2003

The evaluation of Celje communities in terms of $AHSP_m$ is shown in Figure 4. The color of communities depends on the availability of health services for patients. Darker communities have higher health care availability for the population. This representation was well accepted by the experts, as it clearly shows the distribution of the availability of health care resources for patients from the communities.

4 Conclusions

In the MediMap project we have developed methods and tools that can help regional Public Health Institutes and the national Institute of Public Health to perform their tasks more effectively. The knowledge technologies tools developed for the reference case of the PHI Celje were applied to selected problems related to health care organization, the accessibility of health care services to the citizens, and the health care providers network.

The main achievement of applying decision support methods to the problem of planning the development of public health services was the creation of the model of availability and accessibility of health services to the population of a given area. With this model it was possible to identify the regions that differ from the average and to consequently explain the causes for such situations. The developed methodology and tools have proved to be appropriate to support the PHI Celje, serving as a reference model for other regional PHIs.

Acknowledgements

We acknowledge the financial support of the Public Health Institute Celje, the Slovenian Ministry of Education, Science and Sport, and the 6FP integrated project ECOLEAD (European Collaborative Networked Organizations Leadership Initiative).

References

1. Bohanec, M., Rajkovič, V.: DEX: An Expert-System Shell for Decision Support, Sistemica, Vol. 1, No. 1 (1990) 145–157; see also http://www-ai.ijs.si/MarkoBohanec/dexi.html
2. Camarinha-Matos, L.M., Afsarmanesh, H.: Elements of a Base VE Infrastructure. J. Computers in Industry, Vol. 51, No. 2 (2003) 139–163
3. McKenzie, J., van Winkelen, C.: Exploring E-collaboration Space. Henley Knowledge Management Forum (2001)
4. Mladenić, D., Lavrač, N., Bohanec, M., Moyle, S. (eds.): Data Mining and Decision Support: Integration and Collaboration, Kluwer (2003)
5. Pur, A., Bohanec, M., Cestnik, B., Lavrač, N., Debeljak, M., Kopač, T.: Data Mining for Decision Support: An Application in Public Health Care. Proc. of the 18th International Conference on Industrial & Engineering Applications of Artificial Intelligence & Expert Systems, Bari, (2005) in press
6. Smith, R.G., Farquhar, A.: The Road Ahead for Knowledge Management: An AI Perspective. AI Magazine, Vol. 21, No. 4 (2000) 17–40

An Evolutionary Divide and Conquer Method for Long-Term Dietary Menu Planning

Balázs Gaál, István Vassányi, and György Kozmann

University of Veszprém, Department of Information Systems,
Egyetem u. 10, H-8201 Veszprém, Hungary

Abstract. We present a novel Hierarchical Evolutionary Divide and Conquer method for automated, long-term planning of dietary menus. Dietary plans have to satisfy multiple numerical constraints (Reference Daily Intakes and balance on a daily and weekly basis) as well as criteria on the harmony (variety, contrast, color, appeal) of the components. Our multi-level approach solves problems via the decomposition of the search space and uses good solutions for sub-problems on higher levels of the hierarchy. Multi-Objective Genetic Algorithms are used on each level to create nutritionally adequate menus with a linear fitness combination extended with rule-based assessment. We also apply case-based initialization for starting the Genetic Algorithms from a better position of the search space. Results show that this combined strategy can cope with strict numerical constraints in a properly chosen algorithmic setup.

1 Introduction

The research in the field of computer aided nutrition counseling has begun with a linear programming approach for optimizing menus for nutritional adequacy and cost, developed by Balintfy in 1964 [1]. In 1967 Eckstein used random search to satisfy nutritional constraints for meals matching a simple meal pattern [2]. Artificial intelligence methods mostly using Case-Based Reasoning (CBR) combined with other techniques were developed later [3,4]. A hybrid system, CAMPER has been developed recently, using CBR and Rule-Based Reasoning for menu planning [5], that integrates the advantages of two other independent implementations, the case-based menu planner (CAMP) and PRISM [6]. A more recent CBR approach is MIKAS, menu construction using an incremental knowledge acquisition system, developed to handle the menu design problem for an unanticipated client. The system allows the incremental development of a knowledge-base for menu design [7].

Human professionals still surpass computer algorithms on nutrition advice regarding the quality of the generated dietary plan, but computer based methods can be used on demand and in unlimited quantities. Furthermore, with the computational potential of today's computers the gap between human experts and algorithmic methods can be narrowed on this particular field.

The work presented in this paper deals with the problem of planning weekly menus, made up of dishes stored in a database and used to compose meals, daily plans and the weekly plan.

2 Objectives

The evaluation of a dietary plan has at least two aspects. Firstly, we must consider the quantity of nutrients. There are well defined constraints for the intake of nutrient components such as carbohydrate, fat or protein which can be computed, given one's age, gender, body mass, physical activity, age and diseases. Optimal and extreme values can be specified for each nutrient component. The nutritional allowances are given as Dietary Reference Intakes [8]. As for quantity, the task of planning a meal can be formulated as a constraint satisfaction and optimization problem.

Secondly, the harmony of the meal's components should be considered. Plans satisfying nutrition constraints have also to be appetizing. By common sense some dishes or nutrients do not appeal in the way others do. In our approach, this common sense of taste and cuisine may be described by simple rules recording the components that do or do not go together. We must cope with conflicting numerical constraints or harmony rules.

The fact base of the proposed method and our software tool MenuGene is a commercial nutritional database widely used in Hungarian hospitals, that at present contains the recipes of 569 dishes with 1054 ingredients. The nutrients contained in the database for each ingredient are energy, protein, fat, carbohydrates, fiber, salt, water, and ash.

3 Methods

In order to satisfy the numerical constraints and the requirements about harmony on each nutritional level, we divide the weekly menu planning problem into subproblems (daily menu planning and meal planning). Genetic Algorithms (GA) are run on these levels, driven by our C++ framework GSLib, which is also responsible for scheduling the multi-level evolution process. A similar multi-level multi-objective GA was proposed and tested in [9]. On each level, GSLib optimizes a population of solutions (individuals) composed of attributes (genes).

We also maintain a Case-Base for storing dietary plans made by experts or created through adaptation. Whenever a new dietary plan is requested, the Case-Base is searched for plans that were made with similar objectives regarding quantity and harmony.

In our abstract framework, a solution composed of its attributes, represents one possible solution of the problem. An attribute represents either a solution found by a GA, selected from a POOL, or it is predefined as SINGLE. Example solutions and an outline of the hierarchical structure are shown in tables 1 and 2 respectively.

Table 1. Example solutions and their attributes for meal and dish. (pcs: pieces)

Solution for a typical lunch

attribute	minimal	default	maximal
a_{soup}	1pc	1pc	1pc
$a_{garnish}$	1pc	1pc	1pc
$a_{redmeat}$	1pc	1pc	2pcs
a_{drink}	1pc	2pcs	3pcs
$a_{dessert}$	1pc	1pc	2pcs

Solution for a garnish (mashed potato)

attribute	minimal	default	maximal
a_{milk}	120g	120g	120g
a_{potato}	357.1g	357.1g	357.1g
a_{butter}	5g	5g	5g
a_{salt}	5g	5g	5g

Table 2. Solutions and their Attributes in the Multi-Level Hierarcy

solution	attribute	attribute type
weekly plan	daily plan	GA
daily plan	meal plan	GA
meal plan	dish	POOL
dish	foodstuff	SINGLE
foodstuff	nutrient	SINGLE
nutrient	–	–

In each iteration of a population, solutions are recombined and mutated. Recombination involves two solutions and exchanges their attributes from a randomly selected crossover point. If the attribute is GA type, mutation either fires evolution process on the population connected to the attribute (mutation-based scheduling), or reinitializes the population. If the attribute is POOL type, mutation randomly chooses a solution from its pre-defined pool. No mutation occurs on SINGLE type attributes.

Other possible scheduling alternatives include the top-down and the bottom-up strategies. The top-down and bottom-up strategy runs the uppermost/lowest level populations for a given iteration step and continues on the lower/upper level.

Each solution maintains a list storing its underlying hierarchy. For example, a solution for a daily plan knows how much protein, carbohydrate or juice it may contain. So, a solution can be assessed by processing its whole underlying structure.

Numerical constraints (minimal, optimal and maximal values) are given by the nutrition expert for solutions (nutrients, foodstuffs) and solution sets on a weekly basis. These constraints are propagated proportionally to lower levels. We calculate a non-linear, second order penalty function (see Fig. 1.) for each constraint and use linear fitness combination to sum up the fitness of the solutions according to the numerical constraints. The fitness function will provide a non-positive number as a grade where zero is the best. The fitness function does not punish too much small deviations from the optimum (default) but it is strict on values that are not in the interval defined by the minimal and maximal limits. The function is non-symmetric to the optimum, because the effects of the

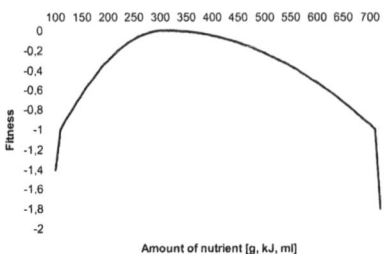 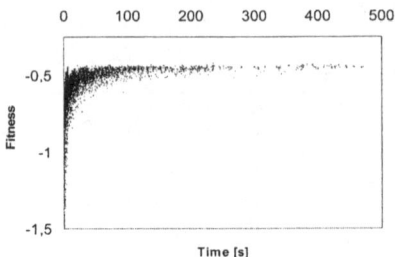

Fig. 1. An example penalty function for a constraint with $min = 100$, $opt = 300$, $max = 700$ parameters.

Fig. 2. Fitness of the best solution in function of runtime

deviations from the optimal value may be different in the negative and positive directions.

Rule-Based Assessment is used to modify the calculated fitness value, if there are rules for harmony that are applicable for the solution being assessed. Rules apply a penalty on the simultaneous occurrence of solutions or solution sets. Only the most appropriate rules are applied. For example if a meal contains tomato soup and orange juice, and we have the rules $r_1 = ([S_{soups}, S_{drinks}], 70\%)$ and $r_2 = ([S_{orangedrinks}, S_{juices}], 45\%)$ then only r_2 is applied, because the set of orange drinks is more specific to orange juice than the set of drinks.

4 Results and Discussion

We found that the plans generated by our tool MenuGene satisfy numerical constraints on the level of meals, daily plans and weekly plans. The multi-level generation was tested with random and real world data. Our tests showed that the rule-based classification method successfully omits components that don't harmonize with each other.

We performed tests to explore the best algorithmic setup. First, we analyzed the effect of the crossover and mutation probabilities on the fitness. The results showed that the probability of the crossover does not influence the fitness too much, but a mutation rate well above 10% is desirable, particularly for smaller populations.

We examined the connection between the runtime and the quality of the solution in a wide range of algorithmic setups. As Fig. 2. shows, although the quality of the solutions improves with runtime, the pace of improvement is very slow after a certain time, and, on the other hand, a solution of quite good quality is produced within this time. This means that it is enough to run the algorithm until the envelope curve starts to saturate.

Using the optimal algorithmic setup, we tested how the algorithm copes with very close upper and lower limits (minimal and maximal values). Minimal and maximal values were gradually increased/decreased to be finally nearly equal.

The results in ca. 150.000 test runs showed that our method is capable of generating nutritional plans, even where the minimal and maximal allowed values of one or two constraints are virtually equal and the algorithm found a nearly optimal solution when there are three or four constraints of this kind. According to our nutritionist, there is no need for constraints with virtually equal minimal and maximal values, and even in most pathological cases the strict regulation of four parameters is sufficient.

5 Conclusions and Future Work

The paper gave a summary on a novel dietary menu planning method that uses a Hierarchical Evolutionary Divide and Conquer strategy for weekly or longer-term dietary menu plan design with a fitness function that assesses menus according to the amount of nutrients and harmony. Algorithmic tests revealed that the method is capable, for non-pathological nutrition, of generating long-term dietary menu plans that satisfy nutritional constraints even with very narrow constraint intervals.

Further work includes the extension of the present rule set to a comprehensive rule base to ensure really harmonic menu plans and the integration of the service into a lifestyle counseling framework.

References

1. Balintfy, J.L.: Menu planning by computer. Commun. ACM **7** (1964) 255–259
2. Eckstein, E.F.: Menu planning by computer: the random approach. Journal of American Dietetic Association **51** (1967) 529–533
3. Yang, N.: An expert system on menu planning. Master's thesis, Department of Computer Engineering and Science Case Western Reserve University, Cleveland, OH. (1989)
4. Hinrichs, T.: Problem solving in open worlds: a case study in design (1992) Erlbaum, Northvale, NJ.
5. Marling, C.R., J., P.G., Sterling, L.: Integrating case-based and rule-based reasoning to meet multiple design constraints. Computational Intelligence **15** (1999) 308–332
6. Kovacic, K.J.: Using common-sense knowledge for computer menu planning. PhD thesis, Cleveland, Ohio: Case Western Reserve University (1995)
7. Khan, A.S., Hoffmann, A.: Building a case-based diet recommendation system without a knowledge engineer. Artif Intell Med. **27** (2003) 155–179
8. Food and Nutrition Board (FNB), Institute of Medicine (IOM): Dietary reference intakes: applications in dietary planning. National Academy Press. Washington, DC. (2003)
9. Gunawan, S., Farhang-Mehr, A., Azarm, S.: Multi-level multi-objective genetic algorithm using entropy to preserve diversity. In: EMO. (2003) 148–161

Human/Computer Interaction to Learn Scenarios from ICU Multivariate Time Series

Thomas Guyet[1], Catherine Garbay[1], and Michel Dojat[2]

[1] Laboratoire TIMC, 38706 La Tronche, France
thomas.guyet@imag.fr
http//www-timc.imag.fr/Thomas.Guyet/
[2] Mixt Unit INSERM/UJF U594

Abstract. In the context of patients hospitalized in intensive care units, we would like to predict the evolution of the patient's condition. We hypothesis that human-computer collaboration could help with the definition of signatures representative of specific situations. We have defined a multi-agent system (*MAS*) to support this assumption. Preliminary results are presented to support our assumption.

1 Introduction

Physiological monitors currently used in high dependency environments such as Intensive Care Units (ICUs) or anaesthesia wards generate a false alarm rate that approximately reaches 86% [1]. This bad score is essentially due to the fact that alarm detection is mono-parametric and based on predefined thresholds. To really assist clinicians in diagnosis and therapy tasks we should design intelligent monitoring systems with capacities of predicting the evolution of the patients state and eventually of triggering alarms in case of probable critical situations.

Several methods have been proposed for false alarm reduction based on data processing algorithms (using trend calculation)[2, 3] or data mining techniques [1]. In general, the methods proposed are based on two steps, first data processing algorithms detect relevant events in time series data and secondly information analysis techniques are used to identify well-known critical patterns. When applied to multivariate time series, these methods can be powerful if patterns to discover are well-known in advance.

In order to predict the evolution of the patient's state, typical high level scenes, combination of several patterns that are representative of specific situations, have to be formalized. Unfortunately, clinicians have some difficulties in defining such situations. We propose an interactive environment for an in-depth exploration by the clinician of the set of physiological data. In the interactive environnement TSW, used in [4], allows to collect overall statistics. Our approach is based on a collaborative work between a computer, which efficiently analyzes a large set of data and classifies information, and a clinician, who has skills and pragmatic knowledge for data interpretation and drives the computerized data exploration. We assume that such a collaboration could facilitate the discovery of signatures representative of specific situations. To test this hypothesis we have designed a collaborative multi-agent system (MAS) with the capacities of segmenting, classifying and learning.

2 Scenarios Construction Based on Clinician/Computer Interaction

The philosophy of the approach is the creation of a self-organized system guided by an clinician. The system dynamically builds its own data representation for scenario discovery. The clinician interacts with the system in introducing annotations, solving ambiguous cases, or introducing specific queries. Consequently, the system should be highly adaptive.

Data, information and knowledge are dynamically managed at several steps during clinician/computer interactions. Data, numeric or symbolic, are represented as multivariate time series. The whole system is an experimental workbench. The clinician can add or delete pieces of information, explore time series by varying the time granularity, using trends computed on various sliding-windows, and in selecting or combining appropriate levels of abstraction. Annotations can be introduced by the clinician generally as binary information (for instance, cough (0 or 1), suction (0 or 1)).

The goal of our method is to learn from time series data the more likely scenario, i.e. a set of events linked by temporal constraints, that explains a specific event. In the following, we distinguish between events, that contribute to the description of a scenario, and specific events that are explained by scenarios. Specific events are characterized by a decision tree that is built from "instantaneous" patient states described by numeric and symbolic time series data and annotated as positive or negative examples. Then the decision tree is used to find new occurrences of the same type of specific events. To explain the so called specific events, scenarios are learned by the MAS (cf. section 3).

A clinician interacts with the MAS to guide the learning and be informed of discoveries. A short example can briefly describe our method

1) Starting from time series data, the clinician annotates some SpO_2 desaturation episodes in specific regions of interest. Annotations are encoded as binary time series data.
2) From data plus annotations, the system learns desaturation episodes, their characteristics (a tree) and possible scenario (learned by the MAS) that explains these episodes (specific events).
3) The system, in browsing a part of time series data, searches for similar characteristics and scenario.
4) Based on similar characteristics, new desaturation episodes can be discovered by the system. They are used as new examples for the decision tree or if they present an atypical signature compared to others, they are shown to the clinician for examination.
5) When similar scenarios not followed by a desaturation episode are discovered, they are provided to the clinician who decides either to keep or reject them.

They are then used respectively as positive or negative examples for the learning phase
6) The system loops to step 2 until no new scenarios or characteristics can be discovered.

Depending on its discoveries and information provided by the clinician, the system continuously adapts its behavior. Its complex self-organisation is masked to the clinician who interacts with the system only via time series data.

3 A Multiagent System

MASs present good properties to implement self-organization and reactivity to user interactions. Our general architecture was inspired by [5]. Three data abstraction levels, namely segments, classes of segments and scenarios, are constructed in parallel with mutual and dynamic adaptations to improve the final result. These levels are associated to a numerical, a symbolic and a semantic level respectively.

The *MAS* ensures an equivalence between what we call specific events and classes of segments. For symbolic time series, like annotations, symbols are associated to some classes of segments. For instance, the clinician can annotate each SpO_2 desaturation episode. Learning a scenario that explains this specific event is equivalent to learning a scenario that explains occurrences of a class of segments (with the corresponding symbol) in the time series "SpO_2 annotations". Other classes of segments discovered by the system should be interpreted by the clinician.

Three types of agents exist in the *MAS*. At the numerical level, reactive agents segment time series. Each reactive agent represents a segment, *i.e.* a time series region bounded by two borders with neighboring agents. Frontiers move, disappear or are created dynamically by interactions between agents based on the approximation error of an SVR[1] model of segment. Then, at the symbolic level, classification agents build classes of segments. To compare segments, we have defined a distance between SVR models that takes into account dilatation and scaling. A vocabulary is then introduced to translate times series into symbolic series.

At the semantic level, learning agents build scenarios that explain classes of segments (or specific events for clinicians). In fact, we consider a scenario that occurs before a specific event e_2 as a possible explanation for e_2. Consequently, learning a scenario that explains e_2 consists in finding common points (signature) in temporal windows preceding examples of the class of e_2. To find such signatures, we have adapted the algorithm presented in [7] to multivariate series inputs. This algorithm takes into account temporal constraints to aggregate frequent relevant information and to progressively suppress noisy information. Then, the learning agent proposes modifications (via feedback) to segmentation and classification agents by focussing on discrepancies found between the learned scenario and the examples. In this way, it improves its global confidence.

---

[1] Support Vector Regression [6].

Interactions are the key of the self-organization capability of the system and are used at three main levels

1) Feedback that dynamically modifies, adds or deletes segmentation agents, thus leading to segmentation modifications.
2) Feedback that adjusts classification.
3) Improvement of the overall learning accuracy (discrimination power) by pointing out, between learning agents, inconsistencies in the resulting associations of scenarios and specific events.

We highlight that at the two first levels, symbolization of all series are performed independently. However, learning agents use multivariate symbolic series to build scenarios and to deliver feedback to obtain a global coherence.

4 Preliminary Results

We used data from ICU patients under weaning from mechanical ventilation. We selected four physiological signals (SpO_2, Respiratory rate, Total expired volume and heart rate) sampled at 1 Hz during at least 4 hours. Each signal was preprocessed by computing sliding-windows means (3 min width) and was abstracted by following a specific methodology [8] into symbolic values and trends. Moreover, we used SpO_2 desaturation annotations inserted at the patient's bedside by a clinician. Consequently, each patient's recordings was a multivariate time series that contained 17 ($4*4+1$) long times series. Presently, the implementation of our *MAS* is partial, feedbacks are not fully implemented. Data acquisition is still undergoing. Thus, the quantity of data currently available is not sufficient to ensure a robust learning.

The figure 1 displays the experimental computer's interface to manage the *MAS*. The panel A) shows the way to access to patient's data and agents classes. The Panel B) shows recordings for 2 patients ($P1$ and $P2$). For each one, we display two time series "Heart Rate data" (numeric) and "SpO_2 Annotations"

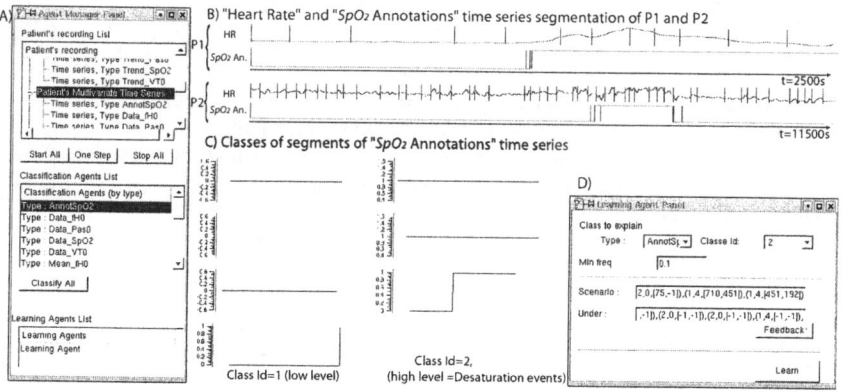

Fig. 1. *MAS* interface. (see text for details)

(symbolic). Vertical bars represent frontiers of segments obtained by segmentation agents. SpO_2 annotations are segmented in 3 (for $P1$) and 5 (for $P2$) segments. Segmentation is not perfect especially for heart rate but will be refined by feedback. In panel C), are displayed the 2 classes of segments that classify the 8 segments (only 7 are shown) of "SpO_2 Annotations" time series. In panel D) the more probable scenario that explains class 2 is indicated as a set of events linked by temporal relations. A clinician interface should be developed to mask technical aspects of this interface and translate scenarios into comprehensible representations.

5 Conclusion and Perspectives

The system we present proposes an experimental workbench to assist clinicians in the exploration of physiological data in poorly formalized domains such as ICUs.

The central concept of our system is to support interactions between a self-organized *MAS*, with data processing, data abstraction and learning capabilities and a clinician, who browses the provided mass of data to guide the learning of scenarios representative of the patient's state evolution. Preliminary results invite us to pursue the implementation and show the necessity to reinforce the *MAS* capabilities to segment, classify and learn from time series data.

References

1. Tsien, C.L., Kohane, I.S., McIntosh, N.: Multiple Signal Integration by Decision Tree Induction to Detect Artifacts in the Neonatal Intensive Care Unit. Art. Intel. in Med. **19** (2000) 189–202
2. Salatian, A., Hunter, J.: Deriving Trends in Historical and Real-Time Continuously Sampled Medical Data. J. Intel. Inf. Syst. **13** (1999) 47–71
3. Lowe, A., Harrison, M.J., Jones, R.W.: Diagnostic Monitoring in Anaesthesia Using Fuzzy Trend Templates for Matching Temporal Patterns. Art. Intel. in Med. **16** (1999) 183–199
4. Hunter, J., Ewing, G., Freer, Y., Logie, F., McCue, P., McIntosh, N.: NEONATE: Decision Support in the Neonatal Intensive Care Unit - A Preliminary Report. In Dojat, M., Keravnou, E.T., Barahona, P., eds.: AIME. Volume 2780 of Lecture Notes in Computer Science., Springer-Verlag, Berlin Heidelberg New York (2003) 41–45
5. Heutte, L., Nosary, A., Paquet, T.: A Multiple Agent Architecture for Handwritten Text Recognition. Pattern Recognition **37** (2004) 665–674
6. Vapnik, V., Golowich, S., Smola, A.: Support Vector Method for Function Approximation, Regression Estimation, and Signal Processing. Ad. in Neural Inf. Proc. Sys. **9** (1997) 281–287
7. Dousson, C., Duong, T.V.: Discovering Chronicles with Numerical Time Constraints from Alarm Logs for Monitoring Dynamic Systems. In Dean, T., ed.: IJCAI, Morgan Kaufmann (1999) 620–626
8. Silvent, A.S., Dojat, M., Garbay, C.: Multi-Level Temporal Abstraction for Medical Scenarios Construction. Int. J. of Adaptive Control Signal Process. (2005) Processing to appear.

Mining Clinical Data: Selecting Decision Support Algorithm for the MET-AP System

Jerzy Blaszczynski[1], Ken Farion[2], Wojtek Michalowski[3], Szymon Wilk[1,*], Steven Rubin[2], and Dawid Weiss[1]

[1] Poznan University of Technology, Institute of Computing Science,
Piotrowo 3a, 60-965 Poznan, Poland
{jurek.blaszczynski, szymon.wilk, dawid.weiss}@cs.put.poznan.pl

[2] Children's Hospital of Eastern Ontario,
401 Smyth Road, Ottawa, ON, K1H 8L1, Canada
{farion, rubin}@cheo.on.ca

[3] University of Ottawa, School of Management,
136 Jean-Jacques Lussier Street, Ottawa, ON, K1N 6N5, Canada
wojtek@management.uottawa.ca

Abstract. We have developed an algorithm for triaging acute pediatric abdominal pain in the Emergency Department using the discovery-driven approach. This algorithm is embedded into the MET-AP (Mobile Emergency Triage - Abdominal Pain) system – a clinical decision support system that assists physicians in making emergency triage decisions. In this paper we describe experimental evaluation of several data mining methods (inductive learning, case-based reasoning and Bayesian reasoning) and results leading to the selection of the rule-based algorithm.

1 Introduction

Quest to provide better quality care to the patients results in supplementing regular procedures with intelligent clinical decision support systems (CDSS) that help to avoid potential mistakes and overcome existing limitations.

A CDSS is "a program designed to help healthcare professionals make clinical decisions" [1]. In our research we concentrate on systems providing patient-specific advice that use clinical decision support algorithms (CDSAs) discovered from data describing past experience. We evaluate various methods of data mining for extracting knowledge and representing it in form of a CDSA. The evaluation is based on the decision accuracy of the CDSA as the outcome measure.

CDSAs discussed in this paper aim at supporting triage of abdominal pain in the pediatric Emergency Department (ED). Triage is one of ED physician's functions that requires the following disposition decisions: discharge (discharge

---
* Corresponding author.

and possible follow-up by a family doctor), observation (further investigation in the ED or hospital), or consult (consult a specialist).

MET-AP [2] is a mobile CDSS that provides support at the point of care for triaging abdominal pain in the ED. It suggests the most appropriate dispositions and their relative strengths.

The paper is organized as follows. We start with a short overview of data mining methodologies used for developing CDSAs. Then, we describe the experiment and conclude with the discussion.

2 CDSA and Data Mining

One of the oldest data mining approaches applied in developing discovery-driven CDSA is Bayesian reasoning [3]. It is a well-understood methodology that is accepted by physicians [3], as it mimics clinical intuition [4]. Bayesian reasoning was adopted in the Leeds system [5] for diagnosing abdominal pain.

Other techniques of data mining, including case-based reasoning [3] and inductive learning [4], have not been as widely accepted in clinical practice [4]. However, some practical applications [3,4] of CDSAs constructed with these techniques have attracted the attention of healthcare professionals.

Case-based reasoning [6] allows arriving at a recommendation by analogy. This approach was employed in the development of CDSA for the CAREPARTNER system [7] designed to support the long-term follow-up of patients with stem-cell transplant.

Inductive learning [4] represents discovered knowledge in the form of decision rules and decision trees that are later used in CDSAs. It is less often used in practice despite some successful clinical applications (e.g., for evaluating coronary disease [8]).

3 Selecting the Most Appropriate CDSA

In order to select the CDSA for triage of abdominal pain we designed and conducted a three-phase computational experiment.

The first phase of the experiment dealt with the development of CDSAs on the basis of learning data transcribed retrospectively from ED charts of patients with abdominal pain, who visited the ED in the Children's Hospital of Eastern Ontario between 1993 and 2002 (see Table 1). Each record was described by values of 13 clinical attributes. Charts were assigned to one of three decision classes by reviewing the full hospital documentation.

The following data mining methods were evaluated: induction of decision rules (LEM2 algorithm [9]); Bayesian reasoning (naive Bayesian reasoning [10]); case-based reasoning (IBL algorithm [11]); and induction of decision trees (C4.5 algorithm [12]).

During the second phase of the experiment we tested performance of the algorithms on new retrospectively collected independent testing data set (see Table 1). There is general consensus among the physicians that it is important

Table 1. Learning and testing data sets

Decision class	Number of charts	
	Learning set	Testing set
Discharge	352	52
Observation	89	15
Consult	165	33
Total	606	100

to differentiate between the classification accuracies obtained for different decision classes (high accuracy for the consult class is more important than for the discharge class). This means than the assessment and selection of the most appropriate CDSA should consider not only its overall classification accuracy, but also performance for critical classes of patients.

The results of the second phase are given in Table 2. Although all CDSAs had very similar overall accuracies, the most promising results considering the observation and consult classes were obtained for case-based CDSA and for the rule-based CDSA. The tree-based CDSA had the same accuracy for the consult class as the rule-based one, however, its performance for the observation class was much lower. Finally, naive Bayesian CDSA offered the highest accuracy for the discharge class, and the lowest accuracy for the consult class, which is unacceptable from the clinical point of view.

Table 2. Classification accuracy of the CDSAs

CDSA	Overall	Discharge	Observation	Consult
Rule-based	59.0%	55.8%	46.7%	69.7%
Naive Bayesian	56.0%	65.4%	20.0%	57.6%
Case-based	58.0%	57.7%	20.0%	75.8%
Tree-based	57.0%	59.6%	20.0%	69.7%

In the third phase of the experiment we tested and compared the CDSAs considering the misclassification costs (in terms of penalizing undesired misclassifications). The costs, given in Table 3, were defined by the physicians participating in the study and introduced into the classification scheme. We excluded rule-based CDSA from this phase, as its classification strategy did not allow cost-based evaluation.

The results of the third phase are given in Table 4. The most remarkable change comparing to the second phase is the increased classification accuracy for the observation class resembling the way a cautious physician would proceed. Such an approach also has drawbacks – the decreased classification accuracy for the consult class.

Table 3. Misclassification costs

Outcome	Recommendation		
	Discharge	Observation	Consult
Discharge	0	5	10
Observation	5	0	5
Consult	15	5	0

Table 4. Classification accuracy of the CDSAs (costs considered)

CDSA	Overall	Discharge	Observation	Consult
Naive Bayesian	56.0%	59.6%	46.7%	54.6%
Case-based	49.0%	42.3%	60.0%	54.6%
Tree-based	55.0%	59.6%	40.0%	54.6%

Comparison of the performance of the cost-based CDSAs with the performance of the rule-based CDSA from the second phase favors the latter one as the preferable solution for MET-AP. This CDSA offers high classification accuracies for crucial decision classes (observation and consult) without decreasing accuracy in the discharge class. It is important to note that a rule-based CDSA represents clinical knowledge similarly to practice guidelines, and thus it is easy for clinicians to understand. Taking all of the above into account, we have chosen to implement the rule-based CDSA in MET-AP.

4 Discussion

Our experiment showed better performance of the rule-based CDSA in terms of classification accuracy for crucial decision classes (observation and consult), even when misclassification costs were introduced. This observation proves the viability and robustness of the rule-based CDSA implemented the MET-AP system.

More detailed evaluation of the results suggested that the learning data did not contain obvious classification patterns. This was confirmed by a large number of rules composing the rule-based CDSA (165 rules) and their relatively weak support – for each class there were only a few stronger rules. This might explain why rule-based CDSA and case-based CDSA that consider cases in an explicit manner (a rule can be viewed as a generalized case) were, in overall, superior to other algorithms.

During further studies we plan to research for more possible dependencies between the characteristics of the analyzed data and data mining methods used to build CDSAs. This should enable us to select the most appropriate CDSA in advance without a need for computational experiments. Moreover, it will be worth checking how the integration of different CDSAs impacts the classification accuracy.

Acknowledgments

Research reported in this paper was supported by the NSERC-CHRP grant. It was conducted when J. Blaszczynski, Sz. Wilk, and D. Weiss were part of the MET Research at the University of Ottawa.

References

1. Musen, M., Shahar, Y., Shortliffe, E.: Clinical decision support systems. In Shortliffe, E., Perreault, L., Wiederhold, G., Fagan, L., eds.: Medical Informatics. Computer Applications in Health Care and Biomedicine. Springer-Verlag (2001) 573–609
2. Michalowski, W., Slowinski, R., Wilk, S., Farion, K., Pike, J., Rubin, S.: Design and development of a mobile system for supporting emergency triage. Methods of Information in Medicine **44** (2005) 14–24
3. Hanson, III, C.W., Marshall, B.E.: Artificial intelligence applications in the intensive care unit. Critical Care Medicine **29** (2001) 427–35
4. Kononenko, I.: Inductive and Bayesian learning in medical diagnosis. Applied Artificial Intelligence **7** (1993) 317–377
5. de Dombal, F.T., Leaper, D.J., Staniland, J.R., McCann, A.P., Horrocks, J.C.: Computer-aided diagnosis of acute abdominal pain. British Medical Journal **2** (1972) 9–13
6. Schmidt, R., Montani, S., Bellazzi, R., Portinale, L., Gierl, L.: Cased-based reasoning for medical knowledge-based systems. International Journal of Medical Informatics **64** (2001) 355–367
7. Bichindaritz, I., Kansu, E., Sullivan, K.: Case-based reasoning in CAREPARTNER: Gathering evidence for evidence-based medical practice. In Smyth, B., Cunningham, P., eds.: Advances in Case-Based Reasoning: 4th European Workshop, Proceedings EWCBR-98, Berlin, Springer-Verlag (1998) 334–345
8. Krstacic, G., Gamberger, D., Smuc, T.: Coronary heart disease patient models based on inductive machine learning. In Quaglini, S., Barahona, P., Andreassen, S., eds.: Proceedings of 8th Conference on Artificial Intelligence in Medicine in Europe (AIME 2001), Berlin, Springer-Verlag (2001) 113–116
9. Grzymala-Busse, J.: LERS - a system for learning from examples based on rough sets. In Sowiski, R., ed.: Intelligent Decision Support - Handbook of Applications and Advances of the Rough Set Theory. Kluwer Academic Publishers, Dordrecht/Boston (1992) 3–18
10. John, G.H., Langley, P.: Estimating continuous distributions in Bayesian classifiers. In: Proceedings of the 11th Conference on Uncertainty in Artificial Intelligence. Morgan Kaufmann, San Mateo (1995) 338–345
11. Aha, D., Kibler, D., Albert, M.: Instance-based learning algorithms. Machine Learning **6** (1991) 37–66
12. Quinlan, R.: C4.5: Programs for Machine Learning. Kaufmann Publishers, San Mateo, CA (1993)

A Data Pre-processing Method to Increase Efficiency and Accuracy in Data Mining

Amir R. Razavi[1], Hans Gill[1], Hans Åhlfeldt[1], and Nosrat Shahsavar[1,2]

[1] Department of Biomedical Engineering, Division of Medical Informatics,
Linköping University, Sweden
[2] Regional Oncology Centre, University Hospital, Linköping, Sweden
{amirreza.razavi, hans.gill, hans.ahlfeldt,
nosrat.shahsavar}@imt.liu.se
http://www.imt.liu.se

Abstract. In medicine, data mining methods such as Decision Tree Induction (DTI) can be trained for extracting rules to predict the outcomes of new patients. However, incompleteness and high dimensionality of stored data are a problem. Canonical Correlation Analysis (CCA) can be used prior to DTI as a dimension reduction technique to preserve the character of the original data by omitting non-essential data. In this study, data from 3949 breast cancer patients were analysed. Raw data were cleaned by running a set of logical rules. Missing values were replaced using the Expectation Maximization algorithm. After dimension reduction with CCA, DTI was employed to analyse the resulting dataset. The validity of the predictive model was confirmed by ten-fold cross validation and the effect of pre-processing was analysed by applying DTI to data without pre-processing. Replacing missing values and using CCA for data reduction dramatically reduced the size of the resulting tree and increased the accuracy of the prediction of breast cancer recurrence.

1 Introduction

In recent years, huge amounts of information in the area of medicine have been saved every day in different electronic forms such as Electronic Health Records (EHRs) [1] and registers. These data are collected and used for different purposes. Data stored in registers are used mainly for monitoring and analysing health and social conditions in the population. In Sweden, the long tradition of collecting information on the health and social conditions of the population has provided an excellent base for monitoring disease and social problems. The unique personal identification number of every inhabitant enables linkage of exposure and outcome data spanning several decades and obtained from different sources [2]. The existence of accurate epidemiological registers is a basic prerequisite for monitoring and analysing health and social conditions in the population. Some registers are nation-wide, cover the whole Swedish population, and have been collecting data for decades. They are frequently used for research, evaluation, planning and other purposes by a variety of users [3].

With the wide availability and comprehensivity of registers, they can be used as a good source for knowledge extraction. Data mining methods can be applied to them in order to extract rules for predicting the outcomes of new patients. Extraction of hidden predictive information from large databases is a potent method with extensive capability to help physicians with their decisions [4].

A Decision Tree is a classifier in the form of a tree structure and is used to classify cases in a dataset [5]. A set of training cases with their correct classifications is used to generate a decision tree that, optimistically, classifies each case in the test set correctly. The resulting tree is a representation that can be verified by humans and can be used by either humans or computer programs [6]. Decision Tree Induction (DTI) has been used in different areas of medicine including oncology [7] and respiratory diseases [8].

Before the data undergo data mining, they must be prepared in a pre-processing step that removes or reduces noise and handles missing values. Relevance analyses for omitting unnecessary and redundant data, as well as data transformation, are needed for generalising the data to higher-level concepts [9]. Pre-processing techniques take the most effort and time, i.e. almost 80% of the whole project time for knowledge discovery in databases (KDD) [10]. However, replacing the missing values and finding a proper method for selecting important variables prior to data mining can make the mining process faster and even more stable and accurate.

In this study the Expectation Maximization (EM) method was used for replacing the missing values. This algorithm is a parameter estimation method that falls within the general framework of maximum likelihood estimation and is an iterative optimisation algorithm [11].

Hotelling (1936) developed Canonical Correlation Analysis (CCA) as a method for evaluating linear correlation between sets of variables [12]. The method allows investigation of the relationship between two sets of variables and identification of the important ones. It can be used as a dimension reduction technique to preserve the character of the original data stored in the registers by omitting data that are nonessential. The objective is to find a subset of variables with predictive performance comparable to the full set of variables [13].

CCA was applied in the pre-processing step of Decision Tree Induction. DTI was trained with the cases with known outcome and the resulting model was validated with ten-fold cross validation. In order to show the benefits of pre-processing, DTI was also applied to the same database without pre-processing, as well as after just handling missing values. For performance evaluation, the accuracy, sensitivity and specificity of the three models were compared.

2 Materials and Methods

Preparing the data for mining consisted of several steps: choosing proper databases, integrating them to one dataset, cleaning and replacing missing values, data transformation and dimension reduction by CCA. To see the effect of the pre-processing, DTI was also applied to the same dataset without prior handling of missing values and dimension reduction.

2.1 Dataset

In this study, data from 3949 female patients, mean age 62.7 years, were analysed. The earliest patient was diagnosed in January 1986 and the last one in September 1995, and the last follow-up was performed in June 2003. The data were retrieved from a regional breast cancer register operating in south-east Sweden.

In order to cover more predictors and obtain a better assessment of the outcomes, data were retrieved and combined from two other registers, namely the tumour markers and cause of death registers. After combining the information from these registers, the data were anonymised for security reasons and to maintain patient confidentiality. If patients developed symptoms following treatment they were referred to the hospital; otherwise follow-up visits occurred at fixed time intervals for all patients.

There were more than 150 variables stored in the resulting dataset after combining the databases. The first criterion for selecting appropriate variables for prediction was consulting domain experts. In this step, sets of suggested predictors and outcomes (Table 1) were selected. Age of the patient and variables regarding tumour specifications based on pathology reports, physical examination, and tumour markers were selected as predictors. There were two variables in the outcome set, distant metastasis and loco-regional recurrence, both observed at different time intervals after diagnosis indicating early and late recurrence.

2.2 Data Pre-processing

After selecting appropriate variables, the raw data were cleaned and outliers were removed by running a set of logical rules. For handling missing values, the Expectation Maximization (EM) algorithm was used. The EM algorithm is a computational method for efficient estimation from incomplete data. In any incomplete dataset, the observed values provide indirect evidence about the likely values of the unobserved values. This evidence, when combined with some assumptions, comprises a predictive probability distribution for the missing values that should be averaged in the statistical analysis. The EM algorithm is a general technique for fitting models to incomplete data. EM capitalises on the relationship between missing data and the unknown parameters of a data model. When the parameters of the data model are known, then it is possible to obtain unbiased predictions for the missing values [14]. All continuous and ordinal variables except for age were transformed to dichotomised variables.

The fundamental principle behind CCA is the creation of a number of canonical solutions [15], each consisting of a linear combination of one set of variables, Ui, and a linear combination of the other set of variables, Vi. The goal is to determine the coefficients that maximise the correlation between canonical variates Ui and Vi.

The number of solutions is equal to the number of variables in the smaller set. The first canonical correlation is the highest possible correlation between any linear combination of the variables in the predictor set and any linear combination of the variables in the outcome set. Only the first CCA solution is used, since it describes most of the variations.

The most important variables in each canonical variate were identified based on the magnitude of the structure coefficients (loadings). Using loadings as the criterion for finding the important variables has some advantages [16]. As a rule of thumb for meaningful loadings, an absolute value equal to or greater than 0.3 is often used [17].

SPSS version 11 was used for transforming, handling missing values, and implementing CCA [18].

Table 1. List of variables in both sets

Predictor Set	Outcome Set [‡]
Age	DM, first five years
Quadrant	DM, more than 5 years
Side	LRR, first five years
Tumor size [*]	LRR, more than 5 years
LN involvement [*]	
LN involvement [†]	
Periglandular growth [*]	
Multiple tumors [*]	
Estrogen receptor	
Progesterone receptor	
S-phase fraction	
DNA index	
DNA ploidy	

Abbreviations: LN: lymph node, DM: Distant Metastasis, LRR: Loco-regional Recurrence
[*] from pathology report, [†] N0: Not palpable LN metastasis,
[‡] all periods are time after diagnosis

2.3 Decision Tree Induction

One of the classification methods in data mining is decision tree induction (DTI). In a decision tree, each internal node denotes a test on variables, each branch stands for an outcome of the test, leaf nodes represent an outcome, and the uppermost node in a tree is the root node [19]. The algorithm uses information gain as a heuristic for selecting the variable that will best separate the cases into each outcome [20]. Understandable results of acquired knowledge and fast processing make decision trees one of the most frequently used data mining techniques [21].

Because of the approach used in constructing decision trees, there is a problem of overfitting the training data, which leads to poor accuracy in future predictions. The solution is pruning of the tree, and the most common method is post-pruning. In this method, the tree grows from a dataset until all possible leaf nodes have been reached, and then particular subtrees are removed. Post-pruning causes smaller and more accurate trees [22]. In this study, DTI was applied to the reduced model resulting from CCA after handling missing values to achieve a predictive model for new cases. For the training phase of DTI, the resulting predictors in CCA with the absolute value of loadings ≥ 0.3 were used as input. As the outcome in DTI, important outcomes with the absolute value of loadings ≥ 0.3 in CCA were used, i.e. the occurrence of distant metastasis during a five-year period after diagnosis.

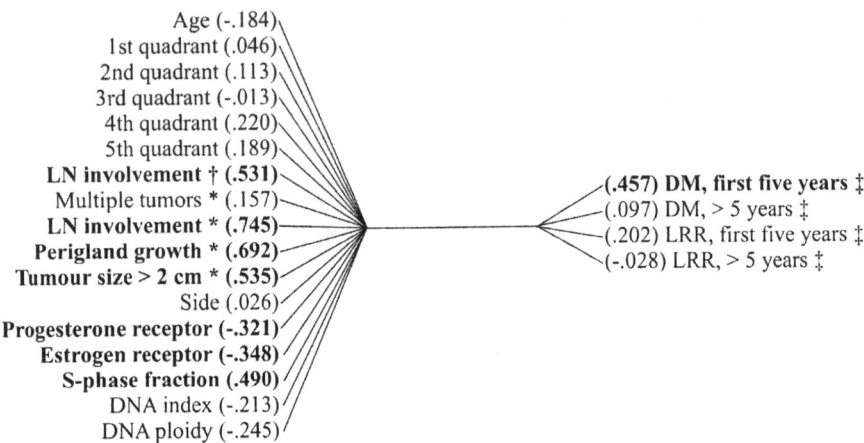

Abbreviations: LN: lymph node, DM: Distant Metastasis, LRR: Loco-regional Recurrence
* from pathology report, † palpable LN metastasis, ‡ all periods are time after diagnosis. If the signs in the sets are the same, then if one increases the other also increases, and vice versa.

Fig. 1. Canonical structure matrix and loadings for the first solution

As a comparison, DTI was also applied to the dataset without handling the missing values and without dimension reduction by CCA (Table 1). In this analysis of outcome, any recurrence (either distant or loco-regional) at any time during the follow-up after diagnosis was used as outcome. Another similar analysis was done after just handling missing values with the EM algorithm. DTI was carried out using the J48 algorithm in WEKA, which is a collection of machine learning algorithms for data mining tasks [23]. Post-pruning was done to trim the resulting tree. The J48 algorithm is the equivalent of the C4.5 algorithm written by Quinlan [5].

2.4 Performance Comparison

Ten-fold cross validation was done to confirm the performance of predictive models. This method estimates the error that would be produced by a model. All cases were randomly re-ordered, and then the set of all cases was divided into ten mutually disjointed subsets of approximately equal size. The model then was trained and tested ten times. Each time it was trained on all but one subset, and tested on the remaining single subset. The estimate of the overall accuracy was the average of the ten individual accuracy measures [24]. The accuracy, sensitivity and specificity were used for comparing the performance of the two DTIs, i.e. the one following pre-processing and the other without any dimension reduction procedure [25]. In addition, the size of the tree and the number of leaf nodes in each tree were also compared.

3 Result

CCA was applied to the dataset and in each solution the loadings for predictor and outcome sets were calculated. The first solution and the loadings (in parentheses) for variables are illustrated in Figure 1. The canonical correlation coefficient (rc) is 0.49 ($p \leq .001$). The important variables are shown in bold type.

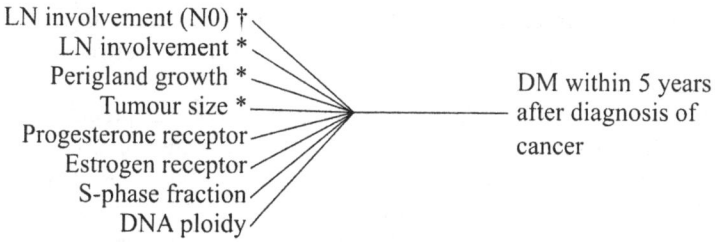

Abbreviation: LN: lymph node, DM: distant metastasis.
† N0: Not palpable LN metastasis, * from pathology report.

Fig. 2. Extracted model from CCA in the pre-processing step

After the primary hypothetical model was refined by CCA and the important variables were found by considering their loadings, then they were ready to be analysed by DTI in the mining step. The important outcome was distant metastasis during the first five years and it was used as a dichotomous outcome in DTI. This model is illustrated in Fig. 2. DTI was also applied without the pre-processing step that included handling missing values and dimension reduction. Three different pre-processing approaches were used before applying DTI, and the accuracy, sensitivity, specificity, number of leaves in the decision tree and the tree size were calculated for predictive models. The results are shown and compared in Table 2.

Table 2. Results for the different approaches

DTI	Without pre-processing	With replacing missing values	With pre-processing
Accuracy	54%	57%	67%
Sensitivity	83%	82%	80%
Specificity	41%	46%	63%
Number of Leaves	137	196	14
Tree Size	273	391	27

In the analysis done after handling missing values and dimension reduction using CCA, the accuracy and specificity show improvement but the sensitivity is lower. The tree size and number of leaves in the decision tree that was made after the pre-processing are smaller and more accurate.

4 Discussion

An important step in discovering the hidden knowledge in databases is effective data pre-processing, since real-world data are usually incomplete, noisy and inconsistent [9]. Data pre-processing consists of several steps, i.e. data cleaning, data integration, data transformation and data reduction. It is often the case that a large amount of information is stored in databases, and the problem is how to analyse this massive quantity of data effectively, especially when the data were not collected for data mining purposes.

For extracting specific knowledge from a database, such as predictions of the recurrence of a disease or of the risk of complications in certain patients, a set of important predictors is assumed to be of central importance, while other variables are not essential. These unimportant variables simply cause problems in the main analysis. They may contain noise and may increase the prediction error and increase the need for computational resources [26]. Dimension reduction results in a subset of the original variables, which simplifies the model and reduces the risk of overfitting.

The first step in reducing the number of unimportant variables is discussion with domain experts who have been involved in collecting the data. Their involvement in the knowledge discovery and data mining process is essential [27].

In this study, the selection by domain experts was based on their knowledge and experience concerning variables related to the recurrence of breast cancer. In this step the number of variables was reduced from more than 150 to 21 (17 in the predictor set and 4 in the outcome set).

One of the problems in real-life databases is low quality data such as where there are missing values. This is frequently encountered in medical databases, since most medical data are collected for purposes other than data mining [28]. One of the most common reasons for missing values is not that they have not been measured or recorded, but that they were not necessary for the main purpose of the database.

There are different methods for replacing missing values, the most common of which is simply to omit any case or patient with missing values. However, this is not a good idea because it causes the lost of information. A case with just one missing value has other variables with valid values that can be useful in the analysis. Deleting a case is implemented as default in most statistical packages. The disadvantage is that this may result in a very small dataset and can lead to serious biases if the data are not missing at random. Methods such as imputations, weighting and model-based techniques can be used to replace the missing values [29]. In this study, replacing the missing values was done after the variables were selected by the domain experts. This results in fewer calculations and less effort, and a better analysis with CCA in the dimension reduction step.

In the CCA, non-important variables were removed from the dataset by considering loadings as criteria. Loadings are not affected by the presence of strong correlations among variables and can also handle two sets of variables. After the dimension reduction by CCA, the number of suggested variables from domain experts was reduced to 9 (8 + 1). The benefits can be more apparent when the number of variables is much higher. This small subset of the initial variables contains most of the information required for predicting recurrence of the cancer.

DTI is a popular classification method because its results can be easily changed to rules or illustrated graphically. In the case of small and simple trees, even a paper copy of the tree can be used for predicting purposes. The results can be presented and explained to domain experts and can be easily modified by them for a higher degree of explainability.

As an important step in KDD, the pre-processing step is vital for successful data mining. In some papers, no specific pre-processing was noted before mining the data with DTI [8], and in others data discretization was performed [21]. We combined different techniques: substituting missing values, categorisation and dimension reduction.

The results of the three DTIs that were performed (Table 2) show that the accuracy and specificity of the analysis with replacement of missing values and CCA prior to DTI are considerably better, but the sensitivity has decreased.

The number of leaves and tree size show a considerable decrease. This simplifies the use of the tree by medical personnel and makes it easier for domain experts to study the tree for probable changes. This simplicity is gained along with an increase in the overall accuracy of the prediction, which shows the benefits of a well-studied pre-processing step. In this study, the role of dimension reduction by CCA in pre-processing is more apparent than that of handling missing values. This is shown by the better accuracy and reduced size of the tree after adding CCA to pre-processing.

Combining proper methods for handling missing values and a dimension reduction technique before analysing the dataset with DTI is an effective approach for predicting the recurrence of breast cancer.

5 Conclusion

High data quality is a primary factor for successful knowledge discovery. Analysing data containing missing values and redundant and irrelevant variables requires a proper pre-processing before application of data mining techniques. In this study, a pre-processing step including CCA is suggested.

Data on breast cancer patients stored in the registers of south-west Sweden have been analaysed. We have presented a method that consists of replacing missing values, consulting with domain experts and dimension reduction prior to applying DTI.

The result shows an increased accuracy for predicting the recurrence of breast cancer.

Using the described pre-processing method prior to DTI results in a simpler decision tree and increases efficiency of predictions. This helps oncologists in identifying high risk patients.

Acknowledgments

This study was performed in the framework of Semantic Mining, a Network of Excellence funded by EC FP6. It was also supported by grant No. F2003-513 from FORSS, the Health Research Council in the South-East of Sweden. Special thanks to the South-East Swedish Breast Cancer Study Group for fruitful collaboration and support in this study.

References

[1] Uckert, F., Ataian, M., Gorz, M., Prokosch, H. U.: Functions of an electronic health record. Int J Comput Dent 5 (2002) 125-32
[2] Sandblom, G., Dufmats, M., Nordenskjold, K., Varenhorst, E.: Prostate carcinoma trends in three counties in Sweden 1987-1996: results from a population-based national cancer register. South-East Region Prostate Cancer Group. Cancer 88 (2000) 1445-53
[3] Rosen, M.: National Health Data Registers: a Nordic heritage to public health. Scand J Public Health 30 (2002) 81-5
[4] Windle, P. E.: Data mining: an excellent research tool. J Perianesth Nurs 19 (2004) 355-6
[5] Quinlan, J. R.: C4.5: Programs for Machine Learning. Morgan Kaufmann, San Mateo, CA (1993)
[6] Podgorelec, V., Kokol, P., Stiglic, B., Rozman, I.: Decision trees: an overview and their use in medicine. J Med Syst 26 (2002) 445-63
[7] Vlahou, A., Schorge, J. O., Gregory, B. W., Coleman, R. L.: Diagnosis of Ovarian Cancer Using Decision Tree Classification of Mass Spectral Data. J Biomed Biotechnol 2003 (2003) 308-314
[8] Gerald, L. B., Tang, S., Bruce, F., Redden, D., Kimerling, M. E., Brook, N., Dunlap, N., Bailey, W. C.: A decision tree for tuberculosis contact investigation. Am J Respir Crit Care Med 166 (2002) 1122-7
[9] Han, J., Kamber, M.: Data Mining Concepts and Techniques. Morgan Kaufmann (2001)
[10] Duhamel, A., Nuttens, M. C., Devos, P., Picavet, M., Beuscart, R.: A preprocessing method for improving data mining techniques. Application to a large medical diabetes database. Stud Health Technol Inform 95 (2003) 269-74
[11] McLachlan, G. J., Krishnan, T.: The EM algorithm and extensions. John Wiley & Sons (1997)
[12] Silva Cardoso, E., Blalock, K., Allen, C. A., Chan, F., Rubin, S. E.: Life skills and subjective well-being of people with disabilities: a canonical correlation analysis. Int J Rehabil Res 27 (2004) 331-4
[13] Antoniadis, A., Lambert-Lacroix, S., Leblanc, F.: Effective dimension reduction methods for tumor classification using gene expression data. Bioinformatics 19 (2003) 563-70
[14] Dempster, A. P., Laird, N. M., Rubin, D. B.: Maximum Likelihood from Incomplete Data via the EM Algorithm. J R Stat Soc Ser B 39 (1977) 1-38
[15] Vogel, R. L., Ackermann, R. J.: Is primary care physician supply correlated with health outcomes? Int J Health Serv 28 (1998) 183-96
[16] Dunlap, W., Landis, R.: Interpretations of multiple regression borrowed from factor analysis and canonical correlation. J Gen Psychol 125 (1998) 397-407
[17] Thompson, B.: Canonical correlation analysis: Uses and interpretation. Sage, Thousand Oaks, CA (1984)
[18] SPSS Inc.: SPSS for Windows. SPSS Inc. (2001)

[19] Pavlopoulos, S. A., Stasis, A. C., Loukis, E. N.: A decision tree--based method for the differential diagnosis of Aortic Stenosis from Mitral Regurgitation using heart sounds. Biomed Eng Online 3 (2004) 21
[20] Luo, Y., Lin, S.: Information gain for genetic parameter estimation with incorporation of marker data. Biometrics 59 (2003) 393-401
[21] Zorman, M., Eich, H. P., Stiglic, B., Ohmann, C., Lenic, M.: Does size really matter--using a decision tree approach for comparison of three different databases from the medical field of acute appendicitis. J Med Syst 26 (2002) 465-77
[22] Esposito, F., Malerba, D., Semeraro, G., Kay, J.: A comparative analysis of methods for pruning decision trees. IEEE Trans Pattern Anal Mach Intell 19 (1997) 476-491
[23] Witten, I. H., Frank, E.: Data Mining: Practical machine learning tools with Java implementations. Morgan Kaufmann, San Francisco (2000)
[24] Kohavi, R.: A Study of Cross-Validation and Bootstrap for Accuracy Estimation and Model Selection. In: Proc. International Joint Conference on Artificial Intelligence (1995) 1137-1145
[25] Delen, D., Walker, G., Kadam, A.: Predicting breast cancer survivability: a comparison of three data mining methods. Artif Intell Med In press (2004)
[26] Pfaff, M., Weller, K., Woetzel, D., Guthke, R., Schroeder, K., Stein, G., Pohlmeier, R., Vienken, J.: Prediction of cardiovascular risk in hemodialysis patients by data mining. Methods Inf Med 43 (2004) 106-113
[27] Babic, A.: Knowledge discovery for advanced clinical data management and analysis. Stud Health Technol Inform 68 (1999) 409-13
[28] Cios, K. J., Moore, G. W.: Uniqueness of medical data mining. Artif Intell Med 26 (2002) 1-24
[29] Myrtveit, I., Stensrud, E., Olsson, U. H.: Analyzing data sets with missing data: an empirical evaluation of imputation methods and likelihood-based methods. IEEE Trans Softw Eng 27 (2001) 999-1013

Rule Discovery in Epidemiologic Surveillance Data Using EpiXCS: An Evolutionary Computation Approach

John H. Holmes[1] and Jennifer A. Sager[2]

[1] University of Pennsylvania School of Medicine, Philadelphia, PA, USA
jholmes@cceb.med.upenn.edu
2 University of New Mexico Department of Computer Science,
Albuquerque, NM, USA
sagerj@cs.unm.edu

Abstract. This paper describes the architecture and application of EpiXCS, a learning classifier system that uses reinforcement learning and the genetic algorithm to discover rule-based knowledge in epidemiologic surveillance databases. EpiXCS implements several additional features that tailor the XCS paradigm to the demands of epidemiologic data and users who are not familiar with learning classifier systems. These include a workbench-style interface for visualization and parameterization and the use of clinically meaningful evaluation metrics. EpiXCS has been applied to a large surveillance database, and shown to discover classification rules similarly to See5, a well-known decision tree inducer.

1 Introduction

Evolutionary computation encompasses a variety of machine learning paradigms that are inspired by Darwinian evolution. The first paradigm was the genetic algorithm which is based on chromosomal knowledge representations and genetic operators to ensure "survival of the fittest" as a means of efficient search and optimization. A number of evolutionary computation paradigms have appeared since John Holland [3] first developed the genetic algorithm.

Of particular interest to this investigation is the learning classifier system (LCS). Its natural, rule-based knowledge representation, accessible components, and easily understood output positions the LCS above other evolutionary computation approaches as a robust knowledge discovery tool. LCSs are rule-based, message-passing systems that learn rules to guide their performance in a given environment. Numerous LCS architectures have been described, starting with CS-1 [3], the first system in the so-called Michigan approach. Another design, Smith's LS-1 system [9], is the first in a series of Pittsburgh approaches to learning classifier systems. Wilson's Animat [10] represents a departure from the Michigan approach. Since these early efforts, LCS and particularly XCS has been a focus of a great deal of recent research activity [2, 6].

XCS is a LCS paradigm first developed by Wilson [11] and refined by others [2, 7] that diverges considerably from traditional Michigan-style LCS. First, classifier fitness is based on the accuracy of the classifiers payoff prediction, rather than the prediction itself. Second, the genetic algorithm is restricted to niches in the action set, rather than applied to the classifier population as a whole. These two features are responsible for XCS's ability to evolve accurate, maximally general classifiers, much more so than earlier LCS paradigms. To date, no one has investigated XCS's possible use as a medical knowledge discovery tool, particularly in epidemiologic surveillance.

As is typical of LCSs, the fundamental unit of knowledge representation in XCS is the *classifier*, which corresponds to an IF-THEN rule represented as a genotype-phenotype pair. The left-hand side, or genotype, is commonly referred to as a *taxon*, and the right-hand side is the *action*. Other components of the classifier include various indicators such as classifier fitness, prediction, birth date, numerosity (number of a classifier's instances in the classifier population), and classifier error. A more complete description of XCS is given in Butz and Wilson [1]. However, it is helpful to consider the schematic of generic XCS architecture as shown in Figure 1.

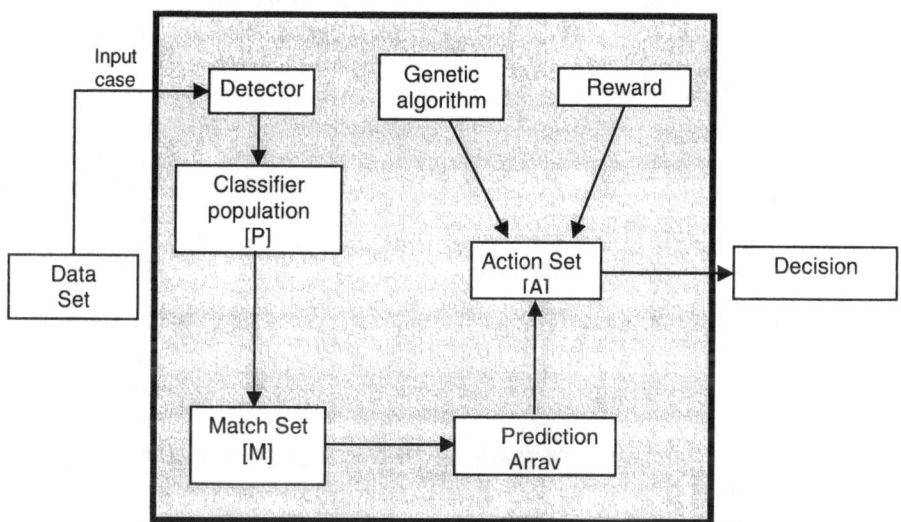

Fig. 1. Schematic of generic XCS architecture

At each time step, or *iteration*, a case is drawn from the data set (either training or testing) and passed through a detection algorithm that performs a matching function against the classifier population to create a Match Set [M]. Classifiers in [M] match the input case only on its taxon, so [M] may contain classifiers advocating any or all classes present in the problem domain. Using the classifiers in [M], a prediction array is created for each action. The values of the prediction array are based on fitness-weighted averages of the classifier predictions for each action; thus, for a two-class problem, there will be two elements in the prediction array, one for each possible action, or class. Actions can be selected from the array based on exploration (randomly) or exploitation (the action with the highest value). Classifiers in [M] with actions similar to the action selected from the prediction array form the Action Set [A], and that action is used as the decision of the system.

Classifiers in [A] are rewarded, using a variety of schemes. For single-step supervised learning problems, such as those found in data mining, the reward is simply some value applied to the prediction of the classifiers in [A]: correct decisions reward classifiers in [A] by adding to their prediction; incorrect decisions receive no reward.

In addition to reward, classifiers in [A] are candidates for reproduction (with or without crossover and/or mutation) using the genetic algorithm (GA). Parents are selected by the GA based on their fitness, weighted by their numerosity. This niche-based approach represents a major departure from other LCS approaches, which apply the GA *panmictally*, or across the entire classifier population. The advantage of the XCS approach is that reproduction occurs within the subset of the classifier population that is relevant to an input case, and therefore it is faster, but also it is also potentially more accurate. If the creation of a new classifier would result in exceeding the population size, a classifier is probablistically deleted from the population, based on fitness. Thus, over time, selection pressure causes low-fitness classifiers to be removed from the population, in favor of high-fitness classifiers, and ultimately, an optimally generalized and accurate population of classifiers emerges, from which classification rules can be derived. During testing, the GA and reward subsystems are turned off, and the system then functions like a forward-chaining expert system.

2 EpiXCS

EpiXCS was developed by the authors to accommodate the needs of epidemiologists and other clinical researchers in performing knowledge discovery tasks on surveillance data [4, 5]. Typically, these data are large, in that they contain many features and/or observations, and in turn, they often contain numerous relationships between predictors and outcomes that can be expressed as rules. EpiXCS adheres to the architectural paradigm of XCS in general, but with several differences that make it more appropriate for epidemiologic research. These features include a workbench-style interface that and the use of clinically relevant evaluation parameters.

The EpiXCS Workbench. EpiXCS is intended to support the needs of LCS researchers as they experiment with such problems as parameterization, as well as epidemiologic researchers as they seek to discover knowledge in surveillance data. The EpiXCS Workbench is shown in Figure 2.

The workbench supports multitasking to allow the user to run several experiments with different learning parameters, data input files, and output files. For example, this feature could be used to compare different learning parameter settings or to run different datasets at the same time. Visual clues convey the difference between experiments and runs to the user. Each simultaneous experiment is displayed in a separate child window. The learning parameters can be set for each individual experiment at run-time by means of a dialog box. Each run is displayed on a separate tab in the parent experiment's window. Each *run tab* displays the evaluation (obtained at each 100th iteration) of accuracy, sensitivity, specificity, area under the receiver operating characteristic curve, indeterminate rate (the proportion of training or testing cases that can't be matched), learning rate, and positive and negative predictive values in both graphical and textual form. These values help the user to determine how well the system is learning and classifying the data. Since the overall results of a batch run may be of interest to the user, additional tabs are provided for the training and testing evaluations. These tables include the mean and standard deviation of the aforementioned metrics calculated for all runs in the experiment.

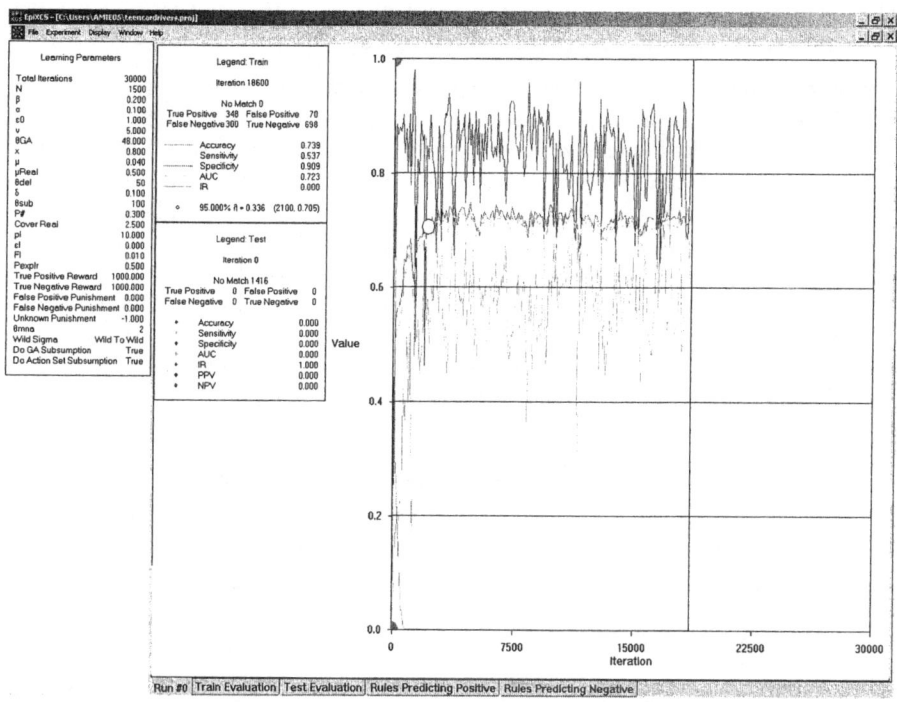

Fig. 2. The EpiXCS Workbench. The left pane is an interface to the learning parameters which are adjustable by the user prior to runtime. The middle pane contains classification metrics, obtained on each 100th iteration and at testing, as well as a legend to the graph in the right pane, which displays classification performance in real time during training (here at iteration 18600). The tabs at the bottom of the figure are described in the text

Rule Visualization. EpiXCS affords the user two means of rule visualization. The first of these is a separate listing of rules predicting positive and negative outcomes, respectively, ranked by their predictive value. Each rule is displayed in easily-read IF-THEN format, with an indication of the number of classifiers in the population which match the rule, as well as the number of those classifiers which predict the opposite outcome. This ratio provides an indication of the relative importance of the rule: even though a rule might have a high predictive value, if it matches only a few of the population classifiers, it is likely to be less general and potentially less important than if it matched multiple classifiers. On the other hand, it is entirely possible that such a rule could be "interesting," in that it represents an anomaly or outlier. As a result, the researcher would do well not to ignore such low-match rules.

The second means of rule visualization provides a graphical representation of each rule's conjunct using an X-Y graph. The X-axis represents the relative value of a specific conjunct as framed by range, from minimum to maximum, associated with the feature represented by the conjunct. The Y-axis represents each feature in the dataset. The user can select any number of rules to visualize. This tool is most useful when visualizing all rules, to develop a sense of the features and their values that seem to cluster for a particular outcome (Figures 3 and 4).

Evaluation Metrics. EpiXCS uses a variety of evaluation metrics, most of which are well-known to the medical decision making community. These include sensitivity, specificity, area under the receiver operating characteristic curve (AUC), and positive and negative predictive values. In addition, two other metrics are employed in EpiXCS: indeterminate rate, or IR, and learning rate, or λ. The IR indicates the proportion of input cases that can't be matched in the current population state. The IR will be relatively high in the early stages of learning, but should decrease as learning progresses and the classifier population becomes more generalized. While important for understanding the degree of generalization, the IR is also used for correcting the other evaluation metrics. The learning rate, λ, indicates the velocity at which 95% of the maximum AUC is attained, relative to the number of iterations.

3 Applying EpiXCS to Epidemiologic Surveillance

Research Questions. This investigation focuses on two research questions. The first is the epidemiologic question: What features are associated with fatality in teenaged (15 to 18 years of age) automobile drivers? To answer this question, EpiXCS was applied to the FARS database and compared with a well-known rule inducer, See5 [8].

Data: Fatality Analysis Reporting System. The Fatality Analysis Reporting System (FARS) is a census of all fatal motor vehicle crashes occurring in the United States

Table 1. Data elements in the final FARS dataset

Age	Age in years, 15 to 18
Sex	Sex of driver
Restraint use	Type of restraint used
Air bag deployment	Air bag deployed in crash, and if so, type of airbag
Ejection	Driver ejection from vehicle: No ejection, partial, complete
Body type	Type of vehicle
Rollover	Vehicle rollover during crash: No; once, multiple rollovers
Impact1	Initial impact, based on clock face (12=head-on)
Impact2	Principal impact, based on clock face
Fire	Fire or explosion at time of crash
Road function	Major artery, minor artery, street, classed by urban/rural
Manner of collision	Front-to-front, front-to-side, sideswipe, front-to-rear
Fatal	Driver died: Yes, No

and Puerto Rico, and is available at http://www-fars.nhtsa.dot.gov/. Records in FARS represent crashes involving a motor vehicle with at least one death.

In order to address the first research question, records were selected from the 2003 FARS Person File (the most recent version of the data available) using the following criteria: drivers of passenger automobiles, aged 15-18 years. Thus drawn, the dataset contained 1,997 fatalities and 2,427 non-fatalities. Additional criteria were applied to select data elements thought to be important for answering the first research question. The final dataset contained the data elements shown in Table 1, and was partitioned into training and testing sets, such that the original class distribution was maintained.

Experimental Procedure. EpiXCS was trained over 30,000 iterations using a population size of 1,000. The values for all other parameters were those described in (Butz and Wilson). See5 was trained using 10 boosting trials. Rules were examined for clinical plausibility and accuracy.

4 Results

4.1 Rule Discovery

Rules Discovered by EpiXCS. A total of 30 rules advocating the positive class and 21 rules advocating the negative class were discovered. The graphic representations

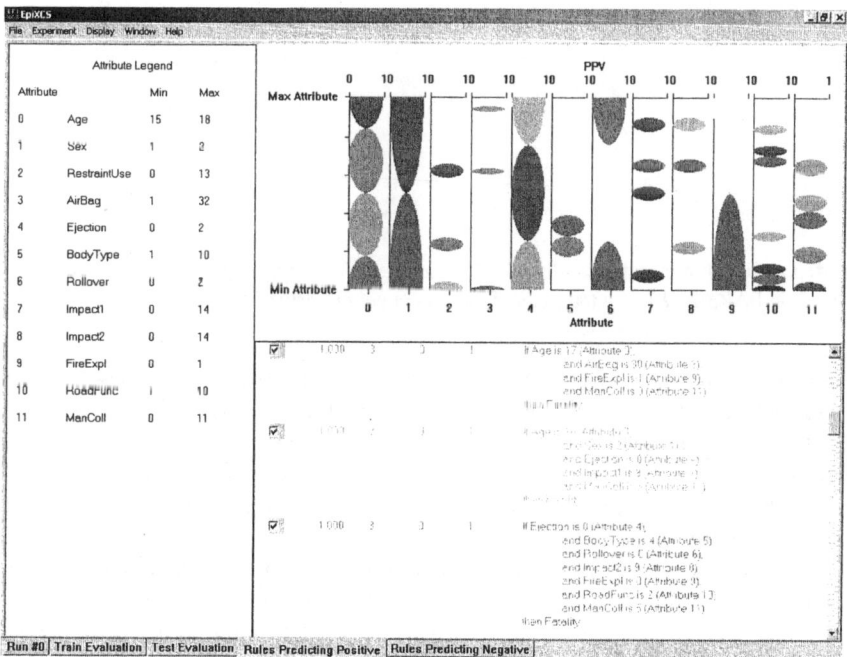

Fig. 3. Graphical representation of all 30 class-positive (fatality) rules discovered by EpiXCS on FARS data restricted to teenaged passenger car drivers. Three sample rules are shown in the bottom pane. Feature values are shown for all 30 rules in the top pane, and the features are referenced in the left-hand pane

of the positive and negative rules are shown in Figures 3 and 4, respectively. Several differences stand out. First, the youngest (15 year-old) drivers do not appear in the non-fatal rules. Second, vehicle fire, and ejection from the vehicle, either partial or total, appear only in the fatal rules. Third, the initial and principal impact points cluster on the driver's side of the vehicle in the fatal class.

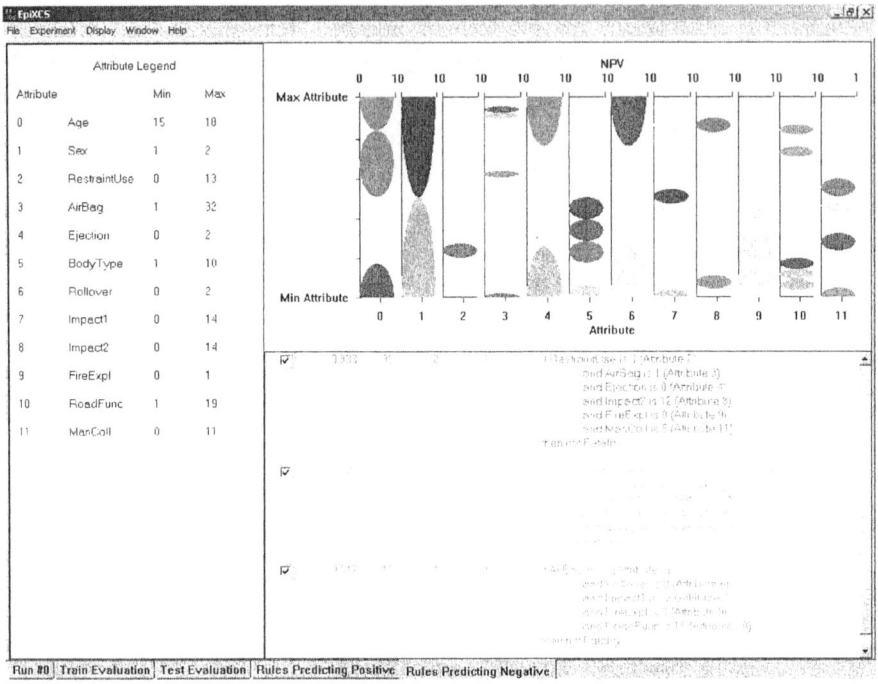

Fig. 4. Graphical representation of all 21 class-negative (non-fatality) rules discovered by EpiXCS on FARS data restricted to teenaged passenger car drivers

Comparison with Rules Discovered by See5. See5 discovered 415 rules, 262 in the fatal class, and 138 in the non-fatal class. Nearly all of the rules (97%) demonstrated predictive values of 1.0, but applied to very small numbers of training cases (<15), indicating that even with rule pruning, See5 required many more rules than EpiXCS to cover the problem domain. This was also evident in the large number of rules that contained conjuncts repeated from rule to rule.

Even though the final See5 rule set was large, an experienced automotive injury epidemiologist would have considerable difficulty identifying rules of importance to the clinical research question. In this rule set, several features emerged as potential associations with the outcome, as shown in Table 2, which compares the prominent features found by the two rule discovery methods, and demonstrates considerable agreement except for driver restraint and the youngest drivers.

Table 2. Key features associated with the classes, as identified by rule set inspection. Discrepancies are shown in boldface

Features	Non-fatal cases		Fatal cases	
	EpiXCS	See5	EpiXCS	See5
Driver restrained	Yes	Yes	**No**	**Yes**
Age=15	Yes	Yes	**Yes**	**No**
Road type: urban	Yes	Yes	**No**	**Yes**
Road type: rural	Yes	Yes	Yes	Yes
Fire or explosion	No	No	Yes	Yes
Ejection from vehicle	No	No	Yes	Yes
Driver's side impact	No	No	Yes	Yes

4.2 Classification of Novel Cases

The classification accuracy of EpiXCS and See5 is comparable, as shown in Table 3. The differences in AUC and NPV are not significant, although PPVs are ($p=0.04$).

Table 3. Classification accuracy metrics for EpiXCS and See5 on the FARS testing set

	AUC	PPV	NPV
EpiXCS	.66	.77	.66
See5	.70	.70	.64

5 Discussion and Conclusion

Both EpiXCS and See5 were able to discover clinically meaningful classification rules in the 2003 FARS dataset. However, there were qualitative differences in the rules, as well as the number of rules discovered. For example, EpiXCS discovered several important feature-outcome relationships that were missed by See5. These included driver restraint status, young driver age, and type of roadway.

EpiXCS discovered a total of 51 rules, comprising 30 fatalities and 21 non-fatalities. This is a manageable number of rules for qualitative analysis, but in order to reach this small rule set, a small tradeoff had to be considered in terms of classification accuracy when applying the rules to novel FARS data. Given that the tradeoff was primarily seen in the positive predictive value, and that the dataset had an unbalanced class distribution in favor of the non-fatal class, opting for a smaller rule set may result in even more compromised predictive values with a larger or different dataset. This issue is clearly one demanding further attention in future work.

In comparison, See5 discovered over 400 rules over 10 boosts, after pruning. While the classification accuracy at the end of the 10th boost is marginally better than that of EpiXCS, one is left with sifting through a very large rule set, the members of which, like those in the EpiXCS rule set, apply to small numbers of cases. This is not to say that See5's rules are not useful. Rather, they would be more useful if visualized through the same type of tool used in EpiXCS, and this too is a line of research for future work.

Finally, there is the fundamental issue of whether or not the rules from EpiXCS or See5 are useful in a clinical sense. Clearly, both systems induced rules that were clinically plausible. For example, it is reasonable to suggest that teen drivers who are not properly restrained are more likely to die in a crash where at least one fatality occurred. In addition, it is reasonable to posit that crashes where the teen driver's vehicle was hit from the driver's side are likely to result in that driver's demise. Finally, fires and ejection of the driver from the vehicle would be plausibly associated with teen driver fatality. However, some of the rules appear to be equivocal, even unnervingly so. For example, one would assume that an airbag exposure would protect the driver, yet there is little difference on this among the EpiXCS rules in either class. The See5 rules on airbag deployment are just as equivocal, although the deployment of side air bags occurred more frequently in these rules, albeit equally in both classes.

In conclusion, EpiXCS and See5 clearly discover rules in epidemiologic surveillance data, and most of these are clinically plausible. However, EpiXCS provides a workbench-style interface with a rule visualization tool that may provide a degree of marginal utility for LCS and epidemiologic researchers alike. Characterizing this utility is a focus of ongoing research by the authors.

References

1. Butz MV and Wilson SW: An algorithmic description of XCS. Soft Computing 6:144-52, 2002.
2. Butz MV, Kovacs T, Lanzi PL, and Wilson SW: Toward a theory of generalization and learning in XCS. IEEE Transactions on Evolutionary Computation, 8(1):28-46, 2004.
3. Holland, JH; Reitman, J: Cognitive systems based in adaptive algorithms. Waterman, D; Hayes-Roth, F (eds.). Pattern-directed inference systems. New York: Academic Press, 1978.
4. Holmes, JH, Lanzi, PL, Stolzmann W, and Wilson SW: Learning classifier systems: new models, successful applications. Information Processing Letters, 82(1), 23-30, 2002.
5. Holmes JH and Bilker WB: The effect of missing data on learning classifier system classification and prediction performance.
6. Advances in Learning Classifier Systems. Lecture Notes in Artificial Intelligence. Lanzi PL, Stolzmann W, and Wilson SW (eds.). Berlin, Springer Verlag, Vol. 2661: 46-60, 2003.
7. Lanzi PL: Learning classifier systems from a reinforcement learning perspective. *Soft Computing*, 6(3-4):162-70, 2002.
8. Rulequest Systems, www.rulequest.com
9. Smith S: A learning system based on genetic algorithms. Ph.D. dissertation, University of Pittsburgh, 1980.
10. Wilson, SW: Knowledge growth in an artificial animal. Grefenstette, JJ. Proceedings of the First International Conference on Genetic Algorithms, Lawrence Erlbaum Associates; 16-23, 1985.
11. Wilson SW: Classifier fitness based on accuracy. Evolutionary Computation. 3(2):149-175, 1995.

Subgroup Mining for Interactive Knowledge Refinement

Martin Atzmueller[1], Joachim Baumeister[1], Achim Hemsing[2],
Ernst-Jürgen Richter[2], and Frank Puppe[1]

[1] Department of Computer Science, University of Würzburg, 97074 Würzburg, Germany
{atzmueller, baumeister, puppe}@informatik.uni-wuerzburg.de
[2] Department of Prosthodontics, University of Würzburg, 97070 Würzburg, Germany
{hemsing_a, richter_e}@klinik.uni-wuerzburg.de

Abstract. When knowledge systems are deployed into a real-world application, then the maintenance of the knowledge is a crucial success factor. In the past, some approaches for the automatic refinement of knowledge bases have been proposed. Many only provide limited control during the modification and refinement process, and often assumptions about the correctness of the knowledge base and case base are made. However, such assumptions do not necessarily hold for real-world applications.

In this paper, we present a novel interactive approach for the user-guided refinement of knowledge bases. Subgroup mining methods are used to discover local patterns that describe factors potentially causing incorrect behavior of the knowledge system. We provide a case study of the presented approach with a fielded system in the medical domain.

1 Introduction

In the medical domain knowledge systems are commonly built manually by domain specialists. When such systems are deployed into a real-world application, then often the correctness needs to be improved according to the practical requirements. In the past, many approaches for the automatic refinement of knowledge bases have been proposed [1, 2, 3, 4]. However, such methods make two important assumptions that do not necessarily hold in a real-world setting. The first assumption states that the considered knowledge base is mainly correct and only requires minor modifications in the refinement step, i.e., the *tweak assumption*. This assumption does not hold, if the development of the knowledge base is in an earlier stage, and if corrections or extensions are still necessary. As the second assumption a collection of correctly solved test cases is expected. These cases are used by the methods for identifying *guilty* (faulty) elements in the knowledge base, that are the target for refinement in a subsequent step. Unfortunately, this assumption is not valid in our setting since the available cases were manually entered. Although the user is guided by an adaptive dialog during the case acquisition phase, and consistency checks are applied, we frequently experienced falsely entered findings in our case study.

In this paper, we present a novel approach for the user-guided refinement of knowledge bases. The proposed method supports the user to perform the correct refinements in an interactive process. This is especially important if the formalized knowledge is still incomplete, i.e., no tweak assumption for the underlying knowledge base can be made. In such circumstances, extensions and not only modifications of the knowledge base are necessary. Furthermore, if manually acquired case bases are used to refine knowledge systems, then the applied case base may contain incorrectly solved cases, e.g., due to incorrectly entered findings or solutions. Additionally, it is possible that automatic methods overfit the learned (refinement) knowledge by over-generalization or over-specialization. This problem is increased by the presence of incorrectly solved cases. Then, automatic refinements may not be acceptable for the expert.

In the presented approach subgroup mining methods are used to discover local patterns that describe factors potentially causing incorrect behavior of the knowledge system. It is important that no global refinement model of the knowledge base is generated but refinement operators are proposed based on a local model. The proposed method keeps the domain specialist in control of all steps of the refinement process. The user is supported by visualization techniques to easily interpret the (intermediate) results.

The rest of the paper is organized as follows: In Section 2 we introduce subgroup mining and its application for the refinement task. In Section 3, we present the subgroup driven interactive refinement process: we discuss the refinement steps, a visualization technique and related work. Finally, we provide a case study of the presented approach with a fielded system in the medical domain in Section 4. A summary of the paper is given in Section 5.

2 Subgroup Mining

In this section, we first introduce our knowledge representation, and we describe the basics of the subgroup mining approach. After that, we introduce the adaptation of subgroup mining to the interactive refinement process.

General Definitions. Let Ω_D be the set of all diagnoses and Ω_A the set of all attributes. For each attribute $a \in \Omega_A$ a range $dom(a)$ of attribute values is defined. Furthermore, we assume $\mathcal{V}_A$ to be the (universal) set of attribute values (*findings, observations*) of the form $(a : v)$, where $a \in \Omega_A$ is an attribute and $v \in dom(a)$ is an assignable value. For each diagnosis $d \in \Omega_D$ we define a (boolean) range

$$dom(d): \forall d \in \Omega_D : dom(d) = \{established, not\ established\}.$$

Let CB be the case base containing all available cases. A case $c \in CB$ is defined as a tuple $c = (\mathcal{V}_c, \mathcal{D}_c)$, where $\mathcal{V}_c \subseteq \mathcal{V}_A$ is the set of attribute values observed in the case c. The set $\mathcal{D}_c \subseteq \Omega_D$ is the set of diagnoses describing the *solution* of this case. The occurrence of a diagnosis d in a case c, indicates the value *established*. The value *not established* does not occur in our case base. Thus, $\mathcal{V}_F = \mathcal{V}_A \cup \Omega_D$ denotes the (universal) set of all possible "generalized" attribute values of the case base CB.

A diagnosis $d \in \Omega_D$ is derived using (heuristic) rules. A rule r can be considered as a triple $(cond(r), conf(r), d)$, where $cond(r)$ is the condition of the rules, $conf(r)$ is the confirmation strength (points), and $d \in \Omega_D$ is a diagnosis. Thus a rule $r = cond(r) \rightarrow d, conf(r)$ is used to derive the diagnosis d, where the rule condition $cond(r)$ contains conjunctions and/or disjunctions of (negated) generalized findings $f_i \in \mathcal{V}_F$. The state of a diagnosis is gradually inferred by summing all the confirmation strengths (points) of the rules that have fired; if the sum is greater than a specific threshold value, then the diagnosis is assumed to be established.

2.1 Basic Subgroup Mining

Subgroup mining [5, 6] is a method to discover "interesting" subgroups of cases, e.g., in the domain of dental medicine the subgroup "teeth with a strong attachmentloss and an increased degree of tooth lax" has a significantly higher share of "extracted teeth" than the total population. The main application areas of subgroup mining are exploration and descriptive induction: subgroups are described by relations between independent (explaining) variables and a dependent (target) variable rated by a certain interestingness measure.

A subgroup mining task mainly relies on the following four main properties: the target variable, the subgroup description language, the quality function, and the search strategy. We will focus on binary target variables.
The description language specifies the individuals from the reference population belonging to the subgroup.

Definition 1 (Subgroup Description). *A subgroup description $sd = \{e_i\}$ consists of a set of selection expressions (selectors) $e_i = (a_i, V_i)$ that are selections on domains of attributes, where $a_i \in \Omega_A, V_i \subseteq dom(a_i)$. A subgroup description is defined as the conjunction of its contained selection expressions. We define Ω_{sd} as the set of all possible subgroup descriptions.*

A quality function measures the interestingness of the subgroup. Several quality functions were proposed, for example in [6, 7].

Definition 2 (Quality Function). *A quality function*

$$q : \Omega_{sd} \times V_F \to R$$

evaluates a subgroup description $sd \in \Omega_{sd}$ given a target variable $t \in V_F$. It is used by the search method to rank the discovered subgroups during search.

For binary target variables, examples for quality functions are given by

$$q_{BT} = \frac{p - p_0}{\sqrt{p_0 \cdot (1 - p_0)}} \sqrt{n} \sqrt{\frac{N}{N-n}}, \quad q_{TP} = \frac{pn}{(1-p)n + g},$$

where p is the relative frequency of the target variable in the subgroup, p_0 is the relative frequency of the target variable in the total population, $N = |CB|$ is the size of the total population, and n denotes the size of the subgroup. For quality function q_{TP} the generalization parameter g trades of the number of true positives (pn) vs. the number of false positives $((1-p)n)$. For a low value of g fewer false positives are tolerated.

Considering an automatic subgroup mining approach an efficient search strategy is necessary, since the search space is exponential concerning all possible selection expressions. Commonly, a beam search strategy is used because of its efficiency. We use a modified beam search strategy, where a subgroup description can be selected as the initial value for the beam. Beam search adds selection expressions to the k best subgroup descriptions in each iteration. Iteration stops, if the quality as evaluated by the quality function q does not improve any further.

For the characterization of the discovered subgroups we have two alternatives: Besides the principal factors contained in the subgroup description there are also supporting factors. These are generalized findings $supp \subseteq \mathcal{V}_F$ contained in the subgroup, which are characteristic for the subgroup, i.e., the value distributions of their corresponding attributes (supporting attributes) differ significantly comparing two populations: the true positive cases contained in the subgroup and non-target class cases contained in the total population. In addition to the principal factors the supporting factors can also be used to statistically characterize a discovered subgroup, as described, e.g. in [8].

2.2 Subgroup Mining for the Refinement Task

For subgroup mining we consider a binary target variable corresponding to a diagnosis d, that is true (established) for incorrectly solved cases. Then, we try to identify subgroups with a high share of this "error" target variable. However, we need to distinguish different *error analysis states* relating to the measures *false positives* $FP_d(CB)$, *false negatives* $FN_d(CB)$, and the total error $ERR_d(CB)$:

$$FP_d(CB) = |\{c \,|\, CD_c \neq \emptyset \land d \in SD_c \land d \notin CD_c\}|,$$
$$FN_d(CB) = |\{c \,|\, CD_c \neq \emptyset \land d \notin SD_c \land d \in CD_c\}|,$$
$$ERR_d(CB) = |\{c \,|\, CD_c \neq \emptyset \land SD_c \neq CD_c\}|,$$

where CD_c are the *correct diagnoses* of the case c, and SD_c are the diagnoses derived by the system. It is easy to see that we want to minimize the measures for the (general) refinement task, while we want to maximize the measures for the discovered subgroups that are then used as candidates for refinement.

To identify the "potential faulty factors" PFF we consider the subgroup descriptions of the discovered subgroups containing a high share of falsely solved cases. Then there are two options: the interesting factors are always the *principal factors* describing the subgroup, i.e., the attribute values contained in the subgroup description. Additionally, also the *supporting factors* of the subgroup can be faulty factors, since their distribution differs significantly considering the incorrectly and correctly solved cases. Then, the potential faulty factors PFF are defined as follows:

$$PFF = \{\, f \mid f \text{ is principal or supporting factor}\,\}.$$

For the refinement task we also apply static test knowledge, i.e., immutable validation constraints, to detect inconsistent behavior of the knowledge system. These constraints are provided by the domain specialist as subgroups for which a specific diagnosis should always be derived. Then, by assessing the distribution of the diagnoses contained in these subgroups, we can validate the state of the knowledge base or the case base directly. Furthermore, after a refinement step has been performed, the test knowledge is always checked again, in order to exclude modifications which degrade the performance of the system. Examples of the static test knowledge are given in the case study in Section 4.

3 The Subgroup-Driven Interactive Refinement Process

In this section, we introduce the process for interactive knowledge refinement and its characteristics. We present the visualization method which provides an easy interpretation of intermediate results. Finally, we discuss related work.

3.1 Subgroup Mining for Interactive Knowledge Refinement – Process Model

For the interactive refinement process we apply the subgroup mining method to discover local patterns describing a set of incorrectly solved cases. We aim to discover subgroup cases with a high share of incorrectly solved cases. The incremental process depicted in Figure 1 mainly consists of six steps:

1. Consider a diagnosis $d \in \Omega_D$, and select an analysis state $e \in \{FP_d, FN_d, ERR_d\}$.
2. A set of subgroups SGS_e is mined, either interactively by the domain specialist, or automatically by the system. Then, for each subgroup $SG_i \in SGS_e$ a set of *potential faulty factors* PFF_i contained in SG_i is retrieved.
3. The subgroup descriptions/factors are interpreted by the domain specialist.
4. Based on the analysis of the potential faulty factors *guilty* (faulty) elements in the knowledge base or the case base are identified, and appropriate modification steps are applied. Then, the solutions of each case in the case base are recomputed.
5. The (changed) state of the system is assessed: the analysis measure e is checked for improvements; similarly the immutable validation constraints, if available, are tested whether they still indicate a valid state.
6. If necessary, restart the process.

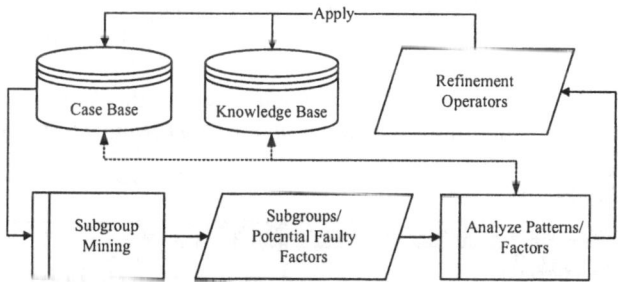

Fig. 1. Process Model: Subgroup Mining for Interactive Knowledge Refinement

Refinement operators can either modify the knowledge base or the applied case base. The knowledge base is usually adapted to fit the available correct cases. The case base is adapted, if particular cases are either wrong or they denote an extraordinary, exceptional state, which should not be modelled in the knowledge base. For the different refinement operators we need to distinguish two cases: if the expert decides that the subgroup descriptions are valid, i.e., they are reasonable, then probably the knowledge base needs to be corrected. Otherwise, if the subgroup descriptions, i.e., the combination of factors are not meaningful, then this can imply that the contained cases need corrections. However, these "doubtful" subgroups could also be caused by random correlations in the case base. In this case, the expert needs to manually assess the subgroups and cases in detail. In summary, the following refinements can be performed:

- **Adapt/modify rules:** generalize or specialize conditions and/or actions. This action is often appropriate if only one selector is contained in the subgroup, and if the subgroup is assessed to be valid.
- **Extend knowledge:** add missing relations to the knowledge base. This operator is often applicable when the subgroup description consists of more than one selector, and if the dependencies between the selectors are meaningful.
- **Fix case:** correct the solution of a single case, or correct the findings of a case, if the domain specialist concludes in a detailed case analysis that the case has been labeled with the wrong solution.
- **Exclude case:** exclude a case completely from the analysis. If the behavior modeled by the case cannot be explained by factors inherent in the knowledge base, e.g., by external decisions, then the case should be removed. This happened in our case study only for a low number of cases.

Examples of the application of the refinement operators are given in Section 4.

3.2 Visualizing Subgroups and Interesting Factors

If the user is not supported by visualization techniques, then an interactive refinement approach typically is not tractable, since the refinement space is usually large. Therefore, we provide visualization methods that enable the user to browse the space of subgroup hypotheses, while testing the hypotheses interactively. This process can also be supported by automatic subgroup mining methods that provide an initial starting point for further interaction. Additionally, visualization techniques simplify the interpretation of the subgroup mining results. Furthermore, they should guide the user to the right direction for refinement.

An examplary visualization is shown in Figure 2 where the distributions of several factors are given. The subgroup *toothlax = minor (Lockerungsgrad = Grad I)* (An-

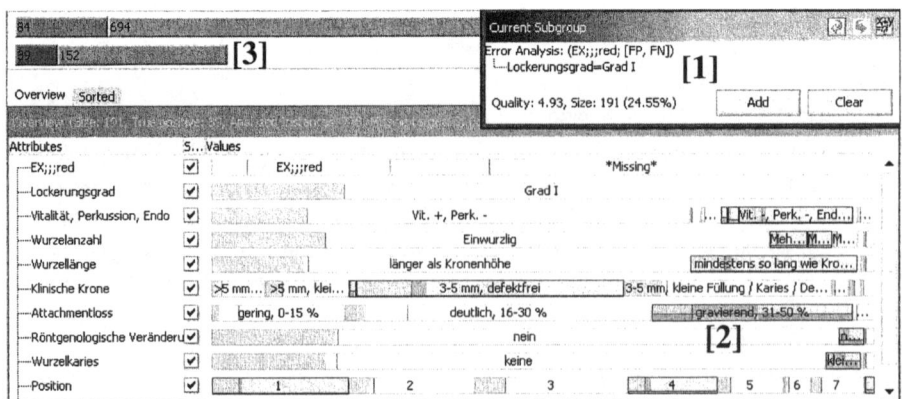

Fig. 2. Visualizing Subgroups and Interesting Factors (in German)

notation 1) is shown with 39 incorrectly solved cases and 152 correctly solved cases; the general population contains 84 incorrectly and 694 correctly solved cases (Annotation 3).

The rows in the table below the subgroup show the value distributions of the other attributes. Labels with a large "dark-gray" (green) sub-label, or a (red) horizontal bar that is close to the top, indicate "interesting" attribute values: the width/height, respectively, of these sub-bars indicates the *improvement* of the target share, if the respective attribute value (selector) would be added to the current subgroup, resulting in a virtual *future* subgroup. The horizontal line indicates the *relative improvement* of the target share: if the line is in the middle of the attribute value bar, then the target share in the future subgroup improves by 50%. In addition to the improvement of the target share of the current subgroup, the (potential) reduction of the subgroup size shown by the width of a attribute value cell also needs to be taken into account. In the example visualization the cell *attachmentloss = strong (Attachmentloss = gravierend, 31-50%)* is the best one considering its size, and also the target share (Annotation 2). Another interesting factor could be *Position = 4* which, however, can be regarded as a random finding.

In this visualization the user is able to inspect different subgroups directly by one click on the corresponding cells. All elements, i.e., subgroups, rules, and cases, can be browsed directly by one click, and changes can be assessed immediately. The changes are also intuitively reflected by the size of the bars (Annotation 3). Therefore, the user-guided integrated method provides direct interaction and instant feedback to the user.

3.3 Discussion

In the past, various approaches for knowledge refinement were proposed, e.g. [1]. More recently, Knauf et al. [4] presented a refinement approach embedded in a complete validation methodology. Carbonara and Sleeman [2] describe an efficient method for selecting effective refinements, and Boswell and Craw [3] introduce a set of general refinement operators that are applicable in various application domains and that can be used within different problem-solving tasks. All these approaches are classified as *automatic refinement techniques* modifying rule based knowledge. The modifications are motivated by a previous analysis step performing a *blame allocation*, i.e., identifying faulty knowledge. Then, alternative strategies are applied in order to automatically generate possible and select suitable refinements of the knowledge base.

However, all automatic methods make the *tweak assumption* [2], which implies that the knowledge base is almost valid and only small improvements need to be performed. In our application scenario the validity of the knowledge base was quite poor (about 86% accuracy) and therefore no tweak assumption could be made. In contrast, we expected that important rules were missing and that we have to acquire additional knowledge during the process. For this reason, we decided to choose a mixed refinement/elicitation process, which emphasizes the interactive analysis and modification of the implemented rules based on found subgroup patterns. Similarly, Carbonara and Sleeman [2] use an inductive approach for generating new rules using the available cases. Additionally, in our application we cannot expect that all cases contain the correct solution, and thus a thorough analysis of the cases within the process was also necessary. In contrast, automatic approaches mainly do assume a correct case base.

4 Case Study

In this section, we introduce the applied medical domain and we present practical experiences with the described approach.

4.1 The Prothetic System

The case study was implemented with a consultation and documentation system for dental findings regarding any kind of prosthetic appliance. The system was developed by the department of prosthodontics at the Würzburg University Hospital in cooperation with the department of computer science VI of the University of Würzburg. The domain specialists used the knowledge system D3 [9] to implement the knowledge base.

The systems aims to decide about a diagnostic plan using the clinical findings to accommodate the patient with denture. In the first level the system proposes the teeth that could be conserved and the teeth that should be extracted. The cases contain always the standard findings acquired in the first consultation with the patient, and additional findings from x-ray examinations, e.g., abnormal x-ray findings (apical, periradicular), grade of tooth lax, endodontic state (root filling, pulp vitality), root quantity, root length, crown length, level of attachment loss, root caries, tooth angulation and elongation/extrusion. The cases are manually entered by the examiners using an interactive dialog. For a given tooth all findings are stored in a single case in a data base.

In the knowledge base each finding obtains a point score depending on its quality. The outcome of the addition of the single scores is the dental score of the examined tooth. If the total dental score is less or equal than 40 points, then the tooth should be conserved. If the dental score is greater than 40 points, then the tooth has to be extracted (EX).

The system tries to support the dentist with time-efficient planning of patients' denture. Additionally, it should increase the efficiency of clinical work by chairside taking findings that are immediately translated to a prosthodontic therapy decision. In the future, it is also envisioned to use the diagnostic decision tool as a knowledge-based system for dental student education in order to train the ensuing diagnostic work up. Then, students can learn recognition and interpretation of symptoms and clinical findings by comparing their diagnosed solutions with the derived solutions of the system.

4.2 Results

To assess the quality of the system we compared the results of the system with the solutions of a domain specialist, both using the same set of findings. The initial case base contained 802 cases. 24 cases were removed from the case base, because the corresponding teeth had been extracted by prosthodontic reasons during planning denture. Although these teeth had a better dental score their extraction (EX) was decided, e.g., to prevent irregular construction in denture which can cause problems in future. Finally, the applied case base contained 778 cases corresponding to 778 examined teeth. We investigated the diagnosis corresponding to tooth extraction/non extraction. Considering this diagnosis the case base contained 108 false positive and 670 correct cases without any refinement of the knowledge base.

First subgroup mining efforts turned out unexpected subgroups with a very high share of incorrectly solved cases. However, some subgroup descriptions were very difficult to interpret by the domain specialist, since they contained finding combinations that should establish the diagnosis *EX* categorically. Therefore, the domain specialist provided immutable test knowledge represented as a set of synthetically generated test cases. Examples are shown in Table 1. The given subgroup descriptions indicate certain knowledge, when the diagnosis *EX* should be categorically established.

Table 1. Examples for immutable test knowledge

No.	Subgroup Description (findings)	Diagnosis
1	tooth lax = medium ∧ attachmentloss = strong	EX
2	attachmentloss = very strong	EX
3	tooth lax = strong ∧ root quantity = 3	EX
4	tooth lax = strong ∧ root caries = deep caries	EX

Using these subgroups the domain specialist was immediately able to locate incorrect cases, due to problems concerning data acquisition, i.e., noise in cases. Either the cases contained a false solution or incorrect findings. In total, 19 cases were corrected: 16 contained false diagnoses, and 3 contained incorrect case descriptions (findings).

Using the refined case base further analysis by automatic subgroup mining turned up several subgroups which were assessed as *dubious* by the expert, e.g., a subgroup described by *tooth lax = medium ∧ tooth position = 2 ∧ tooth quadrant = 2*. However, these subgroups had a high share of incorrectly solved cases. Since the combined potential faulty factors did not indicate anything particular, the domain specialist checked the contained cases. It turned out, that the *false positives* and *false negatives* had a high share of incorrect case descriptions and incorrectly assigned solutions. In total, further 12 cases were fixed.

Table 2. Discovered subgroups indicating a knowledge base refinement

No.	Subgroup Description	Diagnosis	Points
1	abnormal x-ray = only apical	EX	10 → 5
2	tooth lax = medium ∧ root length = longer than crown length	EX	-20
3	tooth lax = minor ∧ attachmentloss = strong	EX	-20

Using subgroup mining for the refinement of the knowledge system we managed to improve the knowledge base by reducing the number of incorrectly solved cases down to 54 cases: the domain specialist assessed several subgroups mined by the system as significant, which were then used for knowledge base refinement. We modified and added several rules, examples are given in Table 2. Subgroup description #1 is an example for a simple modification. For *abnormal x-ray = only apical* we modified the score, such that the rule only contributes 5 points. The last two subgroup descriptions the corresponding rules exemplify two general mechanisms: in rule #2 the condition *root length = longer than crown length* counts as negative for extraction, and relativizes the factor *tooth lax = medium* which is positive for extraction. Such an interaction can also work the other way round, i.e., when a positive factor influences a negative one. Then, for extraction, we would have to add points, e.g., for *tooth lax = medium* and *attachmentloss = minor*. For subgroup description #3 the selectors *tooth lax = minor* and *attachmentloss* = *strong* are both positive for extraction, but since they are assessed independently in the rule base they should not be over-emphasized by being counted twice. Therefore, the score points of the corresponding rules were decreased. The system also discovered some subgroups that could not be interpreted by the experts afterwards and thus were ignored, e.g., *tooth lax* = *medium* ∧ *root quantity* = *1*. In summary, we managed to reduce the number of incorrectly solved cases from 108 to 54 by 50%. In consequence, we increased the precision of the knowledge base from 86% to 93%. The method was very well accepted by the domain specialist, who was able to directly inspect and change the subgroups and cases by himself.

5 Summary and Future Work

In this paper, we presented a novel method using subgroup mining for interactive knowledge refinement. We introduced the application of the mining method, and proposed a process model for the refinement task. Furthermore, we described the identification of potential faulty factors and discussed the applicable refinement operators. We also motivated how the user of the process is supported by visualization techniques that guide the interactive refinement process. In a case study using cases from a fielded medical system we demonstrated the application and the benefit of the proposed techniques.

In the future, we plan to investigate further visualization techniques to support the user during the refinement process. Additionally, a semi-automatic refinement method that is adapted to the used knowledge representation (rules with point scores) is another interesting issue to consider.

References

1. Ginsberg, A.: Automatic Refinement of Expert System Knowledge Bases. Morgan Kaufmann (1988)
2. Carbonara, L., Sleeman, D.: Effective and Efficient Knowledge Base Refinement. Machine Learning 37 (1999) 143–181
3. Boswell, R., Craw, S.: Organizing Knowledge Refinement Operators. In: Validation and Verification of Knowledge Based Systems. Kluwer, Oslo, Norway (1999) 149–161
4. Knauf, R., Philippow, I., Jantke, K.P., Gonzalez, A., Salecker, D.: System Refinement in Practice – Using a Formal Method to Modify Real-Life Knowledge. In: Proceedings of the 15th International Florida Artificial Intelligence Research Society Conference (FLAIRS-2002), AAAI Press (2002)
5. Wrobel, S.: An Algorithm for Multi-Relational Discovery of Subgroups. In Komorowski, J., Zytkow, J., eds.: Proc. First European Symposion on Principles of Data Mining and Knowledge Discovery (PKDD-97), Berlin, Springer Verlag (1997) 78–87
6. Klösgen, W.: Subgroup Discovery. Chapter 16.3. In: Handbook of Data Mining and Knowledge Discovery. Oxford University Press, New York (2002)
7. Gamberger, D., Lavrac, N., Krstacic, G.: Active Subgroup Mining: a Case Study in Coronary Heart Disease Risk Group Detection. Artificial Intelligence in Medicine 28 (2003) 27–57
8. Gamberger, D., Lavrac, N.: Expert-Guided Subgroup Discovery: Methodology and Application. Journal of Artificial Intelligence Research 17 (2002) 501–527
9. Puppe, F.: Knowledge Reuse among Diagnostic Problem-Solving Methods in the Shell-Kit D3. Intl. Journal of Human-Computer Studies 49 (1998) 627–649

Evidence Accumulation to Identify Discriminatory Signatures in Biomedical Spectra

A. Bamgbade[1,2], R. Somorjai[1], B. Dolenko[1], E. Pranckeviciene[1],
A. Nikulin[1], and R. Baumgartner[1]

[1] Institute for Biodiagnostics, National Research Council Canada,
435 Ellice Avenue, Winnipeg, MB, Canada, R3B 1Y6
[2] Department of Computer Science, University of Manitoba,
545 Machray Hall, Winnipeg, MB, Canada, R3T 2N2
{Nike.Bamgbade, Ray.Somorjai, Brion.Dolenko, Erinija.Pranckevie,
Alexander.Nikulin, Richard.Baumgartner}@nrc-cnrc.gc.ca

Abstract. Extraction of meaningful spectral signatures (sets of features) from high-dimensional biomedical datasets is an important stage of biomarker discovery. We present a novel feature extraction algorithm for supervised classification, based on the evidence accumulation framework, originally proposed by Fred and Jain for unsupervised clustering. By taking advantage of the randomness in genetic-algorithm-based feature extraction, we generate interpretable spectral signatures, which serve as hypotheses for corroboration by further research. As a benchmark, we used the state-of-the-art support vector machine classifier. Using external crossvalidation, we were able to obtain candidate biomarkers without sacrificing prediction accuracy.

1 Introduction

Biomedical data (e.g. spectra) are characterized by large numbers of features (e.g., spectral intensities), but by considerably fewer samples. However, neighboring spectral features are strongly correlated, hence highly redundant. It is therefore reasonable to assume that the data do not span the entire high-dimensional input space, but lie near some low-dimensional manifold, representable by contiguous spectral regions that form a *spectral signature* [1,2]. Obtaining a spectral signature (a panel of biomarkers) consisting of a small number of spectral regions is an important step in biomarker discovery and provides the domain expert with interpretable information (hypothesis), usable for further experimental corroboration.

Fred and Jain [3] proposed an evidence accumulation framework (EAF) for unsupervised clustering. In this framework, results of several clusterings are combined to form a final data partition such that the most frequently clustered data points are assigned to the same cluster. A possible way to obtain multiple clusterings is to use clustering algorithms that depend on random initialization. Inspired by this EAF, we propose, in the supervised classification setting, a genetic-algorithm-driven feature extraction procedure for identifying discriminatory signatures in biomedical spectra, in our case magnetic resonance (MR) spectra. We used external crossvalidation to avoid overoptimistic assessment of the feature extraction procedure due to selection bias [4,5]. Our gold standard is a state-of-the-art support vector machine (SVM) classifier [6].

2 Datasets and Methods

We studied two 2-class MR spectral datasets (Dataset 1 and Dataset 2). We used the amplitude spectra. The properties of the datasets, and their original partition into training and independent test sets are presented in Table 1 below.

Table 1. Properties of the datasets

	Dimensionality	Training Samples (Class 1)+(Class 2)	Test Samples (Class 1)+(Class 2)
Dataset 1	1500	(62) + (62)	(42) + (31)
Dataset 2	1500	(70) + (70)	(105) + (59)

2.1 Genetic Algorithm

GA_ORS is a Genetic-Algorithm-based Optimal Region Selector, developed at the Institute for Biodiagnostics (IBD) [1]. In GA_ORS, the fitness function to be optimized for guiding the search for discriminatory spectral regions is the mean square error of the training set classification, using linear discriminant analysis (LDA), with internal leave-one-out (LOO) crossvalidation. The details of the parameters controlling the evolution of the genetic algorithm (GA), and its implementation are given in [1]. In this experiment, three (3) spectral regions are requested, and the probabilities of crossover and mutation of the GA-ORS are set at 0.6600 and 0.00100 respectively. The spectral signature found by the GA depends on the initial random seeds. We use this instability property of the GA in our evidence-accumulation-based feature extraction procedure. Note, that any unstable feature selection/extraction procedure can be used in the evidence accumulation framework. For a discussion of various feature selection algorithms in high-dimensional gene microarray profiling, see for example Ref. [7].

2.2 Evidence-Accumulation-Based Feature Extraction

The experimental procedure is illustrated in the pseudo code in Figure 1. We used N = 100 different random seeds to carry out N feature extractions via the GA. We count the frequency of occurrence of each of the extracted features in the N runs. The more frequently a feature is identified, the more likely that it is important. The final spectral signature (group of features) is obtained at a chosen frequency fraction threshold that we call the *occurrence fraction* (OF) of the feature groups. A 0.25 OF identifies features occurring with a frequency of 0.25N in N selections. We assessed feature occurrences at 0.25, 0.50 and 0.75 OFs. Figure 2 shows the spectral signature obtained from one of K random partitions of one of the datasets using a 0.25 OF.

We also investigated the effect of varying the number of generations of the GA on the accuracy of the evidence-accumulation-based feature extraction.

Input:
  R = Number of regions to be selected
  N = Maximum number of feature extractions
  G = Number of generations
  OF = Occurrence fraction
1. Generate **K** random splits of the dataset.
2. For each random split
   2.1. Do **N** times
      2.1.1. Select initial random seed **r**
      2.1.2. Initialize GA_ORS with seed **r** and **G** then select **R** feature regions from split
      2.1.3. Increment frequency count of selected features
3. Plot histogram of feature frequency counts
4. Select features with **OF** occurrence fraction
5. Compute predictive accuracy for a threshold **OF** features, using external crossvalidation

---

Fig. 1. The evidence-accumulation-based feature extraction pseudo code

2.3 Support Vector Machine Classifier

Support Vector Machines (SVMs) are currently considered state-of-the-art off-the shelf classifiers. To deal with the overfitting problem, SVMs use L_2-norm regularization during training. Typically, SVMs give sparse solutions, using only a small number of support vectors for classification. We applied the SVM to the full p-dimensional data. For the classification experiments, we used LIBSVM [6].

2.4 External Crossvalidation

We partition the dataset K times (K = 10) into training and test sets. The proportions of the samples in the training and test sets were identical to those given in Table 1 (stratification). For each split, we carried out the feature extraction procedure (or SVM) on the training set and then obtained the classification accuracy on the corresponding test set. Note, that each particular test set was used only once after the feature extraction procedure / SVM. We computed the average accuracy and standard deviation over the K splits.

3 Results

The results of the external crossvalidation, using the evidence accumulation framework for Dataset 1 and Dataset 2, are summarized in Table 2. They show that the misclassification error increases for features with higher OFs. We also observed that from 10 to 20 generations of the GA_ORS, the misclassification error provided by the extracted features decreased. However, as the number of generations increased from 30 to 100, the misclassification error increased. This observation suggests that as the number of generations increases, the feature selection procedure starts to adapt to

Table 2. External crossvalidation for Dataset 1 and Dataset 2 with the evidence-accumulation-based feature extraction method

Dataset 1			Dataset 2		
No. of Generations	Occurrence Fraction	Average Misclassification Error	No of Generations	Occurrence Fraction	Average Misclassification Error
20	0.25	0.06	20	0.25	0.14
	0.50	0.08		0.50	0.15
	0.75	0.13		0.75	0.16
40	0.25	0.08	40	0.25	0.15
	0.50	0.11		0.50	0.15
	0.75	0.15		0.75	0.15
60	0.25	0.09	60	0.25	0.15
	0.50	0.10		0.50	0.15
	0.75	0.19		0.75	0.15
100	0.25	0.10	100	0.25	0.15
	0.50	0.08		0.50	0.15
	0.75	0.13		0.75	0.15

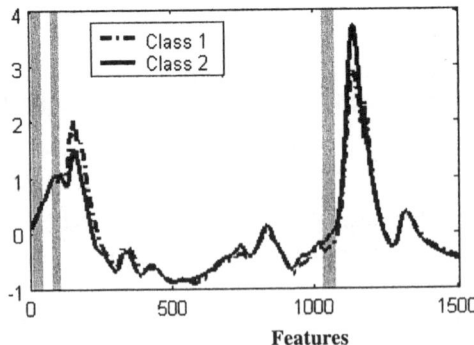

Fig. 2. Spectral signature (shaded regions) with the centroids (means) of Class 1 and Class 2 for Dataset 1 from one of the random splits using a 0.25 OF threshold

the peculiarities of the training set used in the feature selection, and that overfitting commences beyond 30 generations. The results (average misclassification error over the 10 splits ± standard deviation) of using the SVM benchmark, evaluated by external crossvalidation, were 0.053 ± 0.028 and 0.176 ± 0.326 for Dataset 1 and Dataset 2, respectively. Comparing the classification accuracy of SVM with that of the evidence accumulation feature extraction indicates that the latter was able to obtain interpretable candidate biomarkers without sacrificing classification accuracy.

4 Conclusions

We proposed a novel feature extraction method based on an evidence accumulation framework. We took advantage of the inherent randomness of the genetic-algorithm-based feature extraction to generate multiple feature subsets. We used MR spectra, but our method is directly applicable to other spectral modalities as well. We benchmarked our algorithm with the state-of-the-art support vector machine classifier. We were able to find discriminatory spectral signatures or panels of biomarkers with high predictive capability.

Acknowledgements. We acknowledge partial support of this work by NSERC. The first author acknowledges support of the University of Manitoba graduate fellowship.

References

1. Nikulin, A., Dolenko, B., Bezabeh, T., Somorjai, R.: Near-optimal Region Selection for Feature Space Reduction: Novel-preprocessing Methods for Classifying MR Spectra. NMR Biomed. 11 (1998) 209-216
2. Pranckeviciene, E., Baumgartner, R., Somorjai, R.: Consensus-based Identification of Spectral Signatures for Classification of High-dimensional Biomedical Spectra. Proc. ICPR Conf. (2004) 319-322
3. Fred, A., Jain, A.K.: Data Clustering using Evidence Accumulation. Proc. ICPR Conf. (2002) 276-280
4. Ambroise, C., McLachlan, G.: Selection Bias in Gene Extraction on the Basis of Microarray Gene-expression Data. Proc. Natl. Acad. Sci. USA. 99 (2002) 6562-6566
5. Simon, R., Radmacher, M., Dobbin, K., McShane, L.M.: Pitfalls In the Use of DNA Microarray Data for Diagnostic and Prognostic Classification. J.Natl.Cancer Inst. 95 (2003) 14-18
6. Chang, C., Lin, C.J.: LIBSVM: A library for Support Vector Machines, 2001. http://www.csie.ntu.edu.tw/~cjlin/libsvm
7. Inza, I., Larrañaga, P., Blanco, R., Cerrolaza, A.J.: Filter versus Wrapper Gene Selection Approaches in DNA Microarray Domains. Artif. Intell. Med. 31 (2004) 91-102

On Understanding and Assessing Feature Selection Bias

Šarunas Raudys[1], Richard Baumgartner[2], and Ray Somorjai[2]

[1] Vilnius Gediminas Technical University, Sauletekio 11, Vilnius LT-2100, Lithuania 2006
raudys@ktl.mii.lt
[2] Institute for Biodiagnostics, National Research Council Canada,
435 Ellice Avenue, Winnipeg, MB, Canada R3B 1Y6
{Richard.Baumgartner, Ray.Somorjai}@nrc-cnrc.gc.ca

Abstract. Feature selection in high-dimensional biomedical data, such as gene expression arrays or biomedical spectra constitutes and important step towards biomarker discovery. Controlling feature selection bias is considered a major issue for a realistic assessment of the feature selection process. We propose a theoretical, probabilistic framework for the analysis of selection bias. In particular, we derive the means of calculating the true selection error when the performance estimates of the feature subsets are mutually dependent and the distribution density of the true error is arbitrary. We demonstrate in an extensive series of experiments the utility of the theoretical derivations with real-world datasets. We discuss the importance of understanding feature selection bias for the small sample size (n) / high dimensionality (p) situation, typical for biomedical data (genomics, proteomics, spectroscopy).

Keywords: Machine learning, pattern recognition, feature selection bias, biomedical data.

1 Introduction

Feature selection in high-dimensional biomedical data is an important step towards biomarker discovery for disease profiling. The clinician is provided with a practical hypothesis, i.e. a panel of biomarkers (particular genes or spectral peaks) that can be validated by further biomedical tests. Ideally, three datasets are required for a feature selection procedure: a *training* set, a *validation* set and an *independent test* set. The training set is used to estimate the parameters of a classification rule. The validation set aids in evaluating the performance of the classifier obtained, and the selection of the best classifier. The independent test set should be used only after the best features and the optimal classifier have been identified.

Biomedical data (microarrays from genomics, mass spectra from proteomics, magnetic resonance, Raman and infrared spectra of tissues and biofluids), however are characterized by very few samples, $n = (O(10) - O(100))$ and numerous features, $p = (O(1000) - O(10000))$. As a consequence, we are confronted with the twin curses of dimensionality and dataset sparsity [3]. Specific two-class examples include gene microarray data [7] ($n/p = 72/7129$), mass spectra for proteomics [12] ($n/p = 100/15154$), and MR spectra for biofluids [13] ($n/p = 78/3500$).

When training the classifier, we inevitably *adapt to the training set*. The degree of adaptation depends on the size of this set, and the complexity (number of features and number and type of classifier parameters) of the classification algorithm.

When selecting the feature subset, we *adapt to the validation set*. An objective of the present paper is to evaluate how this adaptation occurs when imprecise criteria are used to compare the feature subsets or classification methods when feature selection is carried out. Known as the (model) feature selection bias (FSB) problem [1,4,5], its control is a major issue for any feature selection procedure. We propose a theoretical analysis of FSB when the performance estimates of the feature subsets are mutually dependent and the distribution density of true error rates in a pool of possible feature subsets is arbitrary. Our purpose is to provide theoretical scaffolding, and assess its validity and limitations by computer simulation on artificial and real-life biomedical data.

2 Theoretical Background

We assume m different models (e.g., feature subsets). For each of the models, one obtains validation error estimates, $\hat{\varepsilon}_{val\ 1}, \hat{\varepsilon}_{val\ 2}, \ldots, \hat{\varepsilon}_{val\ m}$. The selection of the best model is based on minimal error estimates. We call the minimal value, $\hat{\varepsilon}_{apparentS} = \min_j (\hat{\varepsilon}_{val\ j}) = \hat{\varepsilon}_{val\ z}, j = 1, \ldots, m$, the *apparent selection error*. An important aspect of the subsequent analysis is the assumption that there exist true error rates, $\varepsilon_{true\ 1}, \varepsilon_{true\ 2}, \varepsilon_{true\ 3}, \ldots, \varepsilon_{true\ m}$. Although these are unknown, assuming their existence helps understand the feature selection problem and its analysis.

For the analysis of adaptation to the validation set, we also need to define the true selection error. Given the estimates $\hat{\varepsilon}_{val\ 1}, \hat{\varepsilon}_{val\ 2}, \ldots, \hat{\varepsilon}_{val\ m}$, we consider the error of the zth feature subset (best according to the above estimates), as the true *selection* error, denoted by $\varepsilon_{trueS} = \varepsilon_{true\ z}$. Assuming further that the m feature subsets were selected randomly, and both sets of estimates $\hat{\varepsilon}_{val\ 1}, \hat{\varepsilon}_{val\ 2}, \ldots, \hat{\varepsilon}_{val\ m}$ and $\varepsilon_{true\ 1}, \varepsilon_{true\ 2}, \varepsilon_{true\ 3}, \ldots, \varepsilon_{true\ m}$ are *independent random variables*, one can obtain theoretically the expected values of $\hat{\varepsilon}_{apparentS}$ and ε_{trueS}. Raudys [9] considered the case when the vectors to be classified derive from spherical Gaussian distributions. He showed that the increase in generalization error due to suboptimal feature selection is larger than that due to imperfect training of the classifier.

Using the statistics of extremes [14], a method was developed [10] to analyze the apparent and true errors in model (feature) selection when considering m randomly selected models. It was assumed that $(\varepsilon_{true}, \hat{\varepsilon}_{val})$ is a bivariate random vector with known (joint) distribution density function, $f_3(\hat{\varepsilon}, \varepsilon) = f_2(\hat{\varepsilon}|\varepsilon) f_1(\varepsilon)$. The analysis assumed either Binomial distributions for both $f_1(\varepsilon)$ and $f_2(\hat{\varepsilon}|\varepsilon)$ [6], or Generalized Beta (Pearson type I) for $f_1(\varepsilon)$ and Binomial for $f_2(\hat{\varepsilon}|\varepsilon)$ [8], where $f_1(\varepsilon)$ is the probability density function of the true error ε and $f_2(\hat{\varepsilon}|\varepsilon)$ is the conditional probability density function of the validation error $\hat{\varepsilon}$, given the true error ε. It was shown that for the given distributions $f_1(\varepsilon)$ and $f_2(\hat{\varepsilon}|\varepsilon)$, the expectation $E(\varepsilon_{trueS})$ first decreases with increasing m, the number of feature subsets (types of classifier models) considered. However, the decrease slows down, and later stops altogether.

One of our objectives is to extend the analysis to more realistic situations, for which the generalization *error increases* when m is sufficiently large.

Here, we consider the situation when the estimates $\hat{\varepsilon}_{\text{val } 1}, \hat{\varepsilon}_{\text{val } 2},..., \hat{\varepsilon}_{\text{val } m}$ may be mutually dependent, and the distribution density $f_1(\varepsilon)$ is arbitrary. To formalize the feature selection process, we follow the framework outlined in Refs. [8,9]. We assume that we are evaluating m competing models (feature subsets), using a validation set. We are particularly interested in the *difference* between the expectations of $\varepsilon_{\text{trueS}}$ and $\hat{\varepsilon}_{\text{apparentS}}$; this can be interpreted as a measure of the selection bias of the feature selection process. We assume that the validation error $\hat{\varepsilon}$ is in the interval [0,1]. We model the *true, validation, apparent selection*, and *true selection* errors ($\varepsilon, \hat{\varepsilon}, \hat{\varepsilon}_{\text{apparentS}}, \varepsilon_{\text{trueS}}$) as random variables.

If estimates $\hat{\varepsilon}_{\text{val } 1}, \hat{\varepsilon}_{\text{val } 2},..., \hat{\varepsilon}_{\text{val } m}$ are obtained using a *single* validation set, they are statistically dependent, and the standard theory of extremes cannot be used. To introduce the dependency between the m validation error estimates, we assume that each estimate is obtained as a weighted sum of two binomially distributed random variables, $\hat{\varepsilon}_{\text{valid } j}^{\text{common}}$ and $\hat{\varepsilon}_{\text{valid } j}^{\text{unique}}$. We assume that $\hat{\varepsilon}_{\text{valid } j}^{\text{common}}$ is obtained while classifying a set of validation vectors $n_{\text{valid } 1}$ that are common to all m feature subsets. It has a binomial distribution. $\hat{\varepsilon}_{\text{valid } j}^{\text{unique}}$ is assumed to be unique to each subset and it is also distributed binomially. With these assumptions, the expectations $E(\hat{\varepsilon}_{\text{apparentS}})$ and $E(\varepsilon_{\text{trueS}})$ for the new generalized model can be found. $E(\hat{\varepsilon}_{\text{apparentS}})$ and $E(\varepsilon_{\text{trueS}})$ can be calculated numerically, provided the parameters of the distributions $f_2(\hat{\varepsilon}|\varepsilon)$ and $f_1(\varepsilon)$ are known a priori. This result is the main theoretical contribution of the paper.

3 Feature Selection Bias: Numerical Analysis

For a rough practical assessment of the accuracy of the above theoretical analysis of feature selection bias, we performed experiments with simulated data, and with three real-world biomedical datasets [7,11] for which the dimensionality of the feature space exceeds hundred-fold the number of samples. Due to space limitations we present here only results for the leukemia dataset [7].

For training, we used 35 samples, and the remaining 37 vectors constituted the test set. Then 500,000 8-dimensional (8d) feature subsets were generated randomly and Fisher linear classifiers were trained and subsequently validated on the 8d subsets. The training errors (resubstitution estimates) were used for feature selection. Since only eighteen 8d vectors per class were available in the training set, the resubstitution error estimate of the Fisher classifier is very optimistically biased. To reduce this bias, we used a surrogate error estimate for each error value, $\overline{\hat{\varepsilon}}_{\text{resubstitutionS}}$, in the graph to interpolate and evaluate the Mahalanobis distance. This correction for resubstitution error estimation was developed in [2].

Fig. 1a displays the histogram that characterizes the distribution of the test errors. Graph N1 (dots) in Fig. 1b shows the apparent mean feature selection error $\overline{\hat{\varepsilon}}_{\text{apparentS}}$ as a function of m. The mean, $\overline{\hat{\varepsilon}}_{\text{apparentS}}$, was calculated as the average of the validation errors for each value of *m*, using a combinatorial algorithm developed in Refs. [2,10]. Graph N2 (bold) shows the mean of the "true" selection error, $\bar{\hat{\varepsilon}}_{\text{resubstitutionS}}$ (in this case, the average of the resubstitution errors for the C^m_{500000} 500000 choose m subsets).

The upper graph N3 (dashed line) in Fig. 1b shows the reduced model selection bias for the true error. The minima in graphs N2 and N3 are approximately at the same location. However, due to the random character of the training and test datasets, the random bias between the two graphs is, in principle, unavoidable. Similar results were obtained using two other real-world biomedical examples (classification of pathogenic fungi [11]).

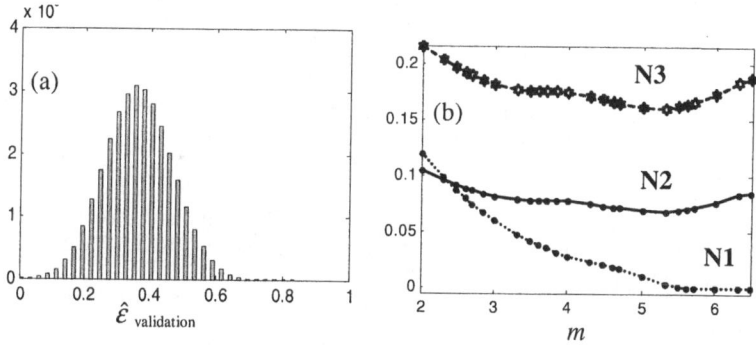

Fig. 1. a) Distribution of the validation error $\hat{\varepsilon}_{\text{validation}}$ in the experiments with the 7129-dimensional leukemia data. b) Means of the *apparent* selection error (N1), *true* selection error (N2) and *corrected* selection error (N3) for the leukemia dataset

4 Concluding Remarks

We presented a theoretical analysis of feature selection bias when the performance estimates of the feature subsets are mutually dependent, and the distribution density of the true error rates, in a pool of possible feature subsets, is arbitrary. Despite the fact that the true performance of a model (e.g., a particular feature subset) is unknown, and has to be evaluated by some "surrogate" estimate, the new approach readily helps appreciate important aspects of feature selection bias, and allows us to quantify more objectively the selection bias problem. This is particularly important in the small sample size/ high feature space dimension situation, for which the selection bias may be considerable.

Based on our results, for a given classification problem, e.g. for classification of high-dimensional biomedical data such as gene microarrays or biomedical spectra, we recommend the following three-step procedure to assess feature selection bias:
First, estimate the probability density function of $\hat{\varepsilon}$ using *m* feature subsets. Then compute $\hat{\varepsilon}_{\text{val }j}$. Finally, calculate the expectation of the true selection error $E(\varepsilon_{\text{trueS}})$.

Theory, numerical study and the experiments carried out with simulated as well as realworld data show that: 1) feature selection bias is very large if the sample size used to evaluate feature subsets is insufficient, 2) the theoretical analysis presented in Section 2 can be used for a rough estimation of feature selection bias.

The assumptions made in our theoretical analysis, i.e., partitioning the validation error into common and unique components, are somewhat restrictive. Development of more general models and constructive estimation of parameters of the distributions $f_1(\varepsilon)$ and $f_2(\hat{\varepsilon}|\varepsilon)$ is a topic for further research.

Acknowledgement. The first author was supported by NATO Expert Visit Grant SST.EAP.EV 980950.

References

1. S. J. Raudys, A. K. Jain. Small sample size effects in statistical pattern recognition: Recommendation for practitioners. IEEE Transactions on Pattern Analysis and Machine Intelligence 13(3) (1991) 242-254
2. S. Raudys. *Statistical and Neural Classifiers - An Integrated Approach to Design*. Springer-Verlag London Ltd. (2001).
3. R. L. Somorjai, B. Dolenko, R. Baumgartner. Class Prediction and Discovery Using Gene Microarray and Proteomics Mass Spectroscopy Data: Curses, Caveats, Cautions. Bioinformatics 19(12) (2003) 1484-1491
4. S.E. Estes. Measurement selection for linear discriminant used in pattern classification. PhD. Thesis, Stanford University, (1965).
5. C. Ambroise, G.J. McLachlan. Selection bias in gene extraction on the basis of microarray gene-expression data. Proc. Natl. Acad. Sci. USA **99** (10) (2002) 6562-6566.
6. S. Raudys. Influence of sample size on the accuracy of model selection in pattern recognition. In *Statistical Problems of Control* (S. Raudys, ed., Institute of Mathematics and Informatics, Vilnius) 50 (1981) 9-30 [in Russian]
7. T.R. Golub et al. Molecular classification of cancer: Class discovery and class prediction by gene expression monitoring. Science 286 (1999) 531-537
8. S. Raudys, V. Pikelis. Collective selection of the best version of a pattern recognition system. Pattern Recognition Letters 1(1) (1982) 7-13
9. S. Raudys. Classification errors when features are selected. In S Raudys (editor), *Statistical Problems of Control*, 38 (1979) 9-26. Institute of Mathematics and Informatics, Vilnius (in Russian).
10. V. Pikelis. (1991) Calculating statistical characteristics of experimental process for selecting the best version. In S Raudys (editor) *Statistical Problems of Control*, **93** 46-56. Institute of Mathematics and Informatics, Vilnius (in Russian).
11. U. Himmelreich et al. Rapid identification of Candida species by using nuclear magnetic resonance spectroscopy and a statistical classification strategy. Appl. Environ. Microbiol. 69(8) (2003) 4566-74
12. E. Petricoin et al. Use of proteomics patterns in serum to identify ovarian cancer. Lancet, 359 (2002) 572-577
13. C. Lean et al. Accurate diagnosis and prognosis of human cancers by proton MRS and a three-stage classification strategy. Annual Reports on NMR Spectroscopy, 48 (2002) 71-111
14. Gumbel E. Statistics of extremes. Dover Publications (2004).

A Model-Based Approach to Visualizing Classification Decisions for Patient Diagnosis*

Keith Marsolo[1], Srinivasan Parthasarathy[1],
Michael Twa[2], and Mark Bullimore[2]

[1] Department of Computer Science and Engineering
[2] College of Optometry, The Ohio State University,
Columbus, OH, USA
srini@cse.ohio-state.edu

Abstract. Automated classification systems are often used for patient diagnosis. In many cases, the rationale behind a decision is as important as the decision itself. Here we detail a method of visualizing the criteria used by a decision tree classifier to provide support for clinicians interested in diagnosing corneal disease. We leverage properties of our data transformation to create surfaces highlighting the details deemed important in classification. Preliminary results indicate that the features illustrated by our visualization method are indeed the criteria that often lead to a correct diagnosis and that our system also seems to find favor with practicing clinicians.

1 Introduction

The field of medicine has benefited greatly from advances in computing. Medical imaging, genetic screening and large-scale clinical trials to determine drug efficacy are just three areas where increased computational power is fueling massive growth in the testing and collection of patient data. With the ability to collect and store large amounts of patient data comes the desire to discover underlying relationships between it. The fields of data mining and bioinformatics have arisen to handle this task. When applied to medical data, traditional data mining applications like classification and clustering can yield commonalities among patients that might be an indicator of a given condition. If such commonalities are found, it is possible to create a type of "signature," where patients who are found to have that signature could be diagnosed with, or classified as potentially having, that condition.

Ideally, one would like a system that can provide more information than a simple *yes* or *no* decision. The criteria used to reach a decision can be just as

---

* This work was partially supported by the following grants: NIH-NEI T32-EY13359, NIH-NEI K23-EY16225 and American Optometric Foundation William Ezell Fellowship, Ocular Sciences Inc. (MT); NSF Career Grant IIS-0347662 (KM, SP); NIH-NEI R01-EY12952 (MB).

important as the decision itself. In some cases, the basis for a diagnosis may be as simple as the presence of a particular antibody in the blood. In diseases that are manifested by the existence or absence of certain physical characteristics, the decision might not be so cut and dry. For instance, keratoconus, a disease affecting the shape of the cornea, is often characterized by a large cone-shaped protrusion rising from the corneal surface. How irregular the cornea must be before the diagnosis of keratoconus is made is arguable. Having a way to visualize the criteria used in classification could provide a great benefit to clinicians, providing a safety check that could limit some of the liability that might arise from relying purely on a single answer from a computer. It is in that spirit that we present our work into developing a system of classifying corneal shape using decision trees to distinguish between several classes of corneas while providing a visualization of the classification criteria to aid in clinical decision support.

Decision tree classifiers are widely used in many applications. The principle behind a decision tree is to select an attribute at each node and divide the feature space into increasingly fine-grained regions. The class label of an object is based on the final region in which it lies. One benefit of decision trees is that they are transparent, meaning the user can inspect the actual tree produced by the classifier to examine the features used in classification.

While accuracy is an important factor in choosing a classification strategy, another attribute that should not be ignored is the interpretability of the final results. Decision trees may be favored over (possibly) more accurate "blackbox" classifiers because they provide more understandable results. In medical image interpretation, decision support for a domain expert is preferable to an automated classification made by an expert system. While it is important for a system to provide a decision, it is often equally important for clinicians to know the basis for an assignment.

Given a dataset containing corneas labeled as diseased, post-operative or non-diseased, we use Zernike polynomials to model the corneal surface. We then use the polynomial coefficients for each geometric mode as an input feature for a decision tree. Part of the rationale behind using Zernike polynomials as a transformation method over other alternatives is that there is a direct correlation between the geometric modes of the polynomials and the surface features of the cornea. Zernike polynomials have been well-studied by the medical community and vision scientists and clinicians are familiar with their use [1]. An added benefit of Zernike polynomials is that *the orthogonality of the series allows us to treat each term independently*. Since the polynomial coefficients used as splitting attributes represent the proportional contributions of specific geometric modes, we are able to create a surface representation that reflects the spatial features deemed "important" in classification. These features discriminate between the patient classes and give an indication as to the specific reasons for a decision.

We have designed and developed a method of visualizing our decision tree results. We partition our dataset based on the path taken through the decision tree and create a surface from the mean values of the polynomial coefficients of all the patients falling into that partition. For each patient, we create an individual polynomial surface from the patient's coefficient values that correspond to the splitting attributes of the decision tree. We contrast this surface against a similar surface containing the mean partition values for the same splitting coefficients and provide a measure to quantify how "close" a patient lies to the mean. *We have shown our results to practicing clinicians and preliminary validation from them indicates there is an anatomic correspondence between the features of these surfaces and corneal aberrations of patients with keratoconus.*

2 Biological Background

Image formation begins when light entering the eye is focused by the cornea, passes through the pupil, and is further focused by the lens, forming an image on the retina at the back of the eye. Since light must pass through the cornea, clear vision depends very much on the optical quality of the corneal surface, which is responsible for nearly 75% of the total optical power of the eye. The normal cornea has an aspheric profile that is more steeply curved in the center relative to the periphery. Subtle distortions in the shape of the cornea can have a dramatic effect on vision. For this reason, the shape of the corneal surface is measured clinically for the treatment and diagnosis of eye disease. The process of mapping the surface features on the cornea is known as *corneal topography*.

2.1 Clinical Use of Corneal Topography

The use of corneal topography has rapidly increased in recent years because of the popularity of refractive surgery and the decreased cost of powerful personal computers. Refractive surgery is an elective surgical treatment intended to reduce one's dependence on glasses or contact lenses. The most common surgical treatment performed for this purpose is laser assisted in-situ keratomileusis (LASIK). Corneal topography is used to screen patients for corneal disease prior to this surgery and to monitor the effects of treatment after surgery.

Another clinical application of corneal topography is the diagnosis and management of keratoconus. Keratoconus, a progressive, non-inflammatory corneal disease, distorts corneal shape and results in poor vision that cannot be corrected with ordinary glasses or contact lenses. Patients with keratoconus frequently seek refractive surgery due to their poor vision. However, such treatment exacerbates their corneal distortion and frequently leads to corneal transplant. Thus, corneal topography is a valuable tool for diagnosis and management of keratoconus as well as for the prevention of inappropriate refractive surgery in this patient group.

2.2 Determination of Corneal Shape

The most common method of determining corneal shape is to record an image of the reflection of a series of concentric rings from the corneal surface. Any distortion in corneal shape will cause a distortion of the concentric rings. By comparing the size and shape of the imaged rings with their known dimensions, it is possible to mathematically derive the topography of the corneal surface.

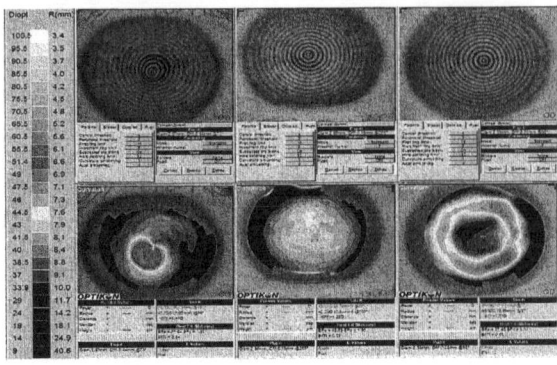

Fig. 1. Example of characteristic corneal shapes for each of the three patient groups. From left to right: Keratoconus, Normal, and post-LASIK. The top image shows a picture of the cornea and reflected concentric rings. The bottom image shows the topographical map representing corneal shape

Figure 1 shows an example of the output produced by a corneal topographer for a member of each patient class. These represent *extreme* examples of each class, i.e. they designed to clearly illustrate the differences between them. The top portion of the figure shows the imaged concentric rings. The bottom portion of the image shows a false color map representing the surface curvature of the cornea. This color map is intended to aid clinicians and the appearance of each map is largely instrument-dependent. Many methods of interpretation exist, but a lack of accepted standards among domain experts and instrument manufacturers usually results in qualitative pattern recognition from the false color maps.

The data files from the corneal topographer consist of a three-dimensional matrix of approximately 7000 spatial coordinates arrayed in a polar grid. The height of each point z is specified by the relation $z = f(\rho, \theta)$, where the height relative to the corneal apex is a function of radial distance from the origin (ρ) and the counter-clockwise angular deviation from the horizontal meridian (θ). The inner and outer borders of each concentric ring consist of a discrete set of 256 data points taken at a known angle θ, but a variable distance ρ, from the origin.

Using the data obtained from a corneal topographer, we can construct a surface to represent the shape of the cornea. It is not possible, however, to use this surface directly in classification. Each surface is represented by thousands of data points and trying to use these points as a feature vector in classification will results in poor performance. Alternatively, using the raw data results in a classifier that is too granular and therefore too specific to provide useful clinical decision support. We transform the raw data to address this problem.

3 Zernike Polynomials

Zernike polynomials are a family of circular polynomial functions that are orthogonal in x and y over a normalized unit circle. Each polynomial term consists of three elements [1]. The first element is a normalization coefficient. The second element is a radial polynomial component and the third, a sinusoidal angular component. The general form for Zernike polynomials is given by:

A Model-Based Approach to Visualizing Classification Decisions 477

Polynomial	Azimuthal Frequency (m)								
Order (n)	-4	-3	-2	-1	0	1	2	3	4
0					0				
1				1		2			
2			3		4		5		
3		6		7		8		9	
4	10		11		12		13		14

(a)

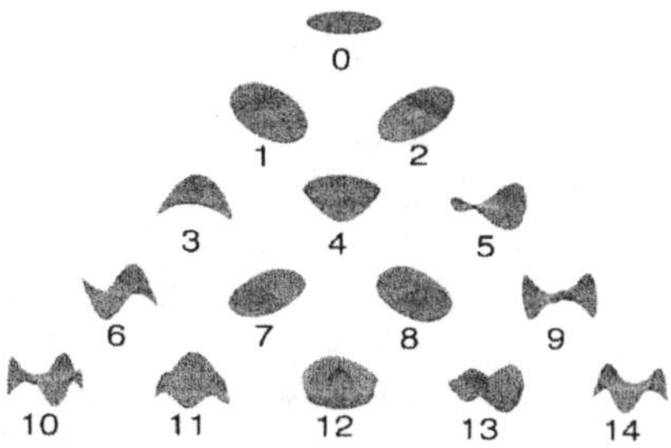

(b)

Fig. 2. (a) Combinations of radial polynomial order (n) and azimuthal frequency (m) that yield the 15 terms comprising a 4th order Zernike polynomial. (b) Graphical representation of the modes

$$Z_n^{\pm m}(\rho, \theta) = \begin{cases} \sqrt{2(n+1)} R_n^m(\rho) \cos(m\theta) & \text{for } m > 0 \\ \sqrt{2(n+1)} R_n^m(\rho) \sin(|m|\theta) & \text{for } m < 0 \\ \sqrt{(n+1)} R_n^m(\rho) & \text{for } m = 0 \end{cases} \quad (1)$$

where n is the radial polynomial order and m represents azimuthal frequency. The normalization coefficient is given by the square root term preceding the radial and azimuthal components. The radial component of the Zernike polynomial is defined as:

$$R_n^m(\rho) = \sum_{s=0}^{(n-|m|)/2} \frac{(-1)^s (n-s)!}{s!(\frac{n+|m|}{2} - s)!(\frac{n-|m|}{2} - s)!} \rho^{n-2s} \quad (2)$$

Please note that the value of n is a positive integer or zero. Only certain combinations of n and m will yield valid polynomials. Any combination that is not valid simply results in a radial component of zero. The table shown in Fig. 2 (a) lists the combinations of n and m that generate the 15 terms comprising a 4th order Zernike polynomial. Rather than refer to each term with the two indexing scheme using n and m, each term is labeled with a number j that is consistent with the single indexing scheme created by the Optical Society of America [1].

Polynomials that result from fitting our raw data with these functions are a collection of orthogonal circular geometric modes. Examples of the modes representing a 4th order Zernike polynomial can be seen in Fig. 2 (b). The label underneath each mode corresponds to the jth term listed in the table to the left. The coefficients of each mode are proportional to their contribution to the overall topography of the original data. As a result, we can effectively reduce the dimensionality of the data to a subset of polynomial coefficients that describe spatial features, or a proportion of specific geometric modes present in the original data.

4 Classification of Corneal Topography

Iskander et al. examined a method of modeling corneal shape using Zernike polynomials with a goal of determining the optimal number of coefficients to use in constructing the model [2]. In a follow-up study, the same group concluded that a 4th order Zernike polynomial was adequate in modeling the majority of corneal surfaces [3]. Twa et al. showed that with Zernike polynomials, lower order transformations were able to capture the general shape of the cornea and were unaffected by noise [4]. They also found that higher order transformations were able to provide a better model fit, but were also more susceptible to noise.

A number of studies on the classification of corneal shape have been produced that use statistical summaries to represent the data [5, 6]. These studies used multi-layer perceptrons or linear discriminant functions in classification. Smolek and Klyce have classified normal and post-operative corneal shapes using wavelets and neural networks with impressive results, but use very few data in their experiments [7, 8]. Twa et al. were the first to use decision trees for corneal classification, reporting classification accuracy around 85% with standard C4.5 and in the mid-90% range with C4.5 and various meta-learning techniques [4]. In our experiments, we achieve roughly the same classification accuracy even though we use a more challenging, multi-class dataset.

5 Visualization of Classification Decisions

Our visualization surfaces are calculated by transforming the patient data using an algorithm detailed by Iskander et al. [2]. It involves calculating a Zernike polynomial for every data point and then computing a least-squares fit between the polynomials and the actual surface data. This results in a set of coefficients which we then use for classification.

Figure 3 shows an example decision tree. In this case, the Z value in each node (diamond) refers to the jth term of a Zernike polynomial. Classification occurs by comparing a patient's Zernike coefficient values against those in the tree. For instance, the value of Z_7 for a patient is compared against the value listed in the top node. If the patient's value is less than or equal to 2.88, we traverse the right branch. If not, we take the left (in all cases, we take the right branch with a *yes* decision and the left with a *no*). With this example, a *no* decision would lead to a classification of K, or Keratoconus. If the

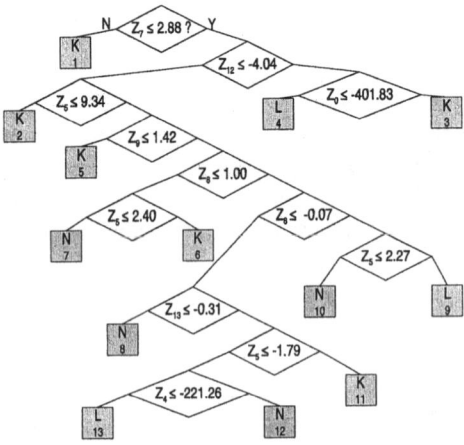

Fig. 3. Decision tree for a 4th order Zernike polynomial

value of Z_7 was less than or equal to 2.88, we would proceed to the next node and continue the process until we reached a leaf and the corresponding classification label (K = Keratoconus, N = Normal, L = LASIK).

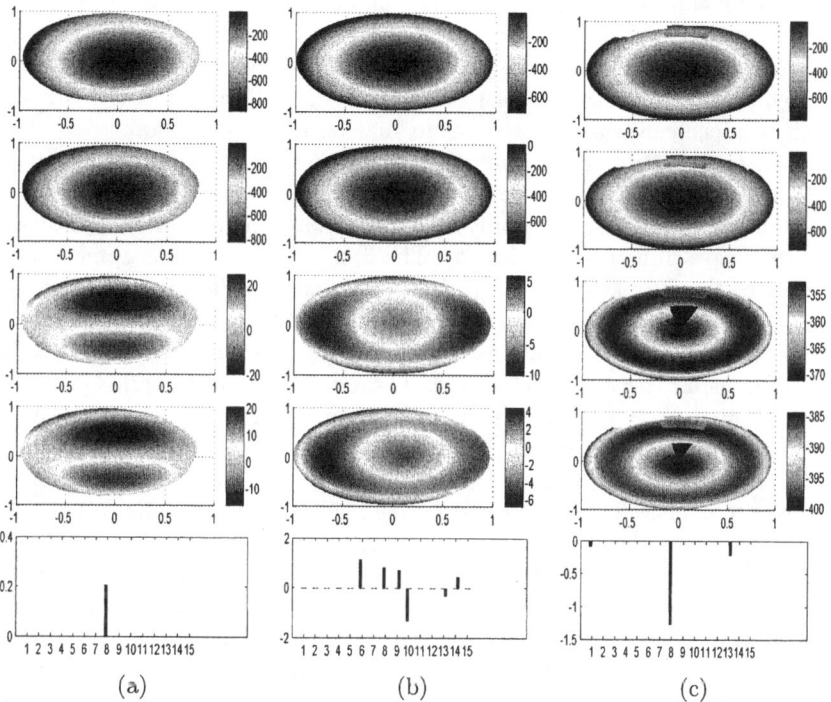

Fig. 4. Example surfaces for the strongest rule in each patient class. Figure (a) represents a Keratoconic eye (Rule 1), (b) a Normal cornea (8), and (c) a post-operative LASIK eye (4). The top panel contains the Zernike representation of the patient. The next panel illustrates the Zernike representation using the $\overline{rule}$ values. The third and fourth panels show the *rule surfaces*, using the patient and $\overline{rule}$ coefficients, respectively. The bottom panel consists of a bar chart showing the deviation between the patient's *rule surface* coefficients and the $\overline{rule}$ values

We can treat each possible path through a decision tree as a rule for classifying an object. Using the tree in Fig. 3, we construct rules for the first four leaves, with the leaf number (arbitrarily assigned) listed below the class label:

1. $Z_7 > 2.88 \to Keratoconus$
2. $Z_7 \leq 2.88 \land Z_{12} > -4.04 \land Z_5 > 9.34 \to Keratoconus$
3. $Z_7 \leq 2.88 \land Z_{12} \leq -4.04 \land Z_0 \leq -401.83 \to Keratoconus$
4. $Z_7 \leq 2.88 \land Z_{12} \leq -4.04 \land Z_0 > -401.83 \to LASIK$

In each rule, the "∧" symbol is the standard *AND* operator and the "→" sign is an implication stating that if the values of the coefficients for a patient satisfy the expression on the left, the patient will be assigned the label on the right. For a given dataset, a certain number of patients will be classified by each rule. These patients will share similar surface features. As a result, one can compare a patient against the mean attribute values of all the other patients who were classified using the same rule. This comparison will give clinicians some indication of how "close" a patient is to the rule average. To compute these "rule mean" coefficients, denoted $\overline{rule}$, we partition the training data and take the average of each coefficient over all the records in that particular partition.

For a new patient, we compute the Zernike transformation and classify the record using the decision tree to determine the rule for that patient. Once this step has been completed, we apply our visualization algorithm, to produce five separate images (illustrated in Fig. 4). The first panel is a topographical surface representing the Zernike model for the patient. It is constructed by plotting the 3-D transformation surface as a 2-D topographical map, with elevation denoted by color. The second section contains a topographical surface created in a similar manner by using the $\overline{rule}$ coefficients. These surfaces are intended to give an overall picture of how the patient's cornea compares to the average cornea of all similarly-classified patients.

The next two panels in Fig. 4 (rows 3 and 4) are intended to highlight the features used in classification, i.e. the distinguishing surface details. We call these surfaces the *rule surfaces*. They are constructed from the value of the coefficients that were part of the classification rule (the rest are zero). For instance, if a patient were classified using the second rule in the list above, we would keep the values of Z_7, Z_{12} and Z_5. The first rule surface (third panel of Fig. 4) is created by using the relevant coefficients, but instead of using the patient-specific values, we use the values of the $\overline{rule}$ coefficients. This surface will represent the mean values of the distinguishing features for that rule. The second rule surface (row 4, Fig. 4) is created in the same fashion, but with the coefficient values from the patient transformation, not the average values.

The actual construction of the surfaces is achieved by running our transformation algorithm in reverse, updating the values in the coefficient matrix depending on the surface being generated. Once the values have been computed, we are left with several 3-D polar surfaces. In the surfaces, the base elevation is green. Increasing elevation is represented by red-shifted colors; decreased elevation is represented by blue-shifted colors.

Finally, we provide a measure to show how close the patient lies to those falling in the same rule partition. For each of the distinguishing coefficients, we compute a relative error between the patient and the $\overline{rule}$. We take the absolute value of the difference between the coefficient value of the patient and the value of the $\overline{rule}$ and divide the result by the $\overline{rule}$ value. We provide a bar chart of these errors for each coefficient (the error values of the the coefficients not used in classification are set to zero). This plot is intended to provide a clinician with an idea of the influence of the specific geometric modes in classification and the degree that the patient deviates from the mean. To provide further detail, if the patient's coefficient value is less than the $\overline{rule}$ coefficient, we color the bar blue. If it is greater, we color it red.

6 Dataset

The dataset for these experiments consists of the examination data of 254 eyes obtained from a clinical corneal topography system. The data were examined by a clinician and divided into three groups based on corneal shape. The divisions are given below, with the number of patients in each group listed in parentheses:

1. Normal ($n = 119$)
2. Post-operative myopic LASIK ($n = 36$)
3. Keratoconus ($n = 99$)

Relative to the corneal shape of normal eyes, post-operative myopic LASIK corneas generally have a flatter center curvature with an annulus of greater curvature in the periphery. Corneas that are diagnosed as having keratoconus are also more distorted than normal corneas. Unlike the LASIK corneas, they generally have localized regions of steeper curvature at the site of tissue degeneration, but often have normal or flatter than normal curvature elsewhere.

7 Visualization of Classification Results

Using a C4.5 decision tree generated from the classification of the dataset on a 4th order Zernike transformation (Fig. 3), we provide an example of our visualization technique on a record from each patient class.

Table 1. Strongest Decision Tree Rules and Support

Rule	Class Label	Expression	Support	Support Percentage
1	K	$Z_7 > 2.88$	47	66.2%
8	N	$Z_7 \leq 2.88 \wedge Z_{12} > -4.04 \wedge Z_5 \leq 9.34 \wedge Z_9 \leq 1.42 \wedge -0.07 > Z_8 \leq 1.00 \wedge Z_{13} > -0.31$	74	89.2%
4	L	$Z_7 \leq 2.88 \wedge Z_{12} \leq -4.04 \wedge Z_0 > -401.83$	19	79.2%

As stated previously, we must reclassify our training data after generating the decision tree in order to partition the data by rule. We expect that certain rules will be *stronger* than others, i.e. a larger portion of the class will fall into those rule's partition. Table 1 provides a list of the strongest rule for each class. Given in the table is the rule number, its class label and *support*, or the number of patients that were classified using that rule. We also provide the *support percentage* of the rule, or the number of patients classified by the rule divided by the total number of patients in that class. These numbers reflect the classification of the training data *only*, not the entire dataset (the data was divided into a 70%/30% training/testing split). Table 1 also provides the expression for each rule.

Using a patient that was classified by each *strong* rule, we execute our visualization algorithm and create a set of surfaces. These surfaces are shown in Fig. 4. Figure 4 (a) shows a Keratoconic patient classified by Rule 1. Figure 4 (b) gives an example of a Normal cornea classified under Rule 8. Finally, Fig. 4 (c) illustrates a LASIK eye falling under Rule 4.

Since these are the strongest, or most discriminating rules for each class, we would expect that the *rule surfaces* would exhibit surface features commonly associated with corneas of that type. Our results are in agreement with expectations of domain experts. For instance, corneas that are diagnosed as Keratoconic often have a cone shape protruding from the surface. This aberration, referred to as "coma" is modeled by terms Z_7 and Z_8 (vertical and horizontal coma, respectively). As a result, we would expect one of these terms to play some role in any Keratoconus diagnosis. Rule 1, the strongest Keratoconus rule, is characterized by the presence of a large Z_7 value. The *rule surfaces* (rows 3 and 4) of Fig. 4 (a) clearly show such a feature. Corneas that have undergone LASIK surgery are characterized by a generally flat, plateau-like center. They often have a very negative spherical aberration mode (Z_{12}). A negative Z_{12} value is part of Rule 4, the strongest LASIK rule. The elevated ring structure shown in the *rule surfaces* (rows 3 and 4) of Fig. 4 (c), is an example of that mode.

8 Conclusions

In order to address malpractice concerns and be trusted by clinicians, a classification system should consistently provide high accuracy (at least 90%, preferably higher). When coupled with meta-learning techniques, decision trees can provide such accuracy. The motivation behind the application presented here was to provide an additional tool that can be used by clinicians to aid in patient diagnosis and decision support. By taking advantage of the unique properties of Zernike polynomials, we are able to create several decision surfaces which reflect the geometric features that discriminate between normal, keratoconic and post-LASIK corneas. We have shown our results to several practicing clinicians who indicated that the important corneal features found in patients with keratoconus were indeed being used in classification and can be seen in the decision surfaces. This creates a degree of trust between the clinician and the system. In addition, the clinicians stated a preference for this technique over several start-of-the-art systems available to them. Most current classification systems diagnosis a patient as either having keratoconus or not. An off-center post-LASIK cornea can present itself as one that has keratoconus and vice versa. Misclassifying the post-LASIK cornea is bad, but misclassifying a keratoconic cornea as normal (in a binary classifier) can be catastrophic. Performing LASIK surgery on a cornea suffering from keratoconus can lead to corneal transplant. Our method can be leveraged by clinicians to serve as a safety check, limiting the liability that results from relying on an automated decision from an expert system.

References

1. Thibos, L., Applegate, R., Schwiegerling, JT Webb, R.: Standards for reporting the optical aberrations of eyes. In: TOPS, Santa Fe, NM, OSA (1999)
2. Iskander, D., Collins, M., Davis, B.: Optimal modeling of corneal surfaces with zernike polynomials. IEEE Trans Biomed Eng **48** (2001) 87–95.
3. Iskander, D.R., Collins, M.J., Davis, B., Franklin, R.: Corneal surface characterization: How many zernike terms should be used? (arvo abstract). Invest Ophthalmol Vis Sci **42** (2001) S896
4. Twa, M., Parthasarathy, S., Raasch, T., Bullimore, M.: Automated classification of keratoconus: A case study in analyzing clinical data. In: SIAM Intl. Conference on Data Mining, San Francisco, CA (2003)
5. Maeda, N., Klyce, S.D., Smolek, M.K., Thompson, H.W.: Automated keratoconus screening with corneal topography analysis. Invest Ophthalmol Vis Sci **35** (1994) 2749–57
6. Rabinowitz, Y.S., Rasheed, K.: Kisaminimal topographic criteria for diagnosing keratoconus. J Cataract Refract Surg **25** (1999) 1327–35
7. Smolek, M.K., Klyce, S.D.: Screening of prior refractive surgery by a wavelet-based neural network. J Cataract Refract Surg **27** (2001) 1926–31.
8. Maeda, N., Klyce, S.D., Smolek, M.K.: Neural network classification of corneal topography. preliminary demonstration. Invest Ophthalmol Vis Sci **36** (1995) 1327–35.

Learning Rules from Multisource Data for Cardiac Monitoring

Élisa Fromont, René Quiniou, and Marie-Odile Cordier

IRISA, Campus de Beaulieu, 35000 Rennes, France
{efromont, quiniou, cordier}@irisa.fr

Abstract. This paper aims at formalizing the concept of learning rules from multisource data in a cardiac monitoring context. Our method has been implemented and evaluated on learning from data describing cardiac behaviors from different viewpoints, here electrocardiograms and arterial blood pressure measures. In order to cope with the dimensionality problems of multisource learning, we propose an Inductive Logic Programming method using a two-step strategy. Firstly, rules are learned independently from each sources. Secondly, the learned rules are used to bias a new learning process from the aggregated data. The results show that the the proposed method is much more efficient than learning directly from the aggregated data. Furthermore, it yields rules having better or equal accuracy than rules obtained by monosource learning.

1 Introduction

Monitoring devices in Cardiac Intensive Care Units (CICU) use only data from electrocardiogram (ECG) channels to diagnose automatically cardiac arrhythmias. However, data from other sources like arterial pressure, phonocardiograms, ventilation, etc. are often available. This additional information could also be used in order to improve the diagnosis and, consequently, to reduce the number of false alarms emitted by monitoring devices. From a practical point of view, only severe arrhythmias (considered as *red alarms*) are diagnosed automatically, and in a conservative manner to avoid missing a problem. The aim of the work that has begun in the Calicot project [1] is to improve the diagnosis of cardiac rhythm disorders in a monitoring context and to extend the set of recognized arrhythmias to non lethal ones if they are detected early enough (considered as *orange alarms*). To achieve this goal, we want to combine information coming from several sources, such as ECG and arterial blood pressure (ABP) channels.

We are particularly interested in learning temporal rules that could enable such a multisource detection scheme. To learn this kind of rules, a relational learning system that uses Inductive Logic Programming (ILP) is well-adapted. ILP not only enables to learn relations between characteristic events occurring on the different channels but also provides rules that are understandable by doctors since the representation method relies on first order logic.

One possible way to combine information coming from difference sources is simply, to aggregate all the learning data and then, to learn as in the monosource (i.e one data source) case. However, in a multisource learning problem, the amount of data and the expressiveness of the language, can increase dramatically and with them, the computation time of ILP algorithms and the size of the hypothesis search space. Many methods have been proposed in ILP to cope with the search space dimensions, one of them is using a declarative bias [2]. This bias aims either at narrowing the search space or at ranking hypotheses to consider first the better ones for a given problem. Designing an efficient bias for a multisource problem is a difficult task. In [3], we have sketched a divide-and-conquer strategy (called biased multisource learning) where symbolic rules are learned independently from each source and then, the learned rules are used to bias automatically and efficiently a new learning process on the aggregated dataset. This proposal is developed here and applied on cardiac monitoring data.

In the first section we give a brief introduction to inductive logic programming. In the second section we expose the proposed method. In the third section we describe the experiments we have done to compare, on learning from cardiac data, the monosource, naive multisource and biased multisource methods. The last section gives conclusions and perspectives.

2 Multisource Learning with ILP

In this section, we make a brief introduction to ILP (see [4] for more details) and we give a formalization of this paradigm applied to multisource learning. We assume familiarity with first order logic (see [5] for an introduction).

2.1 Introduction to ILP

Inductive Logic Programming (ILP) is a supervised machine learning method. Given a set of examples E and a set of general rules B representing the background knowledge, it builds a set of hypotheses H, in the form of classification rules for a set of classes C. B and H are logic programs i.e. sets of rules (also called definite clauses) having the form $h\,:\text{-}\ b_1,\ b_2,\ \ldots,\ b_n$. When $n=0$ such a rule is called a fact. E is a labeled set of ground facts. In a multi-class problem, each example labeled by c is a positive example for the class c and a negative example for the class $c' \in \{C - c\}$. The following definition for a multi-class ILP problem is inspired by Blockeel et al. [6].

Definition 1. *A multi-class ILP problem is described by a tuple* $< L, E, B, C >$ *such that:*

- $E = \{(e_k, c) | k = 1, m; c \in C\}$ *is the set of examples where each e_k is a set of facts expressed in the language L_E.*
- B *is a set of rules expressed in the language L. $L = L_E \cup L_H$ where L_H is the languages of hypotheses.*

The ILP algorithm has to find a set of rules H such that for each $(e, c) \in E$:

$$H \wedge e \wedge B \vDash c \text{ and } \forall\, c' \in C - \{c\},\ H \wedge e \wedge B \nvDash c'$$

The hypotheses in H are searched in a so-called *hypothesis space*. A generalization relation, usually the θ-subsumption [7], can be defined on hypotheses. This relation induces a lattice structure on L_H which enables an efficient exploration of the search space. Different strategies can be used to explore the hypothesis search space. For example, ICL [8], the ILP system we used, explores the search space from the most general clause to more specific clauses. The search stops when a clause that covers no negative example while covering some positive examples is reached. At each step, the best clause is refined by adding new literals to its body, applying variable substitutions, etc. The search space, initially defined by L_H, can be restricted by a so-called *language bias*. ICL uses a declarative bias (DLAB [9]) which allows to define syntactically the subset of clauses from L_H which belong to the search space. A DLAB bias is a grammar which defines exactly which literals are allowed in hypotheses, in which order literals are added to hypotheses and the search depth limit (the clause size). The most specific clauses of the search space that can be generated from a bias specification are called *bottom clauses*. Conversely, a DLAB bias can be constructed from a set of clauses (the method will not be explained in this article).

2.2 Multisource Learning

In a multisource learning problem, examples are bi-dimensional, the first dimension, $i \in [1, s]$, refers to a source, the second one, $k \in [1, m]$, refers to a situation. Examples indexed by the same situation correspond to contemporaneous views of the same phenomenon. Aggregation is the operation consisting in merging examples from different views of the same situations. The aggregation function F_{agg} depends on the learning data type and can be different from one multisource learning problem to another. Here, the aggregation function is simply the set union associated to inconsistency elimination. Inconsistent aggregated examples are eliminated in the multisource learning problem. The aggregation knowledge, such as correspondence between example attributes on different channels and temporal constraints is entirely described in the background knowledge B. Multisource learning for a multi-class ILP problem is then defined as follows:

Definition 2. *Let* $< L_i, E_i, B_i, C >$, $i = 1, s$, *be ILP problems such that* L_i *describes the data from source* i. $E_i = \{(e_{i,k}, c) | k = 1, m; c \in C\}$.
A multisource ILP problem is defined by a tuple $< L, E, B, C >$ *such that:*

- $E = F_{agg}(E_1, E_2, \ldots, E_m) = \{(e_k, c) | e_k = \bigcup_{i=1}^{s} e_{i,k}, k = 1, m\}$
- $L = L_E \cup L_H$ *is the multisource language where*
  $L_E = F_{agg}(L_{E_1}, L_{E_2}, \ldots, L_{E_m})$ *and* $L_H \supseteq \bigcup_{i=1}^{s} L_{H_i}$,
- B *is a set of rules in the language* L.

The ILP algorithm has to find a set of rules H such that for each $(e, c) \in E$:

$$H \wedge e \wedge B \models c \text{ and } \forall\, c' \in C - \{c\},\ H \wedge e \wedge B \not\models c'$$

A *naive* multisource approach consists in learning directly from the aggregated examples and with a global bias that covers the whole search space related to the aggregated language L. The main drawback of this approach is the size of the resulting search space. In many situations the learning algorithm is not able to cope with it or takes too much computation time. The only solution is to specify an efficient language bias, but this is often a difficult task especially when no information describing the relations between sources is provided. In the following section, we propose a new method to create such a bias.

3 Reducing the Multisource Learning Search Space

We propose a multisource learning method that consists in learning rules independently from each source. The resulting clauses, considered as being bottom clauses, are then merged and used to build a bias that will be used for a new learning process on the aggregated data. Algorithm 1 shows the different steps of the method on two source learning. It can be straightforwardly extended to n source learning. We assume that the situations are described using a common reference time. This is seldom the case for raw data, so we assume that the data set have been preprocessed to ensure this property.

A literal that describes an event occurring on some data source, as *qrs(R0,normal)*, is called an *event literal*. Literals of predicates common to the two sources and describing relations between two events, as *suc(R0,R1)* or *rr1(R0,R1,normal)*, are called *relational literals*.

Algorithm 1

1. **Learn** with bias $Bias_1$ on the ILP problem $< L_1, E_1, B_1, C >$. Let H_{c_1} be the set of rules learned for a given class $c \in C$ (rules with head c).
2. **Learn** with bias $Bias_2$ on the ILP problem $< L_2, E_2, B_2, C >$. Let H_{c_2} be the set of rules learned for the class c (rules with head c).
3. **Aggregate** the sets of examples E_1 and E_2 giving E_3.
4. **Generate** from all pairs $(h_{1j}, h_{2k}) \in H_{c_1} \times H_{c_1}$ a set of bottom clauses BT such that each $bt_i \in BT$ built from h_{1j} and h_{2k} is more specific than both h_{1j} and h_{2k}. The literals of bt_i are all the literals of h_{1j} and h_{2k} plus new relational literals that synchronize events in h_{1j} and h_{2k}.
5. For each $c \in C$ **Build** bias $Bias_{c_3}$ from BT. Let $Bias_3 = \{Bias_{c_3} | c \in C\}$.
6. **Learn** with $Bias_3$ on the problem $< L, E_3, B_3, C >$ where :
   - L is the multisource language as defined in section 2
   - B_3 is a set of rules expressed in the language L

One goal of multisource learning is to make relationships between events occurring on different sources explicit. For each pair (h_{1j}, h_{2k}), there are as many bottom clauses as ways to intertwine events from the two sources. A new relational predicate, *suci*, is used to specify this temporal information. The number of bottom clauses generated for one pair (h_{1j}, h_{2k}) is C_{n+p}^n where n is the number of event predicates belonging to h_{1j} and p is the number of event predicates belonging to h_{2k}. The number of clauses in BT is the total number of bottom clauses generated for all possible pairs. This number may be very high if H_{c_1}

and H_{c_2} contain more than one rule and if there are several event predicates in each rule. However, in practice, many bottom clauses can be eliminated because the related event sequences do not make sense for the application. The bias can then be generated automatically from this set of bottom clauses. The multisource search space bounded by this bias has the properties 1, 2 and 3.

Property 1 (Correctness). There exist hypotheses with an equal or higher accuracy than the accuracy of H_{c_1} and H_{c_2} in the search space defined by $Bias_3$ of algorithm 1.

Intuitively, property 1 states that, in the worst case, H_{c_1} and H_{c_2} can also be learned by the biased multisource algorithm. The accuracy[1] is defined as the rate of correctly classified examples.

Property 2 (Optimality). There is no guaranty to find the multisource solution with the best accuracy in the search space defined by $Bias_3$ in algorithm 1.

Property 3 (Search space reduction). The search space defined by $Bias_3$ in algorithm 1 is smaller than the naive multisource search space.

The size of the search space specified by a DLAB bias can be computed by the method given in [9]. The biased multisource search space is smaller than the naive search space since the language used in the first case is a subset of the language used in the second case.

In the next section, this biased multisource method is compared to monosource learning from cardiac data coming from an electrocardiogram for the first source and from measures of arterial blood pressure for the second source. The method is also compared to a naive multisource learning performed on the data aggregated from the two former sources.

4 Experimental Results

4.1 Data

We use the MIMIC database (Multi-parameter Intelligent Monitoring for Intensive Care [10]) which contains 72 patients files recorded in the CICU of the Beth Israel Hospital Arrhythmia Laboratory. Raw data concerning the channel V1 of an ECG and an ABP signal are extracted from the MIMIC database and transformed into symbolic descriptions by signal processing tools. These descriptions are stored into a logical knowledge database as Prolog facts (cf. Figures 1 and 2). Figure 1 shows 7 facts in a ventricular doublet example : 1 *P wave*, 3 *QRSs*,

---

[1] The accuracy is defined by the formula $\frac{TP+TN}{TP+TN+FP+FN}$ where TP (true positive) is the number of positive examples classified as true, TN (true negative) the number of negative examples classified as false, FN (false negative) is the number of positive examples classified as false and FP (false positive), the number of negative examples classified as true.

```
begin(model).
doublet_3_I.
.....
p_wave(p7,4905,normal).
qrs(r7,5026,normal).
suc(r7,p7).
qrs(r8,5638,abnormal).
suc(r8,r7).
qrs(r9,6448,abnormal).
suc(r9,r8).
.....
end(model).
```

Fig. 1. Example representation of a ventricular doublet ECG

```
begin(model).
rs_3_ABP.
.......
diastole(pd4,3406,-882).
suc(pd4,ps3).
systole(ps4,3558,-279).
suc(ps4,pd4).
......
end(model).
```

Fig. 2. Example representation of a normal rhythm pressure channel

Table 1. Number of nodes visited for learning and computation times

	monosource: ECG		monosource: ABP		naive multisource		biased multisource	
	Nodes	Time *	Nodes	Time *	Nodes	Time	Nodes	Time (⊃ *)
sr	2544	176.64	2679	89.49	18789	3851.36	243	438.55
ves	2616	68.15	5467	68.04	29653	3100.00	657	363.86
bige	1063	26.99	1023	14.27	22735	3299.43	98	92.74
doub	2100	52.88	4593	64.11	22281	2417.77	1071	290.17
vt	999	26.40	3747	40.01	8442	724.69	30	70.84
svt	945	29.67	537	17.85	4218	1879.71	20	57.58
af	896	23.78	972	21.47	2319	550.63	19	63.92
TOT	11163	404.51	19018	315.24	108437	15823.59	2138	1377.66

the first one occurring at time *5026* as well as relations describing the order of these waves in the sequence. Additional information such as the wave shapes (normal/abnormal) is also provided. Figure 2 provides a similar description for the pressure channel.

Seven cardiac rhythms (corresponding to seven classes) are investigated in this work: normal rhythm (*sr*), ventricular extra-systole (*ves*), bigeminy (*bige*), ventricular doublet (*doub*), ventricular tachycardia (*vt*) which is considered as being a red alarm in CICU, supra-ventricular tachycardia (*svt*) and atrial fibrillation (*af*). On average, 7 examples were built for each of the 7 classes.

4.2 Method

To verify empirically that the biased multisource learning method is efficient, we have performed three kinds of learning experiments on the same learning data: monosource learning from each sources, multisource learning from aggregated data using a global bias and multisource learning using a bias constructed from rules discovered by monosource learning (first experiment). In order to assess the

Table 2. Results of cross validation for monosource and multisource learnings

	monosource ECG			monosource ABP			naive multisource			biased multisource		
	TrAcc	Acc	Comp	TrAcc	Acc	Comp	TrAcc	Acc	Comp	TrAcc	Acc	Comp
sr	0.84	0.84	9	1	0.98	5	0.98	0.98	3	0.98	0.98	6
ves	1	0.96	5/6	0.963	0.64	3/2/3/2	0.976	0.76	4/3	0.96	0.98	5
bige	1	1	5	0.998	0.84	3/2	0.916	0.7	4/2	1	1	5
doub	1	1	4/5	0.995	0.84	4	0.997	0.8	3/4	0.967	0.9	5
vt	1	1	3	0.981	0.78	3/3/5	0.981	0.94	4	1	1	3
svt	1	1	3	1	0.96	2	1	0.98	2	1	1	2
af	1	1	3	0.981	0.98	2/2	1	1	2	1	1	2

impact of the learning hardness, we have performed two series of experiments: in the first series (4.3) the representation language was expressive enough to give good results for the three kinds of experiments; in the second series (4.4) the expressibility of the representation language was reduced drastically. Three criteria are used to compare the learning results: computational load (CPU time), accuracy and complexity (Comp) of the rules (each number in a cell represents the number of cardiac cycles in each rule produced by the ILP system). As the number of examples is rather low, a *leave-one-out* cross validation method is used to assessed the different criteria. The average accuracy measures obtained during cross-validation training (*TrAcc*) and test (*Acc*) are provided.

4.3 Learning from the Whole Database

Table 1 gives an idea of the computational complexity of each learning method (monosource on ECG and ABP channels, naive and biased multisource on aggregated data). *Nodes* is the number of nodes explored in the search space and *Time* is the learning computation time in CPU seconds on a Sun Ultra-Sparc 5.

Table 1 shows that, on average, from 5 to 10 times more nodes are explored during naive multisource learning than during monosource learning and that about 500 to 1000 times less nodes are explored during biased multisource learning than during naive multisource learning. However the computation time does not grow linearly with the number of explored nodes because the covering tests (determining whether an hypothesis is consistent with the examples) are more complex for multisource learning. Biased multisource learning computation times take into account monosource learning computation times and are still very much smaller than for naive multisource learning (8 to 35 times less).

Table 2 gives the average accuracy and complexity of rules obtained during cross validation for the monosource and the two multisource learning methods. The accuracy of monosource rules is very good for ECG and a bit less for ABP, particularly the test accuracy. The naive multisource rules have also good results. Furthermore, for the seven arrhythmias, these rules combine events and relations occurring on both sources. Only *sr, ves, svt* and *af* got combined biased multisource rules. In the three other cases, the learned rules are the same as the ECG rules. The rules learned for *svt* in the four learning settings are given

```
class(svt):-
  qrs(R0,normal),
  p(P1,normal), qrs(R1,normal),
  suc(P1,R0), suc(R1,P1),
  rr1(R0,R1,short),
  p(P2,normal), qrs(R2,normal),
  suc(P2,R1), suc(R2,P2),
  rythm(R0,R1,R2,regular).
```

Fig. 3. Example of rule learned for class *svt* from ECG data

```
class(svt):-
  cycle_abp(Dias0,_,Sys0,normal),
  cycle_abp(Dias1,normal,Sys1,normal),
  suc(Dias1,Sys0),
  amp_dd(Dias0,Dias1,normal),
  ss1(Sys0,Sys1,short),
  ds1(Dias1,Sys1,long).
```

Fig. 4. Example of rule learned for class *svt* from ABP data

in Figures 3, 4, 5 and 6. All those rules are perfectly accurate. The predicate *cycle_abp(D, ampsd, S, ampds)* is a kind of macro predicate that expresses the succession of a diastole named D, and a systole named S. *ampsd* (resp. *ampds*) expresses the symbolic pressure variation ($\in \{short, normal, long\}$) between a systole and the following diastole D (resp. between the diastole D and the following systole S). The biased multisource rule and the naive multisource rule are very similar but specify different event orders (in the first one the diastole-systole specification occurs before two close-in-time QRS whereas in the second one, the same specification occurs after two close-in-time QRS).

As expected from the theory, the biased multisource rules accuracy is better than or equal to the monosource rules accuracy except for the *doublet*. In this case, the difference between the two accuracy measures comes from a drawback of the cross-validation to evaluate the biased multisource learning rules with respect to the monosource rules. At each cross-validation step, one example is extracted for test from the example database and learning is performed on the remaining database. Sometimes the learned rules differ from one step to another. Since this variation is very small we have chosen to keep the same multisource bias for all the cross-validation steps even if the monosource rules upon which it should be constructed may vary. According to this choice, the small variation between the biased multisource rules accuracy and the monosource rules accuracy is not significant. Table 2 also shows that when the monosource results are good, the biased multisource rules have a better accuracy than the naive multisource rules and rules combining events from different sources can also be learned.

4.4 Learning from a Less Informative Database

The current medical data we are working on are very well known from the cardiologists, so, we have a lot of background information on them. For example, we know which event or which kind of relations between events are interesting for the learning process, which kind of constraints exists between events occurring on the different sources etc. This knowledge is very useful to create the learning bias and can explain partly the very good accuracy results obtained in the learning experiments above. These good results can also be explained by the small number of examples available for each arrhythmia and the fact that our examples are not corrupted. In this context, it is very difficult to evaluate the usefulness of using two data sources to improve the learning performances.

```
class(svt):-
qrs(R0,normal),
cycle_abp(Dias0,_,Sys0,normal),
p(P1,normal),qrs(R1,normal),
suci(P1,Sys0),suc(R1,P1),
systole(Sys1),
rr1(R0,R1,short).
```

Fig. 5. Example of rule learned for class *svt* by naive multisource learning

```
class(svt):-
qrs(R0,normal),
p(P1,normal),qrs(R1,normal),
suc(P1,R0),suc(R1,P1),
rr1(R0,R1,short),
cycle_abp(Dias0,_,Sys0,normal),
suci(Dias0,R1).
```

Fig. 6. Example of rule learned for class *svt* by biased multisource learning

Table 3. Results of cross-validation for monosource and multisource learnings without knowledge on P wave nor QRS shape nor diastole

	monosource ECG			monosource ABP			naive multisource			biased multisource		
	TrAcc	Acc	Comp	TrAcc	Acc	Comp	TrAcc	Acc	Comp	TrAcc	Acc	Comp
sr	0.38	0.36	5	1	0.96	5/4	1	0.92	5	1	0.98	5/4
ves	0.42	0.4	5	0.938	0.76	4/3	0.945	0.64	4/4/6	0.94	0.9	4/3
bige	0.96	0.92	4	1	0.98	4/4	0.98	0.96	4	1	0.98	4/4
doub	0.881	0.78	4/4	0.973	0.86	4/4/5	1	0.92	4/4	0.941	0.9	3/4/5
vt	0.919	0.84	5/5	0.943	0.84	3/4/5	0.977	0.76	6/5	0.96	0.86	3/5/5
svt	0.96	0.94	5	0.962	0.86	4	0.76	0.76	2	0.96	0.94	4
af	0.945	0.86	4/4	1	0.9	3/4/5	0.962	0.82	2/3	1	0.98	3/4/5

We have thus decided to set ourselves in a more realistic situation where information about the sources is reduced. In this experiment we do not take into account the P waves nor the shape of the QRS on the ECG and the diastole on the ABP channel. This experiment makes sense as far as signal processing is concerned since it is still difficult with current signal processing algorithms to detect a P wave on the ECG. Besides, in our symbolic description of the ABP channel, the diastole is simply the lowest point between two systoles. This specific point is also difficult to detect. Note that cardiologists view the diastole as the time period between two systoles (the moment during which the chambers fill with blood).

The results of this second experiment are given in Table 3. This time again, the biased multisource rules have as good or better results than the monosource rules. For arrhythmias *sr*, *bige* and *af* the biased method acts like a voting method and learns the same rules with the same accuracy as the best monosource rules (small variations in accuracies come from the cross validation drawback). For arrhythmias *ves, doublet, vt* and *svt* the biased multisource rules are different from both monosource rules corresponding to the same arrhythmia and accuracy and test are better than for the monosource rules.

5 Conclusion

We have presented a technique to learn rules from multisource data with an inductive logic programming method in order to improve the detection and the recognition of cardiac arrhythmias in a monitoring context. To reduce the computation time of a straightforward multisource learning from aggregated examples, we propose a method to design an efficient bias for multisource learning. This bias is constructed from the results obtained by learning independently from data associated to the different sources. We have shown that this technique provides rules which have always better or equal accuracy results than monosource rules and that it is is much more efficient than a naive multisource learning.

In future work, the method will be test on corrupted data. Besides, since this article only focus on accuracy and performance results, the impact of the multisource rules on the recognition and the diagnosis of cardiac arrhythmias in a clinical context will be more deeply evaluated by experts.

Acknowledgments

Elisa Fromont is supported by the French National Net for Health Technologies as a member of the CEPICA project. This project is in collaboration with LTSI-Université de Rennes1, ELA-Medical and Rennes University Hospital.

References

1. Carrault, G., Cordier, M., Quiniou, R., Wang, F.: Temporal abstraction and inductive logic programming for arrhythmia recognition from ECG. Artificial Intelligence in Medicine **28** (2003) 231–263
2. Nédellec, C., Rouveirol, C., Adé, H., Bergadano, F., Tausend, B.: Declarative bias in ILP. In De Raedt, L., ed.: Advances in Inductive Logic Programming. IOS Press (1996) 82–103
3. Fromont, E., Cordier, M.O., Quiniou, R.: Learning from multi source data. In: PKDD'04 (Knowledge Discovery in Databases), Pisa, Italy (2004)
4. Muggleton, S., De Raedt, L.: Inductive Logic Programming: Theory and methods. The Journal of Logic Programming **19 & 20** (1994) 629–680
5. Lloyd, J.: Foundations of Logic Programming. Springer-Verlag, Heidelberg (1987)
6. Blockeel, H., De Raedt, L., Jacobs, N., Demoen, B.: Scaling up inductive logic programming by learning from interpretations. Data Mining and Knowledge Discovery **3** (1999) 59–93
7. Plotkin, G.: A note on inductive generalisation. In Meltzer, B., Michie, D., eds.: Machine Intelligence 5. Elsevier North Holland, New York (1970) 153–163
8. De Raedt, L., Van Laer, W.: Inductive constraint logic. Lecture Notes in Computer Science **997** (1995) 80–94
9. De Raedt, L., Dehaspe, L.: Clausal discovery. Machine Learning **26** (1997) 99–146
10. Moody, G.B., Mark, R.G.: A database to support development and evaluation of intelligent intensive care monitoring. Computers in Cardiology **23** (1996) 657–660 http://ecg.mit.edu/mimic/mimic.html.

Effective Confidence Region Prediction Using Probability Forecasters

David G. Lindsay[1] and Siân Cox[2]

[1] Computer Learning Research Centre
davidl@cs.rhul.ac.uk
[2] School of Biological Sciences
Royal Holloway, University, Egham, Surrey, TW20 OEX, UK
s.s.e.cox@rhul.ac.uk

Abstract. Confidence region prediction is a practically useful extension to the commonly studied pattern recognition problem. Instead of predicting a single label, the constraint is relaxed to allow prediction of a subset of labels given a desired confidence level $1 - \delta$. Ideally, effective region predictions should be (1) well calibrated - predictive regions at confidence level $1 - \delta$ should err with relative frequency at most δ and (2) be as narrow (or certain) as possible. We present a simple technique to generate confidence region predictions from conditional probability estimates (probability forecasts). We use this 'conversion' technique to generate confidence region predictions from probability forecasts output by standard machine learning algorithms when tested on 15 multi-class datasets. Our results show that approximately 44% of experiments demonstrate well-calibrated confidence region predictions, with the K-Nearest Neighbour algorithm tending to perform consistently well across all data. Our results illustrate the practical benefits of effective confidence region prediction with respect to medical diagnostics, where guarantees of capturing the true disease label can be given.

1 Introduction

Pattern recognition is a well studied area of machine learning, however the equally useful extension of confidence region prediction [1] has to date received little attention from the machine learning community. Confidence region prediction relaxes the traditional constraint on the learner to predict a single label to allow prediction of a subset of labels given a desired confidence level $1 - \delta$. The traditional approach to this problem was to construct region predictions from so-called p-values, often generated from purpose built algorithms such as the Transductive Confidence Machine [1]. Whilst these elegant solutions offer non-asymptotic provenly valid properties, there are significant disadvantages of p-values as their interpretation is less direct than that of *probability forecasts* and they are easy to confuse with probabilities. Probability forecasting is an increasingly popular generalisation of the standard pattern recognition problem; rather than attempting to find the "best" label, the aim is to estimate the conditional probability (otherwise known as a probability forecast) of a possible label given an observed object. Meaningful probability forecasts are vital when learning techniques are involved with cost sensitive decision-making (as in medical diagnostics) [2],[3]. In this study we introduce a simple, yet provably valid technique to generate confidence region predictions from probability forecasts, in order to capitalise on the individual benefits of each classification methodology. There are two intuitive criteria for assessing the effectiveness of region predictions, ideally they should be:

1. **Well calibrated** - Predictive regions at confidence level $1-\delta \in [0, 1]$ will be wrong (not capture the true label) with relative frequency at most δ.
2. **Certain** - The predictive regions should be as narrow as possible.

The first criterion is the priority: without it, the meaning of predictive regions is lost, and it becomes easy to achieve the best possible performance. We have applied our simple conversion technique to the probability forecasts generated by several commonly used machine learning algorithms on 15 standard multi-class datasets. Our results have demonstrated that 44% of experiments produced well-calibrated region predictions, and found at least one well-calibrated region predictor for 12 of the 15 datasets tested. Our results have also demonstrated our main dual motivation that the learners also provide useful probability forecasts for more direct decision making. We discuss the application of this research with respect to medical diagnostics, as several clinical studies have shown that the use of computer-based diagnostics systems [4], [5] can provide valuable insights into patient problems, especially with helping to identify alternative diagnoses. We argue that with the use of effective probability forecasts and confidence region predictions on multi-class diagnostic problems, the end user can have probabilistic guarantees on narrowing down the true disease. Finally, we identify areas of future research.

2 Using Probability Forecasts for Region Prediction

Our notation will extend upon the commonly used supervised learning approach to pattern recognition. Nature outputs information pairs called *examples*. Each example $z_i = (\mathbf{x}_i, y_i) \in \mathbf{X} \times \mathbf{Y} = \mathbf{Z}$ consists of an *object* $\mathbf{x}_i \in \mathbf{X}$ and its *label* $y_i \in \mathbf{Y} = \{1, 2, \ldots, |\mathbf{Y}|\}$. Formally our learner is a function $\Gamma : \mathbf{Z}^n \times \mathbf{X} \to \mathbf{P}(\mathbf{Y})$ of n training examples, and a new test object mapping onto a probability distribution over labels. Let $\hat{P}(y_i = j \mid \mathbf{x}_i)$ represent the estimated conditional probability of the jth label matching the true label for the ith object tested. We will often consider a sequence of N probability forecasts for the $|\mathbf{Y}|$ possible labels output by a learner Γ, to represent our predictions for the test set of objects, where the true label is withheld from the learner.

2.1 Probability Forecasts Versus p-Values

Previous studies [1] have shown that it is possible to create special purpose learning methods to produce valid and asymptotically optimal region predictions via the use of p-values. However these p-values have several disadvantages when compared to probability forecasts; their interpretation is less direct than that of probability forecasts, the p-values do not sum to one (although they often take values between 0 and 1) and they are easy to confuse with probabilities. This misleading nature of p-values and other factors have led some authors [6] to object to any use of p-values.

In contrast, although studies in machine learning tend to concentrate primarily on 'bare' predictions, probability forecasting has become an increasingly popular doctrine. Making *effective* probability forecasts is a well studied problem in statistics and weather forecasting [7][8]. Dawid (1985) details two simple criteria for describing how effective probability forecasts are:

1. **Reliability** - The probability forecasts "should not lie". When a probability $\hat{p}$ is assigned to an label, there should be roughly $1 - \hat{p}$ relative frequency of the label not occurring.
2. **Resolution** - The probability forecasts should be practically useful and enable the observer to easily rank the labels in order of their likelihood of occurring.

These criteria are analogous to that defined earlier for effective confidence region predictions; indeed we argue that the first criterion of reliability should remain the main focus, as the second resolution criterion naturally is ensured by the classification accuracy of learning algorithms (which is a more common focus of empirical studies). At present the most popular techniques for assessing the quality of probability forecasts are *square loss* (a.k.a. Brier score) and *ROC curves* [9]. Recently we developed the *Empirical Reliability Curve* (ERC) as a visual interpretation of the theoretical definition of reliability [3]. Unlike the square loss and ROC plots, the ERC allows visualisation of over- and under-estimation of probability forecasts.

2.2 Converting Probability Forecasts into Region Predictions

The first step in converting the probability forecasts into region predictions is to sort the probability forecasts into increasing order. Let $\hat{y}_i^{(1)}$ and $\hat{y}_i^{(|\mathbf{Y}|)}$ denote the labels corresponding to the smallest and largest probability forecasts respectively

$$\hat{P}(\hat{y}_i^{(1)} \mid \mathbf{x}_i) \leq \hat{P}(\hat{y}_i^{(2)} \mid \mathbf{x}_i) \leq \ldots \leq \hat{P}(\hat{y}_i^{(|\mathbf{Y}|)} \mid \mathbf{x}_i) \ .$$

Using these ordered probability forecasts we can generate the region prediction $\Gamma^{1-\delta}$ at a specific confidence level $1 - \delta \in [0, 1]$ for each test example $\mathbf{x}_i$

$$\Gamma^{1-\delta}(\mathbf{x}_i) = \{\hat{y}_i^{(j)}, \ldots, \hat{y}_i^{(|\mathbf{Y}|)}\} \text{ where } j = \underset{k}{\operatorname{argmax}} \left\{ \sum_{l=1}^{k-1} \hat{P}(\hat{y}_i^{(l)} \mid \mathbf{x}_i) < \delta \right\} \ . \quad (1)$$

Intuitively we are using the fact that the probability forecasts are estimates of conditional probabilities and we assume that the labels are mutually exclusive. Therefore summing these forecasts becomes a conditional probability of a conjunction of labels, which can be used to choose the labels to include in the confidence region predictions at the desired confidence level.

2.3 Assessing the Quality of Region Predictions

Now that we have specified how region predictions are created, how do we assess the quality of them? Taking inspiration from [1], informally we want two criteria to be satisfied: (1) that the region predictions are well-calibrated, i.e. the fraction of errors at confidence level $1 - \delta$ should be at most δ, and (2) that the regions should be as narrow as possible. More formally let $\text{err}_i(\Gamma^{1-\delta}(\mathbf{x}_i))$ be the error incurred by the true label y_i not being in the region prediction of object $\mathbf{x}_i$ at confidence level $1-\delta$

$$\text{err}_i(\Gamma^{1-\delta}(\mathbf{x}_i)) = \begin{cases} 1 \text{ if } y_i \notin \Gamma^{1-\delta}(\mathbf{x}_i) \\ 0 \text{ otherwise} \end{cases}. \quad (2)$$

To assess the second criteria of uncertainty we simply measure the fraction of total labels that are predicted at the desired confidence level $1-\delta$

$$\text{unc}_i(\Gamma^{1-\delta}(\mathbf{x}_i)) = \frac{|\Gamma^{1-\delta}(\mathbf{x}_i)|}{|\mathbf{Y}|}. \quad (3)$$

These terms can then be averaged over all the N test examples

$$\text{Err}_N^{1-\delta} = \frac{1}{N}\sum_{i=1}^{N}\text{err}_i(\Gamma^{1-\delta}(\mathbf{x}_i)), \; \text{Unc}_N^{1-\delta} = \frac{1}{N}\sum_{i=1}^{N}\text{unc}_i(\Gamma^{1-\delta}(\mathbf{x}_i)). \quad (4)$$

It is possible to prove that this technique of converting probability forecasts into region predictions (given earlier in Equation 1) is well-calibrated for a learner that outputs Bayes optimal forecasts, as shown below.

Theorem 1. *Let P be a probability distribution on $\mathbf{Z} = \mathbf{X} \times \mathbf{Y}$. If a learners forecasts are Bayes optimal i.e. $\hat{P}(y_i = j \mid \mathbf{x}_i) = P(y_i = j \mid \mathbf{x}_i), \forall j \in \mathbf{Y}, 1 \leq i \leq N$, then*

$$\mathbf{P}^N\left(\text{Err}_N^{1-\delta} \geq \delta + \varepsilon\right) \leq e^{-2\varepsilon^2 N}.$$

This means if the probability forecasts are Bayes optimal, then even for small finite sequences the confidence region predictor will be well-calibrated with high probability. This proof follows directly from the Hoeffding Azuma inequality [10], and thus justifies our method for generating confidence region predictions.

2.4 An Illustrative Example: Diagnosis of Abdominal Pain

In this example we illustrate our belief that both probability forecasts *and* region predictions are practically useful. Table 1 shows probability forecasts for all possible disease labels made by Naive Bayes and DW13-NN learners when tested on the Abdominal Pain dataset from Edinburgh Hospital, UK [5]. For comparison, the predictions made by both learners are given for the same patient examples in the Abdominal Pain dataset. At a glance it is obvious that the predicted probabilities output by the Naive Bayes learner are far more extreme (i.e. very close to 0 or 1) than those output by the DW13-NN learner. Example 1653 (Table 1 rows 1 and 4) shows a patient object which is predicted correctly by the Naive Bayes learner ($\hat{p}$=0.99) and less emphatically by the DW13-NN learner ($\hat{p}$=0.85).

Example 2490 demonstrates the problem of over- and under- estimation by the Naive Bayes learner where a patient is incorrectly diagnosed with Intestinal obstruction (overestimation), yet the true diagnosis of Dyspepsia is ranked 6th with a very low predicted probability of $\hat{p} = \frac{22}{1000}$ (underestimation). In contrast the DW13-NN learner makes more *reliable* probability forecasts; for example 2490, the true class is

Table 1. This table shows sample predictions output by the Naive Bayes and DW13-NN learners tested on the Abdominal Pain dataset. The 9 possible class labels for the data (left to right in the table) are: Appendicitis, Diverticulitis, Perforated peptic ulcer, Non-specific abdominal pain, Cholisistitis, Intestinal obstruction, Pancreatitis, Renal colic and Dyspepsia. The associated probability of the predicted label is underlined and emboldened, whereas the actual class label is marked with the ✠ symbol

Example #	Probability forecast for each class label								
	Appx.	Div.	Perf.	Non-spec.	Cholis.	Intest.	Pancr.	Renal	Dyspep.
DW13-NN									
1653	0.0	0.0	0.0	0.03	**0.85**✠	0.0	0.01	0.0	0.11
2490	0.0	0.0	0.22	0.0	0.0	0.25	0.04	0.09	**0.4**✠
5831	**0.53**	0.0	0.0	0.425✠	0.001	0.005	0.0	0.0	0.039
Naive Bayes									
1653	3.08e-9	4.5e-6	3.27e-6	4.37e-5	**0.99**✠	4.2e-3	3.38e-3	4.1e-10	1.33e-4
2490	9.36e-5	0.01	0.17	2.26e-5	0.16	**0.46**	0.2	2.17e-7	2.2e-4✠
5831	**0.969**	2.88e-4	1.7e-13	0.03✠	1.33e-9	2.2e-4	4.0e-11	6.3e-10	7.6e-9

correctly predicted albeit with lower predicted probability. Example 5381 demonstrates a situation where both learners encounter an error in their predictions. The Naive Bayes learner gives misleading predicted probabilities of $\hat{p} = 0.969$ for the incorrect diagnosis of Appendicitis, and a mere $\hat{p} = 0.03$ for the true class label of Non-specific abdominal pain. In contrast, even though the DW13-NN learner incorrectly predicts Appendicitis, it is with far less certainty $\hat{p} = 0.53$ and if the user were to look at all probability forecasts it would be clear that the true class label should not be ignored with a predicted probability $\hat{p} = 0.425$.

The results below show region predictions output at 95% and 99% confidence levels by the Naive Bayes and DW13-NN learners for the same Abdominal Pain examples tested in Table 1 using the simple conversion technique (cf. 1). As before, the true label is marked with the ✠ symbol if it is contained in the region prediction.

Conversion of DW13-NN forecasts into region predictions:

Example #	Region at 95% Confidence	Region at 99% Confidence
1653	{Cholis ✠, Dyspep}	{Cholis ✠, Dyspep, Non-spec, Pancr}
2490	{Dyspep ✠, Intest, Perf, Renal}	{Dyspep ✠, Intest, Perf, Renal, Pancr}
5831	{Appx, Non-spec ✠}	{Appx, Non-spec ✠, Dyspep}

Conversion of Naive Bayes forecasts into region predictions:

Example #	Region at 95% Confidence	Region at 99% Confidence
1653	{Cholis ✠}	{Cholis ✠}
2490	{Intest, Pancr, Perf, Cholis}	{Intest, Pancr, Perf, Cholis, Div}
5831	{Appx}	{Appx, Non-spec ✠}

The DW13-NN learner's region predictions are wider, with a total of 20 labels included in all region predictions as opposed to 14 for the Naive Bayes learner. However, despite these narrow predictions, the Naive Bayes's region prediction fails to capture the true label for example 2490, and only captures the true label for example 5831 at a 99% confidence level. In contrast, the DW13-NN's region predictions successfully capture each true label even at a 95% confidence level. This highlights what we believe to be the practical benefit of generating well-calibrated region predictions - the ability to capture or dismiss labels with the guarantee of being correct is highly desirable. In our example, narrowing down the possible diagnosis of abdominal pain could save money and patient anxiety in terms of unnecessary tests to clarify the condition of the patient. It is important to stress that when working with probabilistic classification, classification accuracy should not be the only mechanism of assessment. Table 2 shows that the Naive Bayes learner actually has a slightly lower classification error rate of 29.31% compared with 30.86% of the DW13-NN learner. If other methods of learner assessment had been ignored, the Naive Bayes learner may have been used for prediction by the physician even though Naive Bayes has less reliable probability forecasts and non-calibrated region predictions.

2.5 The Confidence Region Calibration (CRC) Plot Visualisation

The Confidence Region Calibration (CRC) plot is a simple visualisation of the performance criteria detailed earlier (cf. 4). Continuing with our example, figure 1 shows CRC plots for the Naive Bayes and DW13-NN's probability forecasts on the Abdominal pain dataset. The CRC plot displays all possible confidence levels on the horizontal axis, versus the total fraction of objects or class labels on the vertical axis. The dashed line represents the number of errors $\text{Err}_N^{1-\delta}$, and the solid line represents the average region width $\text{Unc}_N^{1-\delta}$ at each confidence level $1 - \delta$ for all N test examples. Informally, as we increase the confidence level, the errors should decrease and the width of region predictions increase. The lines drawn on the CRC plot give the reader at a glance useful information about the learner's region predictions. If the error line never deviates above the upper left-to-bottom right diagonal (i.e. $\text{Err}_N^{1-\delta} \leq \delta$ for all $\delta \in [0,1]$), then the learner's region predictions are *well-calibrated*. The CRC plot also provides a useful measure of the quality of the probability forecasts, we can check if regions are well-calibrated by computing the area between the main diagonal $1 - \delta$ and the error line $\text{Err}_n^{1-\delta}$, and the area under the average region width line $\text{Unc}_n^{1-\delta}$ using simple trapezium and triangle rule estimation (see Table 2). These deviation areas (also seen beneath Figure 1) can enable the user to check the performance of region predictions without any need to check the corresponding CRC plot.

Figure 1 shows that in contrast to the DW13-NN learner, the Naive Bayes learner is not well-calibrated as demonstrated by its large deviation above the left-to-right diagonal. At a 95% confidence level, the Naive Bayes learner makes 18% errors on its confidence region predictions and not $\leq 5\%$ as is usually required. The second line corresponding to the average region width $\text{Unc}_n^{1-\delta}$ shows how useful the learner's region predictions are. The Naive Bayes CRC plot indicates that at 95% confidence, roughly 15% of the 9 possible disease labels (≈ 1.4) are predicted. In contrast, the DW13-NN learner is less certain at this confidence level, predicting 23% of labels (≈ 2.1). However, although the DW13-NN learner's region predictions are slightly wider than those of Naive Bayes, the DW13-NN learner is far closer to being calibrated, which is our

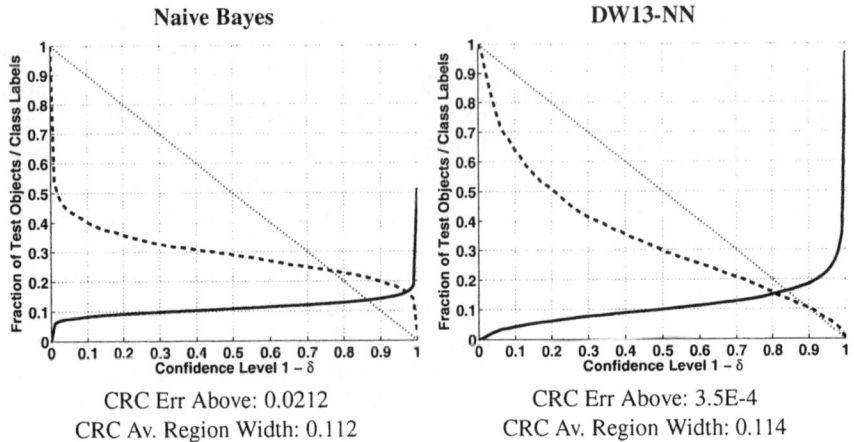

Fig. 1. Confidence Region Calibration (CRC) plots of probability forecasts output by Naive Bayes and DW 13-NN learners on the Abdominal Pain dataset. The dashed line represents the fraction of errors made on the test sets region predictions at each confidence level. The solid line represents the average region width for each confidence level $1 - \delta$. If the dashed error line never deviates above the main left-right diagonal then the region predictions are well-calibrated. The deviation areas of both error and region width lines are given beneath each plot

first priority. Indeed narrowing down the true disease of a patient from 9 to 2 possible disease class labels, whilst guaranteeing less that 5% chance of errors in that region prediction, is a desirable goal. In addition, further information could be provided by referring back to the original probability forecasts to achieve a more direct analysis of the likely disease.

3 Experimental Results

We tested the following algorithms as implemented by the WEKA Data Mining System [9]: Bayes Net, Neural Network, Distance Weighted K-Nearest Neighbours (DWK-NN), C4.5 Decision Tree (with Laplace smoothing), Naive Bayes and Pairwise Coupled + Logistic Regression Sequential Minimisation Optimisation (PC+LR SMO) a computationally efficient version of Support Vector Machines. We tested the following 15 multi-class datasets (number of examples, number of attributes, number of classes): Abdominal Pain (6387,136,9) from [5], and the other datasets from the UCI data repository [11]: Anneal (898,39,5), Glass (214,10,6), Hypothyroid (3772,30,4), Iris (150,5,3), Lymphography (148,19,4), Primary Tumour (339,18,21), Satellite Image (6435,37,6), Segment (2310,20,7), Soy Bean (683,36,19), Splice (3190,62,3), USPS Handwritten Digits (9792,256,10), Vehicle (846,19,4), Vowel (990,14,11) and Waveform (5000,41,3). Each experiment was carried out on 5 randomisations of a 66% Training / 34% Test split of the data. Data was normalised, and missing attributes replaced with mean and mode values for numeric and nominal attributes respectively. Deviation areas for the CRC plots were estimated using 100 equally divided intervals. The stan-

Table 2. Results of CRC Error Above / CRC Av. Region Width (assessing confidence region predictions), Classification Error Rate / Square Loss (assessing probability forecasts), computed from the probability forecasts of several learners on 15 multi-class datasets. Experiments that gave well-calibrated confidence region predictions (where CRC Error Above = 0) are highlighted in grey. Best assessment score of the well-calibrated learners (where available) for each dataset are emboldened

CRC Plot Error Above / CRC Plot Av. Region Width						
Dataset / Learner	Naive Bayes	Bayes Net	Neural Net	C4.5	PC+LR SMO	DW K-NN
Abdominal Pain	0.021 / 0.112	- / -	0.027 / 0.112	0.024 / 0.155	0.002 / 0.113	3.5E-4 / 0.114
Anneal	0.004 / 0.167	0.0 / 0.167	0.0 / 0.169	0.0 / 0.176	0.0 / 0.168	0.0 / 0.169
Glass	0.098 / **0.144**	0.005 / 0.145	0.025 / 0.145	0.017 / 0.202	0.02 / 0.144	**0.004** / 0.146
Hypothyroid	0.0 / **0.250**	0.0 / 0.251	1.6E-4 / 0.252	0.0 / 0.253	0.0 / 0.251	0.0 / 0.252
Iris	0.0 / **0.332**	1.2E-4 / 0.335	1.6E-4 / 0.335	7.5E-4 / 0.339	0.0 / 0.334	0.0 / 0.335
Lymphography	0.002 / 0.251	2.8E-4 / 0.252	0.006 / 0.252	0.004 / 0.284	0.002/ 0.252	0.0 / **0.251**
Primary Tumour	0.146 / **0.048**	0.133 / 0.048	0.156 / 0.048	0.219 / 0.098	0.153 / 0.047	0.24 / 0.048
Satellite Image	0.018 / 0.166	- / -	0.002 / 0.168	0.0 / 0.189	0.0 / **0.169**	0.0 / 0.169
Segment	0.012 / 0.143	0.0 / **0.143**	0.0 / 0.145	0.0 / 0.154	0.0 / 0.145	0.0 / 0.146
Soy Bean	0.001 / 0.053	0.0 / **0.053**	5.5E-4 / 0.056	1.7E-4 / 0.1055	2.9E-4 / 0.055	0.0 / 0.057
Splice	0.0 / **0.334**	- / -	1.2E-4 / 0.333	0.0 / 0.344	0.001 / 0.334	0.0 / 0.334
USPS	0.018 / 0.099	- / -	0.0 / **0.102**	0.0 / 0.121	0.0 / 0.102	0.0 / 0.104
Vehicle	0.083 / 0.251	0.0 / 0.251	0.004 / 0.25142	0.002 / 0.274	0.0 / **0.251**	0.0 / 0.252
Vowel	0.006 / 0.093	2.7E-4 / 0.094	0.001 / 0.093	0.002 / 0.153	0.002 / 0.093	0.0 / **0.094**
Waveform 5000	0.006 / 0.334	0.0 / **0.334**	0.006 / 0.332	0.004 / 0.348	0.0 / 0.335	0.0 / 0.335

Error Rate / Square Loss						
Dataset / Learner	Naive Bayes	Bayes Net	Neural Net	C4.5	PC+LR SMO	DW K-NN
Abdominal Pain	29.309 / 0.494	- / -	30.484 / 0.528	38.779 / 0.597	**26.886 / 0.388**	30.859 / 0.438
Anneal	11.929 / 0.219	4.794 / 0.076	**1.672 / 0.026**	1.895 / 0.051	2.676 / 0.044	2.899 / 0.06
Glass	56.056 / 0.869	**33.521 / 0.47**	37.747 / 0.58	35.775 / 0.579	40.282 / 0.537	37.465 / 0.509
Hypothyroid	4.423 / 0.075	1.002 / 0.016	5.521 / 0.095	**0.461 / 0.009**	2.975 / 0.046	6.858 / 0.118
Iris	4.8 / 0.089	6.8 / 0.1	5.6 / 0.089	7.2 / 0.136	4.8 / 0.068	**3.2 / 0.057**
Lymphography	16.735 / 0.279	15.51 / 0.248	20.0 / 0.346	22.857 / 0.368	22.041 / 0.317	**20.408 / 0.29**
Primary Tumour	53.982 / 0.692	54.867 / **0.695**	59.646 / 0.905	57.699 / 0.855	58.23 / 0.772	**53.628** / 0.721
Satellite Image	20.793 / 0.4	- / -	10.839 / 0.19	14.965 / 0.249	14.382 / 0.194	**9.604 / 0.138**
Segment	19.403 / 0.357	4.364 / 0.071	3.688 / **0.061**	4.156 / 0.078	7.273 / 0.107	**3.61** / 0.066
Soy Bean	9.604 / 0.163	**6.432 / 0.091**	7.489 / 0.125	7.753 / 0.263	8.37 / 0.134	9.779 / 0.142
Splice	**4.365 / 0.068**	- / -	4.774 / 0.079	6.529 / 0.116	7.267 / 0.133	16.764 / 0.269
USPS	19.619 / 0.388	- / -	**3.055 / 0.054**	11.496 / 0.201	4.679 / 0.077	3.162 / 0.055
Vehicle	53.192 / 0.848	29.787 / 0.389	20.213 / 0.319	27.801 / 0.403	**26.312 / 0.363**	29.078 / 0.388
Vowel	40.606 / 0.538	21.455 / 0.308	9.152 / 0.155	24.303 / 0.492	34.909 / 0.452	**1.697 / 0.034**
Waveform 5000	20.12 / 0.342	18.619 / 0.268	16.627 / 0.297	24.658 / 0.407	**13.974 / 0.199**	19.328 / 0.266

dard inner product was used in all SMO experiments. All experiments were carried out on a Pentium 4 1.7Ghz PC with 512Mb RAM.

The values given in Table 2 are the average values computed from each of the 5 repeats of differing randomisations of the data. The standard deviation of these values was negligible of magnitude between E-8 and E-12. It is important to note that all results are given with the default parameter settings of each algorithm as specified by WEKA - there was no need for an exhaustive search of parameters to achieve well-calibrated region predictions. Results with the DWK-NN learners are given for the best value of K for each dataset, which are K = 13, 2, 9, 11, 5, 6, 12, 7, 2, 3, 6, 4, 9, 1, 10 from top to bottom as detailed in Table 2. These choices of K perhaps reflect some underlying noise level or complexity in the data, so a higher value of K corresponds to a noisier, more complex dataset. Results with Bayesian Belief Networks were unavailable due to memory constraints with the following datasets: Abdominal Pain, Satellite Image, Splice and USPS. Results which produced well-calibrated region predictions are highlighted in grey, where 38 out of 86 experiments ($\approx$44%) were calibrated. Figure 1 illustrates that despite DW13-NN not being strictly well-calibrated on the Abdominal Pain dataset with a CRC error above calibration $\approx$3.5E-4, in practice this deviation appears negligible. Indeed, if we loosened our definition of well-calibratedness to small deviations of order $\approx$E-4 then the fraction of well-calibrated experiments would increase to 49 out of 86 ($\approx$57%). All datasets, except Abdominal Pain, Glass and Primary Tumor were found to have at least one calibrated learner, and all learners were found to be well-calibrated for at least one dataset. Some datasets, such as Anneal and Segment, were found to have a choice of 5 calibrated learners. In this instance it is important to consult other performance criteria (i.e. region width or classification error rate) to assess the quality of the probability forecasts and decide which learner's predictions to use. Table 2 shows that the Naive Bayes and Bayes Net confidence region predictions are far narrower (≈ -4%) than the other learners, however this may explain the Naive Bayes learner's poor calibration performance across data. In contrast the C4.5 Decision Tree learner has the widest of all region predictions ($\approx +13$%). The Bayes Net performs best in terms of square loss, whilst the Naive Bayes performs the worst. This reiterates conclusions found in other studies [3], in addition to results in Section 2.4 where the Naive Bayes learner's probability forecasts were found to be unreliable. Interestingly, the K-NN learners give consistently well-calibrated region predictions across datasets - perhaps this behaviour can be attributed to the K-NN learners' guarantee to converge to the Bayes optimal probability distribution [10].

4 Discussion

We believe that using both probability forecasts and region predictions can give the end-users of such learning systems a wealth of information to make effective decisions in cost-sensitive problem domains, such as in medical diagnostics. Medical data often contains a lot of noise and so high classification accuracy is not always possible (as seen here with Abdominal Pain data, see Table 2). In this instance the use of probability forecasts and region predictions can enable the physician to filter out improbable diagnoses, and so choose the best course of action for each patient with safe knowledge of their likelihood of error. In this study we have presented a simple methodology to convert probability forecasts into confidence region predictions. We were surprised at how successful standard learning techniques were at solving this task. It is interesting to consider why it was not possible to obtain exactly calibrated results with the Abdominal Pain, Glass and Primary Tumor datasets. Further research is being conducted to see if meta-learners such as Bagging [12] and Boosting [13] could be used to improve on these initial results and obtain better calibration for these problem datasets.

As previously stated, the Transductive Confidence Machine (TCM) framework has much empirical and theoretical evidence for strong region calibration properties, however these properties are derived from the p-values which can be misleading if read on their own, as they do not have any direct probabilistic interpretation. Indeed, our results have shown that unreliable probability forecasts can be misleading enough, but with

p-values this confusion is compounded. Our current research is to see if the exposition of this study could be done in reverse; namely a method could be developed to convert p-values into effective probability forecasts.

Another interesting extension to this research would be to investigate the problem of multi-label prediction, where class labels are not mutually exclusive [14]. Possibly an adaptation of the confidence region prediction method could be applied for this problem domain. Much of the current research in multi-label prediction is concentrated in document and image classification, however we believe that multi-label prediction in medical diagnostics is an equally important avenue of research, and particularly relevant in instances where a patient may suffer more than one illness at once.

Acknowledgements

We would like to acknowledge Alex Gammerman and Volodya Vovk for their helpful suggestions, and in reviewing our work. This work was supported by EPSRC (grants GR46670, GR/P01311/01), BBSRC (grant B111/B1014428), and MRC (grant S505/65).

References

1. Vovk, V.: On-line Confidence Machines are well-calibrated. In: Proc. of the Forty Third Annual Symposium on Foundations of Computer Science, IEEE Computer Society (2002)
2. Zadrozny, B., Elkan, C.: Transforming Classifier Scores into Accurate Multiclass Probability Estimates. In: Proc. of the 8th ACM SIGKDD, ACM Press (2002) 694–699
3. Lindsay, D., Cox, S.: Improving the Reliability of Decision Tree and Naive Bayes Learners. In: Proc. of the 4th ICDM, IEEE (2004) 459–462
4. Berner, E.S., Wesbter, G.D., Shugerman, A.A., Jackson, J.R., Algina, J., Baker, A.L., Ball, E.V., Cobbs, C.G., Dennis, V.W., Frenkel, E.P., Hudson, L.D., Mancall, E.L., Rackley, C.E., Taunton, O.D.: Performance of four computer-based diagnostic systems. The New England Journal of Medicine **330** (1994) 1792–1796
5. Gammerman, A., Thatcher, A.R.: Bayesian diagnostic probabilities without assuming independence of symptoms. Yearbook of Medical Informatics (1992) 323–330
6. Berger, J.O., Delampady, M.: Testing precise hypotheses. Statistical Science **2** (1987) 317–335 David R. Cox's comment: pp. 335–336.
7. Dawid, A.P.: Calibration-based empirical probability (with discussion). Annals of Statistics **13** (1985) 1251–1285
8. Murphy, A.H.: A New Vector Partition of the Probability Score. Journal of Applied Meteorology **12** (1973) 595–600
9. Witten, I., Frank, E.: Data Mining - Practical Machine Learning Tools and Techniques with Java Implementations. Morgan Kaufmann, San Francisco (2000)
10. Devroye, L., Györfi, L., Lugosi, G.: A Probabilistic Theory of Pattern Recognition. Springer, New York (1996)
11. Blake, C., Merz, C.: UCI repository of machine learning databases (1998)
12. Breiman, L.: Bagging predictors. Machine Learning **24** (1996) 123–140
13. Freund, Y., Schapire, R.E.: Game theory, on-line prediction and boosting. In: Proc. 9th Ann. Conf. on Computational Learning Theory, Assoc. of Comp. Machinery (1996) 325–332
14. Boutell, M.R., Luo, J., Shen, X., Brown, C.M.: Learning multi-label scene classification. Pattern Recognition **37** (2004) 1757–1771

Signature Recognition Methods for Identifying Influenza Sequences

Jitimon Keinduangjun[1], Punpiti Piamsa-nga[1], and Yong Poovorawan[2]

[1] Department of Computer Engineering, Faculty of Engineering,
Kasetsart University, Bangkok, 10900, Thailand
{jitimon.k, punpiti.p}@ku.ac.th
[2] Department of Pediatrics, Faculty of Medicine, Chulalongkorn University,
Bangkok, 10400, Thailand
yong.p@chula.ac.th

Abstract. Basically, one of the most important issues for identifying biological sequences is accuracy; however, since the exponential growth and excessive diversity of biological data, the requirement to compute within considerably appropriate time usually compromises with accuracy. We propose novel approaches for accurately identifying DNA sequences in shorter time by discovering sequence patterns -- signatures, which are enough distinctive information for the sequence identification. The approaches are to find the best combination of n-gram patterns and six statistical scoring algorithms, which are regularly used in the research of Information Retrieval, and then employ the signatures to create a similarity scoring model for identifying the DNA. We generate two approaches to discover the signatures. For the first one, we use only statistical information extracted directly from the sequences to discover the signatures. For the second one, we use prior knowledge of the DNA in the signature discovery process. From our experiments on influenza virus, we found that: 1) our technique can identify the influenza virus at the accuracy of up to 99.69% when 11-gram is used and the prior knowledge is applied; 2) the use of too short or too long signatures produces lower efficiency; and 3) most scoring algorithms are good for identification except the *"Rocchio algorithm"* where its results are approximately 9% lower than the others. Moreover, this technique can be applied for identifying other organisms.

1 Introduction

The rapid growth of genomic and sequencing technologies from past decades has generated an incredibly large size of diverse genome data, such as DNA and protein sequences. However, the biological sequences mostly contain very little known meaning. Therefore, the knowledge is needed to be discovered. Techniques for knowledge acquisition from biological sequences become more important for transforming unknowledgeable, diverse and huge data into useful, concise and compact information. These techniques generally consume long computation time; their accuracy usually depends on data size; and there is no best solution known for any particular circumstances. Many research projects on biological sequence processing still share some stages for their experiments in common. One of important research topics in computational biology is sequence identification.

Ideally, the success of research in sequence identification depends on how we can find some short informative data (signatures) that can efficiently identify types of the sequences. The signature recognition is useful to reduce the computation time since data are more compact and more precise [4]. The existing techniques of biological identification require long computation time as categorized into three groups, namely

Inductive Learning: this technique takes learning tools, such as Neural Network and Bayesians, for deriving rules that are used to identify biological sequences. For instance, gene identification uses a neural network [14] for deriving a rule that identifies whether a sequence is a gene or not. The identification generally uses small contents, such as frequencies of two or three bases, instead of plain sequences as inputs of the learning process. Although the use of the rule derived from the learning process attains low processing time, the procedure used as a pre-process of the systems still consumes too long computation time to succeed in all target concepts.

Sequence Alignment: this technique, such as BLAST [7] and FASTA [10], aligns uncharacterized sequences with the existing sequences in genome database and then assigns the uncharacterized sequences to the same class with one of the sequences in database that gets the best alignment score. The processing time of this alignment technique is much higher than other techniques since the process has to perform directly on the sequences in database, whose sizes are usually huge.

Consensus Discovery: this technique takes multiple alignments [13] as a pre-process of systems for finding a "consensus" sequence, which is used to derive a rule. Then, the rule is used to identify sequences in uncharacterized sequences. The consensus sequence is nearly a signature, but it is created by taking the majority bases in the multiple alignments of a sequence collection. Because of too high computation of the multiple alignments, the consensus sequence is not widely used in any tasks.

Our approaches construct the identifiers on the same way as the pre-processing in the inductive learning and the multiple alignments. However, the proposed approaches have much less pre-processing time than the learning technique and the multiple alignment technique. Firstly, we apply the n-gram method to transform DNA sequences into a pattern set. Then, signatures are discovered from the pattern set using statistical scoring algorithms and used to create identifiers. Finally, the performance of identifiers is estimated by applying on influenza virus sequences.

Our identification framework is described in Section 2. Section 3 describes a pattern generation process of DNA sequences. Section 4 has details on scoring algorithms to discover the signatures. Section 5 describes how to construct the identifiers from the discovered signatures. Section 6 has details on estimating the performance of identifiers. Finally, we summarize our techniques in Section 7.

2 Identification Framework

The identification is a challenge of Bioinformatics since the biological sequences are zero-knowledge based data, unlike the text data of human language. Biological data are totally different from the text data in a case that the text data basically use words as its data representation; while we do not know any "words" of the biological data. Therefore, a process for generating the data representation is needed. Our common identification framework of biological sequences is depicted in Fig. 1:

I: *Pre-process* is to transform the training data into a pattern set as the data representation of biological sequences. In this research, we create the training data from influenza and other virus sequences and use them to generate n-gram patterns.

II: *Construction* is a process of creating identifiers using the n-gram patterns and scoring algorithms. The model construction is divided into two consecutive parts: Signature Discovery and Identifier Construction.

The Signature Discovery is to measure the significance of each pattern, called "Scores" using variously different scoring functions and select a set of the k highest-score patterns as our "Signatures". We then pass the signatures through the Identifier Construction which uses the signatures for formulating a sequence similarity scoring function. If there is a query sequence, the similarity scoring function is to detect whether it is the target (influenza, for our experiments) or not.

III: *Evaluation* is to estimate the performance of identifiers using a set of test data. The performance estimator compares an accuracy of all identifiers to find the best one for identifying unseen data, instances that are not members of training and test sets.

IV: *Usage* uses to identify the unseen data by predicting a value to an actual data and identifying a new object.

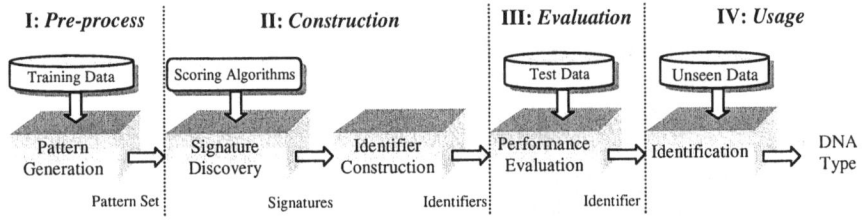

Fig. 1. Common identification framework

3 Pattern Generation

Finding a data representation of DNA sequences is performed in a pre-process of identification using training data. The data representation, called a pattern, is a substring of the DNA sequences. DNA sequences include four symbols {A, C, G, T}; therefore, members of the patterns are also the four symbols. Let Y be a sequence $y_1y_2...y_M$ of length M over the four symbols of DNA. A substring $t_1\ t_2...t_n$ of length n is called an n-gram pattern [3]. The n-gram methodology generates the patterns for representing the DNA sequences using different n-values. There are $M-n+1$ patterns in a sequence of length M for generating the n-gram patterns, but there are only 4^n possible patterns for any n values.

For example, let Y be a 10-base-long sequence ATCGATCGAT. Then, the number of 6-gram patterns generated from the sequence of length 10 is 5 (10-6+1):

ATCGAT, TCGATC, CGATCG, GATCGA, ATCGAT. There are 4,096 (4^6) possible patterns; however, only 4 patterns occur in this example: ATCGAT (2), TCGATC (1), CGATCG (1) and GATCGA (1). From the four patterns, one pattern occurs two times.

Our experiments found that the use of too long patterns (high n-values) will produce poor identifiers. Notice that 3-gram patterns have 64 (4^3) possible patterns; while 24-gram patterns have 2.8×10^{14} (4^{24}) possible patterns. The numbers of possible patterns obviously vary from 64 to 2.8×10^{14} (4^{24}) patterns. Too high n-values may not be necessary because each generated pattern does not occur repeatedly and scoring algorithms cannot discover signatures from the set of n-gram patterns. However, in our experiments, the pattern sets are solely generated from 3- to 24-grams since the higher n-values do not yield the improvement of performance. Discovering the signatures from these n-gram patterns uses the scoring algorithms as discussed next.

4 Signature Discovery

The signature discovery is a process of finding signatures from pattern sets, generated by the n-gram method. We propose statistical scoring algorithms for evaluating significant of each the n-gram pattern to select the best one to be our signatures. The DNA signature discovery uses two different datasets, target and non-target DNA sequences. Section 4.1 has details on the two datasets. The scoring algorithms are performed in Section 4.2. Section 4.3 describes the signature discovery process.

4.1 Datasets

Our datasets are selected from the Genbank genome database of National Center for Biotechnology Information (NCBI) [2]. In this research, we use influenza virus as the target dataset of identification and other viruses, non-influenza virus, as the non-target dataset. The structure of influenza virus is distinctly separated into eight segments. Each segment has different genes. The approximate length of complete sequences of each gene is between 800 and 2,400 bases. We randomly picked 120 complete sequences of each gene of the influenza virus and then insert into the target dataset. The total number of sequences of the target dataset which gathers the eight genes is 960 (120×8) sequences. For the non-target dataset, we randomly picked 960 sequences from other virus sequences, which are not the influenza.

In general, each dataset is divided into two sets, training and test sets. One-third of the dataset (320 sequences) is used for the test set and the rest for the training set (640 sequences). The training set is used for discovering signatures and the test set is used for validation and performance evaluation of discovered signatures.

4.2 Scoring Algorithms

The scoring algorithms are well-known metrics in the research of Information Retrieval [12]. We evaluated the statistical efficiency of six scoring algorithms in their discovery of signatures for identifying biological sequences. The six statistical scoring algorithms are widely categorized into two groups as follows:

Group I: *Based on common patterns*, such as *Term Frequency (TF)* [1] and *Rocchio (TF-IDF)* [5].

Group II: *Based on class distribution*, such as *DIA association factor (Z)* [11], *Mutual Information (MI)* [8], *Cross Entropy (CE)* [8] and *Information Gain (IG)* [11].

The scoring algorithms based on common patterns (Group I) are the simplest techniques for the pattern score computation. They independently compute scores of patterns from frequencies of each pattern; whereas the scoring algorithms based on class distribution (Group II) compute the score of each pattern from a frequency of co-occurrence of a pattern and a class. Each class of identification comprises sequences which are unified to form the same type. Most scoring algorithms based on class distribution consider only the presences (p) of patterns in a class; except the "*Information Gain*" that considers both the presences and absences ($\bar{p}$) of patterns in class [9]. Like the scoring algorithms based on common patterns, they independently compute the score of each pattern. The scoring measures are formulated as follows:

$$TF(p) = Freq(p). \tag{1}$$

$$TF - IDF(p) = TF(p) \cdot \log\left(\frac{|D|}{DF(p)}\right). \tag{2}$$

$$Z(p) = P(C_i \mid p). \tag{3}$$

$$MI(p) = \sum_i P(C_i) \log \frac{P(p \mid C_i)}{P(p)}. \tag{4}$$

$$CE(p) = P(p) \sum_i P(C_i \mid p) \log \frac{P(C_i \mid p)}{P(C_i)}. \tag{5}$$

$$IG(p) = P(p) \sum_i P(C_i \mid p) \log \frac{P(C_i \mid p)}{P(C_i)} + P(\bar{p}) \sum_i P(C_i \mid \bar{p}) \log \frac{P(C_i \mid \bar{p})}{P(C_i)}. \tag{6}$$

Where *Freq(p)* is the Term Frequency (the number of times that pattern p occurred); *IDF* is the Invert Document Frequency; *DF(p)* is the Document Frequency (the number of sequences in which pattern p occurs at least once); $|D|$ is the total number of sequences; $P(p)$ is the probability that pattern p occurred; $\bar{p}$ means that pattern p does not occur; $P(C_i)$ is the probability of the ith class value; $P(C_i \mid p)$ is the conditional probability of the ith class value given that pattern p occurred; and $P(p \mid C_i)$ is the conditional probability of pattern occurrence given the ith class value.

4.3 Signature Discovery Process

The signature discovery process is used to find DNA signatures by measuring the significance (score) of each *n*-gram pattern of DNA sequences, sorting patterns as the scores and selecting the first *k* highest-score patterns to be the "*Signatures*". We use heuristics to select the optimal number of the signatures. Following our previous experiments [6], the identifiers get the highest efficiency when the number of signatures is ten. In this research, we discover the signatures using two different discovery methods, namely *Discovery I* and *Discovery II*.

Discovery I: we divided training data into two classes, influenza virus and non-influenza virus. The scores of each pattern of influenza sequences are computed using the statistical scoring algorithms. The first k highest-score patterns are selected to be the signatures. For instance, let Pattern P represent a set of m members of n-gram patterns $p_1, p_2 \ldots p_m$, generated by the influenza virus sequences. The score of each pattern p_l, denoted $score(p_l)$, is the significance of each pattern evaluated by a pattern scoring measure. Let Signature S be a set of signatures $s_1, s_2 \ldots s_k$, where each signature s_j is selected from the first k highest-score patterns. The Pattern P and the Signature S are defined by the following equations:

$$P = \{\forall_l p_l \mid score(p_{l-1}) \leq score(p_l) \land l = 1,2,\ldots,m\}. \tag{7}$$

$$S = \{\forall_j s_j \mid s_j = p_{m-k+j} \land 1 \leq j \leq k\}. \tag{8}$$

Discovery II: we employed some prior knowledge or characteristics of the target dataset for the signature discovery. In this research, we use the characteristics of distinctly separating into eight segments of influenza virus to discover the signatures. The training data of both influenza and non-influenza virus are divided into eight sub-classes. Each sub-class of influenza virus has different types of segments. Each pair of the influenza and non-influenza sub-class generates a signature subset. The eight signature subsets are gathered into the same set as all signatures of influenza virus.

For instance, there are eight sub-classes of both influenza and non-influenza datasets for generating eight subsets of the separate signatures. Let Pattern P_i represent a set of m members of n-gram patterns $p_1, p_2,\ldots, p_m$, generated by a sub-class i of influenza sequences. The score of each pattern p_l, $score(p_l)$, is the significance of each pattern, evaluated by a scoring algorithm. Let Signature S_i be a subset i of signatures $s_1, s_2 \ldots s_k$, where each signature s_j is selected from the first k highest-score patterns. Each the subset of Pattern P_i and Signature S_i is defined by

$$P_i = \{\forall_l p_l \mid score(p_{l-1}) \leq score(p_l) \land l = 1,2,\ldots,m\}. \tag{9}$$

$$S_i = \{\forall_j s_j \mid s_j = p_{m-k+j} \land 1 \leq j \leq k\}. \tag{10}$$

DNA signatures of the influenza virus with respect to the eight signature subsets, denoted Signature S, are defined to be

$$S = \{S_1, S_2, S_3, S_4, S_5, S_6, S_7, S_8\}. \tag{11}$$

5 Identifier Construction

The identifier construction process uses the signatures to formulate a similarity scoring function. When there is a query sequence, the scoring function is used to measure a similarity value between the query sequence and target sequences, called *SimScore*. If the *SimScore* is higher than a threshold, the query is identified as a member of the target sequences. We use heuristics to select the optimal threshold. In our experiments, we found that the identifiers get the highest efficiency when the threshold is zero. Assume that we pass a query sequence through an identification system; the system is performed according to the four following steps:

Step I: Set the *SimScore* to zero.
Step II: Generate patterns of the query sequence according to the *n*-gram method using the same *n*-value as the one used in the signature generation process.
Step III: Match between patterns of the query sequence and signatures of the target sequences. If one match occurs, the *SimScore* is added one point.
Step IV: Identify the query sequence to the same type of target sequences, if the *SimScore* is more than a threshold.

For example, let X be a query sequence with cardinality m. Let $p_{x_1}, p_{x_2} ... p_{x_d}$ be a set of d $(m-n+1)$ *n*-gram patterns generated by the query sequence. Let Y be a type of target sequences and $s_{y_1}, s_{y_2} ... s_{y_e}$ is a set of its e signatures. Then, $sim(p_x, s_y)$ is a similarity score of a pattern p_x and a signature s_y, where $sim(p_x, s_y)$ is 1, if p_x is similar to s_y, and $sim(p_x, s_y)$ is 0, if not similar. The similarity score between a query sequence X and a type of target sequences Y, denoted $SimScore(X,Y)$, is a summation of similarity scores of every pattern p_x and every signature s_y as

$$SimScore(X,Y) = \sum_{1 \leq i \leq d, 1 \leq j \leq e} sim(p_{x_i}, s_{y_j}). \qquad (12)$$

If $SimScore(X,Y) >$ threshold, the query sequence X is identified to the same type of target sequences Y.

6 Performance Evaluation

Evaluation process is to assess the performance of identifiers over the set of test data. We use Accuracy [12] as a performance estimator for evaluating common strategies. Accuracy is the ratio of the summation of number of target sequences correctly identified and non-target sequences correctly identified to the total number of test sequences. Accuracy is usually expressed as a percentage formulation:

$$Accuracy = \frac{TP + TN}{(TP + FP + TN + FN)} \times 100\%. \qquad (13)$$

Where *True Positive (TP)* is a number of target sequences correctly identified; *False Positive (FP)* is a number of target sequences incorrectly identified; *True Negative (TN)* is a number of non-target sequences correctly identified; and *False Negative (FN)* is a number of non-target sequences incorrectly identified.

In our experiments, we evaluate the performance of two identifiers constructed by the two methods of signature discovery as described earlier. Identifier I is constructed using signatures generated by Discovery I and Identifier II by Discovery II. First, we evaluate the performance of Identifier I as the use of different *n*-grams, where *n* is ranged from 3 to 24, and six different scoring algorithms. Each pair of an *n*-gram and a scoring algorithm generates different signatures for the identifier construction. The results of Identifier I are depicted in Fig. 2. The figure shows that most identifiers have low efficiency, accuracy below 65%. Only few identifiers are successful with accuracy over 80%, i.e., the identifiers are constructed using 7- to 9-gram signatures and almost all scoring algorithms, except the *Rocchio algorithm (TF-IDF)*. The accuracy of the use of *Rocchio algorithm* is approximately 9% lower than the others.

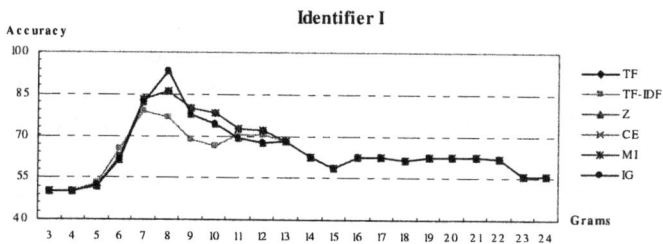

Fig. 2. Accuracy of Identifier I using different *n*-grams and different scoring algorithms

In Fig. 3, we also compare the performance of Identifier II as the use of different *n*-grams and scoring algorithms. Like the experimental results of Identifier I, at the too low and too high *n*-grams, the performance of Identifier II is the lowest, accuracy below 65%. The use of *Rocchio algorithm* also produces 9% lower accuracy than the other algorithms. In contrast to the Identifier I, most experimental results are accomplished with 95% accuracy in average. Moreover, the peak accuracy of Identifier II provides up to 99.69% at 11-gram in several scoring algorithms.

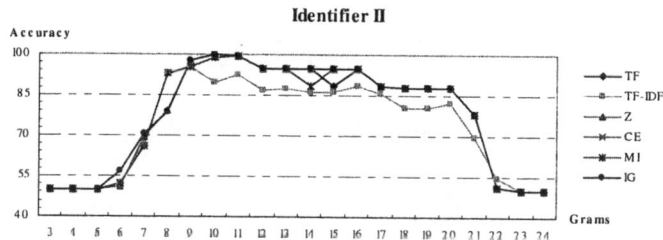

Fig. 3. Accuracy of Identifier II using different *n*-grams and different scoring algorithms

Following all the experimental results, the models based on class distribution, such as *Z*, *CE*, *MI* and *IG*, achieve good results; while the models based on common patterns, such as *TF* and *TF-IDF*, have only *TF* which is achievable. The high efficiency of *TF* indicates that the high-frequency patterns selected to be the signatures are seen in target classes or the influenza dataset only, not seen in the non-influenza dataset. For the *TF-IDF* formula: $TF(p) \cdot \log(\frac{|D|}{DF(p)})$, although the frequency of pattern, $TF(p)$, is high, the score of pattern computed by the *TF-IDF* may be reduced if $\log(\frac{|D|}{DF(p)})$ is low. The formula $\log(\frac{|D|}{DF(p)})$ is low, when the number of sequences in which pattern occurs at least once is high. As discussed above, the high-frequency patterns selected to be signatures are seen in sequences of target classes only; therefore, a large number of the sequences in which patterns occur at least once should also produce high scores. Nevertheless, the *Rocchio algorithm* reduces scores of these patterns. The high-score patterns, evaluated by the Rocchio, are unlikely to be signatures which are good enough for the DNA sequence identification. This is why the use of *Rocchio* gets less performance than the use of the other algorithms.

Finally, we discuss on the four values of Accuracy: *TP*, *FP*, *TN* and *FN*. Table 1 shows that, between 7- and 21-grams, the accuracy of Identifier I and II depends on two values only, *TP* and *FP*, because the other values are quite stable; *TN* is maximal and *FN* is zero. Notice that the identification of non-target sequences is successful since no non-target sequences are identified as the influenza virus. Identifier I produces 70% accuracy in average; whereas Identifier II is higher with 90% accuracy in average. Next, we found that the performance of both identifiers is very low, when the identifiers are constructed using too short or too long n-gram signatures, shorter than 7 and longer than 21. For shorter than 7-gram, both identifiers get accuracy below 65%. Both *TP* and *FN* are nearly maximal; while *FP* and *TN* are nearly zero. The shorter signatures of influenza virus cannot identify any sequences because they are found in almost all sequences. Almost all query sequences get higher score than the threshold; therefore they are identified as influenza virus. This is why both *TP* and *FN* are nearly maximal. For longer than 21-gram, both identifiers also get accuracy below 65%. The longer signatures of influenza virus cannot be found in almost all sequences, including influenza sequences. Most query sequences get lower score than the threshold and they are incorrectly identified. Therefore, *TP* and *FN* are nearly zero, and *FP* and *TN* are maximal.

Table 1. Comparing Accuracy, True Positive (*TP*), False Positive (*FP*), True Negative (*TN*) and False Negative (*FN*) between Identifier I and II using different n-grams

Identifiers	Grams	Accuracy	TP	FP	TN	FN
I	7-21	70% avg.	-	-	max	0
II	7-21	90% avg.	-	-	max	0
I & II	<7	<65%	~max	~0	~0	~max
I & II	>21	<65%	~0	~max	~max	~0

7 Conclusion

The acquisition of an intelligent and low computation method is one of the most significant tasks of identification since the existing research projects apply a high computation method for accomplishing in the target concept of identification, such as projects based on alignments. We propose novel approaches for accurately identifying DNA sequences in shorter time. The approaches apply an n-gram method and statistical scoring algorithms to discover one of intelligent data called "*Signatures*" as inputs of the identification system for reducing the high computation. The experimental results showed that identifiers constructed using almost all scoring algorithms achieve good results, except the use of *Rocchio algorithm* which produces 9% less accuracy than the others. The use of either too short or too long n-gram signatures yields poor efficiency; while other n-gram signatures yield better efficiency. Additionally, the peak accuracy provides up to 99.69%. In conclusion, one of our approaches, based on the n-gram method, the statistical scoring algorithms and the knowledge addition of the target DNA, succeeds in the identifier construction.

Acknowledgements

We would like to thank the precious support provided by Kasetsart University Research and Development Institute (KURDI). We also thank Thailand Research Fund (Senior Research Scholar (Y.P.)) and Center of Excellence, Viral Hepatitis Research Unit, Chulalongkorn University. Finally, we thank Venerable Dr. Mettanando Bhikkhu for reviewing the manuscript.

References

1. Aalbersberg, I.: A Document Retrieval Model Based on Term Frequency Ranks. Proceedings of the 7th Annual International ACM SIGIR Conference on Research and Development in Information Retrieval (1994) 163-172
2. Benson, D.A., Karsch-Mizrachi, I., Lipman, D.J., Ostell, J., Rapp, B.A., Wheeler, D.L.: GenBank. Nucleic Acids Research 28(1) (2000) 15-18
3. Brown, P.F., de Souza, P.V., Della Pietra, V.J., Mercer, R.L.: Class-Based N-Gram Models of Natural Language. Computational Linguistics 18(4) (1992) 467-479
4. Chuzhanova, N.A., Jones, A.J., Margetts, S.: Feature Selection for Genetic Sequence Classification. Bioinformatics Journal 14(2) (1998) 139-143
5. Joachims, T.: A Probabilistic Analysis of the Rocchio Algorithm with TFIDF for Text Categorization. Proceedings of the 14th International Conference on Machine Learning (1997) 143-151
6. Keinduangjun, J., Piamsa-nga, P., Poovorawan, Y.: Models for Discovering Signatures in DNA Sequences. Proceedings of the 3rd IASTED International Conference on Biomedical Engineering, Innsbruck, Austria (2005) 548-553
7. Krauthammer, M., Rzhetsky, A., Morozov, P., Friedman, C.: Using BLAST for Identifying Gene and Protein Names in Journal Articles. Gene 259(1-2) (2000) 245-252
8. Mladenic, D., Grobelnik, M.: Feature Selection for Classification Based on Text Hierarchy. In Working Notes of Learning from Text and the Web. Conference on Automated Learning and Discovery, Carnegie Mellon University, Pittsburgh (1998)
9. Mladenic, D., Grobelnik, M.: Feature Selection for Unbalanced Class Distribution and Naïve Bayes. Proceedings of the 16th International Conference on Machine Learning (1999) 258-267
10. Pearson, W.R.: Using the FASTA Program to Search Protein and DNA Sequence Databases. Methods Molecular Biology 25 (1994) 365-389
11. Sebastiani, F.: Machine Learning in Automated Text Categorization. ACM Computing Surveys 34(1) (2002) 1-47
12. Spitters, M.: Comparing Feature Sets for Learning Text Categorization. Proceedings on RIAO. (2000)
13. Wang, J.T.L., Rozen, S., Shapiro, B.A., Shasha, D., Wang, Z., Yin, M.: New Techniques for DNA Sequence Classification. Journal of Computational Biology 6(2) (1999) 209-218
14. Xu, Y., Mural, R., Einstein, J., Shah, M., Uberbacher, E.: Grail: A Multiagent Neural Network System for Gene Identification. Proceedings of IEEE 84(10) (1996) 1544-1552

Conquering the Curse of Dimensionality in Gene Expression Cancer Diagnosis: Tough Problem, Simple Models

Minca Mramor[1], Gregor Leban[1], Janez Demšar[1], and Blaž Zupan[1,2]

[1] Faculty of Computer and Information Science,
University of Ljubljana, Tržaška 25, Ljubljana, Slovenia
[2] Department of Molecular and Human Genetics,
Baylor College of Medicine, 1 Baylor Plaza, Houston, TX 77030, U.S.A.

Abstract. In the paper we study the properties of cancer gene expression data sets from the perspective of classification and tumor diagnosis. Our findings and case studies are based on several recently published data sets. We find that these data sets typically include a subset of about 100 highly discriminating features of which predictive power can be further enhanced by exploring their interactions. This finding speaks against often used univariate feature selection methods, and may explain the superior performance of support vector machines recently reported in the related work. We argue that a much simpler technique that directly finds visualizations with clear separation of diagnostic classes may be used instead. Furthermore, it may perform better in inference of an understandable classifier that includes only a few relevant features.

1 Introduction

Carcinogenesis is a multi step process in which genetic alterations drive the progressive transformation of normal human cells into malignant derivates. Gene expression microarrays can be used to identify specific genes that are differentially expressed across different tumor types. Classification of clinically heterogeneous cancers using gene expression profiles is an emerging application of microarray technology. Several recent studies of different cancer types, including acute leukemias [1], lymphomas [2], and brain tumors [3] have already demonstrated the utility of gene expression profiles for cancer classification, and reported on the superior classification performance when compared to standard morphological criteria. More accurate classifications based on molecular phenotype can improve and individualize treatment, influence the development of targeted therapeutics, and help in the identification of biomarkers for diagnosis and prognosis.

From the viewpoint of inference of classification models, gene expression data sets are rather peculiar. They most often include thousands of attributes (genes) and a small number of examples (patients). Another problem is a substantial component of noise, resulting from numerous sources of variation affecting expression measurements.

In conquering the curse of dimensionality, the prevailing modelling approaches include gene filtering in the data preprocessing phase, and gene subset selection often coupled with a modelling technique. For instance, in the work reported by Khan et al. [4] to classify four types of tumors in childhood, authors first ignored genes with low expression values throughout the data set, then trained 3750 feed-forward neural networks on different subsets of genes as determined by principal component analysis, analyzed the resulting networks for most informative genes and in this way obtained a subset of 96 genes of which expression clearly separated different cancer types when using multi-dimensional scaling. Other approaches, often similar in complexity of data analysis procedure, include k-nearest neighbors with weighted voting of informative genes [1] and support vector machines (SVM, [5, 6, 7]). In most cases, the resulting prediction models include complex computation over a set of gene expressions (e.g., neural networks, SVM, or principal components models) which are hard to interpret and can not be communicated to the domain experts in a way that would easily reveal the role genes play in separating different cancer types.

While different approaches have been used for selecting marker genes [5, 1, 4, 8] (for a review see [9]), the prevalent approach is based on univariate studies which examine the value of a gene in absence of context, that is, disregarding the expressions of other observed genes. Such an approach, most often used in practice, is for instance signal-to-noise statistics [1]. Since genes interact, one would expect that more information can be gained by observing a set of genes as a group, rather than summing their individual effects. This is confirmed experimentally through a success of non-linear modelling methods that can account for gene interactions [5]. In this respect, the use of univariate scoring for gene subset selection is questionable.

In the paper, we provide a simple alternative to rather complex gene expression diagnostic modelling approaches mentioned above. Namely, we show that a subset of two to five genes can most often provide sufficient information to clearly separate the diagnostic classes when their expression data is visualized either in scatterplot (two genes) or radviz (three genes or more) planar geometric graphs. The paper first introduces gene scoring, visualization, and visual projection search methods we apply in our studies. Our experimental study, together with the data sets used, is described next. The paper finishes with the discussion of results and concluding remarks.

2 Methods

2.1 Gene Ranking

In the paper, we use two in essence very different methods for gene ranking. Signal-to-noise (S2N) [1] is a univariate statistics for scoring of attributes that is derived from the standard parametric t-test statistic and is computed as $\frac{\mu_0 - \mu_1}{\sigma_0 + \sigma_1}$, where μ and σ represent the mean and standard deviation of gene's expression, respectively for each class. To score genes in multi-class problems, we have taken the data for each pair of class values, computed the statistics, and then averaged it across all possible class value pairs.

ReliefF [10, 11] is a feature scoring function that is, in principle, sensitive to feature interactions by being able to detect features that may not provide much information on their own, but could be very useful when used together with some other features. ReliefF scores features according to how well their values distinguish among instances that are similar to each other. Since the similarity is computed based on all features in the data set, they define the context for the feature's score thus providing grounds for revealing the interactions.

2.2 Two-Dimensional Geometric Visualization Methods

In the paper we propose to visualize gene expression data by plotting the examples from the data sets in a two-dimensional graphs. Depending on how many genes we use in the plot, we draw either a scatterplot (two genes) or a radviz (three or more genes). By selecting a suitable set of genes for the plots (see next section), we aspire that either of the two visualization methods would provide for a clear visual separation of diagnostic classes.

For a scatterplot, an example of such a graph is given in Figure 1.a. Figure 1.b shows a radviz with five genes, represented as anchors that are equally spaced around the perimeter of a unit circle. The examples are visualized as points inside the unit circle, where their position depends on gene expression value: the higher the value for a gene, the more the anchor attracts the corresponding point. Finding an attraction equilibria for a visualized set of genes determines the placement of each of examples in the data set [12]. Examples with approximately equal expressions of genes that lie on the opposite sides of the circle will lie close to the center of the circle. On the other hand, if the expression of a single gene in a visualized set prevails, the point will lie close to the corresponding anchor. The radviz projection is defined with the gene subset being visualized, and with the placement of gene anchors. While enabling the visualization of several genes in a single graph, radviz has some deficiencies. For instance, placing two highly correlated genes that are good at discriminating between classes on the opposite side of the circle will make them useless in the visualization, since there joint effect will be cancelled out. On the other hand, they might generate a projection with well separated classes if their anchors are placed adjacently. The "correct" placement of feature anchors was for instance crucial for a nice separation of classes in Figure 1.b, where the two anchors (genes) on the top of the circle (SET and CD19) attract data points from the ALL class and genes APLP2 and LTC4S attract points with AML class value.

2.3 Visualization Scoring and Ranking and Projection Search

In Figure 1 we have shown two data visualizations that utilize only a small number of attributes (genes) but provide a good separation of diagnostic classes. Cancer microarray data includes thousands of genes, and it is therefore not trivial to find a useful projection, that is, a subset of genes to visualize. In fact, we have observed that, for a typical cancer data set, there are only a few among millions of possible projections that exhibit a clear separation of diagnostic classes, making the manual search for a good visualization impossible.

To automate the search for a good projection, we first need to define how to evaluate them. The algorithm we use, VizRank [13], scores a particular projection by training a k-nearest neighbor classifier on two attributes – the x and y positions of points in the projection. The classification accuracy of the classifier is then assessed using 10-fold cross validation and provides for a projection score. When classes in the projection are well separated, the classification accuracy of the k-NN classifier will be high and the projection will be highly ranked. In projections where some points from different classes overlap, the accuracy of the classifier and with it the value of the projection will be accordingly lower.

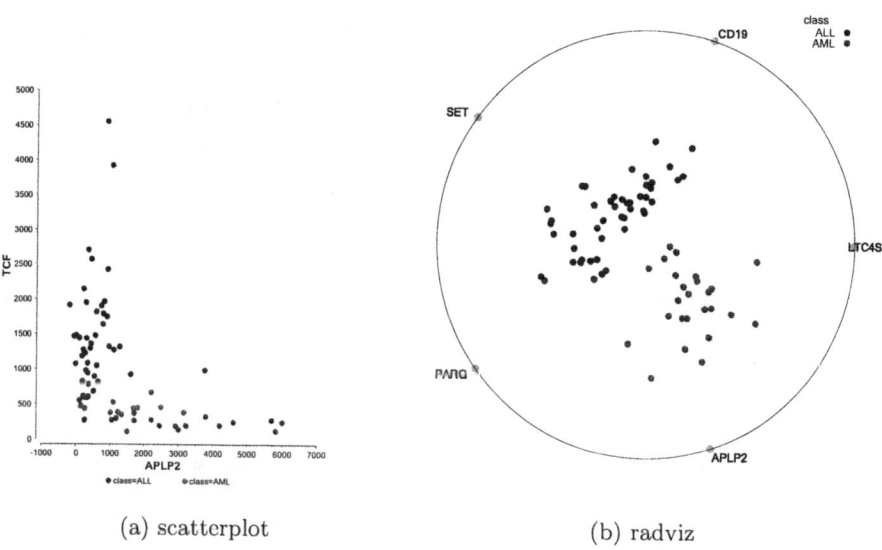

(a) scatterplot   (b) radviz

Fig. 1. Two projections for the leukemia data set (see Section 3.3)

Although VizRank's visualization scoring can be very efficient (more than 2000 projections can be evaluated per minute on a 2.4GHz computer) evaluating all projections in the data sets with several thousands of attributes is not feasible. Instead, VizRank uses an efficient heuristic that first scores the attributes using ReliefF [11], ranks the subsets of attributes to be considered by the sum of ReliefF scores, and evaluates the projections starting with the most likely candidates using this heuristics. Our experiments show that by using this heuristic only a few percents of possible projections have to be assessed in order to find the most interesting ones.

3 Experimental Study

3.1 Data Sets

For experimental analysis reported in this paper we use five publicly available data sets with information on gene expression profiles in different human cancer types (Table 1). Three data sets, leukemia [1], diffuse large B-cell lymphoma (DLBCL) [2] and prostate tumor [14] have two categories. The leukemia data includes 48 acute lymphoblastic leukemia (ALL) samples and 25 acute myeloid leukemia (AML) samples, each with 7074 gene expression values. The DLBCL data set includes 7070 gene expression profiles for 77 patients, 58 with DLBCL and 19 with follicular lymphoma (FL). The prostate tumor data set includes 12533 genes measured for 52 prostate tumor and 50 normal tissue samples. The data for these three data sets and the mixed lineage leukemia (MLL) data set were produced from Affymetrix gene chips and are available at http://www-genome.wi.mit.edu/cancer/.

We additionally analyzed two multi category data sets. The MLL [15] data set includes 12533 gene expression values for 72 samples obtained from the peripheral blood or bone marrow of affected individuals. The ALL samples with a chromosomal translocation involving the mixed lineage gene were diagnosed as MLL, so three different leukemia classes were obtained (AML, ALL and MLL). The SRBCT data set [4] consists of four types of tumors in childhood, including Ewing's sarcoma (EWS), rhabdomyosarcoma (RB), neuroblastoma (NB) and Burkitt's lymphoma (BL). It includes 2308 genes and 83 samples derived from tumor biopsy and cell lines. The data for the SRBCT data set were obtained from cDNA microarrays. The data set is available at http://research.nhgri.nih.gov/microarray/Supplement/.

3.2 Gene Ranking by ReliefF and Signal-to-Noise Statistics

We started our experiments with a comparative study of ReliefF and S2N scores and associated gene ranking. For all five data sets, histograms of ReliefF and S2N scores were qualitatively similar, being skewed to the right, with a group

Table 1. Cancer-related gene expression data sets used in our study. Columns report on number of examples, diagnostic classes and genes included in a data set, and proportion of examples in the majority diagnostic class. Last two columns show the average probability of correct classification ($\overline{P}$) for the top-ranked scatterplot and radviz projection

Data set	Number of Samples	Classes	Genes	Major class	$\overline{P}$ for top projection Scatterplot	Radviz
Leukemia	73	2	7074	52.8%	98.04%	99.55%
MLL	72	3	12533	38.9%	94.82%	99.75%
SRBCT	83	4	2308	34.9%	87.69%	99.74%
Prostate	102	2	12533	51.0%	91.76%	98.27%
DLBCL	77	2	7070	75.3%	96.82%	99.71%

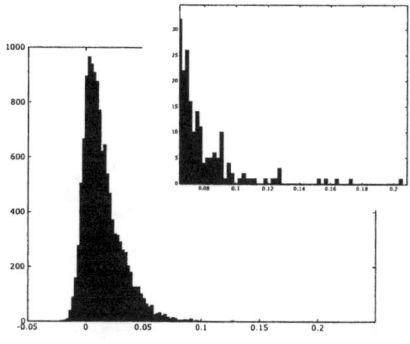 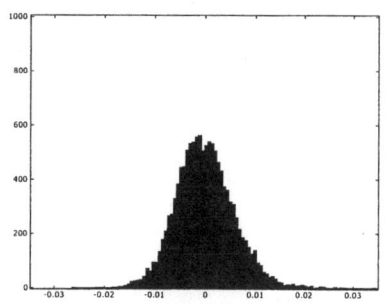

(a) histogram for actual attribute values; the part with the best ranked attributes is magnified in the upper right corner.

(b) histogram for permuted data

Fig. 2. Histograms of ReliefF on actual and permuted values of attributes (Section 3.2)

of about 50 to 100 most discriminating genes in the right tail. A permutation test was used to verify if these highly discriminatory genes were assigned high scores by chance. We used permutation analysis and calculated ReliefF scores after random permutation of expression values for each of the attributes. In the interest of brevity, we here only show a histogram for ReliefF scores on MLL data set and its corresponding histogram on randomly permuted data (Figure 2). Note that the part with the highest scored genes (the magnification in Fig 2.a) is far outside the normal-shaped distribution computed on permuted data (Fig 2.b).

The association between the gene ranks obtained by the univariate S2N and multivariate ReliefF gene ranking methods was obtained by computing the non-parametric Spearman correlation coefficient. The Spearman rank correlation coefficient varied importantly depending on which data set we analyzed. The correlation between ReliefF and S2N was highest (0.89) in the MLL data set but as low as 0.24 in the DLBCL data set, indicating that these two scoring functions would typically yield very different ranking and providing grounds for hypothesis that data includes much interactions between genes.

3.3 Results for the Cancer Gene Expression Data Sets

On all the data sets, VizRank found either scatterplot or radviz visualizations with clear separation of diagnostic classes. If let run for an hour on a standard PC, the number of such projections was in the range of ten to twenty, but most importantly, most of them were found in the first few seconds. The last two columns in Table 1 show Vizrank's scores, the average probability of correct classification, for the top-ranked scatterplot and radviz projections. The best scatterplot projections were scored from 87.64% to 98.04%, with the lowest score assigned to the multiclass SRBCT data set. We found that as the number

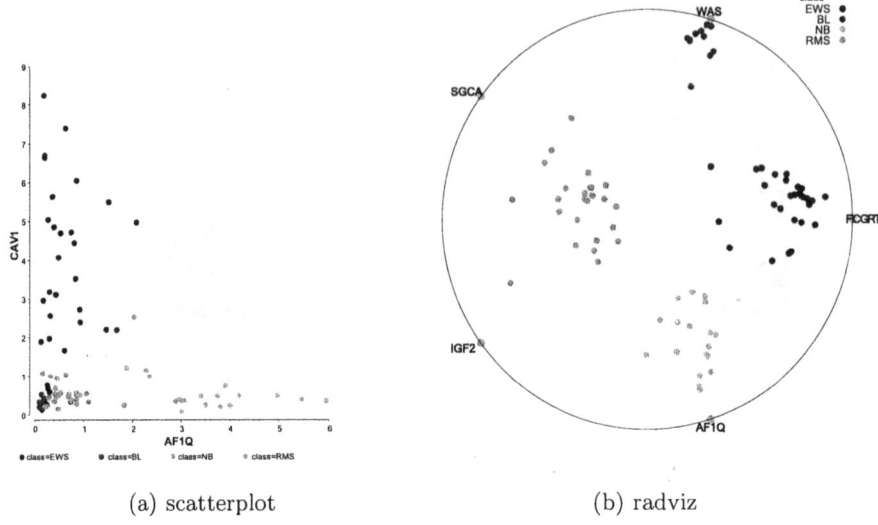

Fig. 3. Projections for the SRBCT data set (Section 3.3)

of classes exceeds two, scatterplot becomes less appropriate and radviz with a number of genes not exceeding five provides for excellent separations. For radviz visualizations the scores shown (from 98.27% to 99.75%) hold for the top-ranked projections using only five genes; increasing the number of genes may yield better separation of instances form different classes and thus a higher score. For reasons of space, we here show the visualizations and provide a corresponding discussion only for one two-valued and one multi-valued class problem.

For the leukemia data set the best scatterplot obtained a score of 98% and included genes APLP2 and TCF (Figure 1.a). Notice a clear separation of instances from the ALL and AML classes with only a few outliers. An example of the radviz visualization with good separation of examples from different classes and a Vizrank score of 98% is shown in Figure 1.b. The five genes used in this projection are CFTR, CD19, LTC4S, IL8 and RNS2.

In Table 2 we show genes appearing in the best scatterplots and the ReliefF and S2N ranks belonging to these genes. Out of the 20 genes represented, two were found to be cancer genes and eleven are cancer related according to the Atlas of genetics and cytogenetics in oncology and haematology (http://www.info-biogen.fr/services/chromcancer/index.html). In the table those genes are marked as C and CR, respectively.

Figure 3 shows the best rated scatterplot and radviz visualization with clear separation of instances from different classes for the multicategory SRBCT data set. While the scatterplot does not provide a good separation between all diagnostic classes, separation in radviz is clear. In Table 2 we show twenty genes appearing in the 41 radviz visualizations with VizRank score of 100%, their Relief and S2N ranks and report on whether they are related to carcinogenesis

Table 2. Twenty best genes from the scatterplot visualizations for the leukemia data set (a) and from the radviz visualization for the SRBCT data set (b). In column 3 and 4 the ReliefF and S2N ranks are shown, respectively. In the cancer column: C = cancer gene, CR = cancer related gene, N = not related to cancer

Gene	name	Rlf	S2N	cancer	Gene	name	Rlf	S2N	cancer
L09209	APLP2	3	3	N	770394	FCGRT	0	1	CR
M31523	TCF3	49	0	C	236282	WAS	26	3	CR
U77948	KAI1	414	26	CR	796258	SGCA	23	104	N
X85116	EPB72	42	62	CR	207274	IGF2	92	39	CR
M91592	ZNF76	578	112	N	812105	AF1Q	5	0	N
U22376	MYB	50	9	CR	183337	HLA-DMA	29	14	N
M62982	ALOX12	143	872	CR	784224	FGFR4	2	44	CR
Y12556	PRKAB1	123	3082	CR	866702	PTPN13	19	54	CR
U82759	HOXA9	9	25	C	786084	CBX1	10	79	CR
U27460	UGP2	588	59	N	814260	FVT1	35	135	CR
L08895	MEF2C	172	72	N	325182	CDH2	66	63	CR
U46499	MGST1	0	2	CR	244618	EST	106	25	
X03663	CSF1R	856	1189	CR	377461	CAV1	4	23	CR
U26312	CBX3	1152	108	CR	296448	IGF2	58	49	CR
X04741	UCHL1	792	4140	CR	629896	MAP1B	117	13	CR
M31211	MYL	57	4	CR	624360	PSMB8	356	18	N
D16469	ATP6AP1	249	341	CR	745019	EHD1	12	5	N
U68063	SFRS10	1070	134	N	1435862	CD99	3	12	CR
U51240	KIAA0085	104	208	N	383188	RCV1	13	2	CR
U09087	TMPO	100	42	N	767183	HCLS1	21	22	N

according to the Atlas of genetics and cytogenetics in oncology and haematology (http://www.infobiogen.fr/services/chromcancer/index.html). One of the genes from this list is an expressed sequence tags (ESTs). Out of the remaining 19 gene products, 13 are cancer related, which is 68%.

4 Discussion

The results from Table 2 show that signal-to-noise and ReliefF measures rank genes very differently. This was expected, as most of our best-scored visualizations show at least a degree of interaction. For instance, in radviz from Figure 3 neither of the genes can provide a clear separation of classes alone, yet when combined all of the cancer categories are perfectly separated.

Contrary to our expectations, though, we would expect a better match between ReliefF ranking and genes included in best set of visualizations. We hypothesize that the problem is in the number of attributes in the data set ReliefF considers as a context. When ReliefF evaluates an attribute it selects some reference examples and searches for the most similar examples from the same class and from the other classes. The context with too many genes can mask the effect of genes in interaction with the estimated gene, thus disabling ReliefF to appropriately account for interactions.

We compared our selection of "marker" genes in the leukemia data set to the genes selected by other methods. The best 20 genes from the scatterplot visualizations are different from the best ranked genes by Golub et al. [1] except for HOXA9 and EPB72. The primary reason is the use of univariate feature selection in their study. Also, in our study, we joined the test and training sets used by Golub et al. and performed the gene ranking and visualization methods on the combined set.

In contrast to the leukemia data set, the selection of our "marker" genes for the SRBCT data set compared with the genes ranked best by other methods is very similar. We found a very high consensus between our selection and the selection based on artificial neural networks [4]. 19 genes from the best scatterplot visualizations and 16 out of 20 from the best radviz visualizations were also selected by the ANN method. Interestingly, there is also a very high consensus (11 and 12 genes out of 20 included in best ranked scatterplot and radviz visualizations) between our method and the method of Fu [7] based on support vector machines.

5 Conclusion

The most striking result from our work is how easy it is to find a simple two-dimensional scatterplot or radviz visualization that clearly, non-ambiguously separates cancer diagnostic classes based on expression measurements for a few selected genes. This holds for all five data set studied, but the same observations also applies to about fifty other publicly available data sets we have studied but not reported in this paper. VizRank, a method we used to find good visualizations, often identifies the best ones within seconds of runtime. This is a significant achievement, especially when compared to hours of required runtime reported in a recent study that uses support vector machines combined with a set of other machine learning and feature selection approaches [5], and considering a clear presentation of results offered by these visualizations.

To a surprise came a relatively poor performance of ReliefF, which was expected to outshine the univariate gene scoring, but instead performed similarly. We have yet to fully understand why this is so, as the finding does not match with those from the systematic study of ReliefF on data sets that contain much fewer attributes [16].

Gene expression data visualizations reported here provide evidence that cancer diagnostic classes can be clearly separated when using the expression data from only a few genes. VizRank also provides a way for robust selection of genes without the need for a particular scoring function. Our future work aims at using top rated visualizations for probabilistic classification, thus also providing grounds for comparison with other, much more complex but nowadays prevailing computational methods in gene expression cancer diagnosis area.

References

1. Golub, T.R., Slonim, D.K., Tamayo, P. et al.: Molecular classification of cancer: Class discovery and class prediction by gene expression monitoring. Science **286** (1999) 531–537
2. Shipp, M.A., Ross, K.N., Tamayo, P. et al.: Diffuse large b-cell lymphoma outcome prediction by gene-expression profiling and supervised machine learning. Nature Medicine **8** (2002) 68–74
3. Nutt, C.L., Mani, D.R., Betensky, R.A. et al.: Gene expression-based classification of malignant gliomas correlates better with survival than histological classification. Cancer Res **63** (2003) 1602–1607
4. Khan, J., Wei, J.S., Ringnr, M. et al.: Classification and diagnostic prediction of cancers using gene expression profiling and artificial neural networks. 7 6 (2001) 673–679
5. Statnikov, A., Aliferis, C.F., Tsamardinos, I., Hardin, D., Levy, S.: A comprehensive evaluation of multicategory classification methods for microarray gene expression cancer diagnosis. Bioinformatics (2004) 33 – 46
6. Su, A.I., Welsh, J.B., Sapinoso, L.M. et al.: Molecular classification of human carcinomas by use of gene expression signatures. Cancer Res **61** (2001) 7388–7393
7. Fu, L.M., Fu-Liu, C.S.: Multi-class cancer subtype classification based on gene expression signatures with reliability analysis. FEBS Letters **561** (2004) 186–190
8. Gamberger, D., Lavrac, N., Zelezny, F., Tolar, J.: Induction of comprehensible models for gene expression datasets by subgroup discovery methodology. Journal of Biomedical Informatics **37** (2004) 269–284
9. Wang, Y., Tetko, I.V., Hall, M.A. et al.: Gene selection from microarray data for cancer classification–a machine learning approach. Computational Biology and Chemistry **29** (2005) 37–46
10. Kira, K., Rendell, L.: A practical approach to feature selection. In: Proceedings of the Ninth International Conference on Machine Learning. (1992) 249–256
11. Kononenko, I., Simec, E.: Induction of decision trees using relieff. In: Mathematical and statistical methods in artificial intelligence. Springer Verlag (1995)
12. Brunsdon, C., Fotheringham, A.S., Charlton, M.: An investigation of methods for visualising highly multivariate datasets. Case Studies of Visualization in the Social Sciences (1998) 55–80
13. Leban, G., Bratko, I., Petrovic, U., Curk, T., Zupan, B.: Vizrank: finding informative data projections in functional genomics by machine learning. Bioinformatics **21** (2005) 413–414
14. Singh, D., Febbo, P.G., Ross, K. et al.: Gene expression correlates of clinical prostate cancer behavior. Cancer Cell **1** (2002) 203–209
15. Armstrong, S.A., Staunton, J.E., Silverman, L.B., Pieters, R. et al.: MLL translocations specify a distinct gene expression profile that distinguishes a unique leukemia. Nature Genetics **30** (2001) 41–47
16. Sikonja, M.R., Kononenko, I.: Theoretical and empirical analysis of relieff and rrelieff. Machine Learning **53** (2003) 23 – 69

An Algorithm to Learn Causal Relations Between Genes from Steady State Data: Simulation and Its Application to Melanoma Dataset

Xin Zhang[1], Chitta Baral[1], and Seungchan Kim[1,2]

[1] Department of Computer Science and Engineering, Arizona State University,
Tempe, AZ 85287, USA
[2] Translational Genomics Research Institute,
445 N. Fifth Street, Phoenix, AZ 85004, USA

Abstract. In recent years, a few researchers have challenged past dogma and suggested methods (such as the IC algorithm) for inferring *causal* relationship among variables using steady state observations. In this paper, we present a modified IC (mIC) algorithm that uses entropy to test conditional independence and combines the steady state data with partial prior knowledge of topological ordering in gene regulatory network, for jointly learning the causal relationship among genes. We evaluate our mIC algorithm using the simulated data. The results show that the precision and recall rates are significantly improved compared with using IC algorithm. Finally, we apply the mIC algorithm to microarray data for melanoma. The algorithm identified the important causal relations associated with WNT5A, a gene playing an important role in melanoma, verified by the literatures.

1 Introduction

The recent development of high-throughput genomic technologies like cDNA microarray and oligonucleotide chips [14] empowers researchers in new ways to study how genes interact with each other. This has led to researchers using mathematical modeling and *in-silico* simulation study to analyze the interaction structure unambiguously and predict the network dynamic behavior in a systematic way [4, 19].

In previous studies on cellular response of genotoxic damage [10] and melanoma data [2, 11, 17], coefficient of determination (CoD) is used to infer gene network structure. CoD provides a normalized measure of the degree to which target variables can be better predicted using the observations in a feature set than it can be in the absence of observations. While CoD provides useful information for network connectivity, the relationships identified via CoD does not necessarily imply causal relations. Bayesian network model, which represents statistical dependencies, also has been proposed to discover interactions between genes [6, 22, 24]. Based on Bayesian model there are some other network inference methods that were evaluated by applying them to biological simulation with known network topology [18]. Bayesian network model considers the maximum likelihood of the observed data given a structure. It is a model associated with statistical probability that does not infer the real *causal* relationships. Other than Bayesian network model, Gardner et al. [5] proposed a linear dynamic network model to infer a gene network from steady state measurement. In addition to above models, several other probabilistic models have been proposed to learn gene networks with multiple data types [7, 15].

In fact none of the earlier research on learning gene networks considers the *causal* relationship between genes. A few researchers in [12, 13, 21] have suggested methods (for example, the IC algorithm) to learn the causal relationships between variables with steady state data, but not in biological domain. The assumption of causal theory is that the distribution of the dataset is faithful[1]. However, the under Boolean gene network model faithful function (we will define formally later) does not implies faithful distribution. Therefore learning gene causal connections with IC algorithms does not yield good result when the distribution of the dataset is not faithful.

In this paper, we present a new algorithm – modified IC (mIC) algorithm for learning causal relations between genes using additional knowledge of topological ordering[2]. We implement the algorithms using entropy to test conditional independence of the genes, and evaluate the causal learning approaches using simulation with the notions of precision and recall. We show that the precision and recall rates of the estimated gene network are significantly improved when using our mIC algorithm than original IC algorithm. In the end, we apply mIC algorithm to gene expression profile for a melanoma data with partial ordering information to learn gene regulatory network. The result shows that the important causal relationships associated with WNT5A gene are identified using mIC algorithm, and those causal connections have been confirmed in the literatures.

2 Learning Gene Causal Relationship

In this section we give a brief background on the difference between simple predictive relationships and causal relationships, and the basic intuition behind learning causal relationship from steady-state data. We also have an introduction to our simulation methodology.

2.1 Learning Causal Relationship with Steady State Data

To understand the difference between the simple and causal relationships between variables consider the propositions *rain* and *falling_barometer* from an example in [12]. When one observes that they are either both true or both false one concludes that they are related. One would then write *rain* = *falling_barometer*. But neither *rain* causes *falling_barometer* nor vice-versa. Thus if one wanted *rain* to be true, one could not achieve it by somehow forcing *falling_barometer* to be true. This would have been possible if *falling_barometer* caused *rain*. We say that the relationship between *rain*

---

[1] A probability distribution P is a faithful/stable distribution if there exist a directed acyclic graph (DAG) D such that the conditional independence relationship in P is also shown in the D, and vice versa.

[2] A topological ordering is an ordering among vertices of a DAG such that all edges are from vertices labeled with a smaller number to vertices labeled with a larger number. Knowledge about topological ordering between genes can be obtained if partial information about the pathways in which the genes (or their products) are involved is known; and also from existing knowledge about homologous genes in other organisms.

and *falling_barometer* is correlation, but not cause. In the context of genes and proteins if one would like to turn on a gene, which cannot be achieved directly, through other genes one would need to know the causal connection between the genes. Thus knowing the causal relationship is very important.

The question then is how to obtain (learn or infer) causal relationship between genes. In wet-labs this can be done by knocking down the possible subsets of genes of a given set and studying its impact on the other genes in the set. This is of course not easy to obtain when the number of genes in the set is more than a handful. An alternative approach is to use time series gene expression data. Unfortunately such data can only be obtained for cells of particular organisms such as yeast. For human tissues high-throughput gene expression data is only available in the steady state observation. Thus the question that begs is how to infer causal relationship between genes from steady state data.

For long it was thought that one can only infer correlations and other statistical measures such as conditional independence from steady state data and there is no way to infer causal relationship from such data. In recent years some researchers have challenged this view and have suggested methods, while not specially for the gene expression data, to infer causal information. The idea is generalized by Pearl in [12] and Spirtes et al in [21], and an Inductive Causation (IC) algorithm is presented where causal relation between variables is learned or inferred by first analyzing independence and dependence between variables and then constructing minimal and stable causal influence graphs that satisfy the independence and dependence information.

The idea behind the inference of causality from steady-state data is based on the principle of finding the simplest explanation of observed phenomena [12]. The causal relationship between a set of genes can be expressed using a causal model which consists of a causal structure (a directed acyclic graph, or a DAG), and parameters that define the value of one node in terms of the value of its parents (in the DAG). The causal theory has an assumption on the distribution called **stability** or **faithfulness**[3] [12]. The assumption is that all the independencies in distribution P are stable, that is P is entailed by a causal structure of a causal model regardless of the parameter. However in microarray dataset, the distribution might not be faithful. Hence the performance of IC algorithm is not good (w.r.t precision and recall) for inferring causal relationship in this case. We propose an modified IC (mIC) algorithm that uses entropy to test conditional independence and combines the steady state data with prior knowledge of gene topological ordering to jointly learn the causal relationship between genes.

2.2 Modelling and Simulation of a Causal Boolean Network

In order to evaluate the performance of the causal algorithms, we perform sets of simulations. We apply Boolean network model, originally introduced by Kauffman [8, 9], for modeling gene regulatory networks. Although Boolean network cannot model quantitative concepts, it provides useful insights in network dynamics [1]. There are two main objectives in modeling and simulation of data-driven Boolean network for the genetic

---

[3] A DAG G and a distribution P are *faithful* to each other if they exhibit the same set of independencies. A distribution P is said to be faithful if it is faithful to some DAG.

regulatory systems. First, we need to infer the model structure and parameters (rules) from observations such as gene expression profiles. Second, we can explore the dynamic behaviors of the system driven by the inferred rules through simulation.

In the simulation, we construct a Boolean network model as a directed acyclic graph (DAG), and obtain the steady-state observations. The model contains n nodes with binary values. The state space has a total of 2^n states. Theoretically there are 2^{2^k} possible functions for a Boolean network, where k is the number of predictors. Among the 2^{2^k} functions, many do not actually reflect the influence of predictors. For example, assume that a gene g_i has two causal parents g_1 and g_2, and a Boolean function f determines the state of g_i at next time step with $g_i = f(g_1, g_2) = (g_1 \wedge g_2) \vee (g_1 \wedge \neg g_2)$. The function f is one of the 2^{2^2} functions, but can be simplified as $g_i = f(g_1, g_2) = g_1$. In this case, function f does not reflect the causal influence of one of its causal parents g_2. Therefore, we define the concepts of *influence* and *proper Boolean function* and only use such functions in our simulation.

Definition 1. *(Influence)*: Let $z = f(x_1, \ldots, x_n)$ be a Boolean function. We say x_i has an influence on z in the function f if there exists two assignment vectors for $x_1, \ldots, x_n$ that only differ on the assignment to x_i, such that the values of f on those two assignments differ.

Definition 2. *(Proper function)*: We say $z = f(x_1, \ldots, x_n)$ is a proper function if for $i = 1 \ldots n$, x_i has an influence on z in the function f.

We did sets of experiments to show that under non-uniform distribution the proper function is faithful function[4], which entails original causal structure.

The simulation process in this study can be summarized as follows:

- Step 1: Generate M Boolean networks with up to three input causal parents for each node in topological ordering.
- Step 2: For each Boolean network connection, generate random proper Boolean functions for each node.
- Step 3: Assign random probabilities for the root gene (gene with no causal parents).
- Step 4: Given one configuration (fixed connection and functions), run the deterministic Boolean network starting from all possible initial states and get the probability distribution of all possible states.
- Step 5: Collect two hundred data points sampled from the probability distribution.
- Step 6: Repeat Step 3 and Step 5 for all M networks with probability distribution and save the configuration file and the data file.

2.3 Entropy and Mutual Information

Given a probability distribution of a dataset, one needs to compute the conditional independence among genes to find the causal information. Shannon [16] developed the concept of entropy to measure the uncertainty of the discrete random variables. In this

---

[4] There exists some special case that under certain non-uniform distribution, proper function might not be faithful function. But those cases are rare and with random generator in the simulation, we may ignore it.

paper we calculate entropy H and mutual information I to obtain uncertainty coefficient U to test conditional independence between genes. The uncertainty coefficient U is range from 0 to 1 and defined as follows:

$$U(X|Y) = I(X,Y)/H(X); \qquad (1)$$

where $H(X) = -\sum_x p(x)\log p(x)$; $H(X,Y) = -\sum_x \sum_y p(x,y)\log p(x,y)$; and $I(X,Y) = H(X) + H(Y) - H(X,Y)$ [25].

3 Algorithms and Criterion for Inferring a Gene Causal Network

3.1 Modified IC (mIC) Algorithm

The IC algorithm [12] examines pairwise conditional independencies between variables to determine the v-structures [5] first, and then applies rules to determine the rest of the network structures. The mIC algorithm is based on the IC algorithm [12], but it incorporates the topological ordering information in the learning step to infer the gene causal relationship from steady state data. It takes as input a probability distribution P generated by a DAG with some gene topological ordering information, and outputs a partially directed DAG. The mIC algorithm is described as follows:

- Step 1: For each pair of gene g_i and g_j in a dataset, test pairwise conditional independence. If they are dependent, search for a set
  $S_{ij} = \{g_k \mid g_i$ and g_j are independent given g_k, with $i < k < j$ or $j < k < i\}$ Construct an undirected graph G such that g_i and g_j are connected with an edge if and only if they are pairwise dependent and no S_{ij} can be found;
- Step 2: For each pair of nonadjacent genes g_i and g_j with common neighbor g_k, if $g_k \notin S_{ij}$, and $k > i, k > j$, add arrowheads pointing at g_k, such as $g_i \rightarrow g_k \leftarrow g_j$;
- Step 3: Orientate the undirected edges without creating new cycles and v-structures.

3.2 Comparing Initial and Obtained Networks - New Definitions for Precision and Recall

For evaluating the learning results, we define the new notions of precision and recall. In comparing the initial and obtained networks one immediate challenge that we faced is in defining recall and precision for the case where the inferred graph may have both directed and undirected edges. (Note that the original graph has only directed edges.) Intuitively, an undirected edge $A - B$ means that we cannot distinguish the directionality between A and B with given dataset.

To deal with this we define the following six categories: FN (false negatives), TP (true positives), PTP (partial true positives), PFN (partial false negatives), TN (true negatives), FP (false positives), PTN (partial true negatives), and PFP (partial false positives) as follows:

---

[5] A v-structure is of the form $a \rightarrow x \leftarrow b$ such that two converging arrows that the tails of a and b are not connected by an arrow.

FN = {X → Y | X → Y is in the original graph and neither X → Y nor X − Y is in the obtained graph}
TP = {X → Y | X → Y is in the original graph and also in the obtained graph}
TN = {X → Y | X → Y is not in the original graph and neither X → Y nor X − Y is in the obtained graph}
FP = {X → Y | X → Y is not in the original graph and X → Y is in the obtained graph}
PFN = PTP = {X → Y | X → Y is in the original graph and X − Y is in the obtained graph}
PTN = PFP = {X → Y | X → Y is not in the original graph and X − Y is in the obtained graph}

Now we can define the values AFP (aggregate number of false positive), ATN (aggregate number of true negatives), AFN (aggregate number of false negatives) and ATP (aggregate number of true positives) in terms of above six categories. $AFN = |FN| + |PFN|/2$; $ATP = |TP| + |PTP|/2$; $AFP = |FP| + |PFP|/2$; $ATN = |TN| + |PTN|/2$.

where $|X|$ is the cardinality of set X. Using the above we can now define Recall and Precision as follows:

$$Recall = \frac{ATP}{(AFN + ATP)}; \quad Precision = \frac{ATP}{(ATP + AFP)}$$

3.3 Precision and Recall with Observational Equivalence

The output of IC algorithm is a pattern, a partially directed DAG, which is a set of DAGs that have equivalence structures. Every edge in the original network is directed, while the edges in obtained graph may be directed or undirected. There might be a case that a directed edge in original graph has a corresponding undirected edge in obtained graph. Therefore with the view of observational equivalence (OE), we should not have penalties for such edges. Here we define the new notions of precision and recall with considering observational equivalence. We transform both original graph and obtained graph into their own observational equivalent classes, called original class and obtained class, using the definition of observational equivalence [12]. Then define the six categories as follows:

FN = {(X, Y) | X → Y or X − Y is in the original class and neither X → Y nor X − Y is in the obtained class}
TP = {(X, Y) | X → Y is in the original class and also in the obtained class or X − Y is in the original class and also in the obtained class}
TN = {(X, Y) | neither X → Y nor X − Y is in the original class and neither X → Y nor X − Y is in the obtained class}
FP = {(X, Y) | neither X → Y Y nor X − Y is in the original class and X → Y is in the obtained class}
PFN = PTP = {(X, Y) | X → Y is in the original class and X − Y is in the obtained class or X − Y is in the original class and X → Y is in the obtained class}
PTN = PFP = {(X, Y) | neither X → Y nor X − Y is in the original class and X − Y is in the obtained class}

The concepts of the AFN, ATP, ATN, AFP, precision and recall are the same as the ones we defined previous section.

3.4 Comparing the Networks Based on Their Transitive Closure

There are many ways for comparing the initial and obtained graphs. We discussed the way for comparing two networks directly, with and without observational equivalence. Transitive closure (TC) is another way for graph comparison. Suppose the initial network that we have is $A \rightarrow B \rightarrow C$ and we obtain the network with the only edge

$A \rightarrow C$. When comparing the obtained network with the initial network we may not treat $A \rightarrow C$ just as a false positive. In fact this obtained network is better than the network that has no edges. To be able to make this conclusion we consider the TC of $\rightarrow$ in the initial network and a similar notion in the obtained network. In the obtained network our definition of TC is based on defining two relations: $cc(x, y)$ and $pcc(x, y)$. Intuitively, $cc(x, y)$, denoting x causally contributes to y, is true if there is a directed or an undirected edge from x to y; and $pcc(x, y)$, denoting x possibly causally contributes to y, is true if there is a path from x to y consisting of properly directed edges and undirected edges such that $pcc(x, y) := cc(x, y) \mid pcc(x, z) \wedge pcc(z, y)$

3.5 Steps of Learning Gene Causal Relationships

The steps for learning gene causal relationships are as follows:

Step 1: Obtain the probability distribution, data sampling and the topological order of the genes;

Step 2: Apply algorithms such as IC or mIC to find causal relations;

Step 3: Compare the original and obtained networks based on the two notions of precision and recall;

Step 4: Repeat step 1-3 for every random network.

4 Experiments, Results and Discussion

We did two sets of experiments for learning gene causal relationships using the IC algorithm and mIC algorithm. Each experiment contains 100 different randomly generated gene networks (DAGs), each of which contains 10 genes, with topological ordering connected by Boolean proper functions. The distribution of the network is generated based on the probability of the root genes, and Monte Carlo sampling is used to generate 200 samples in a dataset for each network based on the probability distribution. We use the uncertainty coefficient (U) to test the conditional independence in step 1 of the algorithm. We choose the of $U = 0.3$ for pairwise and $U = 0.2$ for triplewise conditional independent test. The threshold cut-off values are based on heuristics that we elaborate in [25].

4.1 Learning with IC Algorithm

The first experiment is to use IC algorithm on the learning gene causal relations with steady state data without topological ordering information. The method is applied to derive an obtained graph for every network and then the obtained graphs are compared with their corresponding initial ones. The results with statistical confidence of 95% as the error bar marked are shown in figure 1.

Figure 1(a) shows the precisions of the simulation with IC using two notions: with and without OE and TC. The result shows that the precision rate for inferring causal relations in simulation is 0.3 without OE or TC, 0.45 with OE, around 0.4 with TC, and around 0.5 with OE and TC. Figure 1(b) shows that the recall rate is below 0.3 without OE, and around 0.4 with OE.

From the figure we can see that both precision and recall are significantly improved by using the notion of observational equivalence. However the recall rate is still around

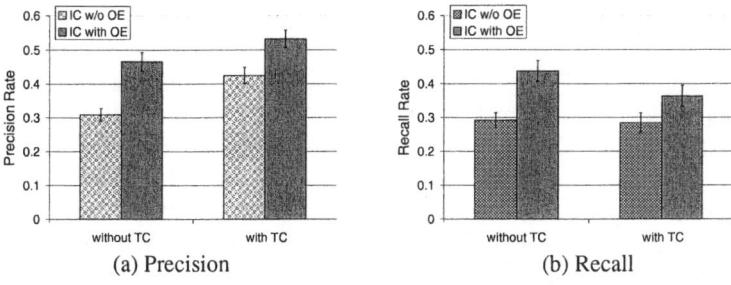

Fig. 1. Precision and Recall for learning by IC algorithm

0.4. From the above simulation results we can see that IC algorithm is not quite good for learning gene regulatory network using only steady state data.

4.2 Learning with Topological Ordering (mIC)

Since using IC algorithm for learning gene causal network from single type of dataset - steady state data did not show a good result, our hypothesis is that a better way is to use additional knowledge such as gene topological ordering. The second simulation we did is jointly learning the gene regulatory network using mIC algorithm combining steady state observation and the background knowledge of gene topological orders. We then compare the results with the ones learned by IC algorithm as shown in Figure 2.

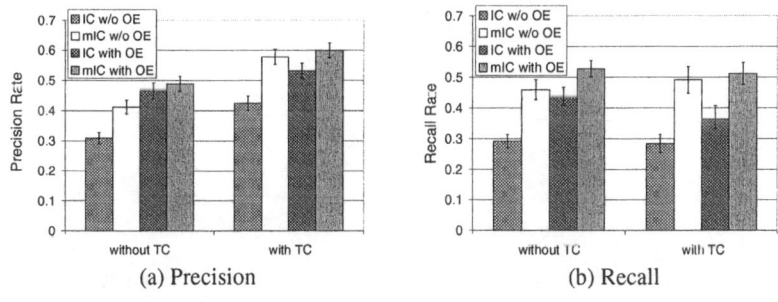

Fig. 2. Precision and Recall for learning by mIC with Ordering

Figure 2(a) shows that with statistical confidence of 95% as the error bar marked, the precision rate is significantly improved with mIC algorithm, and the precision rate is around 0.6 with TC and OE. Figure 2(b) are promising since the recall rates of learning with mIC algorithm are significantly improved from less than 0.3 with IC algorithm to greater than 0.45 by applying mIC algorithm, improved more than 50%, both with and without considering TC or OE. If considering the observational equivalence, the recall rate of learning with mIC algorithm has been significantly improved to above 0.5 with or without TC.

5 Applying mIC Algorithm on Melanoma Dataset

We finally applied mIC algorithm to a gene expression profile used in the study of melanoma [2]. 31 malignant melanoma samples were quantized to ternary format such that the expression level of each gene is assigned to -1(down-regulated), 0(unchanged) or 1 (up-regulated). The 10 genes involved in this study are chosen from 587 genes from the melanoma dataset that have been studied to cross predict each other in a multivariate setting [11]: *pirin*, WNT5A, MART-1, S100, RET-1, MMP-3, PHO-C, synuclein, HADHB and STC2.

In previous expression profiling study, WNT5A has been identified as a gene of interest involved in melanoma[2], and expression level of WNT5A is closely related with metastatic status of melanoma [23]. It was shown that the abundance of messenger RNA for WNT5A can be significantly distinguished between cells with high metastatic competence versus those with low metastatic competence [2]. Later, it was also proved experimentally that increasing the level of WNT5A protein can directly change the cell metastatic competence [23]. It has been also suggested that controlling the influence of WNT5A in the regulation can reduce the chance of melanoma metastasizing [3].

In this study of set of 10-gene network, we have a partial biological prior knowledge that MMP-3 is expected to be at the end of the pathway. We applied mIC algorithm using entropy to test conditional independence among those 10 genes with the above prior knowledge to infer the *causal* regulatory network. The learning results are shown in figure 3.

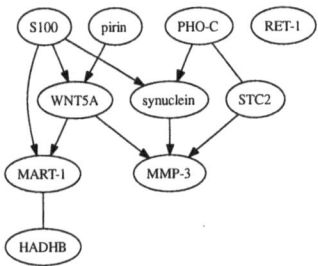

Fig. 3. Learning Melanoma Dataset with prior knowledge that MMP-3 is at the end of gene regulatory network

Figure 3 shows that *pirin* causatively influences WNT5A. This result is consistent with the literature[3] that in order to maintain the level of WNT5A, we need to directly control WNT5A or control WNT5A through *pirin*. The result also shows the causal connection between WNT5A and MART-1 such that WNT5A directly causes MART-1, which has been verified in the literature [20] that WNT5A may actually directly influence the regulation and suppression of MART-1 expression. In Figure 3, there are some causal connects that have not been verified by the scientist yet. However, they are unlikely to be obtained by random chance (see supplement materials http://www.asu.edu/~zhang24/AIME05). mIC algorithm bring up a systematic way to predict the *causal* connections among genes using steady state data with some prior biological knowledge. It could be applied as a guidance for the biologist to verify the causal connections in future experiments.

6 Conclusion

In this paper we presented a modified IC algorithm with entropy that can learn steady state data with gene topological ordering information. We did simulation based on Boolean network to evaluate the performance of the causal algorithms. In the process we developed ways to compare initial networks with obtained networks. From our simulation based evaluation we conclude that (i) IC algorithm does not work well for learning gene regulatory networks from steady state data alone, (ii) a better way for learning the gene causal relationship from steady state data is to use additional knowledge such as gene topological ordering, (iii) the precision and recall rates for mIC algorithm is significantly improved compared with IC algorithm with statistical confidence of 95%. For randomly generated networks, the mIC algorithms work well for joint learning the causal regulatory network by combining steady state data and gene topological ordering knowledge, with precision rate of greater than 60%, and recall rate greater than 50%. We then applied the algorithm to real biological microarray data Melanoma dataset. The result showed that some of the important causal relationships associated with WNT5A gene have been identified using mIC algorithm, and those causal connections have been verified in the literatures.

Acknowledgement

This work was supported by NSF grant number 0412000. The authors acknowledge the valuable comments of the anonymous reviewers of this paper.

References

1. Akutsu, T., et al. Identification of Genetic Networks from A Small Number of Gene Expression Patterns under the Boolean Network Models. *PSB*,1999.
2. Bittner, M. et al. Molecular Classification of Cutaneous Malignant Melanoma by Gene Expression Profiling. *Nature*, 406:536-540, 2000.
3. Datta, A., Bittner, M. and Dougherty. E. External Control in Markovian Genetic Regulatory Networks. *Machine Learning*, Vol 52, 169-191, 2003.
4. De Jong, H. Modeling and Simulation of Genetic Regulatory Systems: A Literature Review. *Journal of Computational Biology, 2002.* 9(1): p. 67–103.
5. Bernardo, T. et al Inferring Genetic Networks and Identifying Compound Mode of Action via Expression Profiling. *Science* 2003.
6. Friedman, N., Linial, L., Nachman, I. and Pe'er D. Using Bayesian Networks to Analyze Expression Data. *RECOMB* 2000.
7. Hartemink, A. et al. Combining Location and Expression Data for Principled Discovery of Genetic Regulatory Network Models. *PSB*, 2002.
8. Kauffman, S.A. Requirements for Evolvability in Complex Systems: Orderly Dynamics and Frozen Components. *Physica D, 1990.* 42: p. 135-152.

9. Kauffman, S.A. The Origins of Order, Self-Organization and Selection in Evolution. *Oxford University Press*, 1993.
10. Kim, S., et al. Multivariate Measurement of Gene-expression Relationships. *Genomics*, vol. 67, pp. 201–209, 2000
11. Kim S., et al. Can Markov Chain Models Mimic Biological Regulation? *Journal of Biological Systems, vol. 10, No. 4* (2002) 337-358.
12. Pearl, J. Causality : Models, Reasoning, and Inference. 2000 *Cambridge, U.K. ; New York: Cambridge University Press*. xvi, 384 p.
13. Scheines, R., Glymour, C. and Meek, C. TETRAD II: Tools for Discovery. *Hillsdale, NJ: Lawrence Erlbaum Associates*, 1994.
14. Schulze, A. and Downward, J. Navigating Gene Expression Using Microarrays - A Technology Review. *Nature Cell Biology, 2002*. 3: p.190-195.
15. Segal, E., et al. From Promoter Sequence to Expression: A Probabilistic Framework. *RECOMB* 2002.
16. Shanon, C. A Mathematical Theory of Communication *The Bell Systems Technical Journal*, 27, 1948.
17. Shmulevich, I. et al Probabilistic Boolean Networks: A Rule-based Uncertainty Model for Gene Regulatory Networks. *Bioinformatics,* 18(2), 2002.
18. Smith, V., Jarvis, E. and Hartemink, A. Influence of Network Topology and Data Collection on Network Inference. *PSB* 2003.
19. Smolen, P. et al. Modeling Transcriptional Control in Gene Networks – Methods, Recent Results, and Future Directions. *Bull Math Biol,* 62(2), 2000.
20. Sosman, J., Weeraratna, A., Sondak, V. When Will Melanoma Vaccines Be Proven Effective? *Journal of Clinical Oncology*, vol. 22, No 3, 2004.
21. Spirtes, P., Glymour, C. and Scheines, R. Causation, Prediction, and Search. *New York, N.Y.: Springer-Verlag*. 2nd Edition, MIT, Press 1993
22. Spirtes, P. et al. Constructing Bayesian Network Models of Gene Expression Networks from Microarray Data. *Proceedings of the Atlantic Symposium on Computational Biology, Genome Information Systems & Technology,* 2000.
23. Weeraratna, A.T., Jiang, Y., et al Wnt5a Signalling Directly Affects Cell Motility and Invasion of Metastatic Melanoma. *Cancer Cell*, 1, 279-288, 2000.
24. Yoo, C. and G.F. Cooper Discovery of Gene-Regulation Pathways Using Local Causal Search. *Proc AMIA Symp*, 2002: p. 914-8.
25. Supplement Materials: http://www.public.asu.edu/~xzhang24/AIME05

Relation Mining over a Corpus of Scientific Literature

Fabio Rinaldi[1], Gerold Schneider[1], Kaarel Kaljurand[1], Michael Hess[1],
Christos Andronis[2], Andreas Persidis[2], and Ourania Konstanti[2]

[1] Institute of Computational Linguistics, IFI,
University of Zurich, Switzerland
{rinaldi, gschneid, kalju, hess}@ifi.unizh.ch
[2] Biovista, Athens, Greece
{candronis, andreasp, okonst}@biovista.com

Abstract. The amount of new discoveries (as published in the scientific literature) in the area of Molecular Biology is currently growing at an exponential rate. This growth makes it very difficult to filter the most relevant results, and the extraction of the core information, for inclusion in one of the knowledge resources being maintained by the research community, becomes very expensive. Therefore, there is a growing interest in text processing approaches that can deliver selected information from scientific publications, which can limit the amount of human intervention normally needed to gather those results.

This paper presents and evaluates an approach aimed at automating the process of extracting semantic relations (e.g. interactions between genes and proteins) from scientific literature in the domain of Molecular Biology. The approach, using a novel dependency-based parser, is based on a complete syntactic analysis of the corpus.[1]

1 Introduction

The amount of research results in the area of molecular biology is growing at such a pace that it is extremely difficult for individual researchers to keep track of them. As such results appear mainly in the form of scientific articles, it is necessary to process them in an efficient manner in order to be able to extract the relevant results. Although many databases aim at consolidating the newly gained knowledge in a format that is easily accessible and searchable (e.g. UMLS, Swiss-Prot, OMIM, Gene Ontology, GenBank, LocusLink), the creation of such resources is a very labour intensive process. Relevant articles have to be selected and accurately read by an human expert looking for the core information.[2]

---

[1] Part of the material contained in this paper has been previously presented at the *Workshop on Data Mining and Text Mining for Bioinformatics*, Pisa, September 2004.

[2] This process is referred to as 'curation' of the article.

The various genome sequencing efforts have resulted in the creation of large databases containing gene sequences. However such information is of little use without the knowledge of the function of each gene and its role in biological pathways. Understanding the relationships between genes and pathways is central to biology research and drug design as they form an array of intricate and interconnected molecular interaction networks which is the basis of normal development and the sustenance of health.

In the context of the OntoGene project[3] we aim at developing and refining methods for discovery of interactions between biological entities (genes, proteins, pathways, etc.) from the scientific literature, based on a complete syntactic analysis of the articles, using a novel high-precision parsing approach.

We consider that advanced parsing techniques combining statistics and human knowledge of linguistics have matured enough to be successfully applied in real settings. OntoGene is intended as a framework for testing this hypotheses in the area of Biomedical Text Mining, where these techniques could have a significant impact.

In section 2, we present the "DepGENIA" corpus upon which our methodology is based. Section 3 describes the Relation Mining approach that we have adopted. Section 4 describes the evaluation of our results and briefly discusses current and future work. We conclude with a survey of related work in section 5.

2 The Corpus

GENIA [1][4] is a corpus of 2000 MEDLINE abstracts which have been annotated for various biological entities, according to the GENIA Ontology.[5] We use version G3.02 of the GENIA corpus, which includes 18546 sentences (average length 9.27 sentences per article) and 490941 words (average of 26.47 words per sentence). The advantage of working over GENIA is that it provides pre-annotated terminological units (Genes, Proteins, etc.), thus removing the need for Terminology Recognition / Entity Detection. This allows attention to be focused on other challenges.

In a first step, we convert the XML annotations of the GENIA corpus into a richer annotation schema [2]. There are two main reasons for performing this step. First, in the new annotation schema all relevant entities are given a unique identifier. As identifiers are preserved during all steps of processing, the existence of a unique identifier for each sentence and each token in the corpus later simplifies the task of presenting the results to the user. The second reason is that the new annotation scheme allows for a neater distinction of different 'layers' of annotations (structural, textual and conceptual) which again simplifies later steps of processing.

---

[3] http://www.ontogene.org/
[4] http://www-tsujii.is.s.u-tokyo.ac.jp/GENIA/
[5] http://www-tsujii.is.s.u-tokyo.ac.jp/~genia/topics/Corpus/genia-ontology.html

We then apply to the resulting modified version of GENIA a pipeline of tools defined as follows:

1. replace terms with their heads
2. lemmatization of all tokens (with morpha)[6]
3. noun group and verb group chunking (LT CHUNK)[7]
4. detection of heads in the group (with two simple rules: take the last noun from the noun group; take the last verb from the verb group)
5. dependency parsing (Pro3Gres)

The pipeline (itself declaratively specified in XML) has been implemented as an Apache Ant build file[8] which supports easy integration or replacement of specific components in the sequence. The end result of the process is a set of dependency relations, which are encoded as (sentence-id, type, head, dependent) tuples (and can be delivered either in CSV or XML). This is a format which is well suited for storage in a relational DB, for further processing with a spreadsheet tool, or for analysis with Data Mining algorithms. We call this modified resource "DepGENIA".[9]

3 Relation Mining

As a first result, we want to show that the availability of domain terminology simplifies and improves the task of parsing the corpus. To this aim we create a corpus which does not contain the original GENIA markup for domain terminology (later we refer to this corpus as the 'NOTERM' corpus).

Second, we want to verify whether the parsing of the corpus can benefit from the existence of semantic tags. The idea is to allow the parser to decide on an ambiguous attachment based on the semantic type of the arguments. For instance the decision of attaching an argument of type 'protein' as the subject of the verb 'bind' could be made on the basis of the type, rather than based purely on the lexical item itself.

The third result that we describe in this paper concerns the detection of specific relations by means of specific lexical classes and a small set of rules that describe specific syntactic patterns. This can be seen as partly similar to [3], which however makes use of surface POS-based patterns, while our patterns apply to the result of syntactic parsing. As an example consider the following GENIA sentence: *NGFI-B/nur77* **binds to** *the response element by monomer or heterodimer with retinoid X receptor (RXR)*.

Based on the interaction with a domain expert, we have identified a set of relations that are of particular interest in this domain. Some examples of relevant

---

[6] http://www.informatics.susx.ac.uk/research/nlp/carroll/morph.html
[7] Available at http://www.ltg.ed.ac.uk/software/chunk/
[8] http://ant.apache.org/
[9] For convenience, we have provided a web interface that allows simplified browsing of the results, see http://www.ontogene.org/

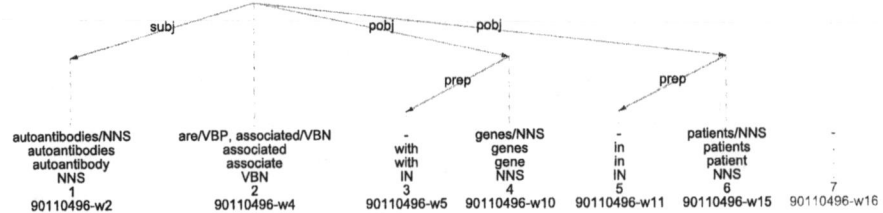

Fig. 1. Analysis of the sentence *"Anti-Ro(SSA) autoantibodies are associated with T cell receptor beta genes in systemic lupus erythematosus patients."*, where each term is represented by a term head

relations are: *activate, bind, interact, regulate, encode, signal* [4]. The use of a lemmatizer allows us to capture with a single pattern all morphological variants of a given verb (e.g. *bind* → *bind, binds, binding, bound*). For each of those relations, we have inspected some of the analysis that we obtained from parsing the corpus (see an example in figure 1).

Table 1. The most important dependency types used by the parser

Relation	Label	Example
verb–subject	subj	he sleeps
verb–first object	obj	sees it
verb–second object	obj2	gave (her) kisses
verb–adjunct	adj	ate yesterday
verb–subord. clause	sentobj	saw (they) came
verb–prep. phrase	pobj	slept in bed
noun–prep. phrase	modpp	draft of paper
noun–participle	modpart	report written
verb–complementizer	compl	to eat apples
noun–preposition	prep	to the house

The deep syntactic analysis builds upon the chunks using a broad-coverage probabilistic Dependency Parser [5] to identify sentence level syntactic relations between the heads of the chunks. The output is a hierarchical structure of syntactic relations — functional dependency structures, represented as the directed arrows in fig. 1. The parser [5,6] uses a hand-written grammar combined with a statistical language model that calculates lexicalized attachment probabilities, similar to [7]. Parsing is seen as a decision process, the probability of a total parse is the product of probabilities of the individual decisions at each ambiguous point in the derivation.

Two supervised models (based on Maximum Likelihood Estimations, MLE) are used. The first is based on lexical probabilities of the heads of phrases, calculating the probability of finding specific syntactic relations (such as subject, sentential object, etc.). The second probability model is a Probabilistic Context Free Grammar (PCFG) for the production of verb phrases. Although Context Free Grammars (CFG) are not a component of dependency grammar, verb phrase PCFG rules can model verb subcategorization frames which are an important component of a dependency grammar.

The parser expresses distinctions that are especially important for a predicate-argument based shallow semantic representation, as far as they are expressed in the Penn Treebank training data, such as PP-attachment, most long distance dependencies, relative clause anaphora, participles, gerunds, and the argument/adjunct distinction for NPs.

In some cases functional relations distinctions that are not expressed in the Penn Treebank are made. Commas are e.g. disambiguated between apposition and conjunction, or the Penn tag *IN* is disambiguated between preposition and subordinating conjunction. Other distinctions that are less relevant or not clearly expressed in the Treebank are left underspecified, such as the distinction between PP arguments and adjuncts, or a number of types of subordinate clauses.

The parser is robust in that it returns the most promising set of partial structures when it fails to find a complete parse for a sentence. Its parsing speed is about 300,000 words per hour.

4 Evaluation

Two different types of evaluation have been performed. First a linguistic evaluation of the parser. Next we focused on the evaluation of the biological significance of the extracted relations.

In order to perform an evaluation on the various experiments mentioned in the previous section we have randomly selected 100 test sentences from the GENIA corpus, which we have manually annotated for the syntactic relations that the parser can detect.

Table 2. Comparison of results of parsing under different conditions

Relation	NOTERM	DepGENIA	semantic
subj (precision)	0.825	0.900	0.888
subj (recall)	0.744	0.862	0.846
obj (precision)	0.701	0.941	0.941
obj (recall)	0.772	0.949	0.949
nounpp (precision)	0.675	0.833	0.808
verbpp (precision)	0.671	0.817	0.770
sentobj (precision)	0.630	0.711	0.692
sentobj (recall)	0.604	0.75	0.729

We have first run the parser over the 100 test sentences as extracted from the NOTERM corpus, containing the chunks as generated by LTCHUNK, but no information on terminology. Later we have performed the analysis over the same 100 sentences, however this time extracted from the "DepGENIA" corpus. A comparison of the results is shown in table 2.[10]

As a second experiment, we have integrated PP-attachment modules [8, 9] using the GENIA corpus, because the original PP-training corpus (the Penn Treebank) is of a different domain. Against sparse data we back off to semantic GENIA classes. Our results do not show any improvement.[11]

In order to evaluate the specific task of Relation Extraction, we have focused on triples of the form (predicate - subject - object). The analysis of the whole GENIA corpus resulted in 10072 such triples (records). For the evaluation of biological relevance we selected only the triples containing the following predicates: *activate, bind* and *block*. This resulted in 487 records.

---

[10] The parser is constantly being improved, results obtained after the publication of this paper will be made available on the OntoGene web site.
[11] This might be attributed to insufficient data or the relative simplicity of the GENIA Ontology.

Table 3. Some examples of expert evaluation

relation	subj	subj type	subj eval	obj	obj type	obj eval
activate	Interleukin-2 (IL-2)	amino acid	Y	Stat5 in fresh PBL, and Stat3 and Stat5 in preactivated PBL	amino acid	A+
activate	IL-5	amino acid	Y	the Jak 2 -STAT 1 signaling pathway	other name	Y
bind	Spi-B	amino acid	Y	DNA sequences	nucleic acid	A-
bind	The higher affinity sites	other name	Pr	CVZ with 20-	other organic compound	N

The extraction algorithm maximally expands the arguments of the predicate, following all their dependencies. Each argument is then assigned a type (a concept of the GENIA Ontology), based on its head. The type assignment depends on the manual annotation performed by the GENIA annotators, so we have taken it as reliable and have not further evaluated it. We then removed all records where a type had not been assigned to either subject or object: this left 169 fully qualified records.[12] This remaining set was inspected by a domain expert.

In order to simplify the process of evaluation, we have created simple visualization tools (based on XML, CSS and CGI scripts), that can display the results in a browser. For instance, for the former type of evaluation, our visualization tool adds a special attribute to the sentences that have been detected by the methodology previously described. All the articles that contain relevant sentences are then automatically collected and displayed in a browser. The extracted relations can also be stored in a DB format for further processing with a spreadsheet tool or for analysis with Data Mining algorithms.

We asked the domain experts to evaluate each argument separately and mark it according to the following codes:

Y the argument is correct and informative
N the argument is completely wrong
Pr the argument is correct, but is anaphoric, and it would need to be resolved to be significant (e.g. "This protein").
A+ the argument is "too large" (which implies that a prepositional phrase has been erroneously attached to it)
A- the argument is "too small" (which implies that an attachment has been omitted)

In table 3 we show as an example the evaluation of the following sentences:

– *Interleukin-2 (IL-2) rapidly activated Stat5 in fresh PBL, and Stat3 and Stat5 in preactivated PBL.*

---

[12] This step is meant to remove records where one of the arguments cannot be clearly assigned a type. This is generally caused by pronouns, which explains why in the error evaluation (see table 4) the number of pronouns appears so low.

- Thus, we demonstrated that IL-5 activated the Jak 2 -STAT 1 signaling pathway in eosinophils.
- Spi-B binds DNA sequences containing a core 5-GGAA-3 and activates transcription through this motif.
- The higher affinity sites bind CVZ with 20- to 50-fold greater affinity, consistent with CVZ's enhanced biological effects.

Table 4. Distribution of errors

	Y	N	Pr	A+	A-
Subject	146	11	4	6	2
Object	99	1	4	59	6

The evaluation resulted in the values shown in table 4. This clearly shows that the biggest source of error is overexpansion of the object, plus there is a little but not insignificant problem in the detection of the subject.[13] Despite the errors, the results can be considered satisfactory, as they show 86.4% and 58.6% correct results in the detection of subjects and objects (respectively). If all loose cases are considered as positive (excluding only the 'N' cases), these results jump to 93.5% and 99.4% (respectively).

As well as improving the parser, currently we are adding facilities for the detection of the polarity and the modality of the relation. Another task being tackled is the treatment of nominalizations (e.g. *"activation"*)[14] and other morphological transformations of the relations of interest (e.g. *"activators"*, *"the activated protein* , *"co-activation"*). Further, some spelling variants should be considered (e.g. *"analyze"* vs. *"analyse"* or *"down-regulate"* vs. *"downregulate"*).

In future we would like to apply Machine Learning Techniques to the task of learning rules that implement transformations from syntactic structures (dependency relations) to domain-relevant semantic relation. We also intend to partner with experts in the task of Bio Entity Identification or use one the available tools (some examples are mentioned in section 5) in order to move from simple experiments over the GENIA corpus to the real-world task of analyzing non-annotated MEDLINE documents. Another advanced application that we are working on is in a Question Answering system over scientific literature in the domain of Genomics [10].

5 Related Work

At present, very few NLP approaches in the Biomedical domain include full parsing. In the following we summarize a number of research projects that include syntactical parsing (to various degrees) for the Biomedical domain.

[11] presents experiments on parsing MEDLINE abstracts with Combinatory Categorial Grammar (CCG). Compared to state-of-the-art parsing speed, the

---

[13] A close inspection of these cases points to problems with conjunctions in subject position, plus a specific problem with the construction *"does not"*.
[14] A simple inspection shows that "activation" makes up almost 50% of the occurrences of the stem "activat*".

system is too slow for practical application (13 minutes for 200 sentences). A small evaluation on 492 sentences containing the anchor verbs yields 80% precision and only 48% recall.

[12] describes a medical IE system that uses a Dependency Grammar. Only German versions of the parser are described. An evaluation with promising results is reported, but only on three low-level relations: auxiliaries, genitives and prepositional phrases.

[13] presents the full parsing approach as entirely novel to the Biomedical domain. "A full parsing approach has not been used in practical application" [ibid.]. The authors belong to the research group that has made the GENIA corpus available, they are currently building the GENIA treebank (which is not claimed to be error-free, but close to the output of their parser). They use a widely established formal grammar, HPSG, and they have shown expertise in robust parsing; [14] is probably the first HPSG parsing approach that scales up to the entire Treebank. [15] use the approach to find anchor verbs in medical corpora.

[4] describes a system (GENIES) which extracts and structures information about cellular pathways from the biological literature. The system relies on a term tagger using rules and external knowledge. The terms are combined in relations using a syntactic grammar and semantic constraints. It attempts to obtain a full parse to achieve high precision, but often backs off to partial parsing to improve recall. It groups the 125 anchor verbs into 14 semantic classes, and it even includes some nominalisations. Only a "pilot evaluation" on a single journal article is reported. The reported precision is 96% and recall 63%.

The PASTA system [16] uses a template-based Information Extraction approach, focusing on the roles of specific amino acid residues in protein molecules. Similar to our approach is the usage of syntactic analysis resulting in a predicate argument representation. On the basis of such representation they also build a domain model which allows inferences based on multiple sentences. PASTA is perhaps the only parsing-based BioNLP system that has been given an extensive and thorough evaluation. Using the MUC-7 scoring system on the hard task or template recognition they report 65% precision and 68% recall.

[17] processes MEDLINE articles (only titles and abstracts) focusing on relation identification. An advantage of their system is the anaphora resolution module, which can resolve many cases of pronominal anaphora and anaphora of the sortal type (e.g. *"the protein"*) including multiple antecedents (e.g. *"both enzymes"*). Their evaluation is based on the **inhibit** relation. They do not use full parsing, but a finite-state cascade approach in which for example many PPs remain unattached. Their shallow parsing is closer to a full parse than most other systems because they include a subordinate clause level, sentential coordination and a flexible relation identification module. On the discourse level, an anaphora resolution module is used.

[18, 19] report their system MedScan which involves full parsing. [18] contains a true broad-coverage evaluation of the coverage of their syntax module, which was tested on 4.6 million sentences from PubMed. Only 1.56 million sentences

of these yield a parse, which is 34 % coverage. Their system is impressive, but the syntactic analysis is not robust. [20] report 91% precision and 21% recall when extracting human protein interactions from MEDLINE using MedScan. In [19], they report that their recall is between 30-50%. A main reason for this relatively low recall is because "the coverage of MedScan grammar is about 51%, which means that information is extracted from only about half of the sentences" [ibid.].

[21] do a formal evaluation of parsing Biomedical texts with the Link Grammar Parser [22], a non-statistical, rule-based broad-coverage parser that does full parsing but delivers highly proprietary structures. [23] have already shown that the performance of Link Grammar is considerably below state-of-the-art. [21] report an overall dependency recall of 73.1%.

6 Conclusions

In this paper we have presented an approach aimed at supporting the process of extraction of core information from scientific literature in the Biomedical Domain. We have first described "DepGENIA", an enhanced version of the GENIA corpus, which has been automatically enriched with syntactic dependencies. The quality of such dependencies has then been evaluated over a randomly selected set of test sentences. We have also described a possible application of our approach to the extraction of semantic relations, suggested by a domain expert. Detailed results of the evaluation and lines of further work have been presented.

References

1. Kim, J., Ohta, T., Tateisi, Y., Tsujii, J.: GENIA Corpus - a Semantically Annotated Corpus for Bio-Textmining. Bioinformatics **19** (2003) 180–182
2. Rinaldi, F., Dowdall, J., Hess, M., Ellman, J., Zarri, G.P., Persidis, A., Bernard, L., Karanikas, H.: Multilayer Annotations in PARMENIDES. In: The K-CAP2003 workshop on "Knowledge Markup and Semantic Annotation". (2003) .
3. Ono, T., Hishigaki, H., Tanigami, A., Takagi, T.: Automated Extraction of Information on Protein-Protein Interactions from the Biological Literature. Bioinformatics **17** (2001) 155–161
4. Friedman, C., Kra, P., Krauthammer, M., H., Rzhetsky, A.: GENIES: a Natural-Language Processing System for the Extraction of Molecular Pathways from Journal Articles. Bioinformatics **17** (2001) 74–82
5. Schneider, G.: Extracting and Using Trace-Free Functional Dependencies from the Penn Treebank to Reduce Parsing Complexity. In: Proceedings of The Second Workshop on Treebanks and Linguistic Theories (TLT 2003), Växjö, Sweden (2003)
6. Schneider, G., Rinaldi, F., Dowdall, J.: Fast, Deep-Linguistic Statistical Minimalist Dependency Parsing. In: COLING-2004 workshop on Recent Advances in Dependency Grammars, August 2004, Geneva, Switzerland. (2004)
7. Collins, M.: Head-Statistical Models for Natural Language Processing. PhD thesis, University of Pennsylvania, Philadelphia, USA (1999)
8. Hindle, D., Rooth, M.: Structural Ambiguity and Lexical Relations. Computational Linguistics **19** (1993) 103–120

9. Volk, M.: Combining Unsupervised and Supervised Methods for PP-Attachment Disambiguation. In: Proceedings of COLING 2002, Taipeh. (2002)
10. Rinaldi, F., Dowdall, J., Schneider, G., Persidis, A.: Answering Questions in the Genomics Domain. In: The ACL 2004 workshop on Question Answering in Restricted Domains, Barcelona, July 2004. (2004)
11. Park, J.C., Kim, H.S., jae Kim, J.: Bidirectional Incremental Parsing for Automatic Pathway Identification with Combinatory Categorial Grammar. In: Proceedings of Pacific Symposium on Biocomputing (PSB), Big Island, Hawaii, USA (2001)
12. Hahn, U., Romacker, M., Schulz, S.: Creating Knowledge Repositories from Biomedical Reports: The medSynDiKATe Text Mining System. In Altman, R.B., Dunker, A.K., Hunter, L., Lauderdale, K., Klein, T.E., eds.: Proceedings of Pacific Symposium on Biocomputing, Kauai, Hawaii, USA (2002) 338–349
13. Yakushiji, A., Tateisi, Y., Miyao, Y.: Event Extraction from Biomedical Papers Using a Full Parser. In: Proceedings of Pacific Symposium on Biocomputing, River Edge, N.J., World Scientific Publishing (2001) 408–419
14. Miyao, Y., Ninomiya, T., Tsujii, J.: Corpus-oriented Grammar Development for Acquiring a Head-driven Phrase Structure Grammar from the Penn Treebank. In: Proceedings of IJCNLP-04. (2004)
15. Yakushiji, A., Tateisi, Y., nad Jun'ichi Tsujii, Y.M.: Finding Anchor Verbs for Biomedical IE using Predicate-Argument Structures. In: Companion Volume to the Proceedings of 42st Annual Meeting of the ACL, Barcelona, Spain (2004) 157–160
16. Gaizauskas, R., Demetriou, G., Artymiuk, P.J., P., W.: Protein Structures and Information Extraction from Biological Texts: The PASTA System. Bioinformatics **19** (2003) 135–143
17. Pustejovsky, J., Castaño, J., Zhang, J., Cochran, B., Kotecki, M.: Robust Relational Parsing over Biomedical Literature: Extracting Inhibit Relations. In: Pacific Symposium on Biocomputing. (2002)
18. Novichkova, S., Egorov, S., Daraselia, N.: MedScan, a Natural Language Processing Engine for MEDLINE Abstracts. Bioinformatics **19** (2003) 1699–1706
19. Daraselia, N., Egorov, S., Yazhuk, A., Novichkova, S., Yuryev, A., Mazo, I.: Extracting Protein Function Information from MEDLINE using a Full-Sentence Parser. In: Proceedings of the Second European Workshop on Data Mining and Text Mining in Bioinformatics, Pisa, Italy (2004)
20. Daraselia, N., Egorov, S., Yazhuk, A., Novichkova, S., Yuryev, A., Mazo, I.: Extracting Human Protein Interactions from MEDLINE using a Full-Sentence Parser. Bioinformatics **19** (2003) 1–8
21. Sampo, P., Ginter, F., Pahikkala, T., Boberg, J., Jrvinen, J., Salakoski, T., Koivula, J.: Analysis of Link Grammar on Biomedical Dependency Corpus Targeted at Protein-Protein Interactions. In: Proceedings of Coling 04 Workshop on Natural Language Proc essing in Biomedicine and its Applications (NLPBA/BioNLP), Geneva, Switzerland (2004)
22. Sleator, D., Temperley, D.: Parsing English with a Link Grammar. Technical Report Technical Report CMU-CS-91-196, Carnegie Mellon University Computer Science (1991)
23. Mollá, D., Hutchinson, B.: Intrinsic versus Extrinsic Evaluations of Parsing Systems. In: Proceedings of EACL03 workshop on Evaluation Initiatives in Natural Language Processing, Budapest (2003) 43–50

Author Index

Abu-Hanna, Ameen 53
Åhlfeldt, Hans 434
Akkaya, Cem 181
Albanèse, Jacques 111
Aleksovski, Zharko 241
Alexopoulou, Dimitra 256
Allart, Laurent 13
Andronis, Christos 535
Antonini, François 111
Atzmueller, Martin 453
Avesani, Paolo 141

Badaloni, Silvana 33
Balcevich, Robert 276
Bamgbade, Adenike 463
Baneyx, Audrey 231
Baral, Chitta 524
Baud, Robert 246
Baumeister, Joachim 453
Baumgartner, Richard 463, 468
Bellazzi, Riccardo 23
Berka, Petr 79
Bisson, Guy 385
Blaszczynski, Jerzy 429
Bohanec, Marko 414
Bonnardel, Nathalie 111
Bonten, Marc 48
Bosman, Robert-Jan 53
Boswell, Brian 375
Bottrighi, Alessio 58, 136, 151
Bouaud, Jacques 131
Bourbellion, Julie 220
Boyer, Célia 251
Bradbrook, Kirsty 171
Bullimore, Mark 473

Castellani, Umberto 315
Cavallini, Anna 89
Cestnik, Bojan 414
Chambrin, Marie-Christine 13
Charlet, Jean 231
Chaudet, Hervé 111
Choi, Soo-Mi 353
Claveau, Vincent 236

Clay, Chris 289
Combi, Carlo 315
Cordier, Marie-Odile 484
Cox, Siân 494
Cristaldi, Gabriele 333

Dailey, Matthew 343
Dankel II, Douglas D. 94
Darmoni, Stéfan J. 251
Dasmahapatra, Srinandan 221
de Jonge, Evert 67
de Mol, Bas 67
Debeljak, Marko 414
Demšar, Janez 514
Distefano, Maria Luisa 333
Dojat, Michel 424
Dolenko, Brion 463
Dupplaw, David 221

Falda, Marco 33
Farion, Ken 429
Faro, Alberto 310
Fox, John 156, 171
Fromont, Élisa 484
Fuchsberger, Christian 101

Gaál, Balázs 419
Garbay, Catherine 226, 424
Gaudinat, Arnaud 251
Geissbühler, Antoine 246
Gill, Hans 434
Giordano, Daniela 310, 333
Giroud, Françoise 226
Glasspool, David 171
Griffiths, Richard 171
Guyet, Thomas 424

Haddawy, Peter 343
Heller, Barbara 266
Hemsing, Achim 453
Herre, Heinrich 266
Hess, Michael 535
Holmes, John H. 444
Hommersom, Arjen 161

Hu, Bo 221
Hunter, Jim 101

Ironi, Liliana 323

Jaulent, Marie-Christine 231
Jermol, Mitja 414
Jorna, René J. 400

Kabanza, Froduald 385
Kaewruen, Ploen 343
Kaiser, Katharina 181
Kaljurand, Kaarel 535
Karkaletsis, Vangelis 256
Kavšek, Branko 414
Keinduangjun, Jitimon 504
Kim, Jeong-Sik 353
Kim, Myoung-Hee 353
Kim, Seungchan 524
Kim, Yong-Guk 353
Klein, Michel 241
Kochin, Dmitry 276, 395
Kononenko, Igor 363
Konstanti, Ourania 535
Kopač, Tadeja 414
Kozmann, György 419
Kristmundsdóttir, María Ósk 94
Kukar, Matjaž 363
Kumar, Anand 213

Larizza, Cristiana 23
Laš, Vladimír 79
Lavrač, Nada 414
Lazarescu, Mihai 289
Leban, Gregor 514
Leonardi, Rosalia 333
Lewis, Paul 221
Lindsay, David G. 494
Lucas, Peter 48, 161
Lukowicz, Paul 7

Magni, Paolo 23
Maiorana, Francesco 333
Marcos, Mar 121, 146, 191
Marsolo, Keith 473
Martin, Claude 111
Marty, Johann 246
Măruşter, Laura 400
Mary, Vincent 251
Marzola, Pasquina 315

McCue, Paul 101
Michalowski, Wojtek 429
Micieli, Giuseppe 89
Miksch, Silvia 126, 146, 181
Milčinski, Metka 363
Molino, Gianpaolo 58, 151
Montani, Stefania 136, 151
Moreno, Antonio 409
Moser, Monika 126
Moskovitch, Robert 141
Mramor, Minca 514
Murino, Vittorio 315

Nannings, Barry 53
Névéol, Aurélie 251
Neville, Ron 375
Nikulin, Alexander 463

Ou, Monica 289

Panzarasa, Silvia 89
Papadimitriou, Elsa 256
Parthasarathy, Srinivasan 473
Patkar, Vivek 156
Peek, Niels 67
Peleg, Mor 156
Pellegrin, Liliane 111
Pennisi, Manuela 310
Pernice, Corrado 89
Persidis, Andreas 535
Piamsa-nga, Punpiti 504
Polo-Conde, Cristina 121, 146, 191
Poovorawan, Yong 504
Porreca, Riccardo 23
Pranckeviciene, Erinija 463
Puppe, Frank 453
Pur, Aleksander 414

Quaglini, Silvana 89
Quiniou, René 484

Ramati, Michael 43
Raudys, Šarunas 468
Razavi, Amir R. 434
Reed, Chris 375
Richter, Ernst-Jürgen 453
Rinaldi, Fabio 535
Rogozan, Alexandrina 251
Rose, Tony 156
Rosenbrand, Kitty 121, 146

Rubin, Steven 429
Ruch, Patrick 246

Sacchi, Lucia 23
Sager, Jennifer A. 444
Šajn, Luka 363
Sánchez, David 409
Sarakhette, Natapope 343
Sbarbati, Andrea 315
Scarciofalo, Giacomo 310
Schmidt, Rainer 300
Schneider, Gerold 535
Schurink, Karin 48
Serban, Radu 121, 191, 201
Séroussi, Brigitte 131
Seyfang, Andreas 146
Shadbolt, Nigel 221
Shahar, Yuval 43, 166
Shahsavar, Nosrat 434
Sharshar, Samir 13
Simony-Lafontaine, Joëlle 226
Sliesoraitiene, Victoria 395
Sliesoraityte, Ieva 276
Smith, Barry 213
Snodgrass, Richard 58
Somorjai, Ray 463, 468
Sona, Diego 141
Spampinato, Concetto 310
Spyropoulos, Constantine D. 256
Steele, Rory 156
Stefanelli, Mario 89

Tbahriti, Imad 246
ten Teije, Annette 121, 191, 201
Tentoni, Stefania 323

Terenziani, Paolo 58, 136, 151
Thomson, Richard 156
Tomečková, Marie 79
Torchio, Mauro 58, 151
Tramontana, Francesco 310
Twa, Michael 473

Urbančič, Tanja 414
Ustinovichius, Leonas 276, 395

Valarakos, Alexandros G. 256
van Bommel, Patrick 161
van Croonenborg, Joyce 121
van der Weide, Theo 161
van Gendt, Marjolein 201
van Harmelen, Frank 3, 191, 201
Vassányi, István 419
Verduijn, Marion 67
Veuthey, Anne-Lise 246
Vieillot, Jean-Jacques 131
Visscher, Stefan 48
Voorbraak, Frans 67
Vorobieva, Olga 300

Weiss, Dawid 429
West, Geoff A.W. 289
Wilk, Szymon 429
Winstanley, Graham 171
Wittenberg, Jolanda 121, 146

Young, Ohad 166

Zampieri, Marco 315
Zhang, Xin 524
Zupan, Blaž 514
Zweigenbaum, Pierre 236

Lecture Notes in Artificial Intelligence (LNAI)

Vol. 3632: R. Nieuwenhuis (Ed.), Automated Deduction – CADE-20. XIII, 459 pages. 2005.

Vol. 3626: B. Ganter, G. Stumme, R. Wille (Eds.), Formal Concept Analysis. X, 349 pages. 2005.

Vol. 3607: J.-D. Zucker, L. Saitta (Eds.), Abstraction, Reformulation and Approximation. XII, 376 pages. 2005.

Vol. 3596: F. Dau, M.-L. Mugnier, G. Stumme (Eds.), Conceptual Structures: Common Semantics for Sharing Knowledge. XI, 467 pages. 2005.

Vol. 3587: P. Perner, A. Imiya (Eds.), Machine Learning and Data Mining in Pattern Recognition. XVII, 695 pages. 2005.

Vol. 3584: X. Li, S. Wang, Z.Y. Dong (Eds.), Advanced Data Mining and Applications. XIX, 835 pages. 2005.

Vol. 3581: S. Miksch, J. Hunter, E. Keravnou (Eds.), Artificial Intelligence in Medicine. XVII, 547 pages. 2005.

Vol. 3575: S. Wermter, G. Palm, M. Elshaw (Eds.), Biomimetic Neural Learning for Intelligent Robots. IX, 383 pages. 2005.

Vol. 3571: L. Godo (Ed.), Symbolic and Quantitative Approaches to Reasoning with Uncertainty. XVI, 1028 pages. 2005.

Vol. 3559: P. Auer, R. Meir (Eds.), Learning Theory. XI, 692 pages. 2005.

Vol. 3558: V. Torra, Y. Narukawa, S. Miyamoto (Eds.), Modeling Decisions for Artificial Intelligence. XII, 470 pages. 2005.

Vol. 3554: A. Dey, B. Kokinov, D. Leake, R. Turner (Eds.), Modeling and Using Context. XIV, 572 pages. 2005.

Vol. 3539: K. Morik, J.-F. Boulicaut, A. Siebes (Eds.), Local Pattern Detection. XI, 233 pages. 2005.

Vol. 3538: L. Ardissono, P. Brna, A. Mitrovic (Eds.), User Modeling 2005. XVI, 533 pages. 2005.

Vol. 3533: M. Ali, F. Esposito (Eds.), Innovations in Applied Artificial Intelligence. XX, 858 pages. 2005.

Vol. 3528: P.S. Szczepaniak, J. Kacprzyk, A. Niewiadomski (Eds.), Advances in Web Intelligence. XVII, 513 pages. 2005.

Vol. 3518: T.B. Ho, D. Cheung, H. Liu (Eds.), Advances in Knowledge Discovery and Data Mining. XXI, 864 pages. 2005.

Vol. 3508: P. Bresciani, P. Giorgini, B. Henderson-Sellers, G. Low, M. Winikoff (Eds.), Agent-Oriented Information Systems II. X, 227 pages. 2005.

Vol. 3505: V. Gorodetsky, J. Liu, V. A. Skormin (Eds.), Autonomous Intelligent Systems: Agents and Data Mining. XIII, 303 pages. 2005.

Vol. 3501: B. Kégl, G. Lapalme (Eds.), Advances in Artificial Intelligence. XV, 458 pages. 2005.

Vol. 3492: P. Blache, E. Stabler, J. Busquets, R. Moot (Eds.), Logical Aspects of Computational Linguistics. X, 363 pages. 2005.

Vol. 3488: M.-S. Hacid, N.V. Murray, Z.W. Raś, S. Tsumoto (Eds.), Foundations of Intelligent Systems. XIII, 700 pages. 2005.

Vol. 3476: J. Leite, A. Omicini, P. Torroni, P. Yolum (Eds.), Declarative Agent Languages and Technologies II. XII, 289 pages. 2005.

Vol. 3464: S.A. Brueckner, G.D.M. Serugendo, A. Karageorgos, R. Nagpal (Eds.), Engineering Self-Organising Systems. XIII, 299 pages. 2005.

Vol. 3452: F. Baader, A. Voronkov (Eds.), Logic for Programming, Artificial Intelligence, and Reasoning. XI, 562 pages. 2005.

Vol. 3451: M.-P. Gleizes, A. Omicini, F. Zambonelli (Eds.), Engineering Societies in the Agents World. XIII, 349 pages. 2005.

Vol. 3446: T. Ishida, L. Gasser, H. Nakashima (Eds.), Massively Multi-Agent Systems I. XI, 349 pages. 2005.

Vol. 3445: G. Chollet, A. Esposito, M. Faundez-Zanuy, M. Marinaro (Eds.), Nonlinear Speech Modeling and Applications. XIII, 433 pages. 2005.

Vol. 3438: H. Christiansen, P.R. Skadhauge, J. Villadsen (Eds.), Constraint Solving and Language Processing. VIII, 205 pages. 2005.

Vol. 3430: S. Tsumoto, T. Yamaguchi, M. Numao, H. Motoda (Eds.), Active Mining. XII, 349 pages. 2005.

Vol. 3419: B. Faltings, A. Petcu, F. Fages, F. Rossi (Eds.), Constraint Satisfaction and Constraint Logic Programming. X, 217 pages. 2005.

Vol. 3416: M. Böhlen, J. Gamper, W. Polasek, M.A. Wimmer (Eds.), E-Government: Towards Electronic Democracy. XIII, 311 pages. 2005.

Vol. 3415: P. Davidsson, B. Logan, K. Takadama (Eds.), Multi-Agent and Multi-Agent-Based Simulation. X, 265 pages. 2005.

Vol. 3403: B. Ganter, R. Godin (Eds.), Formal Concept Analysis. XI, 419 pages. 2005.

Vol. 3398: D.-K. Baik (Ed.), Systems Modeling and Simulation: Theory and Applications. XIV, 733 pages. 2005.

Vol. 3397: T.G. Kim (Ed.), Artificial Intelligence and Simulation. XV, 711 pages. 2005.

Vol. 3396: R.M. van Eijk, M.-P. Huget, F. Dignum (Eds.), Agent Communication. X, 261 pages. 2005.

Vol. 3394: D. Kudenko, D. Kazakov, E. Alonso (Eds.), Adaptive Agents and Multi-Agent Systems II. VIII, 313 pages. 2005.

Vol. 3392: D. Seipel, M. Hanus, U. Geske, O. Bartenstein (Eds.), Applications of Declarative Programming and Knowledge Management. X, 309 pages. 2005.

Vol. 3374: D. Weyns, H. V.D. Parunak, F. Michel (Eds.), Environments for Multi-Agent Systems. X, 279 pages. 2005.

Vol. 3371: M.W. Barley, N. Kasabov (Eds.), Intelligent Agents and Multi-Agent Systems. X, 329 pages. 2005.

Vol. 3369: V. R. Benjamins, P. Casanovas, J. Breuker, A. Gangemi (Eds.), Law and the Semantic Web. XII, 249 pages. 2005.

Vol. 3366: I. Rahwan, P. Moraitis, C. Reed (Eds.), Argumentation in Multi-Agent Systems. XII, 263 pages. 2005.

Vol. 3359: G. Grieser, Y. Tanaka (Eds.), Intuitive Human Interfaces for Organizing and Accessing Intellectual Assets. XIV, 257 pages. 2005.

Vol. 3346: R.H. Bordini, M. Dastani, J. Dix, A.E.F. Seghrouchni (Eds.), Programming Multi-Agent Systems. XIV, 249 pages. 2005.

Vol. 3345: Y. Cai (Ed.), Ambient Intelligence for Scientific Discovery. XII, 311 pages. 2005.

Vol. 3343: C. Freksa, M. Knauff, B. Krieg-Brückner, B. Nebel, T. Barkowsky (Eds.), Spatial Cognition IV. XIII, 519 pages. 2005.

Vol. 3339: G.I. Webb, X. Yu (Eds.), AI 2004: Advances in Artificial Intelligence. XXII, 1272 pages. 2004.

Vol. 3336: D. Karagiannis, U. Reimer (Eds.), Practical Aspects of Knowledge Management. X, 523 pages. 2004.

Vol. 3327: Y. Shi, W. Xu, Z. Chen (Eds.), Data Mining and Knowledge Management. XIII, 263 pages. 2005.

Vol. 3315: C. Lemaître, C.A. Reyes, J.A. González (Eds.), Advances in Artificial Intelligence – IBERAMIA 2004. XX, 987 pages. 2004.

Vol. 3303: J.A. López, E. Benfenati, W. Dubitzky (Eds.), Knowledge Exploration in Life Science Informatics. X, 249 pages. 2004.

Vol. 3301: G. Kern-Isberner, W. Rödder, F. Kulmann (Eds.), Conditionals, Information, and Inference. XII, 219 pages. 2005.

Vol. 3276: D. Nardi, M. Riedmiller, C. Sammut, J. Santos-Victor (Eds.), RoboCup 2004: Robot Soccer World Cup VIII. XVIII, 678 pages. 2005.

Vol. 3275: P. Perner (Ed.), Advances in Data Mining. VIII, 173 pages. 2004.

Vol. 3265: R.E. Frederking, K.B. Taylor (Eds.), Machine Translation: From Real Users to Research. XI, 392 pages. 2004.

Vol. 3264: G. Paliouras, Y. Sakakibara (Eds.), Grammatical Inference: Algorithms and Applications. XI, 291 pages. 2004.

Vol. 3259: J. Dix, J. Leite (Eds.), Computational Logic in Multi-Agent Systems. XII, 251 pages. 2004.

Vol. 3257: E. Motta, N.R. Shadbolt, A. Stutt, N. Gibbins (Eds.), Engineering Knowledge in the Age of the Semantic Web. XVII, 517 pages. 2004.

Vol. 3249: B. Buchberger, J.A. Campbell (Eds.), Artificial Intelligence and Symbolic Computation. X, 285 pages. 2004.

Vol. 3248: K.-Y. Su, J. Tsujii, J.-H. Lee, O.Y. Kwong (Eds.), Natural Language Processing – IJCNLP 2004. XVIII, 817 pages. 2005.

Vol. 3245: E. Suzuki, S. Arikawa (Eds.), Discovery Science. XIV, 430 pages. 2004.

Vol. 3244: S. Ben-David, J. Case, A. Maruoka (Eds.), Algorithmic Learning Theory. XIV, 505 pages. 2004.

Vol. 3238: S. Biundo, T. Frühwirth, G. Palm (Eds.), KI 2004: Advances in Artificial Intelligence. XI, 467 pages. 2004.

Vol. 3230: J.L. Vicedo, P. Martínez-Barco, R. Muñoz, M. Saiz Noeda (Eds.), Advances in Natural Language Processing. XII, 488 pages. 2004.

Vol. 3229: J.J. Alferes, J. Leite (Eds.), Logics in Artificial Intelligence. XIV, 744 pages. 2004.

Vol. 3228: M.G. Hinchey, J.L. Rash, W.F. Truszkowski, C.A. Rouff (Eds.), Formal Approaches to Agent-Based Systems. VIII, 290 pages. 2004.

Vol. 3215: M.G.. Negoita, R.J. Howlett, L.C. Jain (Eds.), Knowledge-Based Intelligent Information and Engineering Systems, Part III. LVII, 906 pages. 2004.

Vol. 3214: M.G.. Negoita, R.J. Howlett, L.C. Jain (Eds.), Knowledge-Based Intelligent Information and Engineering Systems, Part II. LVIII, 1302 pages. 2004.

Vol. 3213: M.G.. Negoita, R.J. Howlett, L.C. Jain (Eds.), Knowledge-Based Intelligent Information and Engineering Systems, Part I. LVIII, 1280 pages. 2004.

Vol. 3209: B. Berendt, A. Hotho, D. Mladenic, M. van Someren, M. Spiliopoulou, G. Stumme (Eds.), Web Mining: From Web to Semantic Web. IX, 201 pages. 2004.

Vol. 3206: P. Sojka, I. Kopecek, K. Pala (Eds.), Text, Speech and Dialogue. XIII, 667 pages. 2004.

Vol. 3202: J.-F. Boulicaut, F. Esposito, F. Giannotti, D. Pedreschi (Eds.), Knowledge Discovery in Databases: PKDD 2004. XIX, 560 pages. 2004.

Vol. 3201: J.-F. Boulicaut, F. Esposito, F. Giannotti, D. Pedreschi (Eds.), Machine Learning: ECML 2004. XVIII, 580 pages. 2004.

Vol. 3194: R. Camacho, R. King, A. Srinivasan (Eds.), Inductive Logic Programming. XI, 361 pages. 2004.

Vol. 3192: C. Bussler, D. Fensel (Eds.), Artificial Intelligence: Methodology, Systems, and Applications. XIII, 522 pages. 2004.

Vol. 3191: M. Klusch, S. Ossowski, V. Kashyap, R. Unland (Eds.), Cooperative Information Agents VIII. XI, 303 pages. 2004.

Vol. 3187: G. Lindemann, J. Denzinger, I.J. Timm, R. Unland (Eds.), Multiagent System Technologies. XIII, 341 pages. 2004.

Vol. 3176: O. Bousquet, U. von Luxburg, G. Rätsch (Eds.), Advanced Lectures on Machine Learning. IX, 241 pages. 2004.

Vol. 3171: A.L. C. Bazzan, S. Labidi (Eds.), Advances in Artificial Intelligence – SBIA 2004. XVII, 548 pages. 2004.

Vol. 3159: U. Visser, Intelligent Information Integration for the Semantic Web. XIV, 150 pages. 2004.